Process Biotechnology Fundamentals

Process Biotechnology Fundamentals

Third Edition, Revised and Updated

S.N. Mukhopadhyay
Ph.D., LMISTE, F.N.A.E., F.I.I.Ch.E

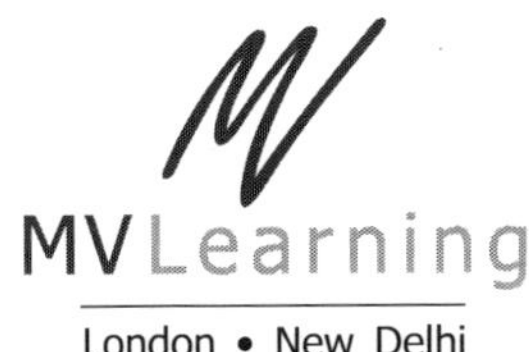

MV Learning
London • New Delhi

MV Learning

3, Henrietta Street
London WC2E 8LU
UK

4737/23, Ansari Road,
Daryaganj, New Delhi 110 002
India

A Viva Books imprint

ISBN: 978-81-309-2959-0

Printed and bound in India.

SUB-0001/SSUB-0004

In loving memories of my
parents, teachers and parents-in-law
&
Respectful homage to
Professor Arabindo Nath Bose
Former Vice-chancellor, Jadavpur University, Kolkata
and to Professor K. Sambamurthy,
Former UGC Emeritus Professor, New Delhi.

CONTENTS

ACKNOWLEDGEMENTS

This edition of the book being in continuation to its first and second editions with addition of newer knowledge and a new chapter, the acknowledgements of the previous editions continue in this edition as well. In writing chapter seventeen for this edition help taken from various published sources is acknowledged. The book being a textbook written for bioengineering and biotechnology students/scholars at the junior and senior levels, I have included additional knowledge in this edition that was gathered through my earlier and recent exposures in academic and research domains in the area. In doing so my revisits to Duke University, Durham, N.C. and Rockefeller University, New York, which is known to be initiator of a landmark in modern biotechnology in 1944 was of great experience and value. After entering in the library of world-renowned Rockefeller University in Founders Building with my son Parag I could see and note some of the valuable research/academic literatures and felt as if my mind has been filled with an inexpressibly large treasure of knowledge which I sincerely acknowledge. For this I appreciate the efforts and time of my son at Rockefeller University and daughter-in-law Pooja at KBI Biopharma Inc., N.C., in organizing such an opportunity for me. Pooja who is currently a scientist in Bristol Meyer and Squibb Co in New Jersey in consultation with Parag made a comprehensive visit programme that enabled me, my wife Sakuntala and my daughter Paramita to acquire an unbounded joy that encouraged me to finish the collation of third edition of the book more quickly. Active coordination of Parag and Pooja for the same is sincerely acknowledged.

As in previous editions I have taken help from various books, journals and other sources in upgrading to the third edition of the book. I sincerely acknowledge these great help without which this third edition would have not appeared.

Sincerely, I acknowledge the cooperation received from BERC/DBEB, Central library and IIT Delhi. I wish to acknowledge also, the patient contributions of the publisher's team during my long association to this enterprise which has occupied us all for a period of nearly ten years.

S.N. Mukhopadhyay

PREFACE TO THE FIRST EDITION

This book has emerged out as a venture of publishing based on long and continuing class room teaching experiences. It is intended to serve the students of undergraduate (UG), postgraduate (PG) and pre-Ph.D. levels in the area. The book has been written for students having basic and heterogeneous educational backgrounds for handling process biotechnology using living organism(s)/cells or biochemicals/chemicals of life. Also, it is intended for students who want to become a special UG and PG degree holders in Biochemical Engineering and Biotechnology and related areas. It has also kept in view of the requirements of students handling environmental engineering systems of biological waste treatments. Major emphasis in the book has been on quantifying character. The students who master this book should have known what he is doing, why he needs to do it and how he should approach to do it in the field. It is the purpose of this book to outline in a concise but comprehensive manner, the fundamentals of process biotechnology. Also it presents the aspect considerations as well as scale up and design approaches providing numerical examples to a large extent. The materials presented in this book can be covered within the scope of four semester course.

The author earnestly requests all teachers, students and readers using this book to communicate to him regarding misprints/errata, erroneous statements, if any and suggestions for improvement of the text unhesitatingly. Also, he considers it a privilege to have the cooperation of all in keeping the text most up-to-date

S.N. Mukhopadhyay

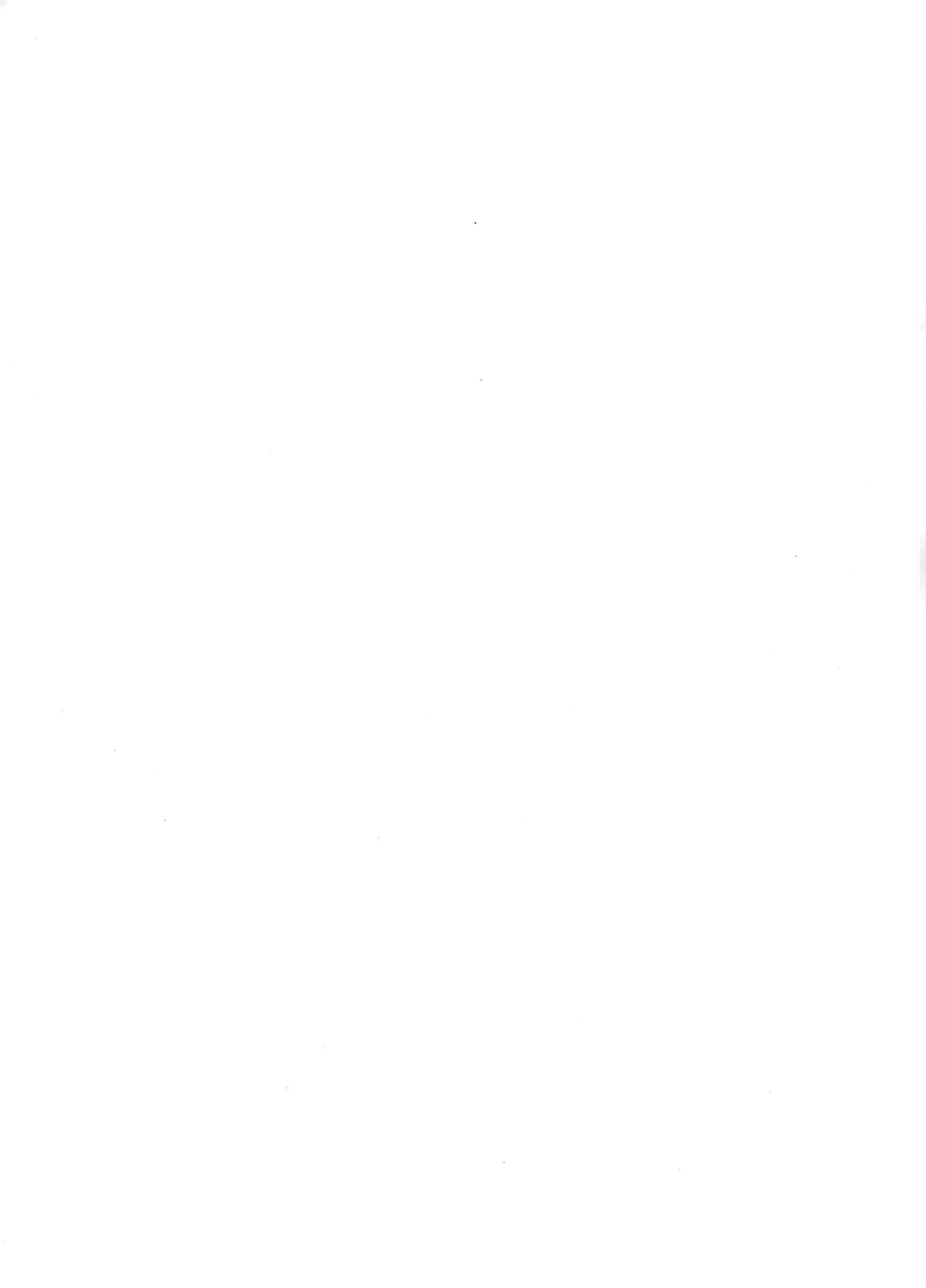

PREFACE TO THE SECOND EDITION

Process biotechnology deals with activity concerned with the exploitation of bioprocessing on indistrial/commercial scale. In recent past the entire field of bioprocess engineering is in the midst of broadening and redefining. So in writing *Process Biotechnology Fundamentals*, I have integrated knowledge of governing biological/biomaterial properties and concerns in a wider perspectives. In doing so, my experiences and exposures as Visiting Scientist/Visiting Associate/ Visiting Professor, study tour scientist, JSPS fellow, Fulbright fellow etc at LANFI/IPN, Mexico; SFIT Zurich; Osaka University, Japan; Caltech, California; UCHC, Farmington; University of Lund, Sweden; Lehigh University, USA; University of Western Ontario/University of Waterloo/ University of Calgary, Canada; University of Compiegn, France; Tomas Bata Universty in Zlin, Czech Republic and participation and presentatioin of papers in international and national conferences/seminars/symposia/workshops/short courses etc. in Mexico, Canada, Singapore, Germany and in India have been very useful.

This new edition, therefore, has been organised to serve better the needs of its readers. I have myself used its contents in teaching UG, PG, and pre Ph.D candidates concerned with process biotechnology and bioprocess engineering at IIT Delhi and have felt the need of inclusion of a few additional chapters and revising the earlier edition. Accordingly, the new edition of the book contains the following considering that it is an introductory book. Chapter 1 provides an introductory description/discussion on the progress of process biotechnology fundamentals. Chapter 2 provides fundamental aspects of engineering biology of cells in terms of the molecules they synthesize. In this chapter an additional subsection on concept of stability and steady state in cell division has been incorporated considering three basis. Chapter 3 provides the readers on the concept of medium engineering required in formulation of medium for a process biotechnology. Chapter 4 is a new addition dealing with provision for supplying contamination free fluid media for process biotechnology. Chapter 5 is also a new addition. It deals with the concerns related to aeration and mixing/agitation in oxic process biotechnology. This chapter with newer additions has been taken from my earlier book published by CRC press, USA. Chapter 6 has provided new bioprocessing aspects and strategies in understanding bioprocess technology with wider perspectives. Chapter 7 describes bioreactors and biosensors required in bioprocessing of cells and enzymes. Chapter 8 brings to readers the concerns and criteria in scaling up of a process biotechnology in general in giving products. Chapter 9 describes modern estimation and bioassay of bioproducts from process biotechnology. Chater 10 deals with conventional and newer methods for recovery of bioproducts obtained from upstream process biotechnology. Chapter 11 describes principles and various treatment biotechnology approaches of liquid wastes and water from various process biotechnology industries. Chapter 12 is also another new addition dealing with control of undesirable microorganisms/contaminants in biosystem using liquids, units and gadgets in process biotechnology. Chapter 13 describes how one can meaningfully utilize the enormous cellulosic resource material of nature using process biotechnology approaches in delivering various high value products. In this chapter a subsection has been added which will help the readers to know how a cocktail enzyme is useful in industry/commerce. Chapter 14 gives a detail account on bioprocessing using cells under stresses to deliver useful high value products. Chapter 15 incorporates to the mind of readers how a bioprocess plant design can be systematically developed giving a typical biosystem example e.g. penicillin production system. The last Chapter 16 has been provided to readers particularly students to get themselves acquainted with the techniques for solving problems and answering questions and multichoice questions (MCQ). In this chapter several new numericals and MCQ have been incorporated. All the chapters are provided with many references at the end of each chapter. These will aid in provoking thoughts in the minds of the readers of this book. Many errors/omissions as observed in the first edition of this book have been rectified as far as possible. In passing, the author again earnestly requests all teachers, researchers, students and readers using this book to communicate to him regarding errata/misprints, erroneous statements, if any and suggestions for improvement of the text unhesitatingly. Also, he considers it a privilege to have the cooperation of all in keeping the text most up-to-date considering amazing advancement in process biotechnology.

Finally, with great pleasure, I come to my pleasant duty to the acknowledgements. I thank Professor Dr. Tarun K. Ghose, Formerly Founding Head, BERC/DBEB, IIT Delhi for his keen interest all the time on my producing research based academic deliverables to serve students. My grateful thanks to my wife Sakuntala for encouragement, to my son Parag at the University of Calgary, Canada, for assisting me to collect some informations for this second edition when I had the opportunity to visit him. Also, my daughter Paramita, who all the time reminded me for the completion of my job, I am really thankful to her. Typographical assistance received from Mr. Rajiv in the Department of Biochemical Engineering and Biotechnology is gratefully acknowledged. Cooperation received from faculty and staff of DBEB, IIT Delhi is also gratefully acknowledged.

Lastly, but not the least I thank members and specially Mr. Nishikant Choudhary of Viva Books, New Delhi and its associated press for taking prompt needful action in its publication.

S.N. Mukhopadhyay

PREFACE TO THE THIRD EDITION

Over many years that have passed since the first and second editions of this book were written and published, explosive progress has been made in the area of process biotechnology. It is difficult to include all these developments in a short book. I have contended myself in this third edition with the inclusion of some new knowledge in several chapters and the addition of a new chapter seventeen, many new MCQ and newer numerical problems. Chapter seventeen deals with refining/pretreatment of renewable substrates for fermentation/bioconversion/ biotransformation industries. As is usual with biochemical engineering and biotechnology, its development takes place through its ever-increasing scope for research. The contributions of scientists and technologists are the chief sources from which the current trend of expansions in the subject can be visualized. The roles of research-based teacher scientists depend upon chances of newer and newer idea developments, discoveries and innovations to imbibe in teaching courses/ subjects. All that needed to be done is to collate new trends, ideas, innovations, discoveries and developments in form of text materials. Taking note of all these aspects in a systematic order in which the subject has been arranged in this book is one of the chief contributions of the present edition. The author hopes that this edition of the book will prove to be more useful to the users and readers.

The few mistakes that had crept in to the previous editions of this book in spite of my best efforts have been corrected in this edition.

Finally, like in previous editions I earnestly requests all teachers, scholars/students and readers using this book to communicate to him regarding misprints/errata, erroneous statements etc., if any, and suggestions for further improvement of the text unhesitatingly. Also, I consider it a previledge to have the cooperation of all in keeping the text most up-to-date.

S.N. Mukhopadhyay

Chapter

1

INTRODUCTION

1.1 PROGRESS OF PROCESS BIOTECHNOLOGY

The process biotechnology practice has made significant contributions through resource utilization towards Biochemical Engineering and Biotechnology progress in contemporary years[1-5]. This progress has strong growth foundations on (a) knowledge acquired through research (b) academic teaching programme development with newer approaches and (c) newer practicing strategies. In bioprocess engineering practice, the knowledge components of basic, physical, chemical, abstract and engineering sciences in association with bioscience domains have been integrated with research and development (R & D) in bioprocesses and biosystems for advancing process biotechnology. The integration objective is to utilize material resource for its biotransformation into high value commercially potential products. In engineering practice if the material resource is of renewable nature it renders availability advantage. However, all renewable and nonrenewable biomaterials have different structural and functional properties. In considering these material resources as a commodity for raw material in process industries education and research based information on the structural and functional properties of these materials will assist to a great extent in practicing technology of their utilization. In realizing progress of process biotechnology many aspects of education, research and training in biochemical engineering and biotechnology have been overviewed[5-9]. In many countries including India, biotechnology has been stated to sprout from engineering discipline. However, prior to nineteen hundred fifties fermentation technology in India has been stated to be confined to the brewing industry and industrial alcohol production although India's position in the traditional fermented foods and distillery industry is amongst the oldest biotechnology like most other Asian countries.

The beginning of process biotechnology may be stated to date back to nearly fifty years of service behind scientists and engineers. In those days the fermentation scientists used to approach mechanical and chemical engineers to construct fermenters for them for the production of penicillin. Although bioscientists knew to produce penicillin by submerged culture method instead of by the laborious and expensive bottle or tray technique, they use to lack the right equipment and technique. The result of the first flirtation with engineers was stated to turn out to be a miserable disappointment.

The bioreaction kettle that was offered by the engineers to the fermentation scientists for penicillin production led to serious and crippling infections. The engineers then tried to solve this problem with steam seals at every possible point[1] where leakage could be expected. This effort also ended up with a hissing and puffing contraption that resembled a noisy old steam engine more than a fermenter. The problems needed eliminations. Gradually over the years by gaining experiences much has progressed in these fifty years. The major progress undoubtedly was that this flirtation of the microbiologists/bioscientists with the persistent engineers resulted a vital hybridization. Out of this hybridization a bioengineer was born to take care for future progress of process biotechnology which had its origins in industrial microbiology, conventional fermentation technology and its related areas.[9-17]

1.2 KNOWLEDGE COLLATION AND EXPANSION

Many countries including India are endowed with raw material resources.[18] Significant noteworthies in India over the last few decades relate to achievements in expanding local manufacture and educational trends for developing indigenously trained human resources. In Indian development trends in Biochemical Engineering and Biotechnology discipline area has taken a significant leap. This is primarily because of the official attitude which has long been favourable to science and technology in totality in the country. One of the best grounds for predicting continued development is the presence in India of a substantial number of scientists and engineers who have been trained not only in-house but also through exposure in several developed countries at higher levels. Their knowledge collation and expansion quality is such that they have been contributing by developing academic, commercial and industrial deliverables, rising to positions of national scientific and technological leadership, advisers and professorship in academic institutions for various activities (Fig.1.1). In the progress of knowledge collation and expansions the contributions of a large number of International and National Symposia, courses, meetings, workshops etc. under the aegis of IUPAC, IOBB, IAMS, GIAM, UNESCO, ICRO Panel of Applied Microbiology, UNDP, UNEP, IFTS/IBS etc served a great role in expanding the "Horizons of Process Biotechnology". India also did not fall behind from this progress. Indo-Swiss collaboration in Biochemical Engineering between the SFIT Zurich and IIT Delhi through the support of DST, GOI was one of the major model footsteps towards progress of Process Biotechnology[15] in India.

1.3 BRIDGING THE GAP: BIOSCIENCES, ENGINEERING AND TECHNOLOGY

As evident from the Fig.1.1 the birth place of modern Biochemical Engineering and Biotechnology and the source of its continuing inspirations from process biotechnology is academia. Researchers in industries and university/institute laboratories funded largely by federal grants developed most of the techniques of fermentation biotechnology, molecular biology,

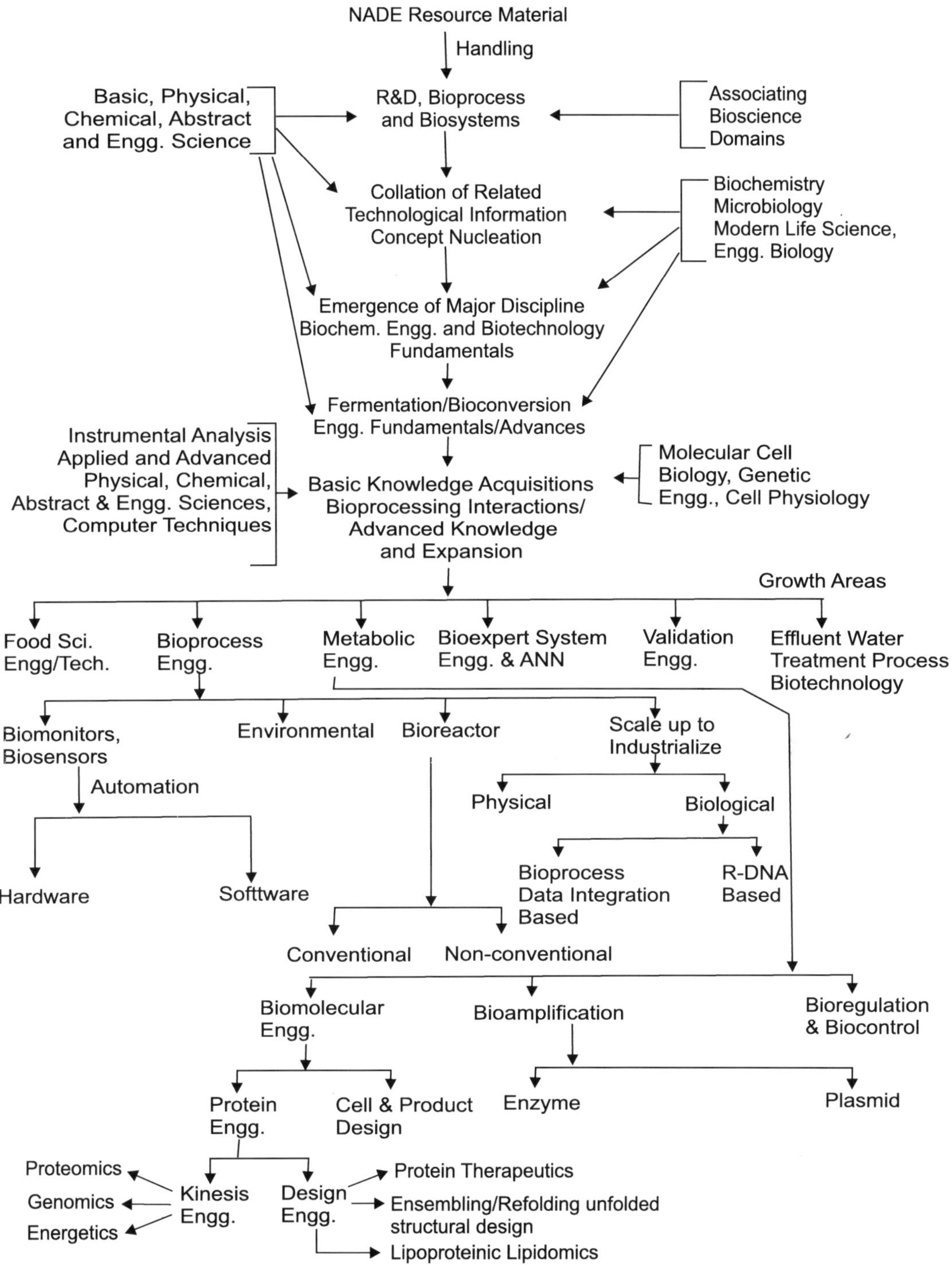

Fig. 1.1 Progressive knowledge collation and expansion areas of process biotechnology (NADE—Naturally Acquired Design Engineering, ANN—Artificial Neural Network)

bimolecular designing/redesigning, monoclonal antibody technology, immunological, mammalian, plant cell culture biotechnology etc. that have given rise to modern bioengineering and biotechnology. In turn academic researchers were among the first to recognize commercial utility and many of them were among the founders, promoters and directors of the new process biotechnology companies. At present the companies involved in process biotechnology remain vitally interested in research being conducted and in progress in institutes and universities and related biotechnology area. The new industry views academia as a reservoir of new ideas and as suppliers of trained human resources and talented consultants. Companies involved in biotechnology realize that one of the best ways to do this is to expose their researchers and development engineers to scientists and academicians working in fundamental and applied research areas. It also provides the new companies with a view of the technology, while not requiring large investment in facilities and personnel. Almost all biochemical industries have now recognized the need for proper biochemical and chemical engineering inputs in setting up of the production units and in their operation. Not only that, there is at present a good deal of emphasis being given to provide adequate inputs in Biochemical Engineering and Biotechnology in setting up of new units as well as in improving and expanding of the existing units. In more contemporary years (late ninteen sixties) fermentation process in biotechnological industries in many countries which represented most of the biochemical industry was set up and expanded primarily using the skills of microbiologists, biochemists and engineers. In those days most of the scientists and technologists employed in industry were trained and obtained working experiences in fermentation biotechnology and techniques from some of the leading universities and institutions abroad, notably in USA, UK, Germany and France.[19-21]

Internationally Biotechnology has been set for a big leap. It required integrated approach to education and research. Besides this the need for gearing towards R & D, evolving and identifying priority areas like agriculture, health care, animal productivity and infrastructure development were emphasized by the Department of Biotechnology, Govt. of India and many of the eminent scientists in the country and involved industrial dignitaries.[22,23] The cause of this big leap of biotechnology is stated to be due to the major revolution in the field of life sciences. Innovations in process biotechnology has primarily been brought about through an increased understanding of biosystems at cellular and molecular levels. These understandings relate to advances in process biotechnology concerns of tissue culture, recombinant DNA cell bioprocessing or genetic engineering, plasmid and gene transfer, immunology, photosynthesis, scale up etc.[23] Even the consumption and demand of antibiotics, the classical industrial biotechnology product in the country is reported to increase fast.[24] Therefore the exciting advances of biotechnology have posed before scientists a challenge of either setting their own priorities guided by logic of science or the rationale governing the industries.[25] Considering all these exciting progress in the area it has been stated that impressive array of accomplishmets in process biotechnology has been amassed and some notable among them have been listed out for a demonstration in bioprocess industry.[26] Rapid advances in present era in molecular cell biology together with the acquisition of important new knowledge in related fields like biochemistry, microbiology, engineering biology and bioengineering sciences have brought about a large potential for process biotechnology industries.[27-29] In the field of biochemical engineering and biotechnology new innovative developments and commercial applications are appearing rapidly in every directions including fermentation industries, enzymes, immobilized cell biotechnology, treatment biotechnology of industrial wastes and bye product utilization. Any integrated successful process biotechnology will be useful to society, attractive to industries for commercial benefits and that will take care of loss prevention, value addition to products and coproducts and minimization of pollution hazard.

1.4 GLOBAL IMPACTS AND SCENARIO[30-36]

1.4.1 Hope in General

The manufacturing of various bioproducts (biocellular and enzymic), being scale factor dependent on process biotechnologies (new and conventional) is controlled by powerful economic and technical forces pointing towards increased levels of interdependence.[30,31] Economy of scale factor being very powerful, engineering concerns play a great role on the technology assessment and overall success of the process biotechnology. Successful process biotechnology will contribute enormously to meet partly the challenges facing society in the future. Of the major challenges for future society six have been stated to be affected by biotechnology. These include: (1) availability of raw material resources and chemical feed stocks, (2) non-conventional energy sources, (3) biological scale up and redesigning to industrial production problems, (4) health care problems, (5) environmental concerns and (6) computer aided automation in biosystems.

Now a global question is when biomass rather than fossil fuels will become the major source of chemical feed stocks. It is revealed by computation that a biomass farm of 5000 acres would be expected to yield approximately 9000 tons or 9×10^6 liters of alcohol per year as feed stock. Clearly, because of raw material cost, total utilization of the biomass is critical to process efficiency. Total biomass utilization is dependent on efficient conversion of cellulose and hemicellulose into alcohol. There are several constraints to achieve this. In order to overcome many of these constraints it will be appropriate to select a process that would simultaneously hydrolyze both cellulose and hemicellulose to sugars, enzymatically convert the xylose and glucose by yeast or bacteria into alcohol.[32]

Less developed countries having enormous tropical rainforests and those which are rich in agriculture products having the presence of a tremendous amount of residual biomass resources have great potential for agroindustrial process biotechnology development.[33]

Developing countries have found biotechnology exciting and it may turn out to be a big business.[34] For this business research and developments in areas of fermentation products, fermented food, biomass production, bioreactors, waste-water treatments, biomethanation, environmental processes, developing academic and research institutionsns,[35] demonstration facilities are noteworthy.

Biotechnology has also a great challenge before it to become a primary producer of organic matter. For this exploitation of microbial photosynthesis overcoming its limitations on conventional agriculture is essential.[27,36] Computer aided bioprocessing control in developing process biotechnology has now become inevitable. Computers will have their greatest effect in process biotechnology with regard to automation, particularly of processes supporting genetic application. Clearly, opportunities for biotechnology for years to come will largely emerge from crisis oriented problems. Raw material resources and qualified and trained human resources will have a great role. Among the crisis the two that are gaining opportunities and that are still very difficult to predict presently are those of genetic engineering and computer aided automation. However, opportunities in biotechnology are expanding.

1.4.2 Raw Material Resources

One of the major needs for development of suitable process biotechnology is the availability of raw material or substrate resources. Industrial raw material resources in most cases being nonrenewable in nature, search for alternate resources has become inevitable all over the globe.

It is to meet the demand of food, feed stock and energy of the world population. The use of biomass/renewable resources, represents a possible long term solution to the problem of dwindling petroleum reserves. Lignocellulose materials are most abundant renewable resources produced by photosynthesis on earth. Thus in agricultural countries crop production forms an integral part in process biotechnology in terms of renewable resource supply.[28] In countries like India 74.5 million hectares of land is under forest covering a total land area of 22.7%. The annual production of cellulose in India is nearly five billion tons.[29-30] Scopes of this abundant resources have been highlighted in several places in terms of developing process biotechnology. Besides cellulose materials many other conventional and indigenous resources have been used either as a substrate or as an enhancer of product formation in process biotechnology. Not only that besides microbial process biotechnology resources,[31-32] plant cell culture and animal cell culture biotechnology are proving their international industrial impact in meeting the needs of mankind. CHEMRAWN conferences focussed on the future sources of organic raw materials, world food supplies, resource material conversions etc. emphasizing impact of Biotechnology.

1.4.3 Human Resources

For adequate human resource power to support programmes in the multidisciplinary activities of process biotechnology, different nations have taken various steps. For example in India the Department of Biotechnology (formerly NBTB) Govt. of India evolved integrated plan comprising several components. Among these components, one is the post-graduate teaching in biotechnology. DBT in cooperation with Ministry of Human Resource Development (MHRD), University Grant Commission, ICAR, ICMR and a few universities including IITs & IISc playing a unique role in the progress of Biotechnology in India. In all these cooperational effort, major objective is to have adequate trained manpower to support programmes in multidisciplinary areas of Biotechnology. Among important areas of Biotechnology, tissue culture application for medicinal and economic plants, fermentation technology and enzyme engineering for chemicals, biochemicals, and antibiotics and other medicinal product developments through process biotechnology including agriculture and forest residues and industrial house wastes utilization, emerging areas like genetic engineering and molecular biology were in the forefront in Indian sixth S & T plan. In order to serve for process biotechnology, besides various academic departments and centers many research laboratories of national importance such as NCL Punae, CDRI Lucknow, CFTRI Mysore, RRL Jorhat, Jammu and Kashmir and Bhubneshwer, Indian Institute of Petroleum, Dehradun, IMT, Chandigarh etc have human resource development programmes through research more in applied microbiology within the framework of their objectives. Likewise

NII, ICGEB, New Delhi, AIIMS, New Delhi and many other centers of DBT, GOI have programmes in their domains of biotechnology activities. Many institutions and universities in overseas countries are deeply concerned to have proper manpower in the area.

1.4.4 Professional Domains of Trained Manpower

With training in Biochemical Engineering and Biotechnology, a person has several fields within industry, academic institutions or research and development (R & D) laboratories to pursue his professional career. These include pharmaceuticals, chemical and biochemical waste and waste water treatments and recycling and food processing biotechnology industries.[35] For examples, to name a few industries in India, Cadila (Pharma), Ahmedabad; India Yeast Co. Ltd., Sreerampur (West Bengal); Alembic Chemicals, Baroda (Gujarat); IDPL, Risikesh (U.P.); Hindustan Antibiotics, Pune (Maharashtra); Unichem Ltd. (Hyderabad); Pfizer (India) Ltd, Chandigarh; Anil Starch, Ahmedabad (Gujarart); Ranbaxy, Delhi; Max India, Chandigarh; Cynamide India, Baroda; Bengal Immunity (West Bengal); SPIC pharmaceutical, Tamil Nadu and many other recent concerns are actively engaged in large scale production of antibiotics, vitamins, steroids, enzymes, vaccines etc. through bioprocesses. Also, several companies are now engaged in production of high value low volume bioproducts like restriction endonucleases, health care diagnostics and many other products. These are in addition to a large number of breweies, distilleries and food industries. These concerns and a large number of industrial waste treatment plants whose activity primarily deals with process biotechnology look for adequately qualified biochemical engineers and biotechnologists. Recently few consultancy and other organizations such as Unique Biochemical Engineering, Bombay; Engineers India Ltd., Delhi; Biotech Consortium India Ltd, Delhi; Vam Organics Pvt. Ltd., Gazraula, U.P.; SPIC, Tamil Nadu; United Breweries, Bangalore; Biocon India, Bangalore etc have plans in the area and are creating job avenues for biochemical engineering and biotechnology personnel. Professional domains of human resources in the area in developed and developing countries are more or less similar.[8,24]

1.4.5 University/Institute–Industry Cooperation

Necessity of strengthening of industry-university/institute linkages and cooperation has been felt in recent years more considerably. There are now a number of technology oriented industries who are appreciative of the linkages and inclined for bilateral cooperation in giving access to the facilities and resources available with them. This is primarily to remove the short comings in both academia and in industry. The objective of creating pilot plant/demonstration facilities in some institutes/ universities was to strengthen this linkage. Pennsylvania State University's Bioprocessing Resource Center opened a pilot plant in May 1990 mainly with this view. The first company to use this facility was Bio Process (Reading, PA) which aimed to developing a process to convert protein bearing wastes into water soluble, high quality predigested proteins for use in animal feeds.[36] In a similar approach a demonstration facility has been opened at IIT Delhi's BERC/Dept. of Biochemical Engineering and Biotechnology for "Bioconversion of lignocellulosies into ethyl alcohol and coproducts" at the beginning. Bigger bioprocessing facility available at Chemical Center of the University of Lund, Sweden, at Leigh University, USA and at a few other places in Europe have similar concepts.

1.5 FORECASTING

In relevance to development of process biotechnology a futurological forecasting of Nobel Laureate Har Govind Khorana need to be kept in mind. It reads as below: "In the years ahead, genes are going to be synthesized. The next step would be to learn to manipulate the information content of genes and to learn to insert them into and delete them from the genetic systems. When, in the distant future, all this comes to pass the temptation to change our biology will be strong."

One of the messages from this is evolutionary findings for revolutionary changes in bioproduct development. It has also been stated that industrial fermentations are money making ventures, and the competition is keen. More than one industrial concern may carry out the same fermentation and even use a similar microorganism. Also the fermentation product may have to compete on the open market with a similar product that is produced by a chemical process. In order to be able to be competitive the essentiality of technologically redesigning the biocells using modern biomolecular redesign engineering principles is obvious. Not only that, in the operation of a 'Biotechnology plant' it is necessary to overcome the weakest link. Also, besides use of indigenous resource material from university and industry interface drive for industrializing 'Biotechnology' in many developing countries would foster the growth of the area. In the envisaged long term plan of the National Biotechnology Board (NBTB), now Department of Biotechnology (DBT) of India, for example the forecasting on the area was encouraging. Accordingly, Biotechnology, viewed as the utilization of biological process based on microbial, plant and animal cells or their constituents to provide the needs of man has been exploited by mankind for centuries[38] through the techniques of fermentation in the areas of alcoholic beverages, food processing and the detoxification of animal and human generated wastes and residues. Realizing biotechnology as one of the major emerging fields, IIT Delhi was the first among IIT educational scenario in India to reorient its curriculum design keeping a balance between liberal arts, basic sciences, engineering arts and sciences and subjects related to the specific field of Biochemical engineering and Biotechnology in the form of a five year integrated M. Tech educational programme to provide the nation and supranation its intellectual property and to foster process biotechnology. Thus, in the modern biotechnological forecasting which involves a systematic quantitative analysis of future technologies the effort is to determine what process biotechnologies should be developed at different times in the future to meet the specific needs of world population and what process biotechnologies are likely to be available at different times in the future in view of the present rate of growth of bioscientific innovations.

This is followed by appropriate resource allocation to ensure that imperative and feasible future biotechnologies are available when they are most needed. Decision makers are thereby able to use future biotechnologies more actively as resources for long range development than is otherwise possible. This is extremely important. It is because in recent years the length of time between the technological developments and the widespread usage of new biotechnologies has been very rapid. Many other technological forecasting and related concerns have been highlighted at various places. These include microbial, plant and mammalian cell and related systems.[39] Since recombinant DNA redesigning researches have revolutionized biology, the common laboratory strains or biocells are now exploited as the factories for producing large amounts of different types of molecules of interest to the mankind for future developments through process biotechnology[40] and renewable resource engineering.[41]

1.6 REFERENCES

1. Steel, R. (ed). "Biochemical Engineering", *Unit Process in Fermentation*, Heywood and Company Ltd., London, 1958.
2. Webb, F.C. *Biochemical Engineering,* D. Van Nostrand Co. Ltd., London, 1964.
3. Aiba, S., A.E. Humphrey and N.F. Millis, *Biochemical Engineering* (Ist Edn.), Acad. Press, N.Y., 1967.
4. Ghose, T.K. and A. Fiechter, *Advances in Biochemical Engineering,* Vol. I, Springer Verlag, Berlin, 1971.
5. Bailey, J.E., D.F. Ollis, *Biochemical Engineering Fundamentals* (Ist Edn.), McGraw Hill Book Co., New York, 1977.
6. Aiba, S. "Some Recent Topics of Research in Biochemical Engineering",*Bioconversionand Biochemical Engineering ,* Vol. I , pp 23-41, BERC, IIT Delhi, (T.K. Ghose ed.), 1980.
7. Moo Young, M.(ed.). "Overview of Biotechnology Activities in Developing Countries", *Adv. in Biotechnology,* Vol. II, pp 679, Pergamon Press, Toronto, Canada, 1981.
8. Moo Young, M (ed.). "Overview of Training Programme in Biotechnology and Biochemical Engineering", *Adv. in Biotechnology,* Vol. I, pp 749-752, Pergamon Press., Toronto, Canada, 1980.
9. Hoogerheide, J.C. *Adv. in Microbial Engineering,* Part II (B. Sikyta, A. Prokop M. Novak, eds.), Address by the Sympo. Co. Chairman, J. Wiley and Sons., New York, 1974.
10. Fiechter, A. *Birth of a Concept in Bioprocess Engineering: The First Generation*, pp 13-19, (T.K. Ghose ed.), Ellis Horwood Ltd., Chichester, U.K. 1989.
11. Mukhopadhyay, S.N. "Biochemical Engineering Education and Research: Past, Present and Future Strategy". *Proc. Twenty Years of Biochemical Engineering Teaching and Research in India*, pp 10-14, Jadavpur Univ., (T.K. Ghose ed.), Calcutta, 1979 .
12. Abelson, P.H.*Indian Development Trends,* Science Editorial, 225,4661, 1984.
13. Elander, R.P. "Biotechnology Bridging the Gap between Fundamental and Applied", *Dev. in Industrial Microbiol,* pp 28, 13-22, (G. Pierce ed.), Elsevier, 1987.
14. Mukhopadhyay, S.N. "Current Status of Biomolecular Design Engineering". *Proc. Jrd AP BioChEC 94,* pp 511-513,W.K. Teo, M.G.S. Yap and S.K.W: Oh (eds.), CHE BTU, NUS, 1994.
15. Ramachandran, S. "How Good is Our Biochemical Industry Progressing without Biochemical Engineering", *Proc. Workhop "Twenty Years of Biochemical Engineering",* pp 35-37, Jadavpur Univ. Calcutta, 1979.
16. Menon, M.G.K. "Basic Research as an Integral Component of a Self Reliant Base of Science and Technology. Its Role, Relevance, Support, and Areas of Thrust", Presidential Address, 69th Session, *Indian Science Congress Association,* Mysore, GOI, DST, New Delhi, 1987 .
17. Gaden Jr, E.L. "Engineering and Biotechnology: Accomplishments and Challenges", *Biotechnology and Bioprocess Engineering,* pp 37-43, (T.K. Ghose ed.), United India Press, New Delhi, 1984.
18. Arber, W. *Future of Recombinant DNA Technology. Ibid,* pp 45-53.
19. Humphrey, A.E. *Biotechnology: Where Do We Go from Here*?, Ibid, pp 55-68.
20. Wiseman, A. "Features of Biotechnology and its Scientific Basis", *Principles of Biotechnology,* pp 1-4, (A. Wiseman ed.), Surrey Univ. Press, Chapman and Hall, New York, 1983 .
21. Ghose, T.K. "Symbiosis of Chemical Engineering and Biology: A Decade Experience", *First J.C. Bose Memorial Award Oration Lecture,* IIT Delhi, Nov. 24, 1983.
22. Heden, C.G. "Global Aspects of Biotechnology", *J. Chem. Tech. Biotechnol,* pp 32, 18-24, 1982.

23. Humphrey, A.E.*Biotechnology*: *The Way Ahead*, *Ibid,* pp 25-23.
24. Rolz, C.E. "Biotechnology in Less Developed Countries", Proc. VIlth IBS, pp 547-550, (T.K. Ghose ed.), United India Press., New Delhi, 1985.
25. King, P.P. "Biotechnology-An Industrial View", *J. Chem. Technol. & Biotechnol,* pp 2-8, 32, 1982.
26. Rehm, H.J. *Biotechnology Research in Europe*, Ibid, pp 9-13.
27. Pirt, S.J. *Microbial Photosynthesis in the Harnessing of Solar Energy*, Ibid, pp 198-202.
28. Chopra, V.L." Biotechnology for Crop Improvement ", *6th Lala Karam Chand Thapar Memorial Lecture,*New Delhi, Feb. 14, 1989.
29. Tilak, B.D. "Prospects of Manufacture of Industrial Chemicals from Cellulose", *Proc. Bioconv. Sympo,*pp 25-36, IIT, Delhi, (T.K. Ghose ed.), 1977 .
30. Ramachandran, A. *Role of Bioconversion in India's Science & Technology,* pp 1-10, IIT Delhi, (T.K. Ghose ed.), 1977 .
31. Banerjee, M., S.N. Mukhopadhyay and N.D. Banerjee, "Utilization of Paddy Soak Water (Parboiling) as a Source of Nutrients for *Penicillium wortmani*, *Ind. Jr. Microbiol,* pp 4, 53-59, 1974.
32. Bose, K. and T.K. Ghose, "Studies on Continuous Fermentation of Indian Care Sugar Molasses by Yeasts", *Process Biochem*, 8(2) 23, 1973.
33. Mukhopadhyay, S.N., E.C. Rubio, A.O. Vale, G.C. Arcos andJ.I. Leon, "Evaluation of SCP from Opuntia Juice", *Biotechnol. Lett* , pp1(7), 276-278, 1979.
34. Cooney, C.L. *Biotechnology and Bioprocess Engineering, Vllth IBS Proc*, pp 5-6, (T.K. Ghose ed.), 1985 .
35. Wang, D.I.C. and A.E. Humphrey, Biochemical Engineering; Chem. Engg., pp 108-116, December 1969.
36. *Bioprocessing Technology,* Pilot Plant Opens at Penn State, Vol. 12(6), 8, 1990.
37. Engels, J. and E. Uhlman, "Gene Synthesis", *Adv. Biochem. Engg./Biotechnol.* Vol. 37, pp 75 (A. Fiechter ed.), Springer-Verlag, 1988.
38. *Biotechnology:Long Term Plan for India,*National Biotechnology Board, DST, 1983.
39. National Paper India, *United Nations Conference on New and Renewable Resources of Energy,* Nairobi, August, 1981.
40. Gopinathan, K.P. "Recombinant DNA Cells and Process Scale up Criteria", *Biotechnology and Bioprocess Engineering.* Proc. *VIIth* IBS, pp 493-498, (T.K. Ghose ed.), 1985.
41. Mukhopadhyay, S.N. and Ajay Srivastava, "Aspects of Cellulose: Synthesis, Conversion, Fabric Bioprocessing and Applications", *Proc. of the IIChE Golden Jubliee Congress,* pp 209-221 (S. Nath ed.) , Vol. 1, Replica Press Pub., New Delhi, 1998 .
42. Plant and Equipment for Biotechnology, Oct. 7, 1988, Biotek India, 88, Oct 4-7, 1988 Ashok Hotel, New Delhi.

Chapter

2

ENGINEERING BIOLOGY OF CELLS AND MOLECULES THEY SYNTHESIZE

2.1 CELL BIOLOGY EVENTS

2.1.1 Introduction

Morphologically prokaryotic cells are bivariant systems in terms of growth processes. Bacterial cells have two links between DNA replication and cell division. In general, it is known that the frequency with which cycles of replication are initiated is adjusted to fit the rate at which the cell is growing. The completion of a replication cycle is connected with the division of a single cell into two. During this divisional course the daughter chromosomes are seggregated. Examples exist to show that the interval between initiation of replication and cell division produce multi- fork chromosome in rapidly growing cells. The cell biology parametric characters of bacteria relates to the classic concept of Cooper and Helmstetter regarding growth parameters. The cell biology parametric characters provide linkage between DNA replication and cell division (Table 2.1). For example in the chromosomal complement of a bacterial cell (*E. coli*) at 5 minutes interval throughout the cell cycle the cell receives a partially replicated chromosome. The replication fork continues to advance. At 10 minutes when the 'old' replication fork has not yet reached the terminus initiation occurs at both origins on partially replicated chromosome. The start and , events of these 'new' replication forks creates a multifork chromosome (Fig. 2.1). However, this concept does not indicate connection of the age of the cell at initiation and interinitiation time (IIT). This connection is important in understanding frequency of initiation from *ori* C as a function of cell growth rate specially in 'technologically designed' cells. In order to understand

Table 2.1 Cell biology parametric characters *vis-a-vis* bacterial growth

	Parameter Components	*Observed Characters*
A.	**Cellbiological**	
	Chromosome (C)	Has single replicon
	Frequency of C	Controlled by a number of initiation action events
	Initiation events	
	(a) replication	Occurs at a single origin
		Coupled to cell cycle by the concentration of Dna A.
	(b) rate of replication	Controlled not by chain elongation
		Controlled by the rate initiation at the origin of replication.
	DNA biosynthesis rate	Invariant at constant temperature
	DNA replication time cycle	Has two phase constants: D & C
B.	**Growth Related**	
	Generation time (t_d)	Value varies (e.g. *E. coli,* 18–180 mins)
	Sum of D and C if > t_d	Replication reinitiates before completion of previous round of replication
		Leads to interinitiation time (IIT) by overlapping D and C periods.

this multifork concept in plasmid system, it has been shown that both chromosomal and plasmid replication are important in the manifestation of cell biology behaviour in cell growth and division.[4] Hence it carried information *ori* the kinetics of cell growth.[1,4] Information of faster or slower growth rate of cells is important in bioprocess engineering design in terms of: (a) transient analysis, (b) maximum specific growth rate or dilution rate, (c) transformations, (d) oxygen responses in transformant cells and (e) bioprocessing strategy. The importance of the engineering biology parameters in developing bacterial process biotechnology is therefore obvious.

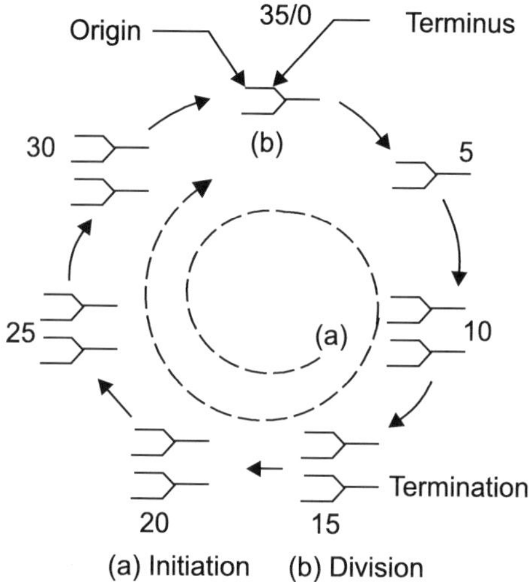

Fig. 2.1 Engineering biology of DNA replication time cycle in *E. coli*

2.1.2 Facts in Biocell Growth in Terms of Engineering Biology

Several facts as given in Table 2.2 are essential in biocell growth. When bacterial cells grow subsequent increase in DNA occurs. As certain antibiotics like chloramphenicol inhibit the proteins required for the initiation of new round of replication, the amount of DNA synthesized should be maximum when the inhibitor is added at the beginning of a round of replication. Highest synthesis occurs when added at appropriate time before cell division. This leads to assume that morphologically prokaryotic cells are bivariant systems in terms of growth processes. Bacterial cells have two links between DNA replication and cell division.[1,2] In general, it has been stated that the frequency with which cycles of replication are initiated, is adjusted to fit the rate at which the cell is growing[3]. The completion of a replication cycle is connected with the division of a single cell into two. During this divisional course the daughter chromosomes are segregated. Examples exist to show that the interval between initiation of replication and cell division produce multiforked chromosome in rapidly growing cells.[2,4,5]

Table 2.2 Facts in bacterial growth in terms of engineering biology

- Protein synthesis needed for initiation event.
- Gene products are necessary for cell division.
- Unit cell with an entity of 1.7 μm long.
- A bacterium has one origin per unit cell.
- Fast growing cell with two origins is > 3.4 μm long.
- Topological link of IIT & cell structure forms site.
- One growth site per unit cell.

2.1.3 Multiforked Model

1. Chromosomal DNA replication & cell division

These events of bacteria relate to the concept of Cooper and Helmstetter[5] regarding growth parameters. Both cell biology and growth parameters display interlinked observed characters which are related to design of process biotechnology.[1,5] For example, it is well known that cells of *E. coli* can grow at a variety of rates. Its doubling time (t_d) accordingly varies widely. It ranges between as quick as 18 minutes to as slow as 180 minutes. As bacterial chromosome is known to be a single replicon, the frequency of its replication cycle is, therefore, controlled by the number of initiation events at the single origin. The biosynthesis rate of DNA is more or less invariant at a constant temperature. The speed of its synthesis reaction remains same unless and until the supply of precursors gets limited. Thus, limiting nutrient parameter of process biotechnology is intimately associated to cell biology.

2. The replication time cycle

The replication time cycle has been defined by two phase constants, namely C phase and D phase. These constants are important in linkage between chromosomal DNA replication phase (C) and cellular divisional phase (D). Besides these several facts are also associated in bacterial growth which are of important concern. In *E. coli* cell, for example, analysis of the replication initiation time to completion of one round of replication in cells growing with generation times between 22 and 60 minutes has revealed these important facts. The time of initiation changed with the growth rate in a definite fashion in rapidly growing cells. The key of this fact is that a round of replication requires nearly 40 minutes. Also, the cell division occurs 20 minutes after the completion of a round of DNA replication. Thus initiation always occurs 60 minutes before the cell division which segregates the daughter chromosomes indicating the linkage between DNA replication and cell division.

2.1.4 Linkage between DNA Replication and Cell Division

1. Cooper-Helmstetter concept [5]

When a bacteria divides more frequently than at 60 minutes intervals, a cycle of replication is initiated before the end of every 35 minutes. This may be taken as an example. The cycle of replication connected with a division must have been initiated 25 minutes before the preceding division. This situation as presented in literature (Fig. 2.1) shows the chromosomal complement of a bacterial cell at 5 minutes intervals throughout the cycle. It has been shown that at division (35/ 0 minutes) the cell receives a partially replicated chromosome. The replication fork continues to advance. At 10 minutes when this old replication fork has not yet reached the terminus, initiation occurs at both origins on partially replicated chromosome. The start of these new replication fork creates a multifork chromosome.[4,5,6]

2. Growth in relation to replication initiation time point

The events of engineering cell biology of a bacteria in growth phases in terms of segregation mechanism of attachment of DNA to membrane in a batch culture could be represented by a pictorial model (Fig. 2.2). This model, however, did not indicate the connection of age of the cell at initiation and inter-initiation time (IIT). This connection is important in understanding frequency of initiation from *ori* C as a function of cell growth rate. Realizing this limitation in the above mentioned pictorial model its extension in terms of cell division cycle time components of a new born cell has been analyzed (Fig. 2.3). Also, bacterial subcellular molecular engineering

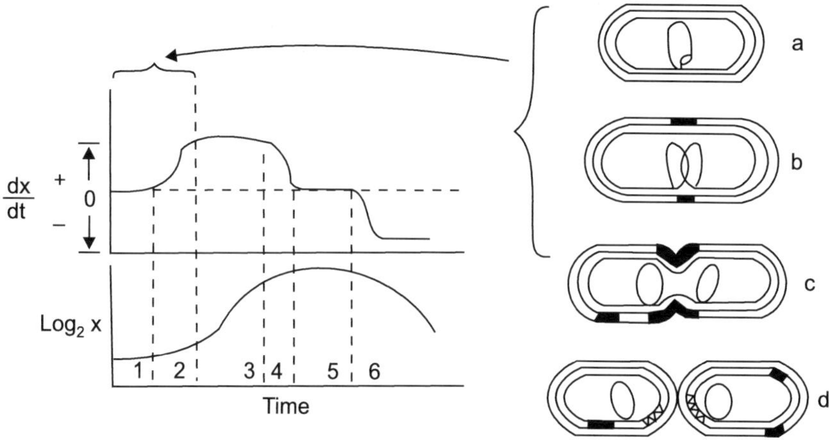

Fig. 2.2 Growth phases in relation to segregation mechanism of attachment of bacterial DNA to the membrane of cell in batch culture (1) lag phase, dx/dt = 0; (2) acceleration phase, dx/dt > 0; (3) exponential phase, dx/dt = constant; (4) retardation phase, dx/dt → 0; (5) stationary phase, dx/dt = 0; (6) declining phase, dx/dt is negative)

biology components, e.g. chromosome and plasmid are contributing significantly in bioprocess engineering by participating in developing technologically redesigned biocells or enzymic protein biocatalysis for specific product formation. Now its examples are many.[6]

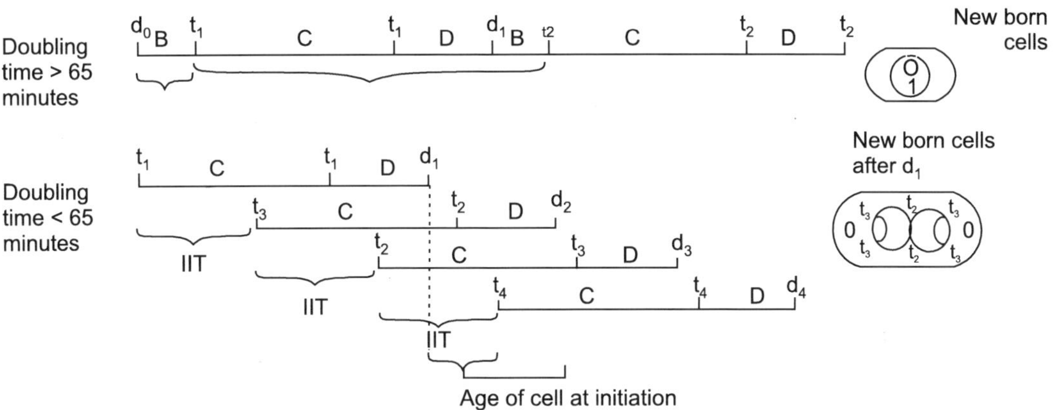

Fig. 2.3 Interinitiation time (IIT) scheme of cell division cycle[6]

3. Translation of replication knowledge to bioprocess engineering

It is evident that both chromosomal and plasmid replication are important in the manifestation of cell biology behaviour in product forming culture. As discussed in preceeding sections replication relates to cell growth and cell division. Hence, it carried information on the kinetics of cell growth. Information of faster or slower growth rate of cells is important in bioprocess engineering design in terms of (a) transient analysis, (b) maximum specific growth rate/dilution rate, (c) optimization of growth related variables, (d) stability of transformant, (e) oxygen responses in transformant cells[7,8] and (f) expression of transformant in scale up system and varying bioprocessing strategy. Analysis of many of these aspects with bacterial cultures are in progress.

4. Concept of stability and steady state in cell division

(*i*) *Physical Basis* : Cell cultures if grown in a batch system is unstable. Non-equilibrium or instability in terms of growth and product formation exhibited for obvious reasons. Also, some organisms grow quickly, some at relatively intermediate rate while others slowly even in the best medium. Cell growth instability however relates to physical, chemical and genetic basis.

For overcoming this instability disadvantage the concept of 'inflow' and 'outflow' for continuous linkage between DNA replication and cell division in nutrients was conceived. As per this concept by inflow of fresh nutrients and concomitantly to the outflow of a portion of culture it would be possible theoretically to maintain the logarithmic growth rate or steady balanced cell division/growth infinitely. In other words 'steady state' growth of cultures is possible. Such 'steady state' cultures have indeed been achieved, if not infinitely, at least for several days in many systems although mostly in laboratory scale by using appropriate cell cultivation strategy. One of the primary factors influencing the logarithmic or steady state growth of the culture relates to the inherent character of the organism. Instability and non-equilibrium condition cause nonuniformity in growth rate and other parameters in the biosystem and is disadvantageous in process biotechnology development.

However, steady state or stability of growth depends on many external factors. The concentration of nutrient(s) at very low levels can limit the rate. If the medium contains all but one of the essential nutrients in excess, both the growth rate and total density of the cell population will then depend on the concentration of this limiting factor in the growth medium. This principle in form of exogenous "differential feeding" can be used to regulate 'steady state' growth of cells. Under such exogenous control both the flow rate and the medium concentration of one essential nutrient are arbitrarily fixed at values that result in less than maximum growth rate of the system. As the culture density increases from the inoculum, the limiting factor is taken up to provide the irreducible individual requirement for more and more cell biomass and the concentration of this factor in the medium become progressively lower and lower. In time, the concentration will reach the very low level at which it limits growth rate, where upon the growth rate will decrease until it just balances the flow rate. At this point the culture is stabilized and will thereafter maintain a constant cell density. This mode of cell cultivation is termed as continuous culture. Stabilized or steady state system is important in kinetic studies on genetic mutation, enzymic adaptation and should offer a valuable approach to the investigation of the synthesis of cell protoplasm. It can also provide larger biomass yield of cells per unit volume of medium than is possible in classical closed system batch method.

(*ii*) *Microbial Engineering Basis :* Two mechanisms for regulation of continuous culture are : (a) internal control or turbidostat/biogen and (b) external control or 'chemostat'. In 'turbidostat' the cell propagation is held constant by a device that measures the culture turbidity and regulates the feed and simultaneously, of course, the withdrawal, accordingly. It means that if the cell population rises above the set levels the proportional speed control pump adds medium at an increased rate until it returns; if the population falls too low the pump adds medium at a reduced rate until it returns to set level. For adequate response it is necessary to operate a turbidostat in or near 'exponential' phase of growth. In bacterial or yeast system by means of a photocell and appropriate electrical connection the turbidostat can maintain a constant culture density easily by adjusting the flow rate of fresh medium in the culture volume. The rate of flow of fresh medium (F) into the culture divided by the volume of the culture (V) in the vessel which is defined as the dilution rate (D) and is equal to the specific growth rate of the cell (μ) depends only on the medium. Thus,

$$D = \frac{F}{v} = m = \frac{\ln 2}{t_g} = \frac{0.693}{t_g} \tag{2.1}$$

When $\mu = \mu_m, \quad t_g = 0.693/\mu_m$

where t_g is the generation time or doubling time of the cells. In 'chemostat' however, feed rate and withdrawl rate are held constant at a value less than maximum specific growth rate. Under such conditions the growth rate is regulated by a limiting nutrient concentration. This constitutes a self regulatory and stable steady state. Although the principle of turbidostat has advantages of three operational allowance in logarithmic phase and nondependence on limiting nutrient except to the extent that some unknown factor limits the growth of a batch culture but it is associated with many weaknesses namely: 1. It involves apparatus for control that is subject to failure and requires extra investment and maintenance. 2. Turbidity measurements are complicated by the clinging of cells to glass surface in the path of the meter's light beam. 3. It must operate further from maximal cell population than chemostat, residual nutrient is necessarily higher than the minimum. This makes turbidostat less efficient. For these reasons chemostat principle is more widely used for continuous cultivations/fermentations.

If the cell population were to grow at a rate μ but without change in the base biomass, a longer time τ would be required for the population to double, which is simply a reciprocal of specific growth rate. Thus

$$\tau = 1/\mu = t_g/0.693 = 1.45t_g \tag{2.2}$$

τ is sometimes referred to as 'birth time' or that time an organism must exist before dividing when in a population that has a particular growth rate μ.

During growth with ample water and nutrients, the resulting growth rate is an inherent characteristics of the organism, μ_{max}, subject to modification by nutrient balance and culture history. Growth proceeds at a maximal rate that increases with temperature until functions are impaired. The change in μ_{max} with temperature is sometimes expressed as a temperature quotient Q_{10}, the temperature rise that causes the rate to double. Alternatively, the change is expressed as an activation energy, E_a, which comes from transition state theory for reversible catalyzed reactions and the assumptions that maximal growth rate is set, as if it were determined by a single rate limiting step. The relationship is

$$\mu_m = A \exp. (E_a/RT) \tag{2.3}$$

Maximal growth rates are used to characterise the specific ability of pouplations to increase under favourable conditions and also to identify the growth rate ($\mu_m/2$) that Michaelis concentration specify. Interpretation of E_a values complicated by multiple interactive phenomena such as sharp change in membrane properties at the transition temperature. However, they remain a convenient way to demonstrate and express the amount of change in rate with temperature.

Cell quota in growth : In some organisms it was noticed that the amout of limiting nutrient per cell decreased with growth rate as it becomes limiting. These observations led to develop the concept of cell quota. As interspecies and chemical comparisons are impossible without knowledge of cell size, the cell quota Q' is sometimes expressed as nutrient per gram of cells. Cell quota approaches some minimum value k_Q.

$$\mu = \mu'_m \, [1 - k_Q/Q'] \tag{2.4}$$

Here $\mu'_{m'}$ is a constant which is considered to be inflated growth rate μ_m. In numerous algal cell systems phosphates, various nitrogen sources, silicon, iron and cobalamine may act as limiting nutrients.

Equation (2.4) was found to hold good in these cases. In the special case where all of the substrate collected is laid down and retained as cell material, then considering Y_G as growth yield.

$$Q' = 1/Y_G \tag{2.5}$$

and substrate uptake is given by the widely used relation

$$q = \mu Q'X \tag{2.6}$$

This equation is appropriate for uptake of substrates when exertion of them is negligible. This is not applicable for hetrotrophic cells because of the large amount of carbon lost to CO_2 and organic products. However, it appears that significant losses occur for other nutrients as well. For example Chan and Campbell could not account for only 40% of the nitrate-nitrogen taken up as particulate material in studies of freshwater phytoplankton. Leakage of both orthophosphate and organic phosphate has been quantified during phosphate limited continuous cultures of *Rhodotorula rubra*. The point that a linear decrease in yield with growth rate gives a good fit to equation (2.4) and can easily be demonstrated graphically. Sometimes Q' is linear rather than hyperbolic with growth rate giving curvature to Y_G vs μ.

(iii) Genetic Basis: It has long been observed that a single species of organism can give rise to variation in terms of development of several types of colonies on the same medium. This variation commonly called culture dissociation give rise to variant strains which exhibit considerable differences not only in colony structure but in cellular morphology and physiology as well. Culture variations is also often observed in repeated subculture. These variation may occur due to genotype or phenotype changes of the culture. Genotype changes are relatively stable alterations of individual genes, of gene assortments, and of the characteristics they control, caused by either automation, sex like processor by lysogenic conversion. However, when genes merely control the reaction range of a cell, the specific expression of a given characteristics is subject to considerable temporary modification by environmental conditions. Such environment dependent instability in the expression of gene-controlled characteristics is known as phenotype variability and the resulting changes are called phenotype changes. Certain bacterial cells possess the genetic potential to form a certain pigment produced by the individual cells, however, is influenced by the nutritional conditions and the H^+ ion concentration of the environment. Although culture variation may be advantageous in providing the basis for effective selection programme for higher yielding cell, continuing phenotype instability is obviously undesirable. In the long term, variability in product yield over successive subcultures is potentially a problem and has often been observed in microbial and plant cells. The mechanisms underlying culture instability is still poorly understood. Genetic factors have been invoked, though the evidence mainly derives from numerous investigation of recognisable phenotype abnormalities in cultured cells. Attempts have been made to link gross genomic changes to altertion in secondary metabolite yield in plant cell cultures.

2.1.5 Cellular Proteolysis Events

1. General

Growth related intracellular events as shown in Fig. 2.4 are the following :

(a) Anabolic aberration and spontaneous mutations.
(b) Biosynthetic error.
(c) Post biosynthetic damage in cells.

During growth of cells intracellular proteins in wild microbial strains are broken down to appropriate rates during starvation or endogenous metabolism. Even in exponential phase of growth of biocells *in vivo* proteolysis has been shown to be possible (Fig. 2.4). It necessitated proper understanding and study of the following :

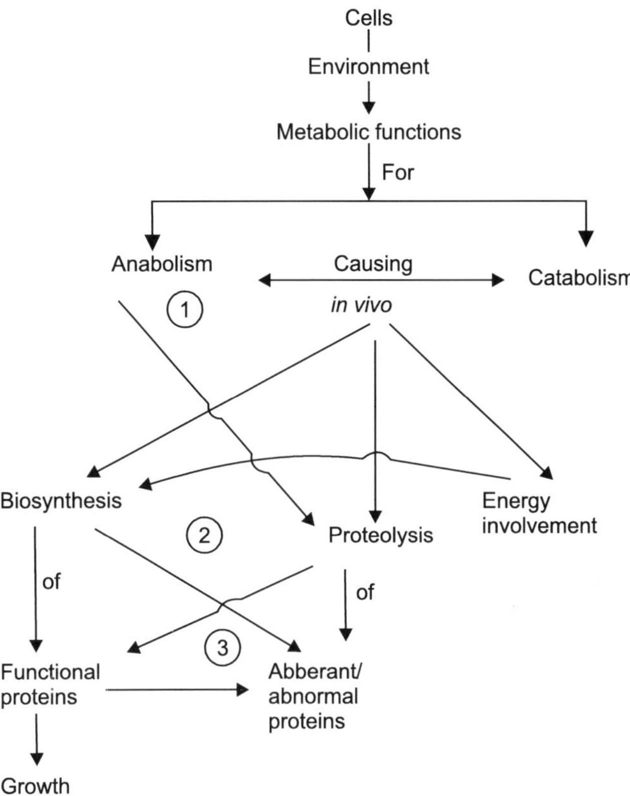

Fig. 2.4 Other events in cell division cycle

- Molecular principles of protein design/biosynthesis vis-a-vis proteolysis in cells.
- *In vivo* proteolysis kinetics.
- Influencial parameters of *in vivo* proteolysis.
- Foreign protein expression and/or secretion in cells.

In microbial cells for obtaining maximum metabolic economy it is essential to minimize and control *in vivo* proteolysis. Among several reasons of aging of cells and reduction in productivity, *in vivo* proteolysis is an important concern. The functional proteins generated through *in vivo* synthesis in cells is the major determinant in reactions, transport and physical and morphological characteristics of the cell. Generally the intracellular proteins in wild strains of microorganisms are broken down at appreciable rates during starvation or endogenous metabolism. Thus *in vivo* proteolysis in cells occurs to prevent the accumulation of highly abnormal proteins that may result from spontaneous mutations, biosynthetic errors or postsynthetic damage in cells. This has direct impact on the bioprocessing objective particularly when the overall objective in a number of contemporary manufacturing biotechnologies and many of those expected in the future is maximal production of a particular protein. In studies with different microorganisms including *E. coli* for proteolysis it appeared that protein label may appear metabolically stable in growing cells sometimes after the label was provided. It necessitated proper estimation of intracellular proteolysis and turnover. The method of steady-state measurement of the turnover of amino acid in the cellular protein of growing cells of *E. coli* has shown the existence of biphasic kinetic regimes in intracellular proteolysis. It has been observed that when exponentially growing bacteria are deprived of nitrogen, a carbon source or a required amino acid the rate of catabolism of cellular protein increases several fold thereby pointing whether intracellular proteolysis need be considered in relation to protein synthesis. Protein synthesis in overall terms has been considered in William's structured growth model. Genetic regulation of synthesis of a particular protein has been studied by several biochemical engineering laboratories. In bacteria as in animal cells *in vivo* proteolysis requires metabolic energy and is an ATP-dependent process. It has been stated that ATP stimulates proteolysis. Continuous culture experiment of Willets[9] could suggest that intracellular proteolysis occurs not only in nongrowing cells but limited proteolysis occurred during exponential phase as well. The mechanism of intracellular proteolysis in microbial cells is not clearly understood. However, participation of enzyme-like processes in the reaction has been shown by various investigators and it necessitates the participation of ATP. Therefore, it is important to understand and to describe in quantitative reaction engineering terms the kinetic, regulatory mechanisms of *in vivo* proteolysis so that protein composition of organisms used in industrial processes can be suitably regulated and controlled.

2. *Molecular principles of protein synthesis and degradation in cells*

The efforts of specialists in the kinetics for increased production capacities of microorganisms in biotechnological industries has been diverted strongly in the optimization of cell culture conditions for intracellular protein synthesis but without considering its *in vivo* degradation. In order to increase the metabolic economy of the cells *in vivo* proteolysis must be regulated. Much experimental data has been accumulated which characterizes the influence of various physical and chemical parameters on the specific cell growth rate on different biosynthetic processes. External character of the influence of temperature, pH, eH values and occasionally pO_2 values is fairly well known. The optimized conditions of these parameters in a well nourished medium lead to cell growth via intracellular protein synthesis based on molecular level principles. Although some simplifying principles may be set forth, exceptions stem from the fact that microbes , particularly bacteria because of extensive inherent control/regulatory mechanisms can adapt to synthesize proteins in many environments and meet diverse challenges in various ways.

Simplifying Principles: The growth of a simple microorganism even as simple as *E. coli* is dependent on numerous reactions and functions of many individual control or regulatory molecular level mechanisms. Molecular level principles of protein synthesis may be ascribed to the following (Fig. 2.5).

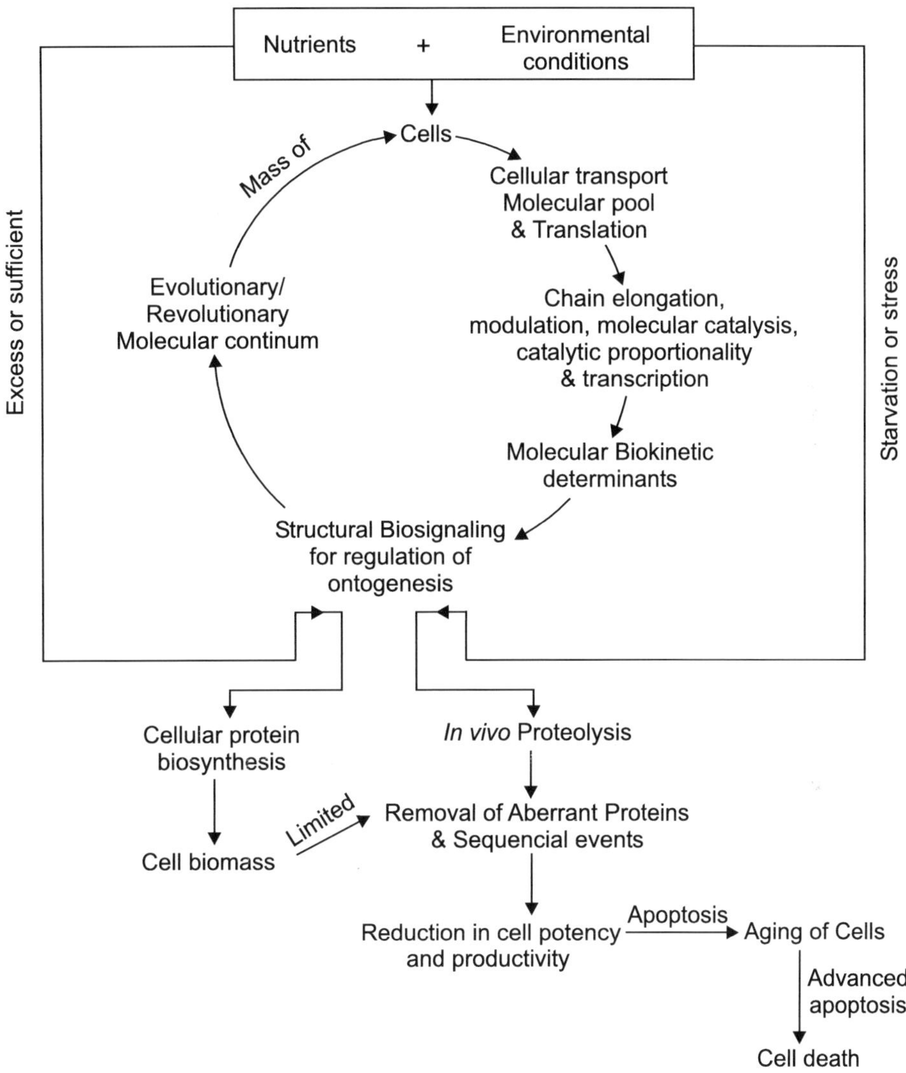

Fig. 2.5 Molecular Principles of cell growth and sequencial events leading to cell death

A. Molecular pool, cellular transport and translation

The microbial regulatory mechanisms function to maintain relatively constant rates of polymerization of macromolecules, e.g., DNA, RNA and protein independent of growth rates. Underlying this are allosteric control mechanisms over metabolic pathways that serve to maintain intracellular pool, active and passive transport mechanisms functioning for the same purpose and regulating the initiation of the synthesis of macromolecules that prevent the inappropriate drain of intermediates.

B. Chain elongation, modulation and molecular catalysis

In rapidly growing cells the available catalytic units for macromolecular synthesis are nearly maximally utilized. Thus a shift to more rapid growth requires the formation of more ribosomes, and possibly more RNA polymerase. In slowly growing cells, the cells have an excess of ribosomes and polymerase and as yet unknown mechanisms limit their initiation of function. Slowly growing cells can respond to shift up by an immediate increase in the rate of RNA and protein synthesis. The controls of slowly growing *E. coli* seem to have evolved to provide rapid adaptability whereas those of rapidly growing cells evolved to provide efficiency.

C. Catalytic proportionality and transcription

In rapidly growing cells, the concentration of ribosomes increases approximately in proportion to the specific growth rate (μ). The rate of rRNA and tRNA synthesis appears coordinated. Their rate is the product of the total rate of cellular RNA synthesis and the viable fraction of the synthesis given to the formation of the stable species. Under certain conditions, turnover of some nascent rRNA has been reported to influence the amount accumulating. This is a feature of normal cell growth as well, at least at low growth rates. Also, tRNA is more stable and increases slightly relative to rRNA at low growth rates. It has also been seen that the synthesis of rRNA *in vivo* is generally correlated with the inverse of concentration of guanosine 5' diphosphate 3' diphosphate (ppGpp) nucleotide (PG). *In vitro* the transcription of rRNA from phage templates is initiated by ppGpp at physiological concentrations and this may be the basis for control over the genes of the protein forming system in cells. In addition or as an alternative to active control over the expression of these genes by ppGpp, a passive mechanism has also been envisaged. The progress that the genes of the protein forming systems are regulated indirectly as a consequence of growth rate depend upon changes in the global pattern of transcription of the genome defined by relative promoter strengths and the effects of repressors and activators operating on the operons. The synthesis of ribosomal and other proteins of the protein forming system follow a pattern of regulations similar to that of rRNA. Underlying this there must be at least partially distinct mechanisms, since the transcription of the r-protein gene is regulated relative to rRNA transcription.

D. Biokinetic determinant

The total rate of RNA synthesis is the most crucial parameter of intracellular protein synthesis and hence of growth as it is a determinant of the rate of rRNA synthesis. Shift up of slowly growing cells indicate the presence of reverse transcriptional capacity, whereas that of already rapidly growing cells do not. It is possible that the concentration of RNA polymerase of ATP and GTP, which are needed for initiation and possibly of ppGpp determine the total rate of synthesis.

E. Signaling and control

It appears that ppGpp plays a significant role in the regulation of enzymatic and transcriptional activities including rRNA formation. The synthesis of ppGpp is related to the differential signal between the rate of provision of aminoacyl tRNA's and the rate at which they are removed in protein synthesis. This takes place through a stringent control system. Presence of ppGpp is also affected by a less well-defined metabolic regulation sensitive to the carbon/energy supply. Function of ribosome, may therefore be considered as sensory organelle and restricted to transients of cell growth.

F. Evolutionary/revolutionary continuum

The growth and protein synthesis in simple bacterium like *E. coli* may be viewed as continuum of ribosomal synthesis and formation of proteins. Genomic replication and cell division may be quasi-independently regulated processes triggered by events in protein synthesis. These two processes and other partially autogenous processes through evolutionary/revolutionary continuity and taxation of intermediary metabolism influence the growth rate. The growth of microorganisms with exquisite and complex life cycles may include alternative modes of signaling and control about which little is known and much evolutionary/revolutionary search is awaited.

Although the above principles of *in vivo* protein synthesis is well known, it is not exactly known whether the same set of principles and parameters of the medium condition and molecular mechanism play a role in *in vivo* proteolysis. It has promoted intensive search in the area. Catabolic intracellular molecular phenomena in *E. coli* has been observed to manifest the following:

(a) *Bioprocessing of proteins*—for cleavage of leader peptides for transported proteins.

(b) *Defective protein and peptide manipulation*—for degradation of non-functional or mutated proteins or protein containing amino acid analogues in order to increase the metabolic efficiency by recycling required amino acids.

(c) *Degradation of functional proteins*—for specific metabolic conditions in growing cells. Most native proteins have half lives much longer than the generation time, but a few are remarkably unstable.

Protein catabolic manifestation in *E. coli* has been shown to depend on the phase of growth rate. Protein catabolism increases several fold in endogenous phase, i.e. on starvation for carbon, nitrogen or amino acids. The above response appeared to be signaled by a lack of complete complement of aminoacyl tRNA. Thus proteolysis is regulated by principles similar to those regulating rRNA synthesis. The high rate of proteolysis during starvation required continued presence of a high level of ppGpp. In amino acid and/or energy deprivation ppGpp level seems to signal the acceleration of proteolysis.

3. Influential factors

(i) Nutrient Limitation : Early Studies of intracellular protein breakdown indicated that proteins were stable to a high extent in growing bacteria although limited proteolysis could be observed in exponentially growing cells of *E. coli* in a defined medium. The cells subjected to starvation, however, exhibited overall proteolysis at rates of 4 to 7% per hour. Enhancements of proteolysis were also observed for batch cultures of *E. coli* entering stationary phase. Organisms like *E.coli*, *Dictyostelium discoideum, Bacillus cerus, B. megaterium, Pseudomonas saccharophila* and many others have proteolysis rates within these limits. Protein turnover in starving yeast is, however, remarkably low and below 1% per hour. It has also been stated that protein synthesized during starvation are much more unstable than the original cell protein. It was seen that 25-35% proteins made under starvation conditions decomposed within 20 minutes.

Pine[10] observed that glucose depletion stimulated intracellular proteolysis and that growth rate influences protein degradation. Cells growing in glycerol limited medium exhibited more rapid breakdown than cells growing more rapidly in medium supplemented with glucose, casein hydrolysate and vitamins. Thus, Goff and Goldberg[11] noted that acceleration of protein catabolism in poor environments is not correlated with a loss of cell viability nor is it an all-or-none response. In fact, rates of breakdown vary in cells growing at different rates. However, to date there has been very little systematic study of parametric influences on protein degradation kinetics of nutrient levels and limitations and other growth parameters such as temperature. A thorough literature review revealed very few investigations on proteolysis in chemostat culture, in spite of the advantage for maintaining a steady-state culture over a long term and for investigation of a broad range of growth rates. Willett[9] observed a small, rapidly degraded proteins fraction of *E. coli* grown in a chemostat. He found identical overall rates of protein degradation at different dilution rates giving generation times of 1,2 and 4 hours, but noted that sudden decreases in dilution rates gave a transient increase in proteolysis. St. John et al.[12] found that 50% of the proteins in a chemostat culture of *E. coli* were degraded within about 48 hours at a dilution rate of 0.0478 h^{-1} (doubling time of 14.5 h). A double labeling protocol showed that a fraction of the cell protein was five times more labile than another fraction. Soluble proteins were apparently those most susceptible to proteolysis. This small dilution rate likely gave very low residual glucose levels in the chemostat.

It is known that limitation or deprivation of different nutrients can influence intracellular proteolysis in different ways. For example, amino acid starvation elicits a response different from deprivation of an energy source. Phosphate or magnesium limitation has different effects on protein degradation than glucose or amino acid limitation. How these degradation rates are influenced by different types of nutrient limitations, and limitations of different degrees, however, has not been shown.

(ii) Temperature : Rates of proteolysis have been observed to increase rapidly as the temperature is increased. In *E. coli* overall intracellular proteolysis at 43-45°C occurs at a rate similar to that observed under nitrogen starvation. Careful experiment has further shown that temperature changes induce transient fluctuations in the relative rates of synthesis of different proteins which greatly vary by as much as a factor of 50. It is likely to be a consequence of a different influence of temperature on synthesis or degradation or both of these intracellular proteins.

(iii) Oxidants : Intracellular protein degradation in presence of oxidants has revealed that oxidative damage to proteins may be an important factor. Stadtman and coworkers[13] have proposed that inactivation by oxidants may be a specific mechanism initiating the breakdown of critical cell proteins such as glutamine synthatase in *E. coli.* This enzyme plays a key role in the flow of ammonia derived nitrbgen into organic compounds and its activity as well as intracellular content is subject to elaborate regulation. Intracellular breakdown of glutamin synthatase has been suggested to occur in the following two steps: (1) the enzyme is first inactivated irreversibly by a mixed function oxidase system as occurs in model *in vitro* studies with ascorbate, iron and oxygen (2) the inactivated enzyme is more susceptible to proteolytic attack and is rapidly degraded by some cellular protease.

4. Current needs[14-19]

For maximization of metabolic economy of cells regulation/control and optimization of *in vivo* proteolysis plays important role in developing newer bioproducts. Also, in relation to metabolic economy *in vivo* proteolysis of aberrant proteins is desirable where as that of functional proteins are undesirable. This is reaction, transport and physical, morphological and ontogenetic characteristics of biocells in producing biocellular products.

It is evident, therefore, that engineering biology's linkage with process biotechnology is inseparable. Close research in these two applied biotechnology areas is ensuing in recent years. In order to understand this intimate linkages between engineering biology and process biotechnology, most advanced techniques of modern age like Artificial Neural Network (ANN), Bio Expert System (BES), Artificial Intelligence (AI) and Advanced computing for life sciences are being used. The major objectives of developing these techniques are for bioprocessing control, on line diagnosis of bioprocessing systems, computer aided design of biomolecules, recognition of specific biomolecular sequence, analysis of biochemical switching etc. Thus, a new wave of technological revolution under the banner of Modern Biotechnology which is hardly twenty years old connotes the use of any living organism or components thereof in the production and processing any of the manufactured products of commercial importance. In the constitution of linkage of engineering biology and process biotechnology through the use of land marks in modern biotechnology, microbial factories, plant agriculture, animal cell culture bioprocessing, medical engineering sciences and technology, energy and environment provide progress foundations.

2.2 STRUCTURAL ENGINEERING OF DNA IN ADVANCING BIOPROCESS ENGINEERING

2.2.1 Introduction

Uniqueness of DNA function in cells is bound by its structural engineering features. With the help of nonclassical engineering tools DNA structural feature is modifiable. The modification relates to its structure-function coordination. DNA structural design modification led to many recent advances in biochemical engineering and process biotechnology[20]. Recent advances in molecular cell biology have provided new approaches to probe the structural and functional bases of DNA associated physiological events. DNA is the fundamental biomolecule of all biosystems. It is a well organised complex biopolymer. Physical, biochemical/chemical, mechanical and electronic configurations of DNA govern its structural engineering features. It will not be exaggerated to say that non-classical engineering modification of structure of DNA has provided a new dimension towards recent advances of biochemical engineering and process biotechnology[20-23.] Structural redesigning of DNA is now a common practice which has revolutionized new biology and is having an ever increasing impact in various arena of biochemical engineering including process biotechnology industry and clinical medicine.

2.2.2 Chromosomal or Genomic and Plasmid DNA

Usually the average number of chromosome per prokaryotic cell cycle may be little more than one. During nuclear division the chromosomes become distinct as individual bodies. They differ in size and in position with primary and secondary constrictions in the cell. The number of chromosomes is characteristic for each species. In cells of higher animals and plants there are two homologous chromosomes. One comes from the mother and the other from the father. It is called diploid set. They look identical with the exception of the sex chromosome. However, most prokaryotes or gamets contain only one chromosome of each pair. It is called a haploid. Fragments of DNA and RNA molecules have been called genes. It is possible to localize single genes on the chromosomes. The genes control the synthesis of proteins. The genes are said to perform "legislative" functions while proteins are "executive" compounds. By means of DNA and its role in above function and execution it has been possible to transform microorganisms.

Bacterial plasmid is a species of non-essential extrachormosomal DNA. It replicates autonomously as a stable component of cell's genome. Naturally occurring plasmids range in size from one to several hundred kilobases and in copy number from one to several hundred per cell. Plasmids self-replication control mechanisms being auto catalytic utilize inhibition as their primary regulatory system. In terms of *in vivo* bioprocess engineering, plasmid replication control is capable of sensing and correcting stochastic fluctuations. This capability is ensured by an inverse proportionality between copy number and replication rate in individual cells.

2.2.3 Structural Engineering of DNA

1. Engineering principles in DNA structure

In 1953 Pauling had observed that physical structure of DNA might be some sort of α-helix. Watson and Crick's model show that by engineering physics DNA is organised as a double helix of nucleotides in which two nucleotide helix were wound around each other. Components were held at certain distances and/or angles to each other. Each full turn structure of the helix follows certain design engineerig dimensional measurement and configurational features. These measurements were in agreement with those obtained from X-ray diffraction pattern of DNA. The DNA double helix can adopt several conformations depending on nucleotide sequence and environmental conditions. Conformational design found in right handed DNA double helix are generally classified into two different types, A and B. The two types differ greatly in their base stacking overlaps and sugar packing modes. Stacking interaction has, therefore, been assumed to play a dominant role in determining the sequence dependent design of double helical DNA. This design analysis has been confirmed by ab initio molecular orbital method. Energies of molecular orbitals of DNA or RNA varied from lowest empty orbitals to highest occupied orbitals. In intra-strand and interstrand stacking interactions these energies have great significance. X-ray studies on single crystals of oligo-nucleotides have shown the detailed geometric design of DNA double helix to change from base to base pair and to be highly dependent on base sequences.

2. Biochemical/chemical structural unit design

The fundamental biochemical/chemical organizational element of DNA is the sequence of purine (adenine A and guanine G) and pyrimidine (cytosine C, thymine T and uracil U) bases. Structurally these bases are attached to the C-1 position of the sugar deoxyribose and the bases are linked together through joining of the sugar moieties at their 3' and 5' positions via a phospho-diester bond (Fig. 2.6). In each turn of the DNA double helix 10 dimer nucleotides are equally spaced from each other. It shows that the four nitrogenous bases of DNA did not occur in equal proportions. The total amount of pyrimidines equalled the total amount of purines (A + G = T + C). In addition the amount of adenine equalled the amount of thymine (A = T) residues and likewise for guanine and cytosine (G = C).

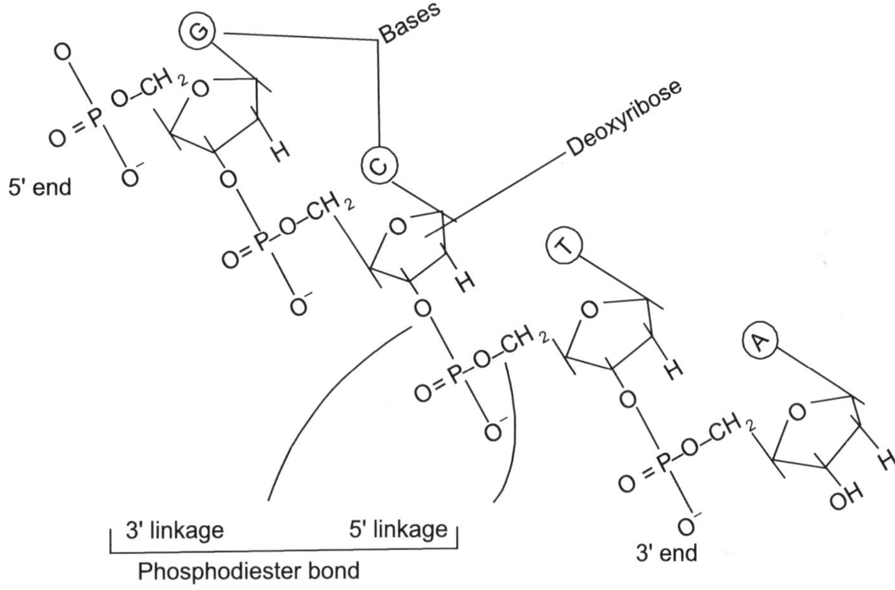

Fig. 2.6 Biochemical/chemical structural unit design of DNA

In order to account for Pauling's observation Watson and Crick proposed that in biochemical/chemical structure of DNA the sugar-phosphate chains should be on the outside and the purines and pyrimidines on the inside, held together by hydrogen bond between bases of opposite chains/strands. When the two chains of the helix were tried to put together it was found that the chains fitted best when they ran in opposite directions. Moreover, because X-ray diffraction studies specified the diameter of the helix to be 20 Å the space could only accommodate one purine and one pyrimidine. The alternating deoxyribose and phosphate groups form the backbone of the double helix.

The 3'-5' linkages of the DNA molecule define the orientation of a given strand of the DNA molecule.

Base pairing is one of the most fundamental bioconcept of DNA structural engineering and function. Adenine (A) and thymine (T) always pair by hydrogen bonding as do guanine (G) and cytosine (C). These base pairs are said to be complimentary.

In structural design of DNA/RNA, therefore, certain design engineering dimensions and conformation nature/feature were followed[11]. For a common DNA these dimensions and conformation nature and feature may be listed as given in Table 2.3.

Table 2.3 Design engineering dimensions and conformation nature/feature of a common DNA

Structural Design Items	*Measurement/Unit*	*Nature/Feature*
• Full turn length	34 A°	Double helix
• Helix radius	10 A°	–
• Distance between two adjacent		
– Sugar molecules	3.4 A°	–
– Phosphates	7.0 A°	–
• Sugar – phosphate-sugar		
– Orientation	–	Angular
– Bond angle	9°	–
• Directional orientation of double strands	Opposite	Anti-parallel
• H-bond length		
G – C	2.98 A°	–
A – T		
• Energy coefficient of molecular orbital	HOMO/* LEMO	Base dependent

* HOMO – Highest occupied molecular orbital
LEMO – Lowest empty molecular orbital

3. Electronic structural features

The electronic spin density distribution in anionic bases of DNA/RNA structures is given in Fig. 2.7. They represent unique character for their interactive role. The double helical structure of DNA has been considered as a polymer construct from ten dinner units of stacked base pairs.

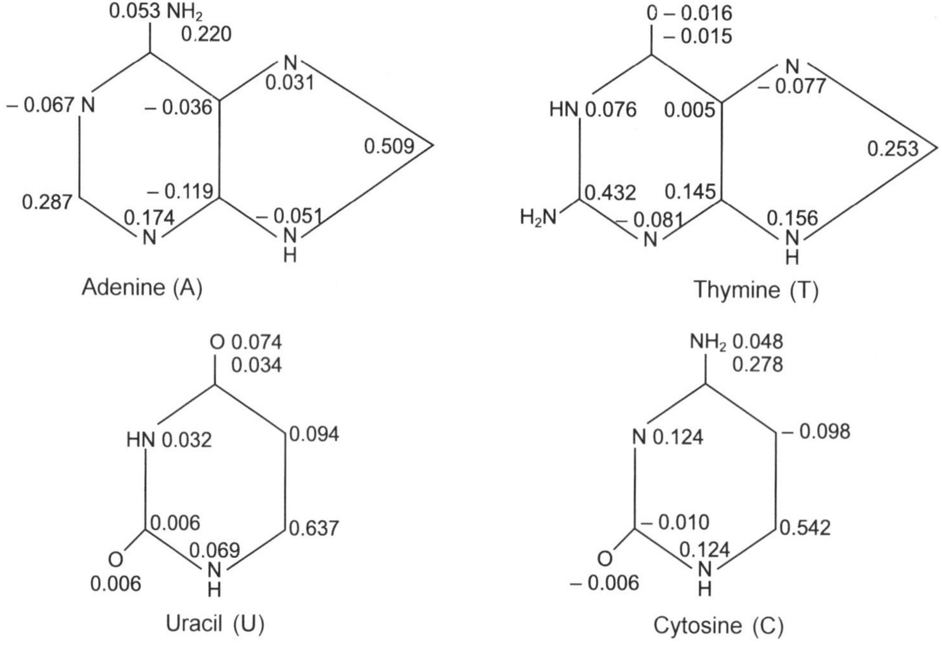

Fig. 2.7 Electron spin density distribution in anionic bases of DNA/RNA

In taking into account both hydrogen bonds and nearest neighbour stacking interaction these units are of the smallest compounds of DNA polymers. Methods are now available to investigate the electronic structures induced by the differences in nearest neighbour stacking interactions.

The electronic spin density distribution in anionic bases of DNA/RNA provides unique character of their interactive role. The double helical structure of DNA has been considered as a polymer constructed from ten dimer units of stacked base pairs. In taking into account both hydrogen bonds and nearest neighbour stacking interaction, these units are the smallest components of DNA polymers. Methods are now available to investigate the electronic structures induced by the differences in nearest-neighbour stacking interactions. Thus electron donor–electron acceptor features of DNA is of great importance. These features relate to resonance stabilization of the base pairing, best possible orientation of the bases, the evolution of the resonance stabilization in the course of the *de novo* synthesis and enhanced activity of phosphate clusters in electrophilic reaction. Therefore, significance of electronic/ionic potential in DNA/RNA molecules bears information in relation to biotechnological implications in terms of mutations and/or genetic engineering or genetic recombination reactions giving transformants.

The electron donor – electron acceptor properties of DNA bases as has to be estimated in terms of energy coefficients of molecular orbitals and given in Table 2.4 below is important. The importance of the energies and features relates to resonance stabilization and enhanced activity of phosphate clusters in electrophilic reaction.

Table 2.4 Energy coefficient of molecular orbitals of base compounds of DNA

	Coefficients for	
Compounds	*Energy of Highest Occupied Molecular Orbital (HOMO Energy)*	*Energy of Least Empty Molecular Orbital (LEMO Energy)*
A	0.49	– 0.37
G	0.31	– 1.05
U	0.60	– 0.96
T	0.51	– 0.96
C	0.60	– 0.80

The estimation of intrinsic energies (Ei) of the molecular orbitals was carried out using the following relation and

$$Ei = \alpha + Ki\beta \quad (2.7)$$

considering the mobile or π electrons of the molecular system. In this relation α is known as Coulomb Constant, β is resonance integration constant of the method and Ki is a factor dependent on the type of molecular orbital. Positive values of Ki corresponds to occupied or bonding type of orbitals. Negative values of Ki corresponds to empty or antibonding type of orbitals. As can be seen from the Table 2.4 that energies of molecular orbitals of DNA varied from lowest empty orbitals to highest occupied orbitals. These energies are concerned with the following importances.

a. Resonance stabilization of the base pairing
b. The specific pairing is based entirely on the best possible orientation of the bases in the DNA double helix
c. The evolution of the resonance stabilization in the course of the *de novo* designing of DNA/RNA

The presence of lone pair (n) and π electrons in DNA bases as given in Table 2.5 bears significance of their electronic or ionic potential as presented in Table 2.6 and implications in biotechnology as listed in Table 2.7.

Table 2.5 Lone pair (n) and π electrons molecular ionisation potential (ev) of DNA bases

Base	*n*	*n(o)*	*n(N)*
G	7.6	9.4	N_7 11.7 N_3 11.6
A	8.4	–	N_1 11.2 N_3 11.3 N_7 11.4
C	8.3	9.8	10.1
U	9.0	10.0C_6O 10.3C_3O	

In general, the double helical structure of DNA has been considered as a polymer constructed from ten dimer units of stacked base pairs. In taking into account both hydrogen bonds and nearest neighbour stacking interaction these units are the smallest components of DNA polymers.

Table 2.6 Significance of the electronic/ionic potential

In DNA/RNA Molecules	*Information in relation to Biotechnological Implications*
All bases	Possess lowest ionisation potential corresponding to ionisation of π electrons
A	Order of increasing ionisation potential: π < n (o) < n (N)
G	π and n (o) donors are the best
U	π and n (o) donor are the worst
C	n(N) donor is the worst

Present available methods for investigations of electrons structures induced by the differences in nearest – neighbour stacking interactions results electron donor – electron acceptor features in DNA molecules. These features relates to resonance stabilization in the course of *de novo* enhanced activity of phosphate clusters in electrophilic reaction. Therefore, significance of electronic/ionic potential in DNA/RNA molecules bear informations in relation to biotechnological implications in terms (Table 2.7) of mutations and/or biomolecular redesign engineering giving transformants.

Table 2.7 Biotechnological implications of electronic character of DNA

In Cellular System	*Implications*
– Lone pair electron of DNA/RNA	Involve some (localized) type of charge transfer
– Tautomeric form of DNA/RNA	Exist and important in redesigning of cell by r-DNA technology
– Biological Scale up	Calculating the electronic characteristics of the miscoupled bases
– Finding that cytosine is the primary target of UV induced mutations in single stranded DNA	Agree with theoretical predicitions

4. Other engineering concerns

Besides above considerations, other engineering inputs like mechanical structural concerns are also very important because in DNA structure one may note the following (Fig. 2.8 A and B)

- Each DNA helix turn is made to slide over the adjacent turn.
- The pitch is held constant.
- The pitch length/turn of the helix may change by an amount equal to the slide per turn.

These are related to the tension in DNA helix.

- Some bacterial pathogen e.g. *Chlamydia trachomatis* contains an enzyme called ribonucleotide reductase that's essential for making and repairing DNA[44].

5. Other molecular engineering concerns

From the above concerns the number of turns in the helix

$$n_o = \frac{L}{2\pi r_o} \tag{2.8}$$

where L is the arc length per turn of the helix, r_o = helix redius. The axial length, h_o of the helix is

$$h_o = n_o p \tag{2.9}$$

Expressing as a function of r by combining (2.8) & (2.9)

$$h = \frac{pL}{2\pi r}, \text{ p is the pitch of the helix} \tag{2.10}$$

Since L is the arc length per turn a decrease in arc represent a decrease in r. If s is the amount of slide to each turn relative to the one below then

$$s = 2\pi (r_o - r) \tag{2.11}$$

Or

$$r = r_o - \frac{s}{2\pi} \tag{2.12}$$

combining (2.10) & (2.12)

$$h = \frac{pL}{2\pi r_o - s} \tag{2.13}$$

The mechanical structural engineering parameter allows one to examine the relationship between a single helix and a system of several coaxial helices (m) of the same sense all lying on the same cylindrical surface. Considering each helix has a radius r_0 equal to the radius of the single helix and the same axial length h_0 and if p be the constant axial spacing separating adjacent helices then every helix in the set will have a pitch mp. It can be seen now that each one has (n_0/m) turns and the length of each helix h_0 must be (L/m). So the relation between h and r for each helix in the multiple helix system may become

$$h = \frac{(mp)\ (L/m)}{2\pi r} = \frac{pL}{2\pi r} \tag{2.14}$$

which being identical to Eqn. (2.4) suggests that the same relation governs the dependence of h upon r in either a single on a multiple helix system. The relation of r and h as function of s considers

$$2\pi r_0 - 2\pi r = ms \tag{2.15}$$

provided there are m helices and s is the slide of one turn over the adjacent turn below. This is valid if

$$r >> mp$$

Thus for multiple helix system

$$r = r_0 - \frac{ms}{2\pi} \tag{2.16}$$

and $$h = \frac{pL}{2\pi r_0 - ms} \tag{2.17}$$

Now by principle of virtual work or by a force triangle analysis

$$T = rF \tag{2.18}$$

Where T = tension in the helix, r = radius of the helix and F is the outward force (Fig. 2.8 B) from the solid per unit arc length along the helix. This needed assumption that

$$r >> n$$

The tension in helix and other *in vivo* DNA design properties are important in multiforked chromosomal replication and division and overcoming plasmid DNA species barriers.

From the above discussion on structural design engineering of DNA and scope of its design modifications one may think of the concerned facets as shown in Fig. 2.9. It also indicates the importance of *in vivo* design modification of DNA where transcription meets repair.

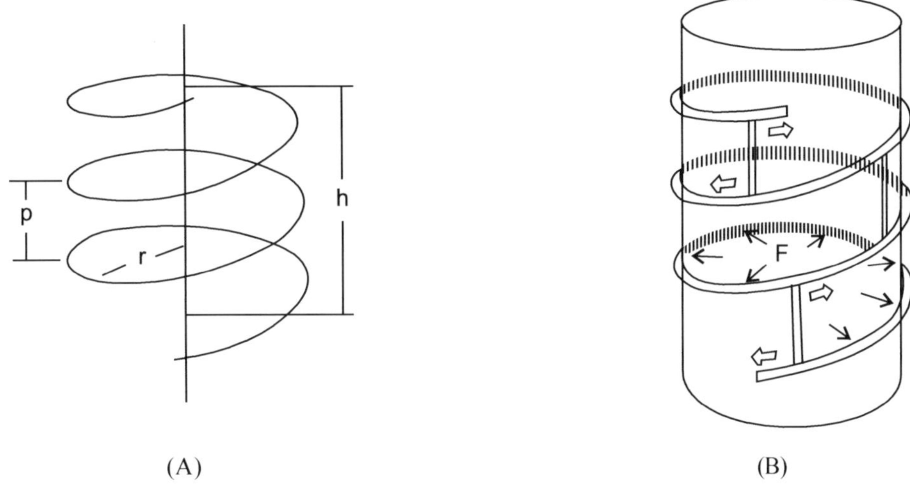

Fig. 2.8 Mechanical structural engineering properties of DNA

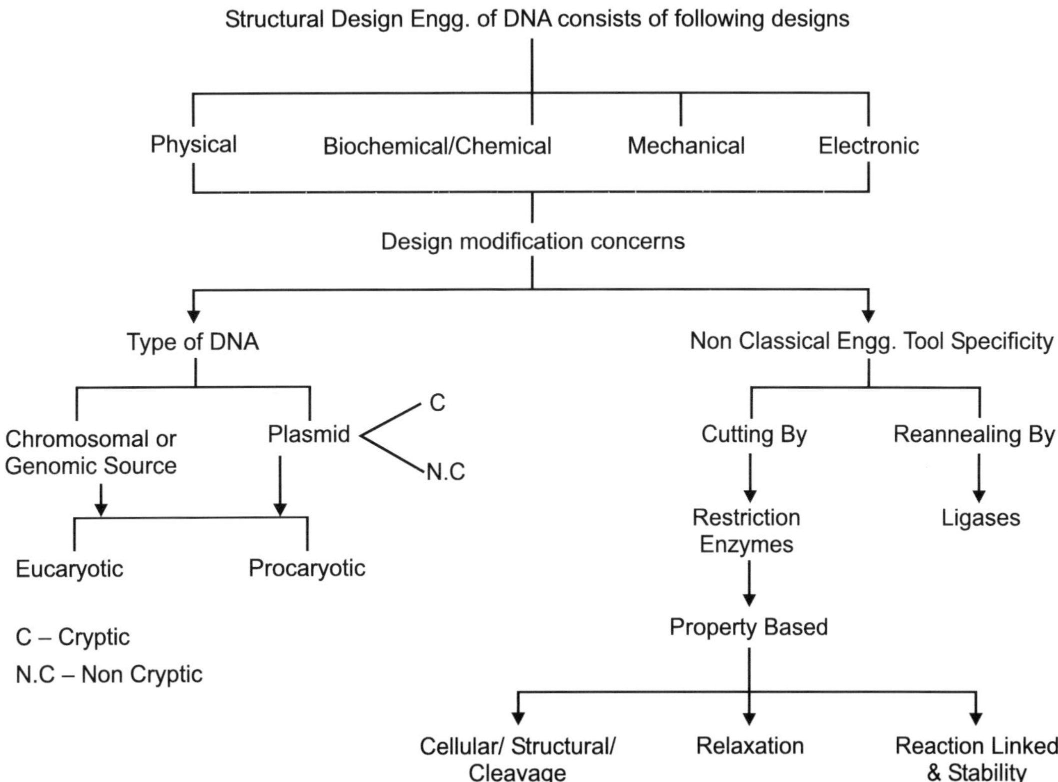

Fig. 2.9 Concerned facets in structural design engineering of DNA

2.2.4 Input to Bioprocess Engineering Advances

In mutational or recombinational design-modification of cells these are important in changing their behaviours. The difference in behaviour between original and modified redesigned strains of biocells has been effected for enhancement of productivity of commercially important bioproducts.

In bioprocess engineering advances, therefore, biomolecular design engineering is contributing significantly. Few well known examples include the following:

(i) In simulating the effect of the plasmid replication of the transformant of thermophillic *Bacillus stearothermophilus* by insertion of penicillinase genes originated from a mesophilic *Bacillus licheniformis.*[21,23,25]

(ii) In optimizing production of recombinant plasmid encoded proteins by recombinant bacteria, plasmid bearing cells may have a growth disadvantage compared to plasmid free cells. It has been known, however, that the presence of a recombinant plasmid can alter the levels of certain metabolites. Also, the presence of plasmid vectors can increase the oxygen demand of cells which harbor it.[23,26] Over the last few years it has been indicated that oxygen may be a nutrient, which when exhausted at the end of logarithmic phase of growth results in decreased growth of cells as plasmid size increases.

Structural or conformational variations in DNA molecule have been shown. It has been possible to redesign DNA molecule structure by molecular replacement using idealized DNA hexamers. Example of one such design is hairpin structure having potential in fundamental research.

2.2.5 Machines and Tools in Biomolecular Design Engineering

Machine : Host biocells (prokaryotic and eukaryotic)
(a) Microbial/Plasmid
(b) Mammalian
(c) Plant

Tools : (a) Restriction enzymes
(b) Ligases etc.

2.2.6 Few Redesigning Methodology

Many important techniques and methodologies have been utilized in empirical and quantitative redesigning of biocells and biomolecules. Some of these methods are:

(a) DNA-DNA hybridization/r DNA technology
(b) Cloning
(c) Conjugation/cell fusion
(d) Transfectional molecular blending.
(e) Stress induced *in vivo* molecular signaling

1. DNA-DNA hybridization/rDNA technology

In general when a double stranded DNA is heated, the two strands separate into single stranded molecules. On cooling reassociation of the two complementary strands slowly takes place, this results in the formation of the original double stranded DNA complex. If single stranded DNAs from two different microorganism are mixed and the nucleotide sequences are identical or nearly identical DNA-DNA hybridization takes place. The DNA-DNA hybridization method has been used for the following purposes:

(a) Detecting relationship of two microorganisms.

(b) Detecting similarities in the base sequence between nucleic acids of two different strains. The schematic as shown in Fig. 2.10 shows that in (a) the two nucleic acids are related where as in (b) only a portion of the nucleic acids are homologous. It appeared that the hybridization procedure becomes easier and works more efficiently if one of the hybridizing nucleic acids is in fairly small pieces, hence one of the nucleic acids is subjected to high speed shearing treatment in a blender.

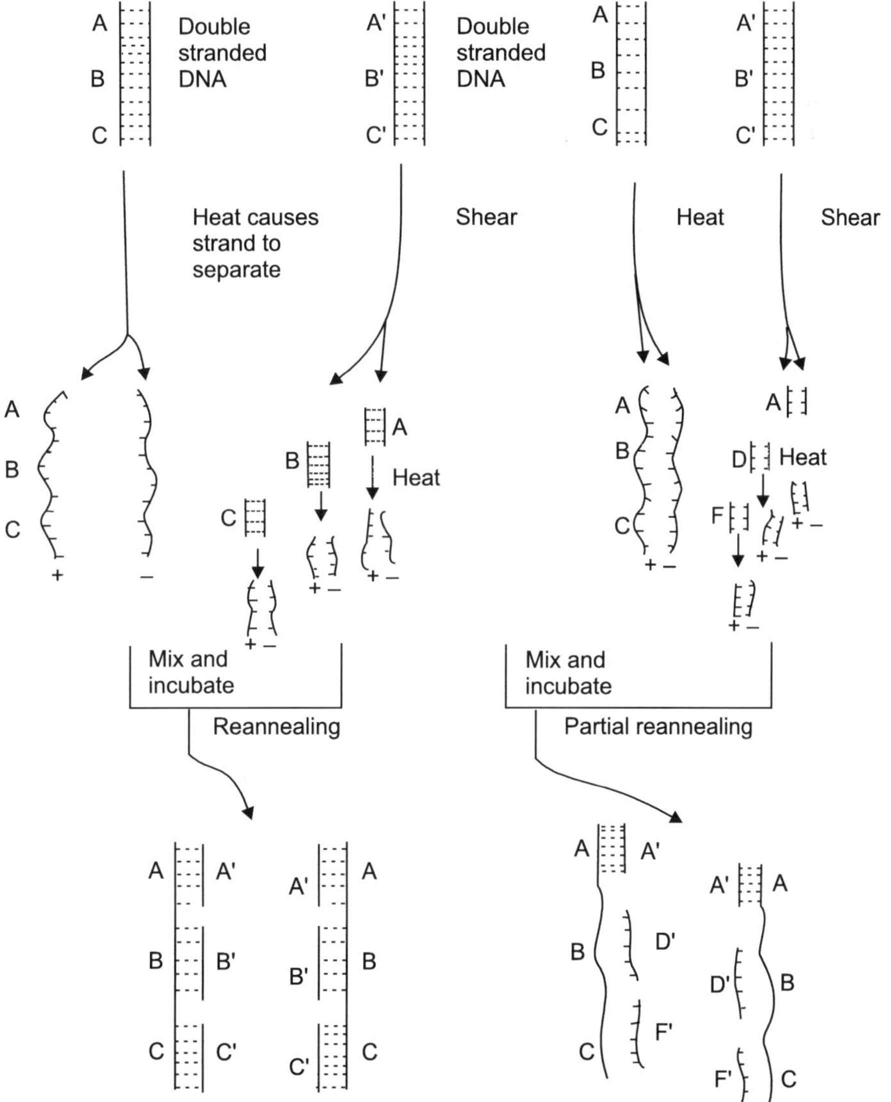

Fig. 2.10 Steps in DNA-DNA hybridization

2. Cloning[24,25]

According to Mendel's rules of inheritance of biological characteristics each inheritable property of an organism is controlled by a factor, called a gene which resides on chromosomes. In practice of molecular cell biology (MCB), cloning refers to gene cloning. The definition of cloning involves following five steps :

1. Selecting and fragmenting proper DNA: The fragmenting of DNA containing the gene to be cloned is inserted into a circular DNA molecule called a vector to produce a chimera or recombinant DNA molecule (r DNA).
2. The constructed vector (vehicle) acts to transport the gene into a host cell to be redesigned which is usually a bacterium, although other type of biocells can be used.
3. The vector multiply inside the host cell producing numerous identical copies not only of itself but also of the gene that it carries.
4. During host cell division copies of the rDNA moleculels are passed to the progeny and further vector replication takes place.
5. On completion of a large number of cell divisions, a colony or clone, of individual identical host cells is produced. Each cell in the clone contains molecule, the gene carried by the redesigned cell is now said to be cloned.

3. Conjugation/Cell fusion[24,25]

This method is one way of bringing together unaccustomed cell partners, i.e. protein coding genes and control regions. This method of redesigning cell system aims at the following:

(a) Attachment of one of the inexpressed genes to a control region.

(b) Turning it on under the conditions prevailing inside the bioreactor/fermentation vessel.

(c) Making provisions for the silent genes became expressed-mRNA being copied from the gene and enzymes being synthesized which the microbe may use to manufacture new and useful product or over production of chemicals like antibiotics and amino acids. A typical cell fusion strategy is as below :

Cells

Remove the outer membrane of the cells by suitable lytic enzyme

Protoplast

Fuse with protoplast of other cell

Hybrid or Recombinant cell

Contains genetic matter of two (or more) cells which is different from the previous individual thus redesigned.

***4. Transfectional molecular blending*[26-28]**

Biochemical engineers have been successful to reconstruct biotoxins by molecular blending for unusual therapeutic application of these molecules in hospitals. Many cells are known to express the desired protein for a period of several days after transfectional molecular blending. In prokaryotic biocells this is spoken of if bacteria forms infectious phage progeny after the uptake of free phage DNA. Two prerequisites have been stated to be required for this: (1) the cells must be able to take up nucleonic acids of high molecular weight (the cells must be competent), (2) one entire phage enter the cell. Sometimes redesigning/reconstruction of an entire genome occur by recombination of overlapping fragments. Transfectional biocell-virus interactive process biotechnological production method of viral vaccines, hormones and interferons are good examples of this method.[29,30]

***5. Stress induced in vivo molecular signaling*[26,30,31]**

In vivo redesigning possibility of newer bioproducts by stressing of biocells are now known. *In vivo* redesigning of biomolecules using interactive stresses has been shown to produce stress proteins of commercial importance. Much more research is under way in producing, designing and promoting stress proteins of commercial beneficial use. Powerful modern instruments and techniques such as NMR, ESR, HPLC, PAGE, 2D-gel chromatography, GCMS etc. in conjunction with modern techniques are being used.

2.3 BIOMOLECULAR DESIGN ENGINEERING TOOLS: PROPERTIES AND FOREFRONT APPLICATIONS

2.3.1 Introduction

DNA and RNA are very key biomolecules of all biocells. For developing biocell to highbiotech, biomolecular design engineering is an important concern. Upgradation of biocells often involves biomolecular redesigning. The redesigning DNA biomolecules for products consists of four major steps. The redesigning of biomolecules may be considered as a non-classical engineering. The tools required in redesigning are called restriction endonucleases or restriction enzymes. As low volume high value microbial products, restriction enzymes have added important dimensions to the development of bioprocess engineering. A more recent review discussed the sources, production, separation and purification of restriction enzymes in general. It emphasized the importance of upstream and downstream processing to obtain pure enzymes for genetic engineering or molecular biology work. Several process engineering variables and state parameters have been found to exert an effect on the maximization of production and many of these biomolecular design engineering tools. The restriction enzyme *Bam*H1 is a typical example of this type of tools. A discussion of the bioprocessing and influence of variables, fundamental molecular properties, physiochemical behaviour and application of these non-classical biomolecular design engineering tools with special reference to *Bam*H1 will, therefore, be useful. In order to maximize production of these tools by bioprocessing, manipulation/optimization of culture conditions is reflected in the behaviour of the cell culture system including its cellular materials. Some important bioprocessing information for production from a biotechnological view point has been provided very recently.[32-35]

Restriction enzymes of living cells are constitutive in nature. *Bacillus amyloliquefaciens* synthesise intracellular restriction enzyme *Bam* H1 during its cultivation.[1] Some information on the behaviour of cellular and cell free native *Bam* H1 in relation to thermotolerence has been reported recently.[33, 34] Thermotolerence of native restriction enzymes, in general, is extremely poor. The lower value of activation energy for denaturation of an enzyme represents its lower heat stability. The unusually low value of activation energy for denaturation of native *Bam*H1 (2.63 kcal/mole), besides confirming its extreme heat labile nature, gives quantitative information on its thermal denaturation. Possibility of inhibition of *Bam*H1 by commercial polysaccharides recently reported by Oishi *et al.*[36] indicated reaction engineering concern of the system.

2.3.2 Perspectives, Results and Discussion in Relation to *Bam*H1

***1. Most suitable in vivo thermotolerence for denovo Bam*H1**

In cell cultivation of *Bacillus amyloliquefaciens* H1 at different temperatures one may simulate microbial cells placed into the cultivation medium as two chambers filled with liquids under constant flow and separated by a cell wall with pores of micron sizes and comparable to the mean free path of the molecules where heat is transferred through the system from T_1 to T_2 ($T_1 > T_2$). Constitutive molecules of the cells on the T_1 side of the cell wall thus have a higher kinetic energy than on the T_2 side of the cell wall with higher velocity and frequency of collision of molecule. This causes transportation of hotter fluid from T_1 side to T_2 side. A steady state in cellular function (not an equilibrium) is reached when total number of collisions of molecules per unit time on the T_1 side and T_2 side of the cell wall are equal. This optimal steady state is not reached until equal optimal cultivation temperature for growth in interior and exterior of cell is established. At this thermal condition it may be expected that biosynthesis of constitutive macromolecular enzyme proteins like *Bam*H1 will take place at highest level. Above this thermal condition, however, the thermoturbulence or thermo collisions increased within the *de novo* *Bam*H1 molecule caused by higher temperature and predominant bulk flow transport in comparison with its thermal diffusive flow at lower temperature. This thermoturbulence might increase the collision within *de novo Bam*H1 molecule thereby causing unwinding and cleavage of its H-bonds. The higher the temperature of cultivation above optimal value the severe is the unfolding and inactivation of thermolabile protein *Bam*H1.

2. Engineering perspectives and concern

The above described concept may be conceivable both in presence or absence of cell wall. In absence of cell wall, however, the average concentration difference is smaller with same energy flow. This means efficiency of the process is lower. When thermal energy flow stops the transport of molecules from T_1 side to T_2 side, it may then be passive. Prevalence of the two possible operative principles may be expected in a cellular system. Thus fluid flow and thermodynamic principles are two concerned perspectives in intracellular bioprocessing.

(i) Intracellular Micro flow Concern : From standard fluid flow concept the bulk flow in the cell may be given by $F_b = v.c.$ where v is the fluid velocity and c is the concentration fluid of the nutrient molecules. However, under the influence of thermal gradient, the diffusive flow (F_d) in

the cell may exist and computable from $F_d = K_l\ \Delta c$ in which K_l is defined as the ratio of diffusivity (D) to the thickness of the resistance layer (x, cell wall thickness). Under thermal influence it could be shown under certain conditions that F_b and F_d have equal influence (i.e $F_b = F_d$) and thus *in vivo* thermolability of *de novo Bam*H1 is of great concern from thermodynamic view point also. In order to illustrate this the relative importance of the flow components F_b and F_d need be characterised from their ratio. This ratio of F_b to F_d is defined as Peclet number (N_{pe}). Thus,

$$N_{pe} = \frac{F_b}{F_d} = \frac{v.c}{\frac{D}{x} \cdot \Delta c} = \frac{v.x}{D}$$

For fluid flow under working temperature across cell wall of the organism if one considers an individual cell as a continuous micro bioreactor placed within a physical bioreactor and assume following reasonable values.

$v \approx 10^{-3}\ ms^{-1}$, $D \approx 10^{-9}\ m^2\ s^{-1}$ and $x = 1$ micron $= 10^{-6}$ m one gets from the above relation

$$N_{pe} = \frac{10^{-3} \times 10^{-6}}{10^{-9}} = 1, \quad \text{or} \quad \frac{F_b}{F_d} = 1 \quad \text{or } F_b = F_d$$

*Experimental support of in vivo thermolability of Bam*H1

Thermal inactivation profile of native *Bam*H1 has been observed in *in vitro* system by incubating it at temperatures ranging from 25 to 50°C for varying target of time ranging from 50 to 240 mins. Ten microliter of *Bam*H1 having 5 units/μl activity were subjected to heat treatment. In each experiment the residual *Bam*H1 activity after heat treatment was determined by serial dilution method using DNA as substrate.[33] Results of serial dilution method are reported. Knowing the thermolability behavior of *Bam*H1 *in vivo* system it was aimed to assess the nature of *in vivo* thermolability of *Bam*H1 during cell cultivation at different temperatures keeping other conditions same in all batch runs. The experimental results support the perspective of fluid flow as discussed in previous section. It can be seen from this figure that till most suitable cultivation temperature has been provided specific *Bam*H1 production has increased. It indicated that binding constitutive molecules of *Bam*H1 take place most suitable by favouring *in vivo* bioreaction system. Above this temperature because of bulk fluid flow mediated higher quantum of thermal energy penetration the units of molecules for constitution of *Bam*H1 presumably got unfolding initiation and attacked by other protein molecules *in vivo*. It rendered hindrance in *de novo* enzyme thereby decreasing the activity depending on the thermal quantum and followed similar pattern as specific growth rate profile.

(ii) Thermodynamic Perspective : Considering Kuhn's[37] concept one may assume that temporary inactivation of restriction enzyme occur, due to separation of broken chain by unwinding of large number of turns (N) of its DNA helix. The separated chains have a higher degree of freedom than similar chain segments bonded within double helix of DNA.[37] Consequently unfolding of

(*Bam*H1 like protein) DNA molecule is accompanied by an increase in entropy or decrease of free energy. This concern is of special significance in computation of decrease in free energy in relation to 'α' which is the ratio of the half life of the enzyme to total thermal exposure time.

(iii) Cell Culture Engineering Parameter in Relation to Unfolding Initiation Time : When N>>1 the initiation time of unfolding of the restriction enzyme in relation to maximum specific growth rate (μ_m) is of great importance in addition to 'α' as defined above.

The variation in the value of μ_m as a function of temperature as in Fig. 2.11 is useful in determining the number of turns unfolded from its initiation time.

(iv) Oxygen Mass Transfer Concern : *Bacillus amyloliquefaciens* H1 is an aerobic organism. During its cultivation for *Bam*H1 synthesis in the cell, the influence of oxygen mass transfer by the aeration-agitation unit operation indicated significant effect on *Bam*H1 specific activity.

The profiles of the influence of cell cultivation variables on production of the restriction enzyme *Bam*H1 have been published.[35] The *Bam*H1 yield in relation to the control variables has been shown. From the results of the influence of cultivation variables it appeared that using a Marubishi bioreacter in bioprocessing for *Bam*H1 production, the most suitable values of the parameters are temperature 37°C, pH 7.0, aeration-agitation 2 vvm-500 rpm with corresponding K_La 260-290 h^{-1}. These results, however, indicated that pH and temperature in the used range did not cause significant change in the specific *Bam*H1 production. However, the existence of optimum pH and temperature for a maximum yield of *Bam*H1 could be seen. Variation of aeration and agitation could show an appreciable increase in specific *Bam*H1 yield upto 500 rpm and 2 vvm aeration. Above K_La 280 h^{-1} the *Bam*H1 yield decreased.

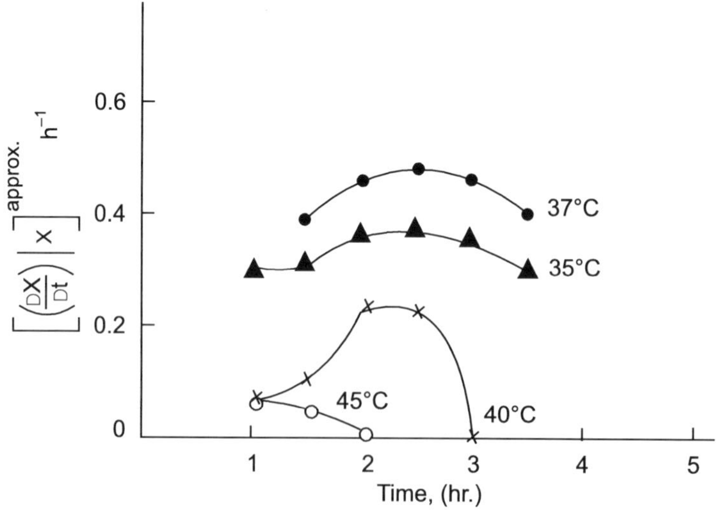

Fig. 2.11 Plot of variation of μ_m (t) with temperature as parameter

Interpretation of the observations

Increase in *Bam*H1 concentration with the increase in aeration-agitation upto certain level (1 vvm, 500rpm, K_La 270 h^{-1} in B.E. Marubishi Bioreactor, 7l) was probably associated with induction of this restriction enzyme in the organism by oxygen. Possibility of induction of microbial enzyme in presence of oxygen has been reported in the literature.[38,39] However, evidence of such induction for constitutive restriction enzyme is scanty. It is, however, stated that superoxide dismutase (SOD) activity is present in practically all aerobes like *Bacillus subtilis, B. stearothermophilus, B. propillae, B.megaterium* etc. It is likely, therefore, that it may also be present in *B. amyloliquefaciens* suggesting the existence of operation of SOD theory of induction-repression in the cell. Exposure of this organism upto certain level as stated above induces *Bam*H1 synthesis mechanism but at elevated oxygen concentration in the cell caused to form more H_2O_2 *in vivo* which perhaps led to the synthesis of more SOD or catalase if insufficient is present to cope with increased 0_2 generation. Exposure of *B.subtilis* to elevated oxygen concentration increases its catalase activity but not SOD and this organism is equally sensitive to high oxygen level whether grown previously in air or 100% pure oxygen. It seems, therefore, below the critical level of oxygen as mentioned above the SOD/catalase level in the cell falls below the level at which *Bam*H1 synthesis is induced. However, on its exposure to above this critical level of oxygen SOD/catalase activity in the cell is promptly resynthesised and cause repression of *Bam*H1 synthesis thereby showing decline in its activity. Until definite evidence is available it may also be due to *in vivo* oxidant mediated DNA damage. When cells are subjected to high extracellular oxygen stress leading to an intracellular micromolar concentration of nascent H_2O_2, temporary DNA strand cleavage may also occur. It is because the oxygen stress leads to activation of some specific DNA cleaving mechanism in monoionic or diionic metal-dependent endonuclease.

(v) Basic Enzyme Reaction Engineering Concern : The restriction enzyme *Bam*H1 has been exploited extensively both for R&D and industrial purposes. In producing important biochemicals/ chemicals through the use of redesigned microorganism *Bam*H1 played a significant role. However, because of the problems associated with stabilizing and making *Bam*H1 reaction inhibition free it has become a task and challenge to the enzyme engineers to stabilize restriction enzymes, in general, at room temperature by some economic process. In order to develop such economic means extensive analysis of the system from reaction engineering perspective has become essential. A preliminary attempt in this regard was made at BERC, IIT Delhi by observing thermotolerence of native and crosslinked *Bam*H1. Reactions were carried out in a volume of 10 μl in 10 mM potassium phosphate buffer (pH 7.0) containing 20μg *Bam*H1 protein at a level of 5 units/ml and cross linking reagents (DMA, DMS and DTBP) at levels ranging from 0.01 to 0.2% (W/V). The temperature of reaction ranged from 25 to 50°C for varying length of time using substrate as stated in earlier literature.[34] The experimental data of the time profile of percent residual activity of native and cross linked *Bam*H1 with temperature as parameter has been reported. Analysis of, these data could show a relationship between K_d and time of exposure at various temperatures (Fig. 2.12). The apparent activation energies required for deactivation of native *Bam*H1 could be computed from these data. This plot in form of a time profile (Fig. 2.12) indicated to involve two stages of deactivation in the temperature range.

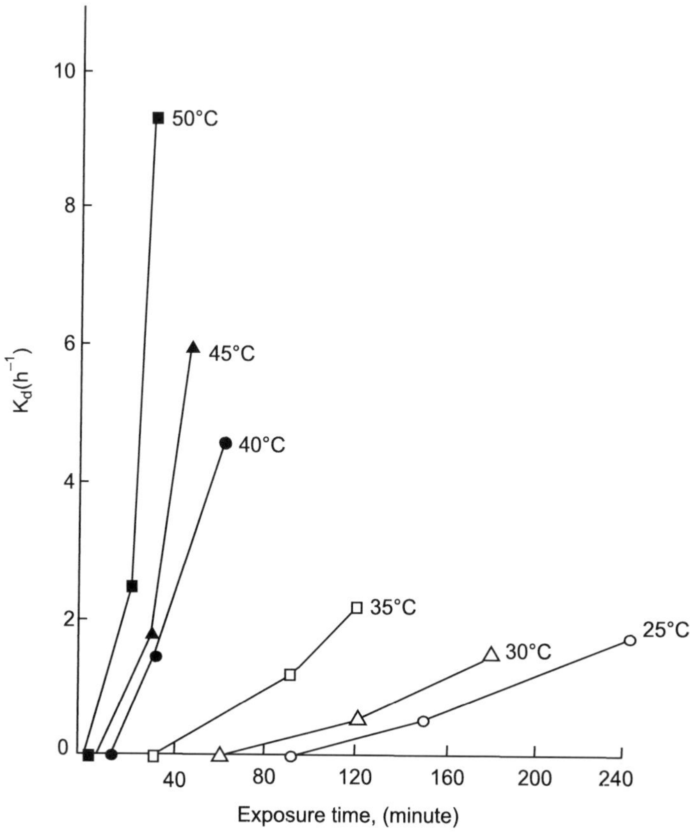

Fig 2.12 Variation of K_d values of native *Bam*H1 with temperature as parameter

2.3.3 Properties of the Biomolecular Cleavage Tools

1. General properties

The biomolecular cleavage tools like restriction endonucleases are strain specific and site specific enzymes which cleave double stranded DNA. Because of their unique nature of controllable, predictable, infrequent and site specific cleavage, restriction endonucleases have been proved to be extremely important tools in dissecting, analysing, and inserting newer genetic information by cloning at molecular level. Based on their cleavage requirements and properties, these tools have been grouped under four types as type I, II, III and IV. The type I or deoxyribonuclease I is the most commonly known endonuclease. This type has very little specificity and cleaves phosphodiester linkages in a DNA molecule indiscriminately. However, the type II or restriction enzymes would never do that but would attack a DNA molecule only at the specific sequence. Like type I the deoxyribonuclease type III cleave away from the recognition sequence and are not of much use to recombinant DNA technology. *EcoRI, Bam*H1 etc are examples of type II restriction endonucleases produced by culturing microorganism (s). Their general properties have been discussed in the literature and in a more recent book.[40]

2. Stability considerations

The interaction of cross-linkers with *Bam*H1 to impart resistance to thermal unfolding has been considered as a suitable strategy in stabilizing *Bam*H1. The most suitable cross-linking reagent will be that which causes minimum inactivation of *Bam*H1. Also the concentration of this suitable reagent at which it will cause maximum stabilization should be taken into account from an economic viewpoint. On the basis of this consideration the effect of different concentrations of three crosslinking reagents, namely glutaraldehyde and dimethyl adipimidate (DMA), dimethyl suberimidate (DMS) and dimethyl 3,3-dithiobispropionimidate (DTBP) on the activity of *Bam*H1 has been observed in the BERC Laboratory. The preparation of these cross-linked *Bam*H1 compounds has been described. From the experimental results it was seen that the activation energies (E) required for native and DMA. DMS and DTBP cross-linked preparations were 2.63, 5.21, 6.55 and 9.2 kcal/mol, respectively. This increase in E values of cross-linked preparations over native *Bam*H1 indicated that stabilization against thermal inactivation was achieved by cross-linking with a suitable reagent.

2.3.4 Forefront Application Areas

Some of the forefront application areas with special reference to *Bam*H1 have been discussed in a recent literature.[33] Other possible application areas of restriction enzymes are discussed below.

1. Agriculture

Characterization and modification of genetic make up of plants has been made possible with the help of recombinant DNA technology. Many plant proteins are deficient in aminoacids that are essential for human health. Genes coding for the synthesis of a protein rich in essential aminoacids could be introduced to improve the quality of plant protein. It might also be possible to transfer genes for resistance to pests, herbicides, microbial toxins and for nitrogen fixation from *Rhizobium* strains which cause nodulation on many different leguminous plants such as peanut, soybean, mungbean and a few others. *Rhizobium* also forms nodules on non-leguminous plants called Troma. Many nitrogen fixing trees such as Alnus, possess nodule formed by an *Actinomycete frankia*. These bacteria may be for nodule formation on nonleguminous plants. Nitrogen fixing capability could also be conferred on many free living bacteria that are abundant in soil and plant rhizospheres. Recently, cloning and expression of whole 'nif' genes of *Klebsiella oxytoca* in *E. coli* is reported.

Resistance to pests and disease to plants is often conferred by a single gene. Resistance based on a single major gene or few such genes becomes ineffective against new races of pathogens and pests a few years of its introduction into a crop-plant. Therefore, novel strategies are needed for obtaining crop resistance to pests and pathogens.

2. Industry

A large number of industrial and academic R & D laboratories are working on gene technology for several industrially important microorganisms. Animal genes responsible for insulin, interferon and human growth hormone have been successfully cloned in *E. coli* in an effort towards their commercialization. Production of human insulin by engineered *E. coli* cells from laboratory scale (10L) is known. Costly media constitutents for fermentation might be replaced by inexpensive naturally occurring abundant substrates such as cellulose. Genes for efficient utilization of cellulose and other substrates can be isolated and cloned into organisms of commercial interest. With development of such genetically engineered microbes that utilize inexpensive media constituents more and more natural products will be produced by fermentation biotransformation replacing their expensive chemical synthesis or isolation from natural sources.

3. Medical sciences

Gene therapy is well known in more recent years. A number of approaches were described envisaging the use of *E. coli* for production of antigenic material, extra-cellular secretion of the antigenic protein, production of antigen inserted in the surface of bacteria or intracellular production of immunogenic protein.

Recombinant DNA technology is being used to develop vaccines against deadly viral diseases. Segments of viral genome may be used to produce appropriate viral antigen in alternative hosts like *Saccharomyces cerevisiae* or *Bacillus subtilis*. The core antigen gene is expressed in *E. coli* and when injected into rabbits, the antigen produced by *E. coli* induces antibody that reacts with human serum core antigen. Genes that code for surface protein of foot and mouth disease virus, can be identified employing rDNA technology. Such genes can be introduced into appropriate host to produce protein that may be an effective vaccine. A DNA sequence from foul plaque virus was inserted into an *E. coli* plasmid. The recombinant plasmid directed the synthesis of a protein that is 0.75% of total cell protein and reacts with antisera to FOV hemaglutinin. Hopes are also raised to cure hereditary diseases like *Haemophilia* and colour blindness. Antibiotics producing genes can be cloned in multicopy plasmids in suitatble microbes leading to economical production of medicines.

4. Pollution control

Metals aromatics, hydrocarbons and other rotting organic wastes which cause pollution can be effectively controlled using genetically manipulated microbes. Many bacteria harbour plasmids that carry genes for transformation of metals, aromatics, and other hydrocarbons. Since they are located on plasmids, such genes can be isolated and introduced into organism like *Azotobacter*. *Azotobacter* can fix nitrogen and utilize the excessive carbon present in the municipal sewage. The microbially treated sewage can be used as fertilizer. Genes responsible for dehalogenase activity can be introduced into organisms that grow in sewage polluted with halogenated chemicals.

5. Nucleic acid research

In addition to the above mentioned applied uses, restriction enzymes are also extensively used to reveal the mysterious facts contained in nucleic acids.

6. Miscellaneous

(i) Complementation Test : Small pieces of genomes of industrially important organisms can be ligated to appropriate vectors that replicate in such organisms as well as in *E. coli* which allows application of complementation test for understanding regulatory mechanisms. Such vectors that replicate in *E. coli* as well as in some other organisms such *B. subtilis* or yeast are already being used to shuttle genes between two different host organisms.

(ii) In Vitro Localized Mutagensis : Introducing small deletions or insertions with the help of restriction enzymes, *in vitro* mutagensis may be caused *in vitro* mutagenesis offers the possibility of mutating isolated purified DNA sequences to obtain enzymes with altered modified properties.

(iii) Genome Organisation : Physical mapping of chromosome or gene
Application of a series of restriction enzymes helps in physical mapping of gene or chromosome. Availability of cloned probes will speed up chromosome mapping. Using labelled probes of complimentary RNA prepared from cloned sea urchin genes, five human histone genes have been localized to the leg arm of chromosome VII.

(iv) Gene Structure : Gene structure principally refers to DNA sequencing through which gene structure can be described in terms of intervening sequences, overlapping genes and location of promoter. As restriction enzymes are capable of generating limited specific cuts, they can be used as the first step in DNA sequencing.

(v) Origin of DNA Replication : The origin and direction of replication of several viral chromosomes and plasmids has been revealed using restriction enzymes, particularly *EcoRI.*

(vi) Protein-DNA Interaction : The type II restriction endonucleases[7] appear to be excellent models for the study of sequence- specific protein DNA interactions whose mechanism has not been elucidated clearly.

2.3.5 Future Scope

Due to their unique nature of controllable, predictable, infrequent and site specific cleavage of DNA, restriction enzymes are proved to be extremely important tools in dissecting, analysing and reconstructing genetic information at the molecular level. To make their use economical, convenient and most effective, their enzymology has to be investigated more thoroughly to reveal their behaviour in terms of kinetics and dynamics to enhance new stability. Considerable emphasis on optimization of culture conditions and harvest period are also needed to increase their productivity. Though, several restriction enzymes are being overproduced by genetically redesigned strains, the optimization of their productivities still remains to be achieved to get maximum recovery and in large scale. A great potential for R&D efforts, therefore, remains as future scope in this field.

2.4 REFERENCES

1. Lewin, B. *Multiforked Chromosome Concept In Gene,* pp 299 , WIE Ltd., 1985.
2. Knempel, P.L. "Bacterial Chromosome Replication", *Adv. Cell Biol.* Vol. 1, pp 3–56, (Prescott, D.M. Goldstein, K and McConky eds.), Appleton-Century-Crafts Edu. Div. (ACC), Meredeth, Corp, N. Y. 1970.
3. Erlich, S.D. "Illegitimate Recombination in Bacteria", *Mobile DNA*, Chapt. 38, pp 799-832, (D.E. Berg and M.M. Howe.eds.) Am. Assoc. of Microbiologists, Washington, DC, 1989 .
4. Aiba, S. "Effect of Temperature on Plasmid Stability and Pencillinase Productivity in a Transformant of Bacillus Stearothermophilus ", *Biotechnology and Bioprocess Engineering Proc.* 7th IBS, pp 471-484, (T.K. Ghose ed.), IIT Delhi, United India Press, New Delhi, 1985 .
5. Cooper, S. and C.E. Helmstetter, " Chromosome Replication and the Division Cycle of *E. coli",* Blr. *J. Mol. Biol*., pp 31,519, 1968.
6. Zyskind, J.N. and D. W. Smith, "DNA Replication: The Bacterial Cell Cycle, and Cell Growth", *Cell*, pp 69, 5-8, 1992.
7. Mukhopadhyay, S.N. and D.K. Das, " Replication and Copy Number", *Oxygen Responses, Reactivities and Measurements in Biosystems* , pp 22 , CRC Press, Boca Raton, Florida, 1994 .

8. Khoshravi, M., W. Ryan, D.A. Webster and B.C. Starl, "Variation of Oxygen Requirement with Plasmid Size in Recombinant", *Escherichia coli. Plasmid,* pp 23, 138, 1966.
9. Willetts, N.S., *Biochem. Journal*, pp 103, 462, 1967.
10. Pine, M.J., *Journal Bacterop* pp 92, 847-850, 1966.
11. Goff S.A.and A.L.Goldberg, *J.Biol.Chem.*, pp 262(10), 4506-4515,1987.
12. St. John, A.C. K. Jakubas and D. Beim., *Biochem. Biophys. Acta.* pp 586, 1979
13. Stadtman, E.R., P.B. Chock and S.G. Rohe, *FEBS Sympo.*, pp 60, 57, 1980.
14. Yoshida T. and K.B. Konstantinov, "Application of AI Techniques on Bioreactor Systems", *Proc. Int. Sympo. on Advanced Computing for Life Sciences*, pp. 49- 54, Kyushu Inst. of Technol, Iizuka, Japan, 1992.
15. Nakajima, M., T. Siimo, H. Yada, H. Asama, T. Nagamune, P. Linko and I. Endo "On Line Diagnosis System in Lactic Acid Process", *Ibid,* pp 281-283.
16. Kitura, K. "New Intermolecular Potential Functions for Molecular Simulations". *Ibid*, pp 220-221.
17. Hakamura, H."Computer Aided Protein Design", *Ibid,* pp13-18.
18. Hitzmann, B., A. Lubbert and K. Schugerl, "An Expert System Approach for the Control of a Bioprocess", "Knowledge Representation and Processing", *Biotechnol*, Bioeng, pp 39, 33-43, 1992
19. Yoshida, T. " Computer Control of Fermentation Processes by AI Techniques". I *CHEME Sympo. Series No. 137: Bioproducts Processing Technology for the Tropics,* (M.A. Hashim ed.), I CHE, Rugby, U.K., pp 227-236, 1994.
20. Arber, W. "Future of Recombinant DNA Technology", *Biotechnology and Bioprocess Engineering,* pp. 45-53 (T.K. Ghose,ed.), Proc. VIIth IBS, BERC IIT Delhi, Feb 19-25, 1984.
21. Bailey, J.E., M. Hjortso, S.B. Lee and F. Sriene "Kinetics of Product Formation and Plasmid Segregation in Recombinant Microbial Populations" *Annuals. N.Y. Acad. Sci., Biochem. Engg. III*, 19 pp 71-87, 1987.
22. Aiba, S., T. Imanaka, and J. I. Koizumi, "Transformation of *Bacillus stearothermophilus* with Plasmid DNA and its Application to Molecular Cloning", *Annuals, N.Y. Acad. Sci.*, pp 57-70, 1985 .
23. Khosla, C. and J.E. Bailey, "Heterologous Expression of Bacterial Haemoglobin Improves the Growth Properties of Recombinant *E. coli", Nature* (London) pp 331, 633-635, 1988.
24. Fuji, M., M. Takagi, T. Imanaka, and S. Aiba *J. Bacteriol.* pp 154 (2), 831-837,1983.
25. Howe, *C. Gene Cloning and Manipulation*, Chapter 7, Cambridge Univ. Press, 1995.
26. Mukhopadhyay, S.N. "Current Status of Biomolecular Design Engineering Science in Better Living through , Innovative Biochemical Engineering", *Proc. 3rd AP BioCh* EC, pp 511- 513, (W.K. Teo Yap, M.G.S and Oh, S.K. W eds.), N.S.U. 1994.
27. Blasey H.D. and R. Alain, "Transient Exprssion with cos Cells on Spiner Scale", "Animal Cell Technology", *Products of Today- Prospects for Tomorrow,* pp. 331 (R.E. Spier, *et al.* eds.). Butterworth-Heinemann, Oxford, 1994.
28. Winkler, U., W. Ringer, and W. Walkernagel, *Bacteria, Phage and Molecular Experimental Course*, pp 36, Springer International Student Edition, 1976.
29. Shevitz, J ., T.L. Laporte and T.E. Stinnett, " Production of Viral Vaccines in Stivred Bioreactors", *Adv. in Biotechnol. Process* Vol. 14, pp 1-55 (A Mizrahi, ed.), Wiley-Liss Inc., 1990 .
30. Mukhopadhyay, A., S.N. Mukhopadhyay and G.P. Talwar, *Biotechnol*, Bioceng, pp 48, 158-68, 1995.
31. Nover, L. *Heat Shock Responses*, pp. 5-40 CRC Press, Boca Raton, Florida, 1991.
32. Dubey, A.K., S.N. Mukhopadhyay, V.S. Bisaria, and T.K. Ghose, *Process Biochem*, pp 22,25, 1987.
33. Mukhopadhyay, S.N., *Bioprocess Engineering—The First Generation*, (T.K.Ghose ed.), pp 220-231, Ellis Horwood, West Sussex, UK, 1989.
34. Dubey, A.K., V.S. Bisaria, S.N. Mukhopadhyay, and T.K, Ghose,*Biotechnol & Bioeng,* pp 33, 1311, 1989.
35. Dubey, A.K., S.N. Mukhopadhyay, V.S. Bisaria, and T.K. Ghose, *Ind. Chem. Engg*, pp 16-21, 33, 1991.

36. Oishi, K. *et al; J. Ferment and Biotechnol.*, pp 69(6), 360, 1990.
37. Kuhn, W. *Experientia,* pp 13, 301, 1957.
38. Biruboin, H.C, *Biochem. Cell Bioi.*, pp 66, 374, 1988
39. McConkey, D.J. *et al., Toxicol. Lett.*, pp 42, 123, 1988.
40. Mukhopadhyay, S.N, D.K. Das, "Oxygen Responses, Reactivities and Measurements in Biosystems", pp 18-22, CRC Press, Boca Raton, Florida, 1994.
41. G. Chin, Cell Biol., Science 305, 452, 2004.
42. E. Danchin *et al*, Public Information, From Noisy Neighbours to Cultural Evolution Science, 305, 487, 2004.
43. O. Levenspiel, Chemical Reaction Engineering, 3rd End., John Wiley & Sons (Asia), Pte. Ltd, Singapore, 2003.
44. A. Yarnell, Enzyme Boasts A Radical Makeover, CEP, July 26, 2004, pp 42-43.
45. C.S. Tsai, An Introduction to Computational Biochemistry, Wiley-Liss, A John Wiley & Sons, Inc., Pub., Brijbasi Art Press Ltd., Noida, U.P., India 2004.
46. JDWatson and FH Crick, A structure for deoxyribonucleic acid, Nature 171, 737-738, 1953.

Chapter

3

MEDIUM ENGINEERING FOR CELL CULTIVATION AND BIOREACTIONS

3.1 INTRODUCTION

In fermentation or bioprocessing, microbial/enzymic or biochemical reactions need appropriate designing of the medium in which reactions occur. Many technological concerns are involved in medium design engineering (Fig. 3.1) in bioprocessing. For fermentative processing this need is to establish the most economic medium for any particular fermentation taking care of certain basic requirements to be met by any nutritional medium. The medium design engineering for fermentation should take care of (a) source of energy (b) source of carbon (c) source of nitrogen (d) source of minerals and (e) source of growth factors in relation to technological concerns.[1, 2] On the other hand biocatalytic medium engineering takes care of micro environments consisting of a thin layer of water around the biocatalyst and an interfacial region, which forms the transition between the biocatalytic and continuous phases.

In recent years an increasing important development in the field of synthetic bioinorganic and bioorganic chemistry relates to application of biocatalysts to chemical reactions. This is not surprising. Biocatalysts are known to perform catalysis very effectively a wide variety of organic and inorganic reactions under relatively mild conditions in a stereo and/or regio-selective way.[3-5] So medium design engineering has many concerns. One of the most important concerns is optimization of a fermentation process in the design of the growth and production medium. Besides meeting nutritional and environmental requirements of the fermenting microorganism, the medium must also minimize several technoeconomic constraints.

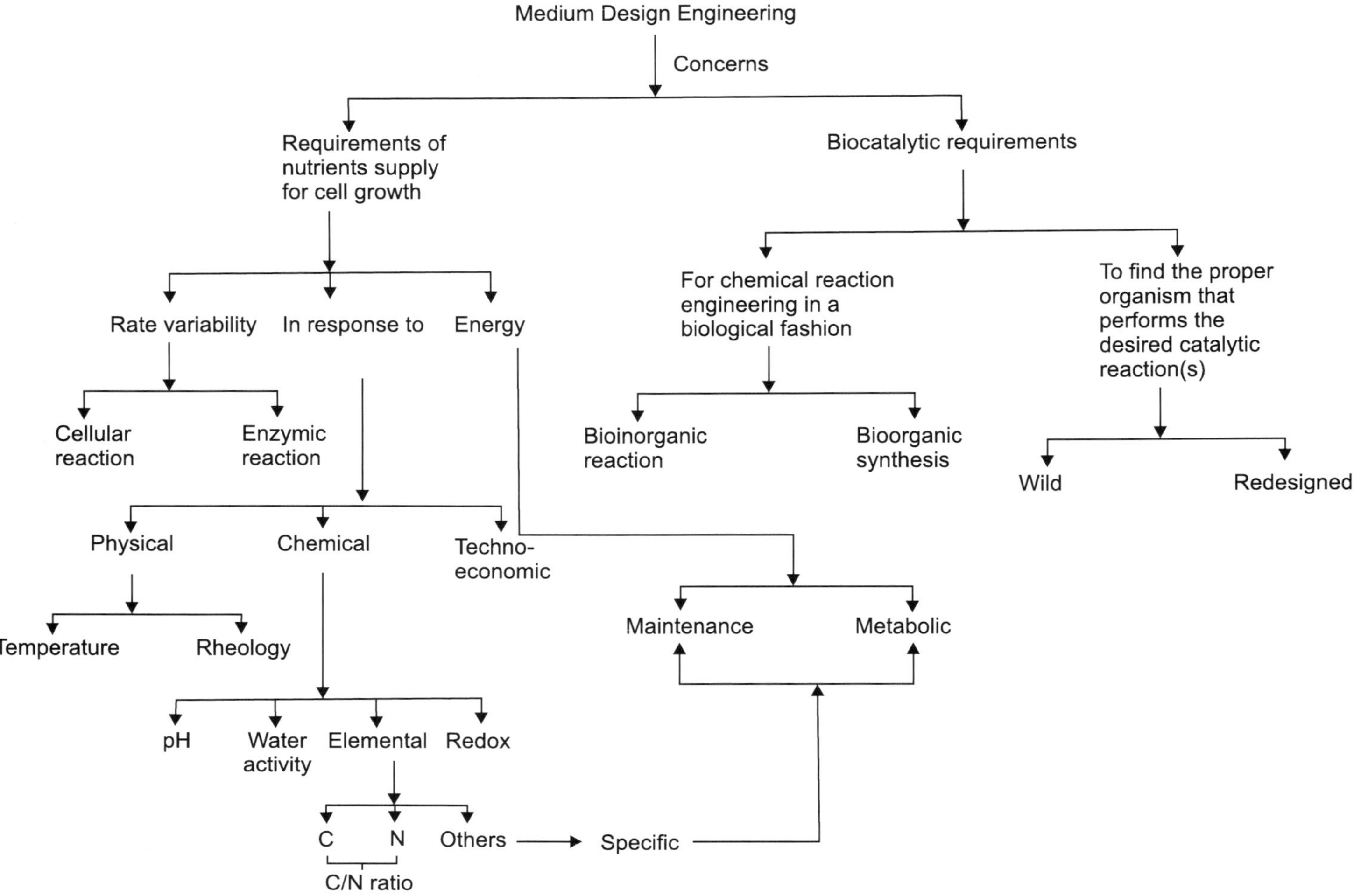

Fig. 3.1 Technological concerns of medium design engineering in bioprocessing

3.2 BASIC CONCEPT IN MEDIUM DESIGN

3.2.1 Fermentation

In meeting nutritional and environmental requirements the first approximation is the minimal medium design, minimal medium design is based on the simple stoichiometry for growth and products formation as given below.[1,2]

$$\text{C-source} + \text{N-source} + O_2 + \text{Minerals} + \text{Growth factors/Specific nutrients} \rightarrow \text{Cell biomass} + \text{Product} + CO_2 + 2H_2O + Q \text{ cals.}$$

The basic concept in such design is simply a material balance and energy balance.

3.2.2. Chemical Reactions in Biological Fashion

In chemical reactions like bioorganic synthesis or bioinorganic transformations, medium engineering concerns[3,5] designing microenvironments for the biocatalyst. The basic objective of this is to reach maximal activity, stability and productivity.

Reactant substrate containing liquid medium + Biocatalyst
Surrounded by Microenvironments
Products + Coproducts + Biocatalysts if any

Medium design engineering in such systems, therefore, involves aspects such as stabilizing the essential liquid layer around the biocatalyst, controlling electrostatic and hydrophobic interactions between substrate(s) and biocatalyst.

3.3 DESIGN PROCEDURE

Design of medium is carried out on the basis of the objective set for.

3.3.1. Growth and Production Medium

All growth processes are endergonic.[1] In the course of cellular growth, organic and inorganic molecules like glucose, NH_3, water and CO_2 may be synthesised to form biomass product. Supply of energy is needed for growth. It must come from chemical energy of oxidation of medium nutrients or from light energy. In medium design procedure the first and foremost importance is to provide suitable and sufficient nutrients (reactants) and in appropriate proportions for a specified amount of biomass (products) to be synthesised.

The most suitable energy and/or carbonaceous nutrient source is selected on the basis of experimental results performed with different energy/carbon source. Present day industrial bioprocessing uses starch or molasses as the commonest carbon or energy source. For computing the necessary amounts of various substrates reaction stoichiometry is useful. It requires the knowledge of the elemental composition of the product biomass (e.g. microorganism). Besides biomass, if fermentative production of other materials occur, the chemical composition of the major products are also required in ascertaining nutrient medium composition. Design of nutrient medium composition is not only important in microbial cell culture system but also the nutrient regime is an important factor in mammalian and plant cell culture bio-processing. Its regime may affect both growth and product synthesis. For cultivations of plant cells most of the used medium has a defined design of chemical composition.[6, 7] The media design for the growth of plant tissue/cells are more complex and costly. This is due to the inclusion of plant growth regulators in the media. Optimization in media design in case of plant cell culture mostly confines to carbon and mineral nutrients. However, media supporting good biomass growth do not necessarily provide maximal yields of natural products. It necessitated defining 'maintenance media' and 'production media'. Maintenance media supports enhanced cell yield and cell division with reduced product yield. Production media on the other hand gives enhanced product yield at the expense of growth.

So in the medium engineering stoichiometric design based and experimental requirement based media formulation approaches have been used in bioprocessing.

3.3.2. Stoichiometric Design Approach: Material and Energy Balances

This approach is entirely based on laws of conservation of mass of each element taking part in the bioreaction. It is essential to balance the elemental requirements for growth and product formation. For example, in hetero-fermentative anaerobic bioreaction for production of propionic acid by *Propionibacter acidipropionici* ATCC 25562 (at 30°C, pH 6.8 for 34 hrs.) the minimum carbon requirement in the medium may be determined stoichiometrically. In this bioprocessing the carbon content of substrate (glucose) was found to be distributed mainly in products propionic acid, acetic acid, CO_2 and cell mass. On elemental analysis the carbon content in the cell mass was found to be 44%. The stoichiometric carbon balance in this bioprocessing at the end of fermentation (34 hrs.) period was as below. Propionic acid is rarely formed as a sole product in an acidogenic bioprocessing. It is usually accompanied by formation of acetic acid. This occurs for stoichiometric reasons and to maintain hydrogen and redox balance.[8, 9]

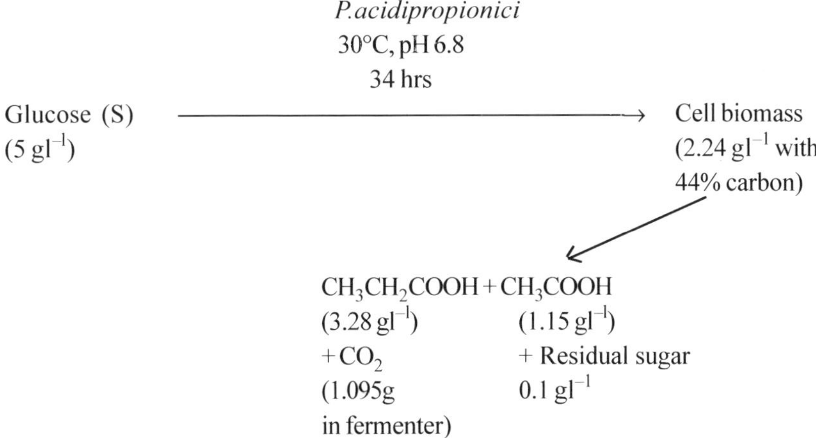

About 95% of the initial substrate carbon present could be accounted in various products. Trace amounts of succinic and isovaleric acids as reported by some workers requiring very sensitive methods of estimation could probably account for the rest of the 5% carbon. In anoxic bioprocessing every oxidation is accompanied by a reduction that yield product(s) formed from the substrate. Thus the balance between the oxidized and reduced product provides an important criterion for evaluation of the accuracy of the analysis. An oxidation-reduction (O/R) balance in propionic acid production by the above stated microorganism revealed the values[10] as shown in Table 3.1 and 3.2.

Table 3.1 Substrate carbon distribution in propionic acid fermentation by *P. acidipropionici* (Substrate carbon distribution at the end of 34 h. gC in fermentor at zero hour = 4.75)

	g/l	*g in Fermentor*	*gC*
CO_2	—	1.095	0.298
Propionic acid	3.28	4.52	2.198
Acetic acid	1.15	1.587	0.634
Cell mass	2.24	3.09	1.359
Residual sugar	0.1	0.138	0.055
			4.544

Table 3.2 Oxidation-reduction balance in propionic acid fermentation based on 100 m Moles of Glucose (30°C, initial pH 6.8)

Products	*m Moles of Product Per 100 m Mole of Glucose*	*O/R Number*	*Milli-equivalent of Oxidized*	*Reduced*
Acetic acid	32.95	0	—	—
Propionic acid	92.0	–1	—	92.00
Carbondioxide	43.26	+2	86.52	—
			86.52	92.00
O/R Index = 0.94				

The balance of hydrogen and oxygen were obtained by comparing their ratio in the substrate and product. When in a substrate 2H = 0, its oxidation value is zero. Every additional pair of hydrogen atom constitutes O/R number of –1 and every additional oxygen atom constitutes O/R number of +1. From Table 3.2 O/R index of 0.94 is observed.

An O/R index close to 1 indicated that all products were accounted for in the right proportions. The deviation from unity accounted for experimental error.

Cell composition and product composition data availability can enable one to assess the elemental requirements in medium design considering requirements and constraints[1,11] (Table 3.3).

Thus mass and energy balances associated with growing cultures play a great role in media design. The heat of reaction per election transferred to oxygen for a wide variety of organic molecules, the number of available electrons per carbon atom in biomass and the weight fraction of carbon in biomass have been found to be relatively constant.

Table 3.3 Nutritional and environmental requirements and techno- economic constraints in medium design

A. Nutritional and Environmental Requirements
   1. Elemental requirements
   2. Specific nutrient requirements
   3. Energy requirements
   4. Environmental needs (culture)

B. Fermentation Process Objectives
   1. Cell mass
   2. Product
   3. Maintenance
   4. Special growth conditions
      (a) avoid catabolite repression
      (b) avoid phosphate repression
      (c) limit a specific nutrient

C. Technoeconomic Constraints
   1. Cost
   2. Availability of raw materials
   3. Requirements of specific C– or N– sources
   4. Recovery
   5. Pollution control

3.4 BASICS OF MATERIAL BALANCE

In any process biotechnology consideration, material balance is essential for the sake of metabolic economy. Frameworks using material balances in metabolic pathways to study cellular metabolism has been investigated by various researchers[1–3]. From material balances the concept of stoichiometric coefficients for the over all reaction representing the biological system has been introduced and were determined on line to provide information about yield factors, substrate consumption and, product formation rates. Despite the excellent performance and the suitability of this approach for on line bioprocess monitoring and control, its application to infer cellular behavior is limited, however. This is because the model does not contain any intracellular mechanisms and is therefore unable to provide essential information at the cellular level. Several researchers have paid attentions on this limitations. In their studies, material balances on the extra cellular compounds were employed to deduce most probable metabolic model for citrate production from glucose. Also, fermentation balance equation for the acetone-butanol using metabolic biochemistry to describe intracellular reactions have been provided.[3]

3.4.4 Concepts

1. Simple representations in simple medium

On the basis of elemental balancing technique a simple material balance in oxic growth is represented as below.

$$\underset{\text{(Substrate)}}{a\,C_x H_y O_Z} + bO_2 + \underset{\text{(Base)}}{cNH_3} \xrightarrow{\text{Cells}} \underset{\text{(Biomass)}}{C_\alpha H_\beta O_\gamma N_\delta} + dH_2O + eCO_2 + \underset{\text{(Product)}}{fC_s H_u O_v N_w} \quad (3.1)$$

For determining the unknown stoichiometric coefficients, the four elements (C, H, 0, N) can be balanced, and three independent measurements must therefore be found. In some cases oxygen uptake rate (OUR), CO_2 evolution rate (CER) and base addition rate (BAR) have been used.[5] If the pH of the culture is constant, the latter can be related to nitrogen uptake rate (NUR) as below.

$$BAR = NUR + kPFR \tag{3.2}$$

where k is a function of the products acidic equilibrium and PFR is the abbreviation of product formation rate.

The nitrogen balance gives

$$NUR = \delta\ BPR + \omega\ PFR \tag{3.3}$$

in which BPR is the biomass production rate. Eliminating the other three balances leads to

$$[a\ (r_B - r_S) + 3\delta]\ BPR = r_S\ CER - 4\ OUR + 3\ NUR + [S(s_s - r_p) + 3W]\ PFR \tag{3.4}$$

In these relations r_B, r_S, r_P are the degrees of reductance of biomass, substrate and product respectively. Here

$$r_B = \frac{4\alpha + \beta - 2v - 3\delta}{\alpha} \tag{3.5}$$

Special case: Product formation is negligible. Growth is calculated by following basis.

(i) Using BAR and equations (3.2) and (3.3). This is very sensitive to even slight organic acid production and to δ.

(ii) Using all the balances, which eliminates NUR, this has been shown to be very sensitive to measurement errors, when r_B is close to r_S and RQ to one.

(iii) Not using the nitrogen balance. This provides a natural way of combining the three measurements and reduces the sensitivity problem as stated in earlier cases.

In this case rate of growth, R_x is

$$R_x = \frac{mwb}{\left[a\ (r_B - r_S) + 3\delta\right]}\ (r_S\ CER - 4\ OUR + 3\ BAR) \tag{3.6}$$

where mwb is the molecular weight (approximate) of biomass.

The advantage of base measurement is apparent from equation (3.6) since r_B is generally close to 4, thereby sensitivity problems are avoided.[6] However, the other two contribute significantly to R_X. This balance analysis is especially important in the contaminant detection case.

2. Biochemical engineering aspects

(i) Material Balance : In an aerobic fermentation one may consider that a microbial system exhibits during a small increase of time Δt cell growth ΔX, product formation ΔC_P as a result of consumption of small amount of dissolved oxygen ΔO_2 and carbonaceous substrate ΔS. Here each term of cell, product, dissolved oxygen and substrate pertains to the amount in moles per unit volume. For this system oxygen balance equation may be written as below.

$$A\ (-\Delta S) = B(\Delta X) + \Delta O_2 + C\ \Delta C_P \tag{3.7}$$

In this equation A, B and C are coefficients. A has been defined as oxygen required for complete combustion of carbonaceous substrate, mole O_2/mole substrate. B is the amount of oxygen required for complete combustion of cell (assuming nitrogen content of the cell to turn out to ammonia) which is equal to 0.042 mole O_2/g. cell, C is the amount of oxygen required for complete combustion of product, mole O_2/mole product and ΔO_2 indicates accumulated dissolved oxygen in fermentation liquid, mole O_2/l.

If and only if the product other than CO_2 and water in fermentation system is not appreciable, equation (3.7) is reduced to the following.

$$A(-\Delta S) = B(\Delta X) + \Delta O_2 \tag{3.8}$$

In parallel with equation (3.8) it is possible to assume the following on the fate of adenosine triphosphate (ATP) synthesized during Δt period.

$$(\Delta\ ATP)_S = (\Delta\ ATP)_M + (\Delta ATP)_G \tag{3.9}$$

Here the subscripts S is for synthesized, M for maintenance and G for cellular growth. It is assumed that

$$\left.\begin{aligned}(\Delta\ ATP)_M &= m_A \times \Delta t\\ (\Delta\ ATP)_G &= \frac{1}{Y_{ATP}^{Max}} \cdot \Delta X\end{aligned}\right\} \tag{3.10}$$

in which m_A is the maintenance coefficient, mole ATP/g cells hr. and Y_{ATP}^{Max} is the growth yield constant for ATP; maximal value of Y_{ATP} for energy-coupled growth, implying the maximum value, g cell/mole ATP.

By substituting equation (3.10) into (3.9) and rearranging one has the following equation.

$$Q_{ATP} = m_A + \frac{1}{Y_{ATP}^{Max}}\ \mu \tag{3.11}$$

In this equation Q_{ATP} is the specific rate of ATP synthesis, mole ATP/g. cell. hr and μ is the specific rate of cell growth, l/hr.

Similar to equations (3.8) and (3.9) the mass balance equation for carbonaceous substrate consumption $-\Delta S$ may be written as below.

$$-\ \Delta S = (-\Delta S)_M + (-\Delta S)_G \tag{3.12}$$

For terms on the right hand side similar to equation (3.10) the following equations are assumed.

$$\left.\begin{aligned}(-\Delta S)_M &= m \times \Delta t\\ (-\Delta S)_G &= \frac{1}{Y_G} \cdot \Delta X\end{aligned}\right\} \tag{3.13}$$

Here m is the maintenance coefficient, mole substrate/g. cell. hr. and Y_G is the growth yield constant for carbonaceous substrate. Substituting equation (3.13) into equation (3.12) and rearranging,

$$v = m + \frac{1}{Y_G} \cdot \mu \tag{3.14}$$

In this equation v is the specific rate of consumption of carbonaceous substrate, mole substrate/g. cell hr. In order to coordinate $(\Delta ATP)_S$ synthesized with the fate of carbonaceous substrate via oxygen consumption one may assume that

$$(\Delta ATP)_S = (Y_{A/O}) (\Delta O_2) \tag{3.15}$$

provided $Y_{A/O}$ = 2(P/0) = ATP yield in respiration, mole ATP/mole oxygen, where (P/O) is the ratio of phosphate to oxygen.

On substituting equation (3.15) into the left hand side of equation (3.9), while the terms on the right-hand side of the equation are substituted by equation (3.10) and then rearranging,

$$Q_{O_2} = \frac{m_A}{Y_{A/O}} + \frac{1}{Y_{A/O}\, Y_{ATP}^{Max}} \mu \tag{3.16}$$

$$= m_O + \frac{1}{Y_{GO}} \mu \tag{3.17}$$

Where

Q_{O_2} = Specific rate of oxygen consumption (respiration), mole O_2/g cell hr.

m_O = $m_A/Y_{A/O}$ Maintenance coefficient, mole O_2/g cell hr. (3.18)

Y_{GO} = $Y_{A/O}\, Y_{ATP}^{Max}$ Growth yield constant for oxygen, g cell/mole O_2

Dividing both sides of equation (3.8) with X Δt, the equation turns out to be:

$$Av = B\mu + Q_{O_2} \tag{3.19}$$

Substitution of equation (3.17) into the second term on the right-hand side of Eq. (3.19) and rearranging,

$$v = \frac{m_O}{A} + \frac{1}{A}\left[B + \frac{1}{Y_{GO}}\right] \mu \tag{3.20}$$

It is clear from equation (3.17) and (3.20) that

$$m = m_O/A,\ 1/Y_G = (l/A)\,[B + (l/Y_{GO})] \tag{3.21}$$

(ii) Energy (enthalpy) Balance : Multiplying each term on both sides of equation (3.7) with enthalpy change ($-\Delta\ H^*_O$) for oxygen,

$$A(-\Delta H^*_O)(-\Delta S) = B(-\Delta H^*_O)(\Delta X) + (-\Delta H^*_O)(\Delta O_2) + C(-\Delta H^*_O)(\Delta C_p) \tag{3.22}$$

Since 4 electrons are commensurable to mole O_2 and the enthalpy change, $-\Delta H^*_{av.e^-}$ with respect to available electron has been claimed to be

$$-\Delta H^*_{av.e^-} = 26.5 \text{ kcal/av. electron}$$

$$-\Delta H^*_O = 26.5 \times 4 = 106 \text{ kcal/mole } O_2$$

The value of $-\ \Delta H^*_{av.e^-}$ (= 26.5 kcal/av. electron) has no theoretical background and in fact, the average value has been assessed from quite a few data on combustion heat of various substances wherein the number of electrons participating in the combustion is assumed to be available. In this context, the concept of $-\Delta H^*_O$, though difficult to envisage, has been introduced to have an easy access to the enthalpy change of a given material whose combustion heat having not always been made available from the references.

Here, some comparison will be made between values of $A(-\Delta H^*_O)$ or $B(-\Delta H^*_O)$ etc. and those available from the data on combustion.

For glucose,

$$A = 6 \text{ mole } O_2/\text{mole glucose}$$

$$-\Delta H^*_O = 106 \text{ kcal/mole } O_2$$

$$A(-\Delta H^*_O) = 6 \times 106 = 636 \text{ kcal/mole glucose}$$

$$-\Delta H \text{ (measured)} = 673 \text{ kcal/mole glucose}$$

$$\text{Difference} = (673 - 636)\ /\ 673 = 5.5\%$$

For dry cell,

$$B = 0.042 \text{ mole } O_2/\text{g cell}$$

$$-\Delta H^*_O = 106 \text{ kcal/mole } O_2$$

$$B(-\Delta H^*_O) = 0.042 \times 106 = 4.5 \text{ kcal/g cell}$$

$$-\Delta H^*_O\text{(measured)} = 5.3 \text{ kcal/g cell}$$

$$\text{Difference} = (5.3 - 4.5)/5.3 = 15\%$$

Accordingly, the difference

$$A(-\Delta H^*_O)\ (-\Delta S) - \{B(-\Delta H^*_O)\ (\Delta X) + C(-\Delta H^*_O)\ (\Delta C_p)\}$$

may be assumed to represent that in enthalpies between the original (initial) and resulting (final) states; i.e.,

$$\begin{aligned} &A(-\Delta H^*_O)\ (-\Delta S) - \{B(-\Delta H^*_O)\ (\Delta X) + C\ (-\Delta H^*_O)\ (\Delta C_p)\} \\ &= -\Delta H_1 - (-\Delta H_2) \\ &= -\Delta H \end{aligned} \tag{3.23}$$

where

$-\Delta H$ = enthalpy change (heat of reaction) subscripts : 1 and 2 : initial and final states.

The right-hand side of equation (3.23) is obviously equated to $(-\Delta H^*_O)\ (\Delta O_2)$ in aerobic system; i.e.

$$\begin{aligned} A(-\Delta H^*_O)\ (-\Delta S) - \{B(-\Delta H^*_O)\ (\Delta X) + C(-\Delta H^*_O)\ (\Delta C_P)\} &= (-\Delta H^*_O)\ (\Delta O_2) \\ &= -\Delta H \end{aligned} \tag{3.24}$$

However, this overall approach to the energy balance remains to be discussed further in the next section to derive a versatile equation for estimating the heat of reaction in microbial systems.

(iii) Heat of Reaction : Although heat of reaction for a microbial system is already referred to in equation (3.23) or in equation (3.24), some additional comment is deemed necessary for a better insight into the fate of carbon—catabolism and anabolism—, because they are already mentioned, in equations (3.23) and (3.24) and are derived solely on oxygen balance of the system.

A. Minimal medium

The cellular carbon assumed to have originated entirely from energy substrate is partly used for anabolism. Accordingly, the heat of reaction Q is expressed by the following equation.

$$\begin{aligned} Q &= -\Delta H_1 - (-\Delta H_2) \\ &= (-\Delta H_s)(-\Delta S) - \{(-\Delta H_c)(\Delta X) + \Sigma\,(-\Delta H_p)(\Delta C_p)\} \\ &= (-\Delta H_s)(-\Delta S) - \{\alpha_1/\alpha_2)(-\Delta H_s)(\Delta X) + \Sigma\,(-\Delta H_p)(\Delta C_p)\} \\ &= (-\Delta H_s)\{(-\Delta S) - (\alpha_1/\alpha_2)(\Delta X)\} - \Sigma\,(-\Delta H_p)(\Delta C_p) \\ &= (-\Delta H_s)\{(-\Delta S) - (\Delta S)_a\} - \Sigma\,(-\Delta H_p)(\Delta C_p) \end{aligned} \quad (3.25)$$

where

$-\Delta H_1$ = Enthalpy change of initial state, kcal/liter

$-\Delta H_2$ = Enthalpy change of final state, kcal/liter

$-\Delta H$ = Enthalpy change, kcal/mole

α_1 = Carbon content in cell, g carbon/g cell

α_2 = Carbon content in carbonaceous substrate, g carbon/mole substrate

Subscripts : a : Anabolism

c : Cell

p : Product

s : Carbonaceous substrate

It is evident that the first term on the right-hand side of equation (3.25) represents the enthalpy expended for catabolism, whereas the second one corrects for that due to product formation.

B. Complex medium

Complex medium here is assumed to comprise carbonaceous substrate (energy source), various natural products such as meat extract, soybean meal, peptone, etc. Although the latter materials serve also as carbon source, the carbonaceous substrate *per se* such as glucose and other sugars do not contribute to the carbon content of the cells, serving solely as energy source. Briefly, the materials to constitute the cells are assumed to exist abundantly in the original medium rather than in sugars.

Heat of reaction, Q in this particular case is:

$$Q = (-\Delta H_1) - (-\Delta H_2)$$

$$= (-\Delta H_s)(-\Delta S) + (-\Delta H_{SN})(-\Delta S_N) - \{(-\Delta H_c)(\Delta X) + \Sigma\ (-\Delta H_p)(\Delta C_p)\} \tag{3.26}$$

$$= (-\Delta H_s)(-\Delta S) - \Sigma\ (-\Delta H_p)(\Delta C_p)$$

$$(-\Delta H_{SN})(-\Delta S_N) \doteqdot (-\Delta H_c)(\Delta X) \tag{3.27}$$

provided:

$-\Delta S_N$ = Concentration change of natural product serving partly as energy source

$-\Delta H_{SN}$ = Enthalpy change of natural product

Eq. (3.27) presumes that the cellular constituents originate entirely from the natural products impregnated initially in the complex medium and that the chemical structure of these products as medium ingredients is akin to that of cells.

From above discussions one may write

$$Q = (-\Delta H_1) - (-\Delta H_2)$$

$$= (-\Delta H_s)(-\Delta S) - \{\xi(-\Delta H_c)(\Delta X) + \Sigma\ (-\Delta H_p)(\Delta C_p)\} \tag{3.28}$$

$$= (-\Delta H_s)(-\Delta S) - \{\xi\ (\alpha_1/\alpha_2)(-\Delta H_s)(\Delta X) + \Sigma(-\Delta H_p)(\Delta C_p))$$

$$= (-\Delta H_s)\ \{(-\Delta S) - \Sigma\ (-\Delta S)_a\} - \Sigma(-\Delta H_p)(\Delta C_p))$$

$$= A\ (-\ \Delta H^*_O)\ \{(-\Delta S) - \xi\ (-\Delta S)_a\ \}\ (\Delta X) + \Sigma C(-\ \Delta H^*_O)(\Delta C_p) \tag{3.29}$$

$$= (-\ \Delta H^*_O)(\Delta O_2) \tag{3.30}$$

where

$\xi = 0$ for complex medium

$\xi = 1$ for minimal medium

Usually, $0 < \xi < 1$

It goes without saying that equation (3.30) is exclusively for aerobic culture and that equations (3.28) to (3.30) are reduced to equations (3.23) and (3.24), if ξ and $(-\Delta H_c)$ in equations (3.28) are taken as unity and $B(-\ \Delta H^*_O)$, respectively.

Conversely speaking, equations appearing in the preceding section have implicit background of minimal medium ($\xi = 1$ in equation (3.28) to (3.30). Though the above-mentioned implication sounds a bit intriguing, the fact that the heat of reaction in aerobic systems can be approximated to $(-\ \Delta H^*_O)\Delta O_2$ regardless of the minimal or complex medium is considered to be useful from practice. The idea of "approximate estimation of reaction heat" by $(-\ \Delta H^*_O)\Delta O_2$ comes firstly from the approximate nature of $(-\ \Delta H^*_O)$ *per se* and secondly from another approximation of equation (3.27) for complex medium, albeit there is no room of "approximation" so far as oxygen and enthalpy balances, equation (3.7) and (3.22) are concerned *in situ*.

3.4.2 Experiment Based Media Formulations

In the absence of cell composition data, it is possible to experimentally determine the requirements by carrying out a series of batch fermentations in which the nutrient of interest is available in limiting supply while all other nutrients are available in excess. So in medium design it is essential to identify the growth limiting nutrient and wheather the product formation is growth associated product formation system in synthetic medium. Since cell composition was unknown to design the medium batch experiments were carried out to find the nutrients essential in synthetic medium. Next fermentation experiments need be done in the same synthetic medium in ascertaining the most optimum concentration of a specific nutrient. For this fermentations were carried out in this medium containing all components excepting the one whose effect is to be observed. In designing medium for gluconic acid fermentation such experiments produced results[1,2] as given in Table 3.4. It showed that in this synthetic medium no growth of *Ps. ovalis* occurred in absence of glucose and ammonium acetate. It was obviously due to the absence of carbon and nitrogen source. In absence of other mineral nutrients growth and gluconic acid production took place although not to the same extent as it was observed in their presence. It appeared, therefore, that in the designed synthetic medium either glucose or ammonium acetate might be serving as limiting nutrient for the growth of *Ps. ovalis* B1486.

3.5 GROWTH LIMITING NUTRIENT IN THE DESIGNED MEDIUM

Identification of growth limiting nutrient is essential since bioprocess design criteria in pure culture system is primarily centred around it. In gluconic acid fermentation in order to know the limiting nutrient between glucose and ammonium acetate two sets of fermentations were conducted to observe the effect of different concentrations of glucose and ammonium acetate on the growth of this organism and its gluconic acid production. In the first set the fermentation medium contained all other nutrients and varying concentrations of ammonium acetate. Similarly in the second set the effect of varying concentrations of glucose was noticed, other conditions of fermentation remaining same as described before. Results are provided in Fig. 3.2 and 3.3. It can be seen from these figures that when other nutrients were at the desired level the optimum concentration of ammonium acetate giving optimum cell growth and gluconic acid yield was 1.0 mg ml^{-1}. Increasing concentration of it showed neither the decrease nor the increase of cell growth and gluconic acid yield. In the case of glucose it was observed that other nutrients remaining at the desired level optimum cell growth and gluconic acid yield was achieved at a glucose concentration of 51.0 mg ml^{-1}. However, unlike the case of ammonia acetate above 51.0 mg ml^{-1} of glucose concentration in the medium showed detrimental effect on both cell growth and gluconic acid yield.[12]

To see whether end product gluconic acid has any effect on the cell growth and glucose utilization by *Ps. ovalis* B1486 fermentation & were conducted adding various concentrations (1– 50 mg ml^{-1}) of sodium gluconate (BDH, Anal R) in the medium. However, no inhibition effect on cell growth as well as gluconic acid yield was observed by such additions. It is consistent with the literature information that the development of acidity due to the formation of gluconic acid was not directly related to the enzyme action in glucose oxidation[13]. It then needs interpretation of the inhibition of gluconic acid formation by glucose concentration above 51.0 mg ml^{-1}.

3.5.1 Inhibition Aspects and Interpretation

One explanation of the above inhibition may be forwarded as discussed below. It is an established fact that if cells are immersed in sugar solution with higher osmotic pressure than that of the cell content water will be drawn out of the cells causing them to shrink in size[14] since the surrounding

Table 3.4 Effect of components of the synthetic medium on cell growth of *Ps. ovalis* B1486 and gluconic acid yield

Fermentation Time	Growth on Medium					Gluconic Acid Production on Medium				
	With all nutrients	Devoid of $MgSO_4.7H_2O$	Devoid of KH_2PO_4	Devoid of ammonium acetate	Devoid of glucose	With all nutrients	Devoid of $MgSO_4.7H_2O$	Devoid of KH_2PO_4	Devoid of ammonium acetate	Devoid of glucose
hrs.	$UODml^{-1}$	$UODml^{-1}$	$UODml^{-1}$	$UODml^{-1}$	$UODml^{-1}$	$UODml^{-1}$	mg ml^{-1}	mg ml^{-1}	mg ml^{-1}	mg ml^{-1}
0	0.10	0.10	0.08	0.08	0.08	–	–	–	–	–
1	0.11	0.10	0.08	No growth	No growth	0.12	–	–	No	No yield
yield										
2	0.169	0.12	0.10	"	"	0.60	0.08	0.28	"	"
3	0.215	0.14	0.12	"	"	1.08	0.22	0.52	"	"
4	0.315	0.16	0.16	"	"	1.92	0.33	0.93	0.80	"
5	0.480	0.20	0.22	"	"	3.27	0.62	2.12	–	"
6	0.873	0.34	0.35	"	"	5.68	1.28	4.25	1.50	"
7	1.25	0.48	0.42	"	"	9.72	–	5.38	–	"
8	1.732	0.56	0.48	"	"	15.08	3.35	–	2.00	"
9	2.203	0.62	0.52	"	"	22.10	–	11.25	–	"
10	2.20	0.62	0.52	"	"	30.86	8.48	–	–	"
11	2.20	0.62	0.52	"	"	37.00	–	17.33	–	"
12	2.20	–	–	"	"	42.14	15.49	–	2.08	"
13	–	–	–	"	"	45.68	–	23.28	–	"
14	–	–	–	"	"	46.82	20.25	25.11	3.00	"

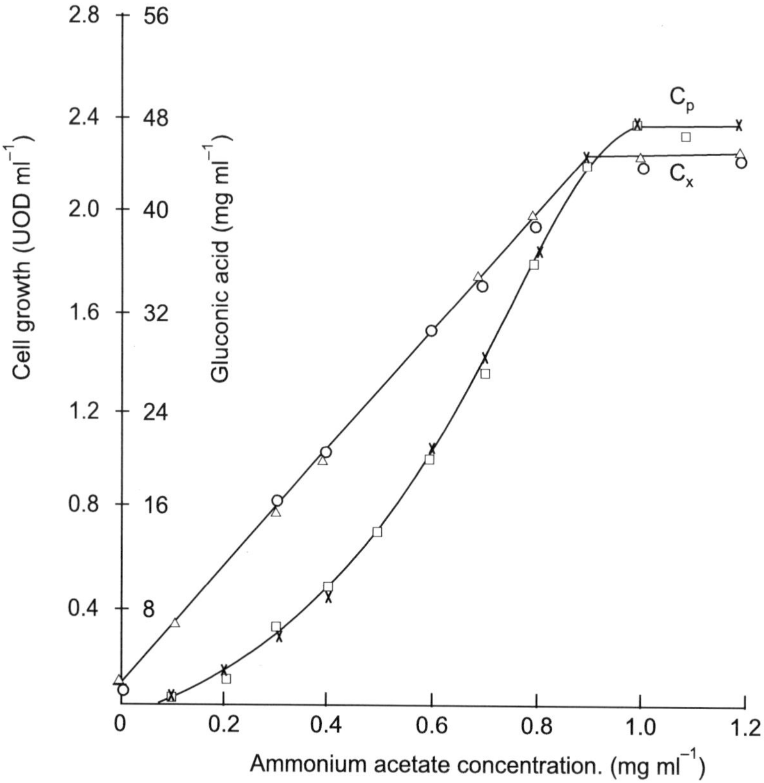

Fig. 3.2 Effect of ammonium acetate on cell growth and gluconic acid yield

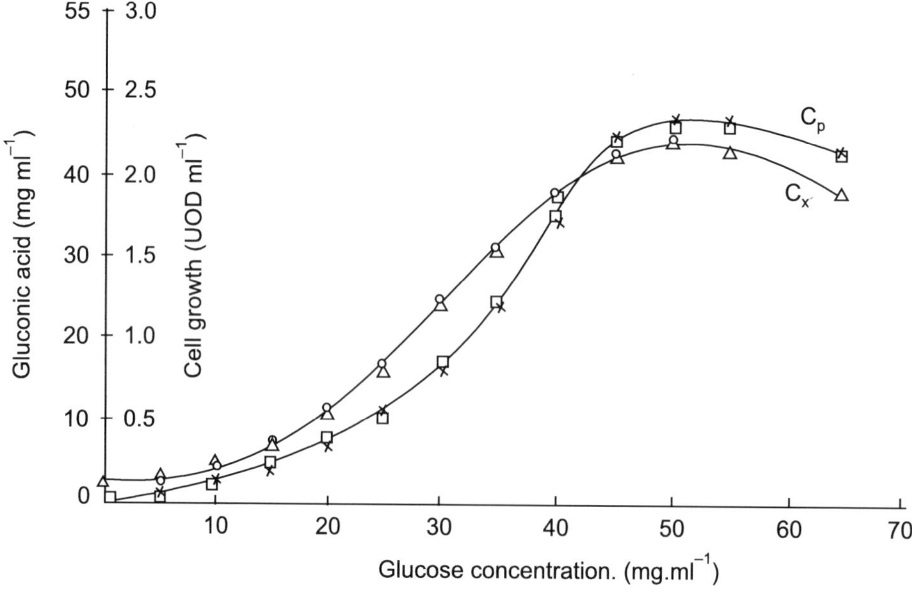

Fig. 3.3 Effect of glucose concentration on cell growth and gluconic acid yield

liquid is hypertonic with respect to the cell (a phenomenon known as plasmolysis). Such hypertonic solutions act as an inhibitor to the cell growth by a desication effect and altering cellular activity[15]. It is plausible, therefore, that glucose solution above 51.0 mg ml^{-1} concentration acts as hypertonic solution with respect to the growth of *Ps. ovalis* B 1486. Due to desication its cell wall shrinked in size and activity was reduced due to lower nutrient uptake of the cells. This in turn inhibited the growth of this organism and oxidation of glucose to gluconolactone. The overall manifestation being inhibition in gluconic acid yield.

3.6 ENGINEERED MEDIUM IN CELL GROWTH AND PRODUCT FORMATION

As medium engineering means designing (micro) environments for biocells/biocatalyst with the objective of reaching maximal activity, stability and hence productivity it exerts, therefore, great influence on bioreaction kinetics.

Production of gluconic acid as discussed above provides a good example of the same. The scheme of this bioreaction is as below.

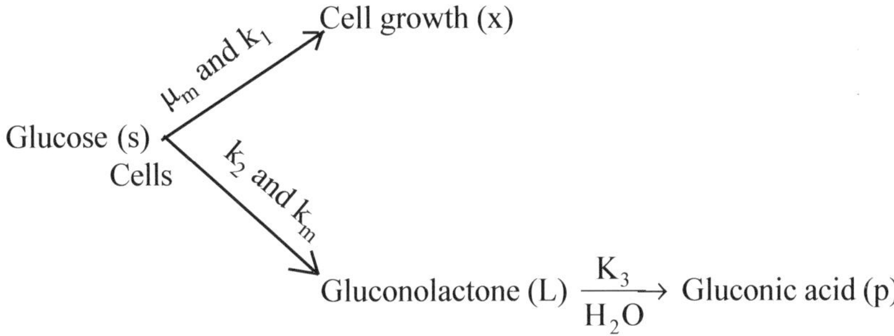

As found experimentally[16,17] one mole of glucose gives one mole of intermediate (gluconolactone) which on hydrolysis gives one mole of product (gluconic acid). From this bioreaction stoichiometry one may write the following equality.

Rate of glucose/substrate consumption = Rate of intermediate accumulation/formation = Rate of product formation.

Thus

$$-\left(\frac{ds}{dt}\right)_{total} = -\left(\frac{dL}{dt}\right) = \frac{dp}{dt} \tag{3.31}$$

However,

$$-\left(\frac{ds}{dt}\right)_{total} = -\left(\frac{ds}{dt}\right)_{growth} + \left(-\frac{ds}{dt}\right)_{product}$$

and

$$-\left(\frac{ds}{dt}\right)_{growth} \propto \left(\frac{k_1 sx}{k_s + s}\right) = f_1 \left(\frac{k_1 sx}{k_s + s}\right)$$

$$-\left(\frac{ds}{dt}\right)_{product} \propto \left(\frac{k_2 sx}{k_L + s}\right) = f_2 \left(\frac{k_2 sx}{k_L + s}\right)$$

So,
$$-\left(\frac{ds}{dt}\right)_{total} = f_1\left(\frac{k_1sx}{k_s+s}\right) + f_2\left(\frac{k_2sx}{k_L+s}\right) \quad (3.32)$$

Here, k_1, k_2, k_L, k_s, f_1 and f_2 are constants.

Since
$$-\frac{dL}{dt} = \frac{dp}{dt}$$

From stoichiometry,
$$-\frac{1}{M_L}\cdot\frac{dL}{dt} = \frac{1}{M_P}\cdot\frac{dp}{dt}$$

or
$$\frac{dp}{dt} = \frac{M_P}{M_L} - \left(\frac{dL}{dt}\right) \quad (3.33)$$

where M_p is the molecular weight of product (gluconic acid) and M_L is the molecular weight of the intermediate lactone. Therefore, the ratio M_P/M_L is a constant. f_3

Now
$$-\frac{dL}{dt} \propto [L] = -k_3L \quad (3.34)$$

From equations (3.33) and (3.34) one has
$$\frac{dp}{dt} = -\frac{M_P}{M_L}(-k_3L) = k_3\frac{M_P}{M_L}.L$$

So,
$$\frac{dp}{dt} \propto L$$

or
$$\frac{dp}{dt} = k_3 f_3 . L \quad (3.35)$$

It indicated that rate of production of gluconic acid by *Ps. ovalis* B1486 is directly proportional to the concentration of accumulated gluconolactone. Following above dynamics of the bioreactions the kinetics of this cell growth associated product formation as has been observed in batch fermentation in CSTBR as follows.

Substrate uptake rate :
$$-\frac{ds}{dt} = f_1\frac{\mu_m s}{k_s+s}x + f_2\frac{k_m s}{k_L+s}x \quad (3.36)$$

Cell growth rate :
$$\frac{dx}{dt} = \frac{\mu_m s}{k_s+s}x \quad (3.37)$$

Lactone accumulation rate :
$$\frac{dL}{dt} = \frac{k_m s}{k_L+s}x - k_3L \quad (3.38)$$

Product formation rate :
$$\frac{dp}{dt} = k_4 L \quad (3.39)$$

Appropriateness of these kinetic equations could be checked by computer simulation of the models with IBM 7040 system I computer using MIDAS program (Modified Integration Digital Analog Simulator). Further investigations on this batch fermentation in a horizontal rotary thin film bioreactor (HRTFB) had indicated a time dependent variation of k_m value, and ammonium acetate as a limiting nutrient (s_s). Kinetics of batch gluconic acid fermentation in HRTFB using a cell concentration of 0.10 UOD ml^{-1} as inoculum was proposed by the following equations :

$$\frac{ds_s}{dt} = -\frac{1}{Y_s}\left(\frac{dx}{dt}\right) \tag{3.40}$$

$$\frac{dx}{dt} = \frac{\mu_m s}{k_s + s} x \tag{3.41}$$

$$-\frac{ds}{dt} = \frac{k_m(t)\, s}{k_l + s} x \tag{3.42}$$

$$\frac{dL}{dt} = \alpha'\left(\frac{ds}{dt}\right) - bL \tag{3.43}$$

$$\frac{dp}{dt} = aL \tag{3.44}$$

Since it was not possible to solve the simultaneous nonlinear differential equation in an analytical manner numerical solution was approached. IIT Delhi's ICL 1909 digital computer was used with fourth order Runge-Kutta programmer for simulating the fermentation kinetic model developed as given above. The kinetic parameters, determined by graphical analysis of batch fermentation data were used in computer simulation. An abrupt variation of k_m in the time range 9.0 to 9.5 hours and then its linear fall from 9.5 to 14 hours led two linear equations with time (by least square method)

$$k_m = -3.8\,t + 7.0 \; (9.0 < t < 9.5 \text{ hrs.})$$

and

$$k_m = -1.13\,t + 5.665 \; (t > 9.5 \text{ hrs.})$$

These equations were considered in computational process and the values of slopes and intercepts of the above k_m relations were used in analysis. A value of k_L/k_m of 1.13 was used throughout the computational process.

Comparison between computed and experimental results as observed by Humphery and his associate[18] in their simulation with MIDAS program in IBM and by Ghose and Mukhopadhyay[17] in their simulation by ICL 1906 using fourth order Runge Kutta Method have shown an excellent fit between the two values. It was therefore obvious that adequate modelling of bioreactions in a process biotechnology can enable the production personnel in a fermentation plant to select a set of operating conditions, which may well be time variant that will produce maximal yield, in minimal time. Engineered medium make it easier for modelling of bioprocessing and its computer simulation.

3.7 METABOLIC ENGINEERING

3.7.1 Introduction

One of the major aims in medium engineering is to make maximal conversion of the designed medium into useful product through cellular metabolic network (Fig. 3.4).

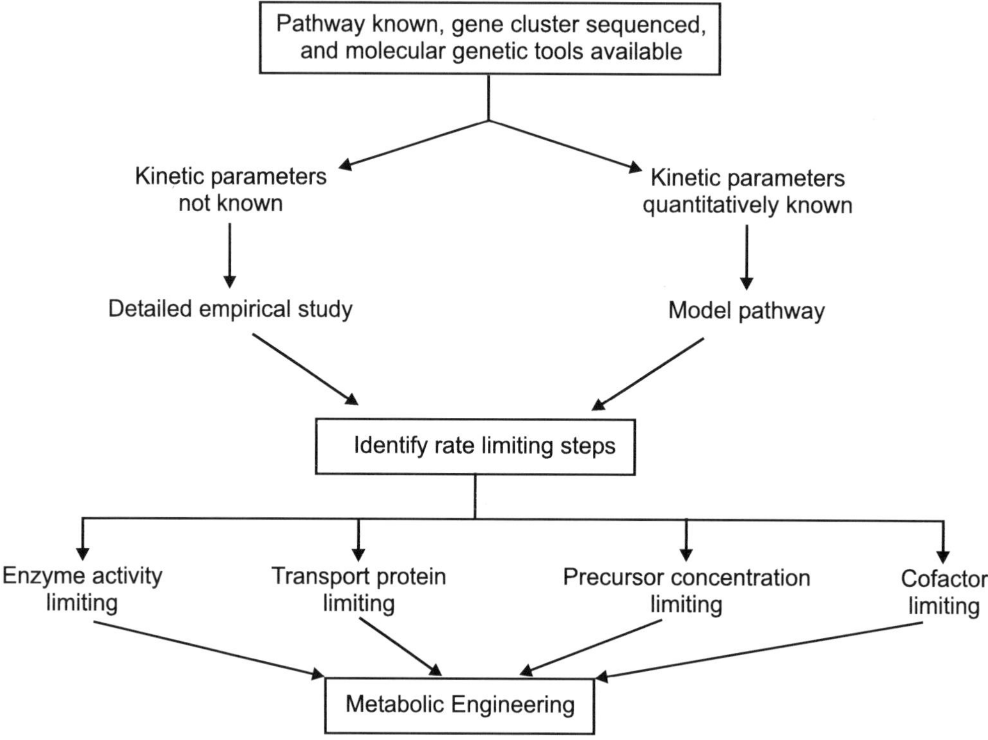

Fig. 3.4 Rational metabolic engineering. A well-characterzed biosynthetic pathway allows prediction of the rate-limiting steps

In more recent years based on microbial biochemistry pathways of metabolism attempts have been laid to set up metabolic network stoichiometric models. For example, based on a review of the *Penicillium chrysogenum* biochemical pathways Jorgensen[19] (1995) and his associates have set up its stoichiometric models. Biochemical engineering analysis of these stoichiometric pathway models providing measures of individual step rates and metabolic fluxes have been defined by the name metabolic engineering. Recombinant methods have further enhanced the study of metabolic engineering. Application of recombinant DNA methods to restructure metabolic networks can improve production of metabolite and protein products by altering pathway distribution and rates, cell functions can also be modified through precisely targeted alterations in normal cellular activities. Recruitment of heterologous proteins enables extension of existing pathways to obtain new chemical products, alter post translational protein processing, and degrade recalcitrant wastes. The experimental and mathematical tool, required for rational metabolic engineering are becoming available more and more. However, complex cellular responses to genetic perturbations can complicate predictive designs. Thus, metabolic engineering naturally acquired design engineering (NADE)/redesigning of DNA that deals with metabolic pathway network in a way that changes metabolic process of the cell. The cell manufactures more of the desired product as a result of the changes in several metabolic reactions.

Advantages of metabolic engineering have been noticed from cloning and expression of heterologous genes. These can serve several useful purpose, including extending an existing pathway to obtain a new product, creating arrays of enzymatic activities that synthesize a novel structure, shifting metabolic flow towards a desired product, and accelerating a rate determining step. So far the usefulness of metabolic engineering includes the following.[20,21]

1. In recruiting heterologous activities for strain improvement

In such recruitment activities metabolic engineering is concerned with the following.

1. Synthesis of new products is enabled by completion of partial pathways.
2. Transferring multistep pathways: Hybrid metabolic networks.
3. Creating new products and new reactants.
4. Transfer of promising natural motifs.

2. Redirecting metabolic flow

The routes of reactions in a metabolic pathway is directed towards maximizing useful product formation by the following means :

1. Directing traffic towards the desired branch.
2. Reducing competition for a limiting resource.
3. Revising metabolic regulation.

Thus consequence of completing metabolic engineering cycle may exhibit potentials and perils of rational design through:

1. Cloning in industrial strains.
2. Dissecting physiological responses.
3. Design principles and cell models; coping with complexity and coupling.

3.7.2 Metabolic Engineering Case Examples

1. Penicillin fermentation

Through ages production of penicillin by *Penicillium chrysogenum* has been improved through the development of modified strains by repeated rounds of mutations and selections on the same parental strain *P. chrysogenum* NRRL 1951. The current estimated report of production of penicillin from mutant strain from NRRL 1951 is around 40-50 g/L penicillin V after 200 h of cultivation. It is hoped that the present production strains of *P. chrysogenum* could be further improved with respect to penicillin production, and with the development of recombinant DNA technology it has become possible to use the more rational approach i.e. metabolic engineering to strain improvement than traditional mutation and selection.

In order to use metabolic engineering successfully the primary requirement of a map of the rate controlling step(s) in the metabolic pathway leading to penicillin production has been fulfilled.[19]

2. Lysine fermentation

Lysine is an important essential amino acid. Its over production has been achieved using metabolic engineering principles.[20, 21] This was done by significant flux alterations in the primary metabolism of *Corynebacterium glutamicum* ATCC 21253 in its metabolic networks. In the new biotechnology area, chemical and biochemical engineers are more likely to find newer roles in quantification of fermentation processes based on metabolic engineering. It will enable them to alter genetic character of the amino acid or other product forming normal catabolic pathways of a cell so that new substrates can be used or new or enhanced chemical products can be formed by that cell.

3. Plant cell culture fermentation

In more recent years metabolic engineering has provided a new promishing avenue for enhancing product formation in a plant or plant cell culture. Metabolic engineering of plant secondary metabolite pathways in the production of fine chemicals has been reported to be a possible approach to increase yields[22]. Several ways of application of metabolic engineering to improve yields have been reported. Compartmentation strategy used for alkaloid biosynthesis in *Cantharanthus roseus* is one of the classical example of the same.

4. Solventogenic clostridial fermentation

By developing suitable software appropriate experiments of *Clostridium acetobutylicum* ATCC 824 fermentation was designed for metabolic flux distribution analysis in the biochemical pathway of acetone-butanol solvent production.[23] This software development served, therefore, as a tool for the metabolic engineering of solventogenic, *Clostridial* fermentation and was useful in stoichiometric modeling of the fermentation process.

3.7.3 Engineering Science Foundations of Metabolic Engineering

1. Molecular stoichiometric model

For such a model a knowledge of the *in vivo* fluxes involved in associated reactions in metabolic pathway is essential. This is because metabolic engineering seeks to replace the shotgun random mutagenic approach with a more rational effort. It is an integrative procedure involving identification of metabolic bottlenecks or limitations followed by manipulation to alter metabolic fluxes. Many powerful molecular biology techniques have been developed in more recent years to manipulate the genetics of an organism. Also, these techniques enabled cloning and sequencing of genes for enzymes associated with the desired product. The resultant genetic repertoire served as an useful tool in redesigning of an organism to enhance product yields. The task of engineering science here is to devise process conditions so as to maintain stable cultures and to realize the full genetic potential of the used culture.[24] Thus, thorough mapping of biosynthetic pathways is a prerequisite for any metabolic engineering programme. Such mapping is necessary to develop a so called fermentation equation to verify fermentation process data consistency, to develop gateway sensors and to predict maximum theoretical yields.[23]

2. Appropriate computational software development

In metabolic engineering for assessing *in vivo* fluxes, various strategies are now available to resolve singularities. Many investigators have incorporated optimality concepts to promote linear programming methods of resolving singularities. This was done for general utility of reformulating any stoichiometric model as a nonlinear constrained minimization system. It is therefore, essential that appropriate computer software be constructed. Also, it should be able to process and/or act on data and make calculations which are beyond human comprehension. In metabolic engineering the calculation of *in vivo* fluxes becomes a nontrivial issue due to interactions of fermentation pathways.

3.8 BIOORGANIC REACTION MEDIUM ENGINEERING[25]

In bioorganic reactions a biocatalyst in a liquid medium is surrounded by various micro environments. The biocatalyst may be an enzyme, or more complex systems such as microorganisms, eucaryotic cells or parts thereof. The micro-environments consist of a thin layer of water around the biocatalyst and an interfacial region. This forms the transition between the biocatalytic and continuous phases. Medium engineering in such cases involves modification of the micro-environment of the biocatalyst either by introducing additives or solid matrices into an existing medium or by varying the composition of the liquid medium itself. Presently medium engineering is a rapidly expanding area of research in which the objectives of biocatalyst engineering viz an increased biocatalytic reactivity, stability and hence productivity are pursued. The nature of different phases and their effects on biocatalysis are therefore investigated intensively. In bioorganic reactions generally each biocatalyst is surrounded by a thin layer of tightly bound water. This aqueous layer is believed to be essential for biocatalytic activity.[4,5] Based on research findings following two important rules in aqueous medium engineering of bioorganic reactions have been laid down.

Rule 1: Do not distort the essential water-around the biocatalyst.

Rule 2: Try to stabilize the biocatalyst conformation by strengthening the essential water-biocatalyst interactions.

The first rule assuring the integrity of the biocatalyst provides expectation of full activity. Second rule on the other hand leads to possible way to achieve the goal in this rule.

In such reactions systems immediately adjacent to the essential water layer surrounding the biocatalyst is the interfacial region. Here the associated problem remains that it is difficult to predict for any given combination of properties of microenvironment what the effect of the matrix will be on the biocatalyst activity, stability and/or productivity. Also, electrostatic interaction effects of organic solvents on biocatalysts, the mutual hydrophobic interactions between matrix, reactants and biocatalyst are far less specific imposing another difficulty in medium design engineering. However for various biocatalytic systems a trend has been observed between biocatalytic activity and polarity of the interphase/bulk phase, when the latter was expressed as the logarithm of the partition coefficient (logp). The unique feature of this trend is that it is completely system and biocatalyst independent. For biocatalytic systems in organic solvents forming continuous phase like enzymes entrapped in reversed micelles the medium engineering principle should be such that optimal activities were reached when the concentration of substrate in the interphase is maximal. One way of achieving this is by matching the polarity of the interphase to that of the substrate, and/or vice versa, by increasing the difference in the polarity between the continuous phase and the substrate.

In medium engineering other considerations involved are solvent toxicity, viscosity, cost, reusability, case of product isolation and bioreactor design.

Additives are also important in medium engineering. These are compounds capable of stabilizing the biocatalyst against denaturation without affecting the activity to a great extent. Few examples of additives are various sugars, glycerol, ethylene glycol and polyhydric polymers. They are important to stabilize various enzymes. However, practical use of additives seems to be restricted to biocatalyst.

The findings that enzymes can function in apolar solvents like heptane dramatically expanded the range of reactions which can be approached through biocatalytic medium engineering. The influencial factors for activity and stability of enzymes in organic solvents include the ionic state of the enzyme, support characteristics and the extent of hydration of biocatalyst and solvent. In bioprocessing of oils and fats through esterification and inter esterification for industrial application medium design engineering served a potential role. Commercialization of cocoa butter is a classical example.[26]

3.9 NOVEL MEDIA

In the search of microorganisms capable of utilising cellulose and hemicellulose materials effectively and to transform them into useful chemicals has prompted the designing and devising of various media. Also it has been done for rapid screening and detection of microbial producers of cellulases and xylanases. One such novel medium was agar nutrient medium containing 0.2% soluble hydroxyethyl cellulose covalently dyed with Ostazin Brilliant Red H-3B or soluble beech wood 4-0-methyl-D-glucurono-D-xylan dyed with Rewazol Brilliant Blue R. They were used for sensitive detection of microorganisms producing and secreting into the medium endo^{1,4} β glucanase and endo-1,4-β-xylanase.[27] In the powdered tissue culture media for mutations for plants important instructions for preparation are available.[28]

In medium design engineering for cell cultivation it is to note that cell function may be regarded as emerging from changes in the dynamics of metabolism, energetics and gene expression. It is therefore, very important to ensure that spatiotemporal responses upon different stimuli e.g. hormones, and pH seemed messengers. Thus medium design in cell cultivation is a crucial task. That is why many novel effector media have been designed for different types of cells.[15,18] The intracellular levels of these effectors fluctuate depending on changes in environmental conditions of cells initial milieu. In order to investigate to what extent cellular metabolism and energetic influence cell function e.g. growth and differentiation, it is crucial to quantitatively assess intracellular fluxes through the main anabolic and catabolic pathways in the used designed medium. The experimental strategy that is chosen to induce different cells metabolic status is to vary primarily carbon and energy sources. Substrate features such as its degree of reduction with respect to biomass, enthalpy of combustion and the metabolic pathways that are activated to assimilate the carbon source drive the cell to different energetic status. For example, *Saccharomyces cerevisiae* displays a variety of growth rates on different carbon sources which can not be solely attributed to differences in thermodynamic properties e.g. the heat of combustion. One may expect carbon and energy balances to change along with fluxes through the central amphibolic pathways. In the designed medium the rate at which metabolic pathways should operate in order to sustain a certain growth rate will also be dependent on the nature of the carbon source.

The media originally used in cultivation of mammalian cells for their growth were based entirely on biological fluids such as plasma and embryonic extracts. They were chemically undefined complex media. Their use suffers from the disadvantages of batch variation and vulnerability to contamination. So need of designed and chemically defined culture media became obvious. The present strategy followed in mammalian cell culture media design is to reduce the number of components to the minimum shown to be essential for cell growth. Later the media were redesigned through modification and improvements as per requirement. In this way the design composition of commonly used media formulations for mammalian cell cultures as given by Butler[29] were ascertained.

It appears from the above discussions that medium design engineering for cell cultivation has two major technological concerns as given in Fig. 3.1 each of which in turn relates to various factors for cell function.

For achieving best performance of biocells as well as enzymes in reactors and to minimize the influence of inhibition and/or deactivation medium design engineering is an important consideration. The influence of inter and intra particle diffusion in immobilized cell or enzyme bioreactors relating to deactivation and on effectiveness factor has been analysed to highlight different concepts.[30]

3.10 REFERENCES

1. Aiba, S., A.E. Humphrey, and N.F. Millis, *Formulation of Media, in Biochemical Engineering*, 2nd edn., pp 28-30, Univ. of Tokyo Press, Tokyo,1973.
2. Bailey, J.E. and D.F. Ollis, *Design and Analysis of Biological Reactors in Biochemical Engineering Fundamentals* 2nd edn. pp 533-657, McGraw Hill Book Co., New York, 1986.
3. Laane, C., S. Baeren, and K. Vos, "On Optimizing Organic Solvents in Multiliquid Phase Biocatalysis", *Trends in Biotechnol* , pp 3 251-52, 1985.
4. Laane, C., S. Boeren, K. Vos. and C. Veeger, "Rules for the Optimization of Biocatalysts in Organic Solvents", *Biotechnol and Bioeng,* pp 30, 81-87, 1987.
5. Zaks, A. and A.M. Klibanov "Enzyme Catalysed Processes in Organic Solvents", *Proc. Natl. Acad. Sci.* USA, pp 3192-96, 1985.
6. Gamborg, O.L., T. Murashige, T.A. Thorpe and K. Vasil, *Plant Tissue Culture Media, In vitro,* pp 12, 473, 1976.
7. Kato, A., A.Fukusawa,Y.Shmizu, Y.Soh and S.Nagai. "Requirements of PO_4^{-3}, NO SO_4^{2-}, K^+ and Ca^{2+} for the Growth of Tobacco Cells in Suspension Culture", *J. Fermnt. Technol*, pp 55, 207.
8. Plyne, M.J. "Microbial Conversion of Straw and Bran into Volatile Fatty Acids, Key Intermediates in the Production of Liquid Fuels", *Food Technol,* pp 31, 451-56, 1980.

9. Seshadri,N.and S.N. Mukhopadhyay, "Influence of Environmental Paramenters on Propionic Acid Upstream Bioprocessing by Propionibacterium Acidi-propionici", *J. Biotechnol,* pp 29, 321-28, 1993.
10. Seshadri, N. " Regulation of an Anaerobic Mixed Acid Fermentation to Accumulate Propionic Acid", *Ph.D. Thesis*, IIT Delhi, 1989.
11. Cooney, C.L. "Growth of Microorganisms", *Biotechnology* Vol. 1, pp 97-112, (Rehm H.J. and G. Reed eds.), Verlag Chemie, Weinheim, 1987 .
12. Mukhopadhyay, S.N. "Studies on the Kinetics of Gluconic Acid Fermentation and Assessment of Volumetric Oxygen Transfer Coefficient by Oxygen Balance Technique", *Ph.D.Thesis*, IIT Delhi, 1976.
13. Bentley. R., *The Enzymes*, Vol. 7, pp 567-72, (P.D. Boyer *et al*. eds.) Acad. Press, N.Y., 1963.
14. Davis, B.D., R. Dulbecco, H.N. Eisen, H.S. Ginsberg and W.B. Wood Jr., *Principles of Microbiology and Immunnology*, pp 28A, Harper International edn., Harper and Row, New York, 1969
15. Frobisher, *M. Fundamentals of Microbiology*, 3rd edn. W.B. Saunders Co., Philadelphia, 1969.
16. Humphrey, A.E. and P.J. Reilly, " Kinetic Studies of Gluconic Acid Fermentations", *Biotechnol & Bioeng,* pp 7, 229, 1965.
17. Ghose, T.K. and S.N. Mukhopadhyay, " Kinetic Studies of Gluconic Acid Fermentation in Horizontal Rotary Fermenter" *Pseudomonas ovalis. J. Ferment. Technol,* pp 54, 738, 1976.
18. Koga, S., C.R. Burg and A.E. Humphrey " Computer Simulation of Fermentation Systems", *Applied Microbiol*, pp 15, 683-89, 1967.
19. Jorgensen. H., J. Nielsen, J. Villadsen and H. Mollgaard, "Metabolic Flux Distributions in Penicillium Chrysogenum during Fed Batch Cultivations", *Biotechnol. & Bioeng*, pp 46, 117-131, 1995.
20. Bailey, J.E. "Towards a Science of Metabolic Engineering", *Science*, pp 252, 1668-75, 1991.
21. Stephanopoulos, G. and J. Vallino, "Network Rigidity and Metabolic Engineering in Metabolic Overproduction", *Ibid*, pp 1675-81.
22. Verpoorte, R., R. Vender Heijden, H.J.G. Ten Hoopen and J. Memelink; "Metabolic Engineering of Plant Secondary Metabolite Pathways for Production of Fine Chemicals", *Biotechnol. Letts.* pp 21, 467-79, 1999.
23. Desai, R.P., L.K. Nielsen and E. T. Popoutsaki, "Stoichiometric Modeling of *Clostridium acetobutylicum* Fermentations with Nonlinear Constants", *J. Biotechnol,* pp 71, 191-205, 1999.
24. Finn, R.K. "New Challenges in Metabolic Engineering", *Bioprocess Engineering :The First Generation*, pp 20-29, (T.K. Ghose ed.), Ellis Horwood Ltd, Pub. Chichester, U.K., 1989.
25. Laane,C. "Midium Engineering for Bioorganic Synthesis", *Biocatalysis,* pp 1, 17-22, 1987.
26. Aldercrentz, P. and Bo, Mattiasson, "Aspects of Biocatalyst Stability in Organic Solvents", *Biocatalysis*, pp 1, 99-108, 1987.
27. Fakas, V., M. Lisková and P. Bieley, *FEMS Microbiol Letters*, pp 28, 137-140, 1985.
28. *Carolina Plant Tissue Culture Media Formulation Booklet,* 1986.
29. Butler, M. *Mammalian Cell Biotechnology: A Practical Approach*, pp 1-25, IRL Press, Oxford, 1991.
30. Sadana, A. *Biocatalysis,* pp 2, 175-216, 1989.

Chapter

4

CONTAMINATION FREE FLUIDS FOR PROCESS BIOTECHNOLOGY

4.1 INTRODUCTION

Air and medium are two fluids that are required in oxic process biotechnology. In monoculture process biotechnology contamination free fluid is a must.

In cellular process biotechnology a contamination free fluid flow refers to air and media sterilization/filtration for supply to bioreactor or in a positive pressure chamber. Air sterilization in aerobic monoculture bioprocessing may be defined as the destruction or removal of all forms of particles or viable organisms from the air.

Aerobic fermentation process requires a continuous supply of large quantities of sterile air. Sterilization of this air is a mandatory requirement in all oxic mono/pure culture fermentation. For pure culture operation incomplete destruction or inadequate removal of undesirable microorganisms carried in the air may preclude unsuccessful bioprocess operations.

4.2 CONTAMINATION FREE AIR SUPPLY[1–5]

The methods destroying microorganisms from air to supply contamination free air in bioprocess which however are not in practice now include the following :

1. Dry heating by gas fired or electrically heated system
2. Adiabatic–compression
3. Irradiation

The methods which remove particles or microbial load from air stream and of which one of them being industrially/commercially practiced include :

4. Scrubbing
5. Electrostatic precipitation in cyclone separator
6. Sieving
7. Filtration through fibrous beds
8. Filtration through granular beds

Of these methods industrially applicable and fruitful are those of (2), (7) and (8). Filtration through fibrous materials such as glass wool is by far the most common of the three.

4.2.1 Basic Requirements of an Air Sterilizer

For sterilization of air for industrial fermentation practices the sterlizer must satisfy the following major requirements :

(a) Design of the system should be simple.
(b) The operation cost of the equipment should be cheap.
(c) It should remove or destroy air-borne contaminants to the extent necessary for satisfactory fermentation performance.
(d) In case of repeated steam or chemical vapour sterilization it should be stable.
(e) It should condition the air i.e. it should remove any oil entrained during compression and adjusting the temperature and humidity to a satisfactory range for fermentation.
(f) It should be able to supply sterile air continuously.

4.2.2 Air Sterilization Using Heat

Many years ago many investigators showed that *Bacillus subtilis* spores can be sterilized by a passage through an electrically heated furnace. They also concluded that the exit air temperature of 225°C from the furnace was sufficient to kill all the spores of a strain of *B. subtilis* with an exposure time of 0.4 – 0.6 secs.

Disadvantage : Very costly method. Also it requires proper cooling of air before sending to fermenter which imparts extra cost.

4.2.3 Sterilization by Air Compressor

In some fermentation processes the air sterilized by adiabatic compression was used. Stark and Pohler[4] designed a small reciprocating compressor to compress the air to 100 p.s.i for supplying sterile air for seed tank fermenter, for pilot plant studies of the aerobic 2,3 butylene glycol process, for aerobic culture of *A. oryzae* and for some other purposes. They demanded reciprocating compressors operated at pressure upto 100 psi. might be preferable for smaller installations but at low pressure turbo-compressors with suitable filters would be more economical for large capacities.

Chain *et al.* also investigated the sterility of air compressed to 3–4 atm. by a reciprocating piston compressor and reported it to be practically sterile, in agreement with the findings of

Stark and Pohler. They used this air in conjunction with glass wool for laboratory scale fermenter and claimed not to have experienced any contamination.

Disadvantage : Very costly method to be applied to large industrial fermentation.

4.2.4 Air Sterilization by Granular Filters

Amongst all the granular materials granular carbon has been found to be the best granular filter material for air sterilization. Adsorptive power of charcoal may be the cause of its selection to filtering medium.

A typical carbon filter size for 20,000 gallons fermentor was as follows :

Material of construction = Steel cylinder
Diameter = 6' to 9'
Packed depth = 6'
Granular carbon particle size = 6 to 30 mesh

Usually carbon particles are supported on a bed of graded gravel which rests on a perforated plate. Another perforated plate or screen rests atop the bed.

Pressure drop across this filter = 1 to 5 psi.

Disadvantages :
1. Inlet air temperature cannot be raised above 120°F otherwise carbon may ignite.
2. Although carbon is screened to a coarse mesh size a certain amount of fine carbon dust still adheres to the coarse material. So if steam sterilization under pressure is started spontaneous ignition frequently occurs since the unit behaves like a water gas plant.

4.2.5 Air Sterilization by Fibrous Filters

1. Basic requirements

At present most commercial air sterilization units are deep beds of glass wool or similar fibrous materials. The reason for choosing the fibrous materials are the following :

(a) Their design and operation is extremely simple.
(b) If they are periodically checked and replaced then their reliability is extremely good.
(c) Lower bed diameter and height is required compared to carbon filters for the same sterilization capacity operating at comparable pressure drops.
(d) Glass wool do not pose any hazard.
(e) Collection efficiency is high.
(f) Low pressure drop of air flow through the fibrous filter bed.

2. Filtration effectiveness of fibrous filters

It was revealed from earlier observations that penetration of microorganisms into a filter was logarithmic in nature. That is, the log ratio of the number of organisms entering a filter (N_1) to those leaving (N_2) a particular depth of filter, L, was a function of the depth, i.e.

$$\ln \frac{N_1}{N_2} = \phi\,(L) \tag{4.1}$$

and it has been found that

$$\ln \frac{N_1}{N_2} = kL$$

$$\text{or } \log \frac{N_1}{N_2} = \frac{k}{2.303}\,L \tag{4.2}$$

where k = filtration constant and is a function of the following factors :

(a) Air velocity
(b) Filter density
(c) Filter size
(d) Density of organisms to be removed.

The filtration constant, k, is usually expressed in terms of the depth of filter necessary to remove 90% of the entering organism (L_{90}) :

$$\log \frac{N_1}{N_2} = \frac{2.303}{L_{90}}\,L \tag{4.3}$$

where $$k = \frac{2.303}{L_{90}}$$

$$\log \frac{N_1}{N_2} = \frac{L}{L_{90}} \tag{4.4}$$

This way of representation makes it easier to visualise the filter performance in terms of physical size.

3. Effect of air velocity on filtration

Various workers performed experiments in terms of L_{90} and the significances of their experimental data are illustrated in Fig. 4.1.

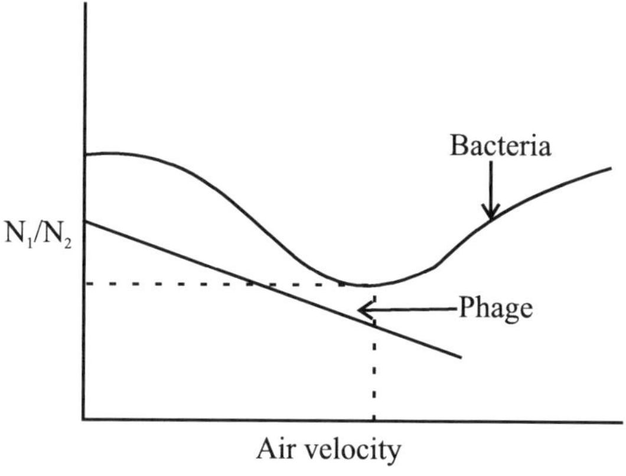

Fig. 4.1 Influence of air velocity on air filtration

From this it is seen that the nature of bacterial collection is such that for a particular filter there is an air velocity at which filtration efficiency (N_1/N_2) is a minimum.

For glass fiber, 16 μ diameter.

When air velocity = 1 fps

then N_1/N_2 = minimum

Minimal efficiency occuring at intermedial air velocity is due to the action of different forces in collecting air borne particles at different air velocities.

Effect of Low Air Velocity : At low air velocities particles are exerted by gravitational, diffusional and electrostatic forces and their effect is inversely proportional to the air velocity.

Effect of High Air Velocity : At high air velocities inertial forces act on the particles. These inertial forces are directly proportional to the air velocity. The nature of inertial effects is such that below a certain critical air velocity collection due to inertial forces is zero. Workers have reported that this air velocity corresponding to inertial impaction is given by

$$V_C = \frac{1.25\,\mu_a\, d_f}{C.\rho_p.d_p^2} \tag{4.5}$$

where

V_C = Critical superficial air velocity

μ_a = Air viscosity
d_f = Fiber diameter
ρ_p = Density of air borne organism
d_p = Particle diameter
C = A correction factor for deviation from Stoke's law called slip flow factor.

For collection of unit density, 1μ bacterial particles from air stream, at room temperature and pressure the velocity is equal to

$$V_{inertial}\ \text{effect} \longrightarrow 0 = 0.066\, d_f \tag{4.6}$$

Regardless of air velocity, some collection always occurs due to the fact that air borne particles possess a finite size and will be intercepted by some fiber blocking an air stream along with which a particle moves. Collection must always be greater than that due to interception as it represents the minimum collection physically possible.

In case of collection of phage only diffusional effects are important at reasonable air velocities. So phage are most efficiently collected at low velocities. Collection of phage are not as efficient as bacteria. But, if phage are unusually small i.e. less than 0.05 μ or the filter fiber are quite small, less than 2μ in diameter, their efficiency of collection approaches that of bacteria.

Now question may arise whether the filter design be based on bacteria or on phage ?

Since little is known about the loading of microorganisms in air stream and since loading can be determined for any plant location, it seems most practical for the present to base filter design on collecting bacteria.

4. Design procedure

The current thinking on the design of a packed filter for sterilizing air includes the following steps:

(a) Proper assessment of filtration job
(b) Estimation of the filter effectiveness for the particular filter medium
(c) Choice of filter size from cost consideration

Assessment : It involves

(i) Determination or setting of contaminant loading of air,
(ii) Choice of what allowable penetration of these contaminants permit.
(iii) Contaminant loading of air varies depending on various factors. A good sound design figure, when experimental observations are lacking might be 50 microorganism (m.o) per cubic foot of air.
(iv) The allowable penetration of m.o. must be less than one m.o. during the course of fermentation. A figure involving 1 to 1,000 chance of single m.o. penetrating the filter during particular fermentation should be amply safe.

5. Economic design of fiber filter

Design should be based on :

(i) Fixed height to diameter ratio of a filter bed i.e. height should be fixed for a given diameter.
(ii) Constant height where diameter is variable.

Basic equation of log penetration law for designing of a fiber filter for air sterilization is as given by equations 4.7 to 4.9

$$\ln \frac{N_1}{N_2} = kL$$

or

$$\log \frac{N_1}{N_2} = \frac{k}{2.303} L \quad \ldots (4.7)$$

When height of the filter bed is taken for 90% collection then

$$\log \frac{N_1}{N_2} = \frac{L}{L_{90}} \quad \ldots (4.8)$$

where L_{90} = height of bed for 90% collection of m.o. or decimal reduction depth.

From equations (4.7) and (4.8) we get

$$\frac{k}{2.3} L = \frac{L}{L_{90}}$$

or

$$k = \frac{2.3}{L_{90}}$$

Therefore $$\ln \frac{N_1}{N_2} = 2.3 \frac{L}{L_{90}} \tag{4.9}$$

6. Evaluation of bed depth for sterilization

One way of expressing the efficiency of air filter is

$$\frac{N_1}{N_2} = \frac{C.Q.t}{p} \tag{4.10}$$

where

N_1 = No. of organisms in entering air

N_2 = No. of organisms in leaving air

C = Concentration of microorganisms in incoming air

Q = Vol. flow rate of air in ft^3/minute

t = Period of operation, minute

p = Allowable chance of penetrating the filter

Combining equations (4.9) and (4.10) one gets

$$\frac{L}{L_{90}} = \log \frac{N_1}{N_2} = \log \frac{C.Q.t}{p} \tag{4.11}$$

7. Log penetration law and its assessment

If air borne microbes number, N_1 passing through a cylindrical bed of fibrous materials are collected uniformly along the bed depth (collection efficiency = η_∞) of single fiber whose vol. fraction in the bed is α and leaving N_2 number of microbes in aerosol, the relation between overall collection efficiency, $\overline{\eta}$ and bed depth L is logarithmic and is expressed as

$$\overline{\eta} = \frac{N_1 - N_2}{N_1} \tag{4.12}$$

$$\eta_\infty = \frac{\lambda d_f (1-\alpha)}{4 L \alpha} \ln \frac{N_1}{N_2} \tag{4.13}$$

$$= \frac{\lambda d_f (1-\alpha)}{4 L \alpha} \ln (1 - 1/\overline{\eta}) \tag{4.14}$$

In addition the following correlation was used by Aiba based on the empirial correlation presented below

$$\eta_\infty = \eta_O (1 + 4.5\ \alpha) \tag{4.15}$$

where η_O is overall collection efficiency of a single fibre and the value of α being bound in the limit $O < \alpha < 0.10$.

8. Single fibre efficiency

In collection of air borne particles/microbes by a single fibre the following mechanisms are presented and supported by experimentation to play major role.

(a) Inertial impaction
(b) Interception
(c) Diffusion

If η_O', η_O'' and η_O''' are collection efficiencies of a single fibre due to above mechanisms respectively, then

$$\eta_O' = 0.16\ [N_R + (1/2 + 0.8\ N_R)\ \psi - 0.1052\ N_R\ \psi^2]$$

in which N_R is the diametral ratio, d_p/d_f (4.16)

$$\eta_O'' \propto N_R^2\ N_{Re}^{1/6} \tag{4.17}$$

where N_{Re} is given by $\dfrac{d_f\ v\ \rho_a}{\mu_a}$

and $$\eta_O''' \propto N_{sc}^{-2/3}\ N_{Re}^{-11/18} \tag{4.18}$$

having N_{Sc} as ρ_a / D_{BM} provided air flow around cylindrical fibre is laminar.
So in equation (4.15) the value of η_O is actually given by

$$\eta_O = \eta_O' + \eta_O'' + \eta_O''' \tag{4.19}$$

The values of η_O', η_O'', and η_O''' have been computed in the following way.

According to Langmuir the value of η_O' depends on the value of inertial parameter (ψ) which is defined as

$$\psi = \frac{C\,\rho_p\,d_p^2\,v_0}{18\,\mu_a\,d_f} \tag{4.20}$$

In the relation C is Cunnigham's factor for slip flow, ρ_p is the density of the particle, d_p is its diameter, v_0 is the velocity of upsteam air, μ_a is air viscosity and d_f is fibre dimeter. It has been observed by Longmuir that when $\psi = 1/16$, the value of η' is zero at the critical air velocity for this condition to exist is given in equations 4.5 and 4.6.

It shows the relationship of radius of d_p with V_C with μ_a as a parameter for a given d_f.

However, if the flowing air borne particles had no mass the flow of air across the fibre would have been closed to streamline. The entrained particles in this streamline air would have been collected by direct contact or interception with the fibres. For such condition Longmuir provides the approximate relation to compute η_O'' (the single fibre efficiency due to interception) as

$$\eta_O'' = \frac{1}{2\,(2 - \ln N_{Re})}\left(2\,(1 + N_R)\ln(1 + N_R) - (1 + N_R) + \frac{1}{1 + N_R}\right) \tag{4.21}$$

In addition since the airborne submicron particles are likely to display Brownian motion it is conceivable that they will be collected by diffusion displacement. This collection efficiency of a single fibre η_O''' due to diffusion has been computed as

$$\eta_O''' = \frac{1}{2(2 - \ln N_{Re})}\left(2(1+B)\ln(1+B) - (1+B) + \frac{1}{1+B}\right) \quad (4.22)$$

in which particle upstream velocity has been assumed to be equal to its downstream velocity i.e. $v_o = v$ with particle diffusivity D_{BM} and thereby

$$B = 1.12\left(\frac{2(2 - \ln N_{Re})D_{BM}}{v\,d_f}\right)^{1/3} \quad (4.23)$$

where $D_{BM} = \frac{Ck\,T}{3\,\pi\mu_a\,d_p}$, k is Boltzmann constant and T is absolute temperature.

So by evaluation of η', η'' and η''' as discussed above the value of overall fibre efficiency η_O could be obtained from equation (4.19).

Later a general equation for computation of η_{si} has been provided by Shuttle as given below.

$$\eta_{si} = 0.01518\left(\frac{C_D\,N_{Re}}{2}\right)(N_R)^{1.5} + 0.16\,(0.25 + 0.4\,N_R)\,N_I - .0268\,N_R \quad (4.24)$$

where $N_1 = \frac{\rho_a\,d_p^2 v}{\pi\mu_a\,d_f}$

The standard relation between C_D and N_{Re} as shown in Fig. 4.2 could be used under experimental condition. From this value of η_{si} the value of overall efficiency of the filter could be obtained as

$$\eta_O = 1 - \exp\left(\frac{4}{\pi}\,n_{si}\,\frac{(\alpha)}{1-\alpha}\,\frac{L}{d_f}\right) \quad \ldots (4.25)$$

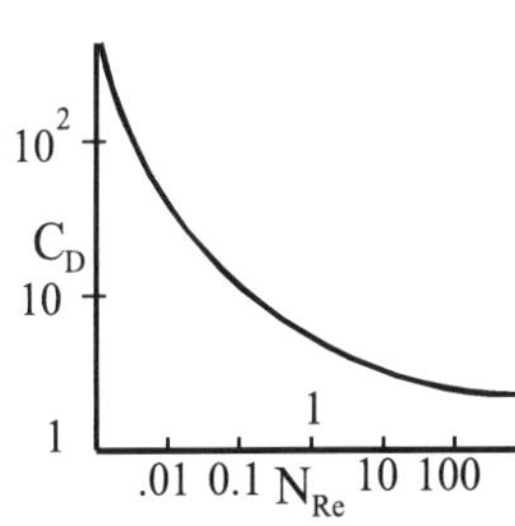

Fig. 4.2. Variation of C_D as a function of N_{Re}

In the operation the pressure drop ΔP across the filter bed could be evaluated by the following relation:

$$\Delta P = \frac{Pv^2}{2g}\,\frac{4L\alpha}{\pi d_f}\,C_D\,f^n(\alpha) \quad (4.26)$$

In this relation the term $f^n(\alpha)$ includes the effect of interference and is given by

$$f^n(\alpha) = 1 + k\,\alpha \quad (4.27)$$

Here k is a proportionality constant. Usually the value of k ranges between 15 to 80.

The value of diffusion coefficient or diffusivity of the particles could also be determined by the relation

$$D_{BM} = \frac{RT}{N}\left(\frac{1 + 1.7\lambda\,d_p}{3\pi\mu_a\,d_p}\right) \quad \ldots (4.28)$$

where R is universal gas constant, N is Avogadro number (6.02×10^{23} molecules/g.mol) and λ is mean free path of the particles.

9. Packing of the filter

The size of the filter may be ascertained using the following relation.

$$V = L.A \tag{4.29}$$

where V is filter bed volume, L is its height and A is cross sectional area of the bed. The amount of fibre material (W) to be packed in this bed volume is computed by the following equation.

$$W = \rho_f \left[2A + \left(l_f + f\sqrt{4\pi A} \right) \right] \tag{4.30}$$

In which W = Weight of the housing fibre material ρ_f = Density of fibre material, l_f = Thickness of fibre and f = Allowable free space above and below the packing material.

10. Cost considerations

An economical fibre filter design as one in which total cost will be minimum. The total cost (C) for the filtration job may be expressed by

$$C = C_1 + C_2 + C_3 + C_4 + \ldots . \tag{4.31}$$

The components of the total cost C are

C_1 = Depreciation cost = $a\, C_e \left[K_3\, A_l + K_4 \sqrt{A_l} \right]$

C_2 = Material cost = $C_f\, \rho_f \propto L\, A_r$

C_3 = Labour cost = $C_m\, L\, A_r$

C_4 = Cost of power for air compression.

In these relations C_e = Cost of equipment/Unit weight, A_l = Annual depreciation allowance, C_f = Cost per unit weight of fibre material, A_r = Annual frequency of packing the filter and C_m = Charge per man-hour.

Design should be based on minimum cost. Minimum load corresponding to minimum cost must be taken into consideration for design purpose. The minimum cost is ascertained as shown in the Fig. 4.3.

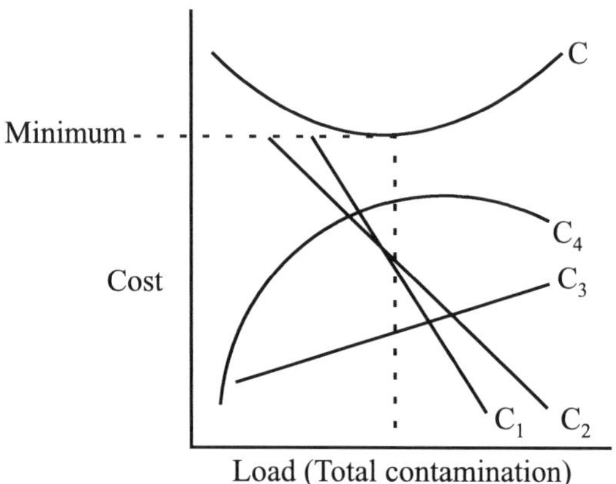

Fig. 4.3. Cost variation relation as a function of load

4.3 FEW NON-CONVENTIONAL AIR BORNE PARTICLE REMOVAL METHODS

4.3.1 Electrostatic Precipitation

Air borne particles can be removed by the principle of electrostatic precipitation into Cotrell precipitator. Its application in sterilizing air for aerobic fermentation has been recommended since airborne microorganisms commonly adhere to small dust particles. In this equipment a core of discharge is applied to particles using a charging field of sufficient strength so that under the influence of drag force the particles get collected. The schematic of this system is shown in the Fig. 4.4. Resisting range is usually 10^4 Ohm sec.

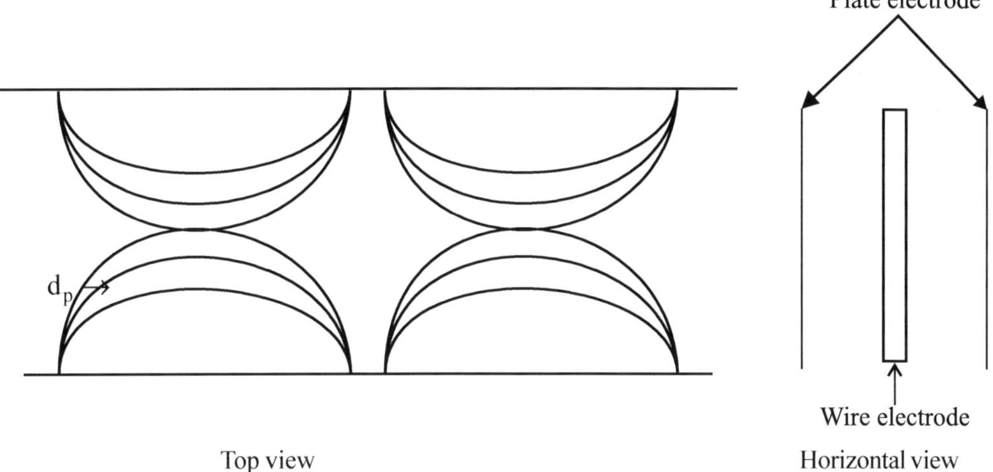

Fig. 4.4 Schematic of an electrostatic precipitator

Charge (q) given to the particles having diameter d_p (>1μ) is given by

$$q = \frac{p_1 E_c dp^2}{4} \tag{4.32}$$

Where $p_1 = \frac{3D}{D+2}$, D is the dielectric constant for the particles. E_c is the strength of charging field. The electrostatic force, F_c is proportional to the charge E_p on the particles and collecting field strength.

So

$$F_c = q \cdot E_p$$

$$= \frac{p_1 E_c E_p dp^2}{4} \tag{4.33}$$

Drag force on the particles is

$$F_d = 3\pi\mu_a d_p W \tag{4.34}$$

where the drift velocity W as given in equation (4.34)

$$W = \frac{p_l\, E_c\, E_p^2}{12\pi\mu_a} \tag{4.35}$$

For 100% theoretical collection efficiency the length (L) of the precipitator passage required for removal is

$$L = \frac{SV_a}{W} \tag{4.36}$$

where S = Distance between charging and collecting electrode.
V_a = Air velocity in the flow passage
The efficiency of collection

$$\eta = 1 - \exp\left(\frac{AW}{Q}\right) \tag{4.37}$$

A = Area of the collection electrode, Q = Volumetric air flow rate.

4.3.2 Cyclone Separator

Fractional collection efficiency

$$D_{P\,50} = \left(\frac{9\,\mu_a\, W_i}{2\pi\, N_i\, V_i\, (\rho_p - \rho_a)}\right)^{1/2} \tag{4.38}$$

where $D_{P\,50}$ = Particle size collected with 50% efficiency
μ_a = Air viscosity
W_i = Inlet width of cyclone
N_i = Effective number of turns in cyclone
V_i = Inlet air velocity
ρ_p = Density of the particles
ρ_a = Air density

Centrifugal force on the particles

$$F_c = \frac{m_p\, v_p^2}{R} \approx \frac{\rho_p\, d_p^3\, v_p^2}{R} \tag{4.39}$$

R = Radius of rotation in the cyclone.

Drag force on the particles

$$F_D = K_c\, d_p\, \mu_a\, V_p\ (d_p < 100\mu) \tag{4.40}$$

where K_c is given by

$$K_c = 1 + \frac{0.172}{d_p} \tag{4.41}$$

and is known as Cunningham correlation.

Collection efficiency

$$\eta = \frac{\text{Centrifugal force}}{\text{Drag force}} \approx \frac{V_P \rho_p dp^2}{K_C R \mu_a} \quad (4.42)$$

Pressure drop $$\Delta P = \frac{KQ^n P \rho_a}{T} \quad (4.43)$$

where Q is volumetric air flow rate, P is air pressure and T is air temperature.

4.3.3 Venturi Scrubber

$$\frac{x_1}{x_2} = \frac{2d_1}{d_2} \quad (4.44)$$

in which x is the distance required to accelerate a particle 90% air velocity, 1 and 2 designate two different sizes, $d_1 > d_2$.

Pressure drops across venturi is

$$\Delta P = 1.03 \times 10^{-6} V_{at}^2 L \quad (4.45)$$

$$\text{Collection efficiency} = (1 - P_t) . 100 \quad (4.46)$$

and $$P_t = \exp\left(\frac{6.1 \times 10^{-9} \rho_L \rho_p K_c d_p^2 f^2 \Delta P}{\mu_a^2}\right) \quad (4.47)$$

in which f is experimental coefficient (0.1 to 0.4). The equation (4.46) is useful when particle size is > 5 microns. However for particles < 5 micron size

$$P_t = \frac{C_0}{C_1} = 3.47 (\Delta P)^{-1.43} \quad \text{... (4.48)}$$

where C_1 = Weight concentration of particles in inlet.
C_0 = Weight concentration of particles in outlet.
and ΔP = Pressure drop in inches of water.

4.4 CONTAMINATION FREE MEDIUM BY STERILIZATION

4.4.1 Introduction

Sterilization of liquid medium may be defined as the destruction or removal of undesirable microbial contaminants in the medium. Proper sterilization of fermentation medium plays an important role in guaranteeing the success of industrial pure culture fermentation/bioprocessing.

Available techniques of medium sterilization include the following.

— Irradiation
— Freezing
— Shear
— High frequency sonic vibrations
— Heating
— Chemical treatment
— Microfiltration

Among all the techniques the most widely practised technique is the destruction of undesignable microbial contaminants through the application of heat for medium containing less thermolabile components. However, for thermolabile media sterilization microfiltration has been used in practice.

4.4.2 Sterilization Methods

Media in fermentation industry can be sterilized either by batch or by continuous mode.

Usually most media in bioprocessing/fermentation industry are sterilized by batch method.

1. Batch sterilization of media

Different types of equipment system for batch sterilization of media have been reported in the literature. Figures below show some typical type of equipment schematics for this purpose.

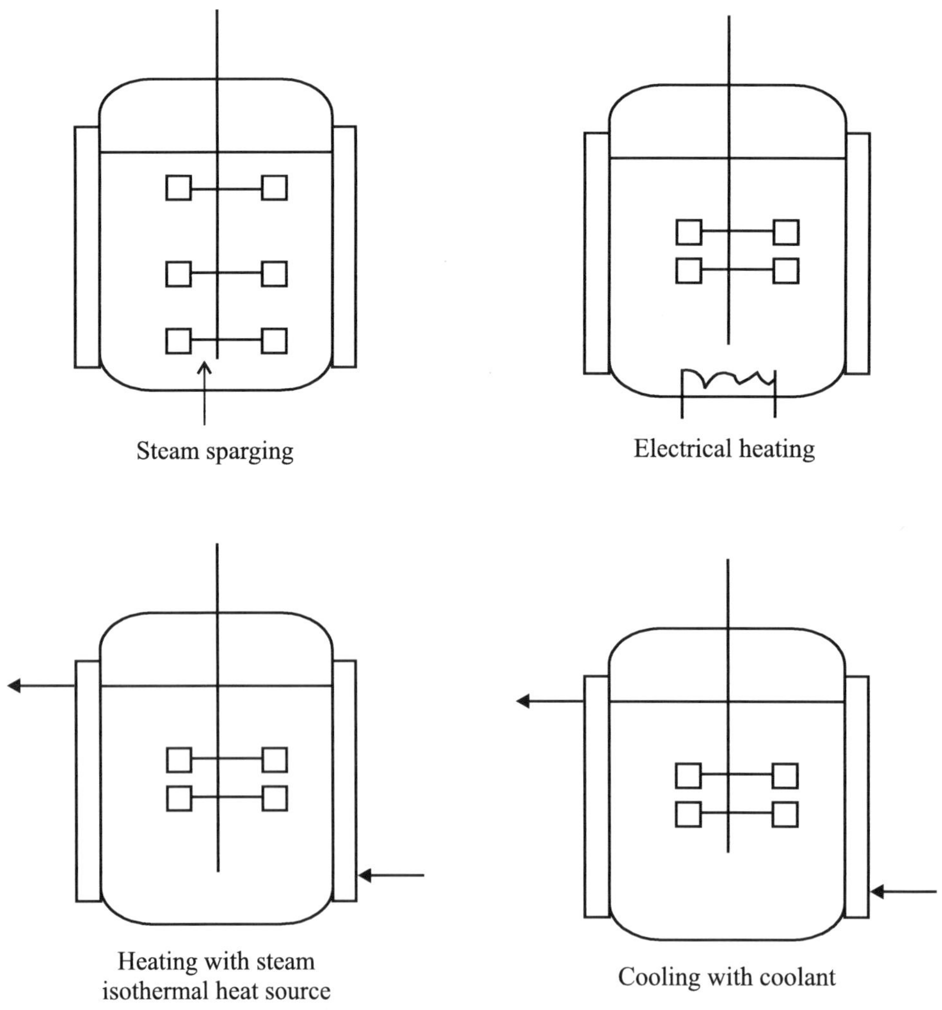

Fig. 4.5 Sterilization type

Methodology : In current practice thermal sterilization of media is carried out by moist heat of saturated steam. In batch the content is heated by saturated pressurised steam flow through the jacket to the design sterilization temperature (121°C at 15 psig). When the design sterilization temperature is reached, the medium is held at that temperature for the required design time and then cooled abruptly by flowing chilled water through the jacket instead of steam.

2. Steam sterilization of equipment

Fermenters and other equipments are routinely sterilized by direct steam to reduce any contaminating organism load. Typical conditions are 121°C (15 – 20 psig steam) for 30 – 60 minutes. Fermenters must be sterilized empty with steam for use with continuous sterilizers, however this is commonly also done in batch sterilization processes to reduce incidental load. Pending use, sterilized vessels should be kept under positive pressure using sterile air.

Steam is also used to sterilize air and solution, sterilizing filters and associated transfer piping.

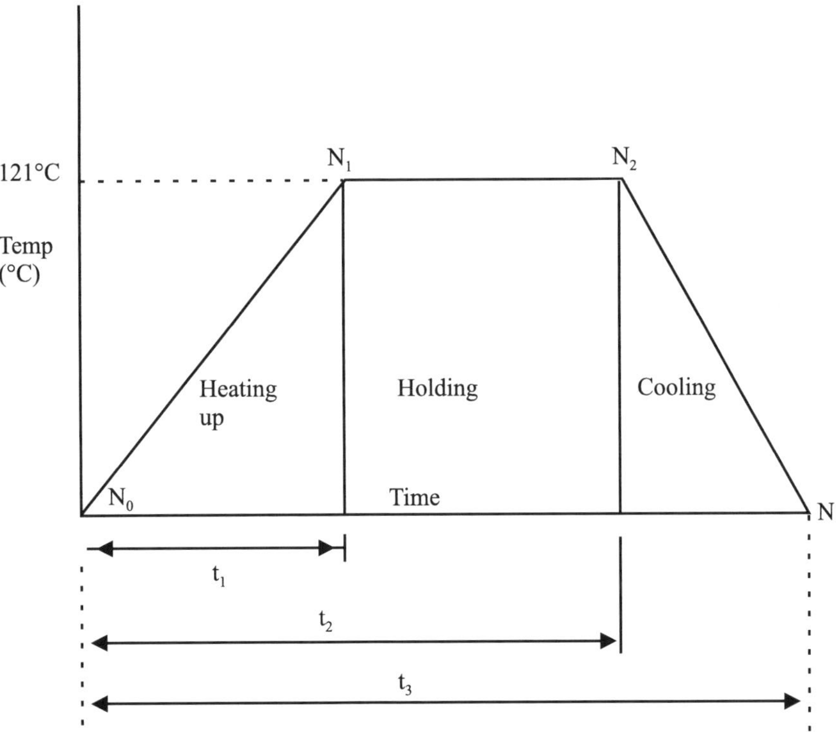

Fig. 4.6. Time-temperature profile in batch sterilization

From the experimental time-temperature profile of batch sterilization it can be seen that there are three distinct periods in total sterilization cycle mainly heating up period, holding period and cooling period. In this cycle the initial number of cells (N_0) present at the initiation of heating is reduced to N_1 at the end of heat up period. Next is the holding period at design sterilization temperature N_1 and it is reduced to N_2, which is finally brought down to zero or safe number level at the end of abrupt cooling period as shown in the above figure.

It can be seen in the figure that there is continuous decrease in number of viable cells during the sterilization cycle. Therefore destruction of microorganisms by heat implies loss of viability, not destruction in physical sense. It is therefore, necessary to understand the nature of thermal death kinetics of microorganisms in media sterilization.

4.4.3 Thermal Death of Microorganisms

Destruction or death of vegetative microbial cells by heating at a specific temperature follows a monomolecular rate of reaction as follows.

$$\frac{dN}{dt} = -KN \tag{4.49}$$

where N = Concentration of viable cells no./ml.
K = Specific death rate constant, min^{-1}
t = Time, min.

Integrating between limits

$N = N_0, t = o$ $$\left(\int_{N_0}^{N} \frac{dN}{N} = -K\int_0^t dt\right)$$

$$\ln \frac{N}{N_0} = -Kt \tag{4.50}$$

$$\text{or } N = N_0 e^{-Kt}$$

If $N = 1$, $N_0 = 10$, $t = D$

$$\therefore \quad \frac{N}{N_0} = \frac{1}{10} = e^{-KD}$$

$$\therefore \quad D = \frac{2.303}{K} \tag{4.51}$$

D is defined as decimal reduction time.

From equation 4.50 if one plots on a semilogarithmic scale $\frac{N}{N_0}$ against time with temperature as parameter gets the most representative form of linear profile for vegetative cells as shown below.

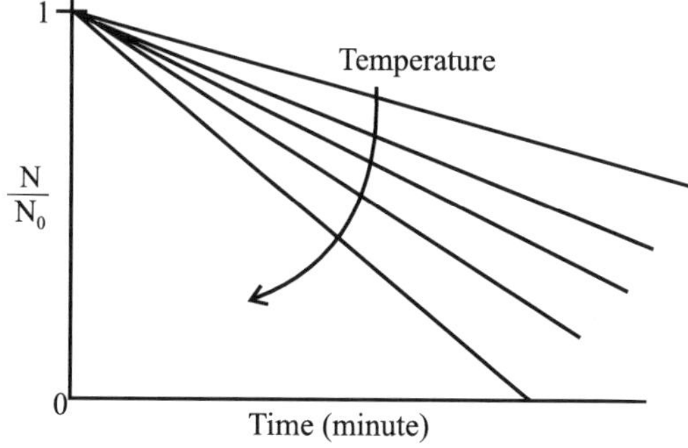

Fig. 4.7 Semilogarithmic variation of N/N_0 as a function of time with temperature as parameter

Slope of this plot is numerically equal to K. Smaller the value of K more resistant the organisms is to thermal death.

However, microbial medium may contain spore as well as contaminants, which need also to be destroyed by heating. It has been proposed by Prokop and Humphery that a sequential step for inactivation of spores occur during thermal sterilization. A representation of these sequential steps has been given by

$$N_R \xrightarrow{K_R} N_S \xrightarrow{K_S} N_D \tag{4.52}$$

in which N_R, N_S and N_D are concentrations of resistant, sensitive and dead spores. The differential equations depicting this model are

$$\frac{d\,N_R}{dt} = -\,K_R\,N_R \tag{4.53}$$

$$\frac{d\,N_S}{dt} = K_R\,N_R - \;K_S\,N_S \tag{4.54}$$

where K_R is specific inactivation rate of resistant spores (min^{-1}) and K_S is the specific inactivation rate of sensitive spores (min^{-1}). Solving this simultaneous differential equations one gets

$$\frac{N}{N_0} = \frac{K_R}{K_R - K_S}\left(e^{-K_S t} - \frac{K_S}{K_R}\,e^{-K_R t}\right) \tag{4.55}$$

In this solution $N = N_S + N_R$ = recoverable viable cell concentration at any time, N_0 is the initial viable cell concentration. Non-linear plot of equation (4.55) has been given in literature as shown in figure below which interpretes experimental survival data.

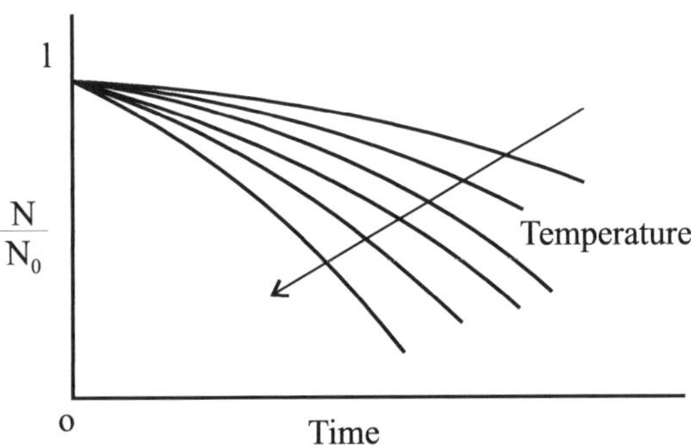

Fig. 4.8 Non-linear relation of equation (4.55)

It can be seen from above figure that the kinetics of death of microbial cells varies with temperature i.e. the value of k is dependent of temperature following Arrhenius relation

$$K = A\;e^{-\frac{E}{RT}} \tag{4.56}$$

where A is Arrhenius constant, E is activation energy, T is absolute temperature and R is universal gas constant. Combining equations 4.50 and 4.56 one gets

$$\ln (N/N_o) = \nabla = A \cdot e^{-E/RT} \cdot t = Kt \tag{4.57}$$

in which ∇ is known as design criteria of sterilization. The temperature relationship of thermal resistances is usually expressed in terms of decimal reduction time (DRT, D) . D value is defined as the time required to reduce the microbial population by one log 10 cycle.

Now considering batch sterilization profile of Fig. 4.6 we have

$$\nabla_{total} = \nabla_{heating} + \nabla_{holding} + \nabla_{cooling}$$

$$\nabla_{heating} = \ln \frac{N_0}{N_1} = a \int_0^{t_1} e^{-E/RT(t)}\, dt \tag{4.58}$$

$$\nabla_{holding} = \ln \frac{N_1}{N_2} = a\, e^{-E/RT}\ t_2 \tag{4.59}$$

$$\nabla_{cooling} = \ln \frac{N_2}{N} = a \int_0^{t_3} e^{-E/RT(t)}\, dt \tag{4.60}$$

where t_1 is the time to reach sterilization temp. t_S, t_2 is the holding time at sterilization temp. t_S and t_3 is the time to cool from t_S to cultivation temperature t_3, N_0 is the initial number of organisms = V_L . N_0; in which V_L is the volume of the liquid in the fermenter and N_0 is the number of organism per unit volume. The drawbacks of batch sterilization relate to scale dependence of ∇_{heat} and ∇_{cool}. Larger fermenters typically have less heat exchange surface per unit volume and so require longer heat up and cool down times.

Consequences of long heat up and cool down time can be severe if the medium components are heat labile. This is because *B. stearothermophilus* is only significantly inactivated above 110°C due to its high activation energy of 67.7 kcal/mole. On the other hand many organic nutrients which also follow the Arrhenius relationship for thermal degradation, have a much lower activation energy of around 25-30 kcal/mole. This implies that longer exposure to lower sterilization temperature, dut to slow heat-up or cool-down can cause proportionately more damage to nutrients. Table 4.1 summarizes the effect of a 1 minute exposure to various temperature on *B. stearothermophilus* compared to a typical nutrient (E = 25 kcal/mole.)

Table 4.1 : Relative degradation rate constants of *B. stearothermophilus* and typical heat labile nutrient

	Relative K Value	
Temperature (°C)	Spore (E = 67.7 kcal/mole)	Nutrient (E = 25 kcal / mole)
80	0.001	0.03
90	0.008	0.07
100	0.009	0.18
110	0.1	0.43
120	1	1
130	8.65	2.22
140	67.7	4.75

4.4.5 Residence Time Concept in Continuous Sterilization

Residence time concept in the pipe flow of continuous sterilizer is important in order to avoid over heating of the medium causing nutritional devaluation. Flow pattern and type are important in ascertaining pipe length and dispersion of fluid (Fig. 4.9). One way to reduce heatup time is to inject steam directly into the medium during sterilization. This will improve the heatup time, but will result in dilution of the media by W factor. The factor W is computable by the following

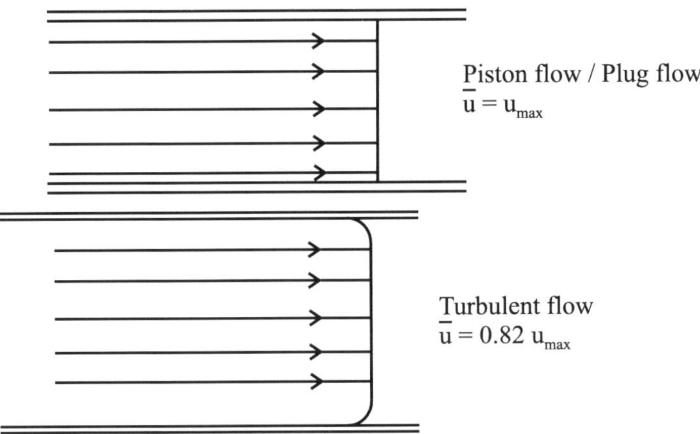

relation, $W = \dfrac{V_L \Delta T}{\Delta H_S}$, where W is the weight of steam condensate, kg; ΔT°C is the temperature rise of the batch heated, V_L is the batch volume (liters) and ΔH_S is the latent heat of steam (556 kcal/kg). This dilution must be compensated for reducing the initial charge by this amount.

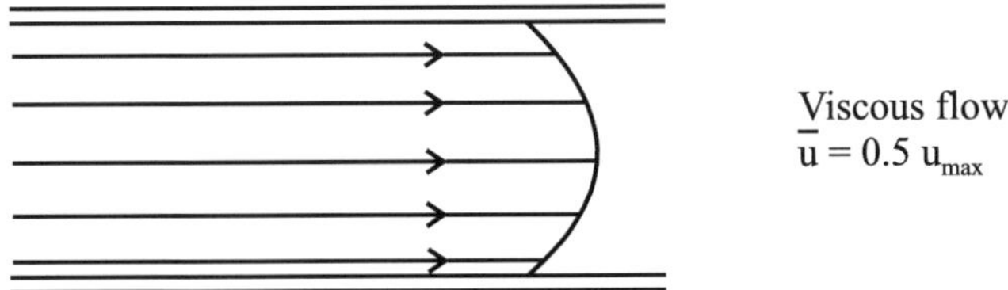

Fig. 4.9 Flow pattern and type in the pipe of continuous sterilizer

The best alternative for heat sensitive materials is to use continuous sterilization. The basic process is shown in (Fig. 4.10) below. Here the raw medium is slurried in water, and then continuously pumped through the sterilizer to a previously sterilized, empty, fermentor vessel. In the sterilizer the media is instantaneously heated by either direct or indirect steam and held at a very high temperature, typically 140°C, for a short time (typically 30–120 seconds). This residence time or holding time of the media is fixed by adjusting the flow rate and length of insulated holding pipe. The hot stream from the sterilizer is rapidly cooled by a heat exchanger, (with or without heat recovery) and/or by flash-cooling before it enters the fermentor vessel.

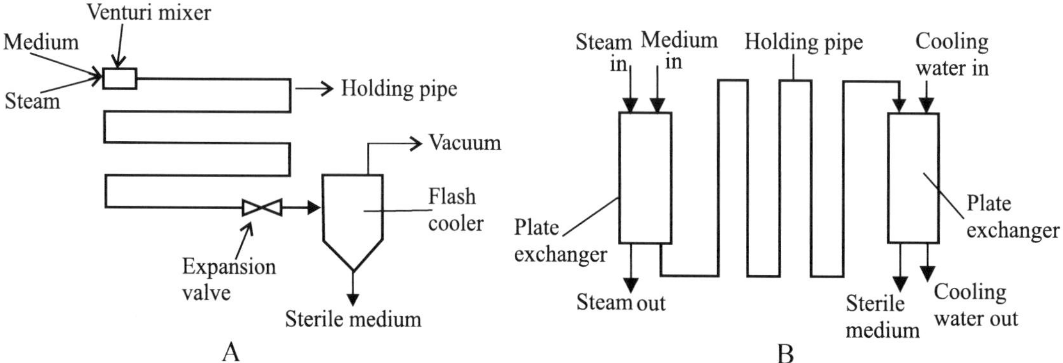

Fig. 4.10 Continuous sterilization : A – with flash cooling; B – with heat exchanger

The continuous sterilization process has several advantages: (1) The temperature profile of the medium (Fig. 4.11) is almost one of instant heating and cooling allowing an easy estimate of the Del factor (∇) required. This makes scale-up very simple. (2) The medium is exposed to high temperatures for short times, thereby minimizing nutrient degradation, and (3) The energy requirements of the sterilization process can be dramatically reduced by using the incoming raw medium to cool the hot sterile media. The difficulties with continuous sterilizers are typically opertional due to exchanger fouling or control instability. In general, media containing solids or starches require attention for continuous sterilization.

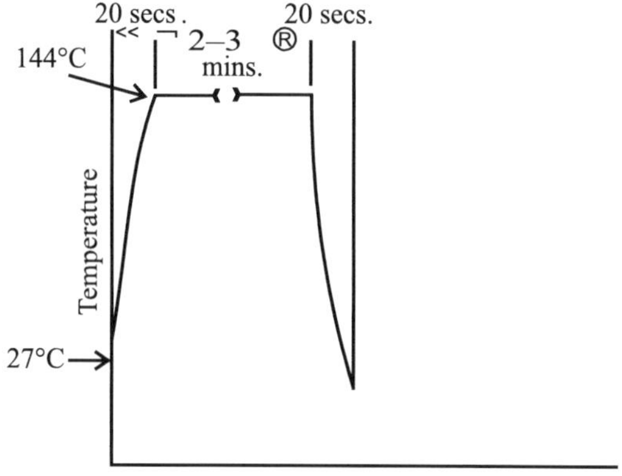

Fig. 4.11 Temperature profile in continuous sterilization

The design of continuous sterilizer must allow some flexibility in operating conditions to adapt the system to different media. The system must incorporate automatic recycle to recirculate media if temperature falls below the design value. The design objectives should include 1. ability to fill the fermentor within 2-3 hours, 2. the recovery of 60-70% of the heat, 3. plug flow in the holding section, and 4. the option of either direct or indirect heating. Essential components of a continuous sterilizer are shown in Fig. 4.12 and include the batching system, solids separator, batch feed tank, heating section, sterilizing section, cooling system, and back pressure valve. Selection of the heat exchanger is critical to successful operation. Typically double pipe, spiral or plate-frame exchangers are used.

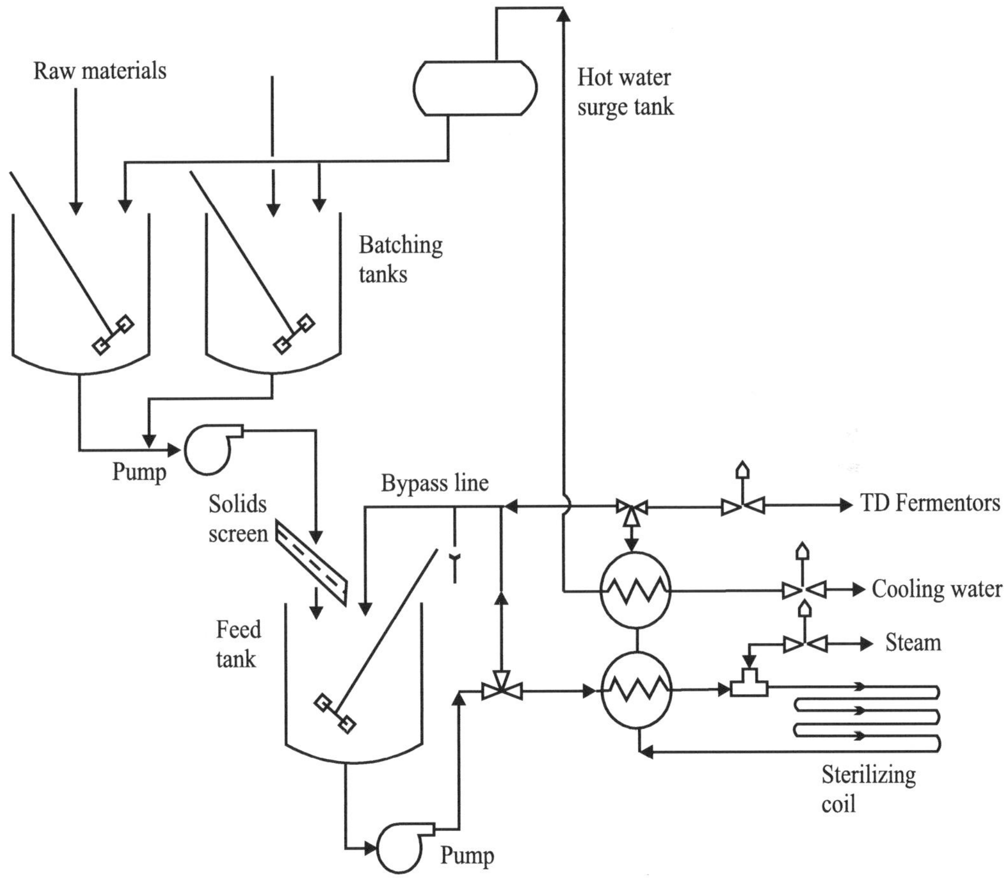

Fig. 4.12 Continuous sterilizer process flow diagram

The major design variables in the design of a continuous sterilizer are the sterilization temperature T_S, the fluid velocity u, and the length L and diameter d of pipe in the holding section. For minor deviation from plug flow the Del factor for continuous sterilization is given by :

$$\nabla_{STFR} = \ln \frac{N_0}{N} = D_a - \frac{D_a^2}{P_e} \tag{4.61}$$

where D_a is the Damkohler number = kL/U
P_e is the Peclet number = ρC_p ud/k
ρ is the liquid density
C_p is the specific heat
k is the thermal conductivity

Continuous sterilizers are typically sterilized by recirculating water for an hour. Then batch components are batched and added separately one after the other. Finally the equipment is cleaned by recirculating cleaning solutions. In continuous sterilization in the equipment flow pipe one may consider a liquid element as depicted in the Fig. 4.13.

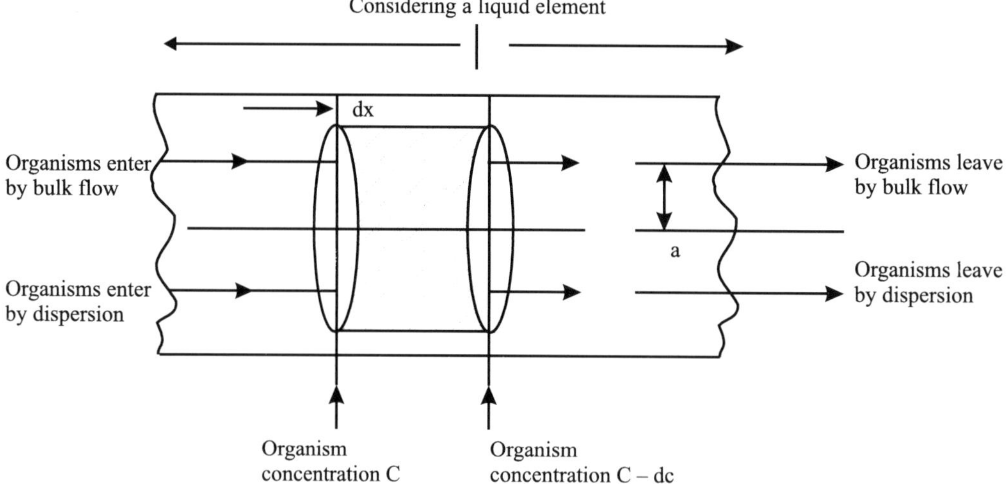

Fig. 4.13 Inflow and outflow in a liquid element

The equation of flow of a microbial suspension through a tube considering both radial and axial dispersions is given by

$$\frac{\partial C}{\partial t} = D^1 \left(\frac{\partial^2 C}{\partial r^2} + \frac{1}{r} \frac{\partial C}{\partial r} \right) + D \frac{\partial^2 C}{\partial Z^2} - U \frac{\partial C}{\partial Z} - KC \tag{4.62}$$

Radial diffusion (Diffusion gradient) Axial Velocity Reaction

Assuming that microbes behave like molecule as far as diffusion is concerned the solution of equation (4.62) may be obtained considering following two cases.

Case 1 : Fraction of material overheated only and no reaction takes place (i.e. KC = 0). When $D^1 > 10^{-5}$ cm^2/sec.

Radial diffusion effects can be neglected provided

$$\frac{\pi D^1}{2F} < 1.95 \times 10^{-3}$$

Where F is the flow rate.

$$\therefore \qquad D\frac{\partial^2 C}{\partial Z^2} - U\frac{\partial C}{\partial Z} = \frac{\partial C}{\partial t} \tag{4.63}$$

Calculation of exit concentration

Let
$$\overline{C} = \frac{C}{C_0}$$

$$x = \frac{Z}{L}$$

$$N_{Pe} = B_0 = \frac{UL}{D}$$

$$q = \frac{t}{t_T}$$

Putting these dimensionless terms in above equation (4.63) one may obtain

$$C = C_0 \,.\, \overline{C}$$

$$\therefore \qquad \frac{\partial C}{\partial Z} = C_0\frac{\partial \overline{C}}{\partial x} = C_0\frac{\partial \overline{C}}{\partial x}\cdot\frac{\partial x}{\partial z} = C_0\frac{\partial \overline{C}}{\partial x}\cdot\frac{\partial}{\partial z}\left(\frac{Z}{L}\right)$$

$$= \frac{C_0}{L}\cdot\frac{\partial \overline{C}}{\partial x}$$

$$\therefore \qquad \frac{\partial^2 C}{\partial Z^2} = \frac{\partial}{\partial Z}\left(\frac{\partial C}{\partial Z}\right)$$

$$= \frac{\partial}{\partial Z}\left[\frac{C_0}{L}\cdot\left(\frac{\partial \overline{C}}{\partial x}\right)\right]$$

$$= \frac{C_0}{L}\,\frac{\partial}{L\partial x}\left(\frac{\partial \overline{C}}{\partial x}\right)$$

$$= \frac{C_0}{L^2}\,\frac{\partial^2 \overline{C}}{\partial x^2}$$

And
$$\frac{\partial C}{\partial t} = C_0\left(\frac{\partial \overline{C}}{\partial t}\right) = C_0\left(\frac{\partial \overline{C}}{\partial \theta}\right)\left(\frac{\partial \theta}{\partial t}\right)$$

$$= C_0 \left(\frac{\partial \overline{C}}{\partial \theta}\right) \frac{\partial}{\partial t}\left(\frac{t}{t_T}\right) \qquad \left[\because \frac{\phi}{t} = \frac{1}{t_T}\right] \qquad \therefore \frac{\partial \theta}{\partial t} = \frac{1}{\phi r}$$

$$= \frac{C_0}{t_T} \quad \frac{\partial \overline{C}}{\partial \phi}$$

Now putting the values of $\frac{\partial^2 \overline{C}}{\partial Z^2}$, $\frac{\partial C}{\partial Z}$ and $\frac{\partial C}{\partial t}$ in equation (4.63) one gets

$$D \cdot \frac{C_0}{L^2} \frac{\partial^2 \overline{C}}{\partial x^2} - U \frac{C_0}{L} \frac{\partial \overline{C}}{\partial x} = \frac{C_0}{t_T} \cdot \frac{\partial \overline{C}}{\partial \phi}$$

or $$\frac{\partial^2 \overline{C}}{\partial x^2} - \frac{UL}{D} \cdot \frac{\partial \overline{C}}{\partial x} = \frac{L^2}{D} \frac{1}{t_T} \frac{\partial \overline{C}}{\partial \phi} \qquad \left(\begin{array}{l}\text{Multiplying both sides} \\ \text{by } L^2 \text{and dividing by } C_o\end{array}\right)$$

or $$\frac{\partial^2 \overline{C}}{\partial x^2} - \frac{UL}{D} \cdot \frac{\partial \overline{C}}{\partial x} = \frac{L}{D} \cdot \frac{L}{t_T} \cdot \frac{\partial \overline{C}}{\partial \phi} = \frac{L}{D} \cdot U \cdot \frac{\partial C}{\partial \theta}$$

or $$\frac{\partial^2 \overline{C}}{\partial x^2} - \frac{UL}{D} \cdot \frac{\partial \overline{C}}{\partial x} = \frac{UL}{D} \cdot \frac{\partial \overline{C}}{\partial \phi}$$

or $$\frac{\partial^2 \overline{C}}{\partial x^2} - B_0 \frac{\partial \overline{C}}{\partial x} = B_0 \frac{\partial \overline{C}}{\partial \phi} \qquad \left(\because \frac{UL}{D} = B_0 \text{ or } P_e\right)$$

or $$\frac{\partial^2 \overline{C}}{\partial x^2} - B_0 \frac{\partial \overline{C}}{\partial x} - B_0 \frac{\partial \overline{C}}{\partial \phi} = O \qquad (4.64)$$

The initial conditions are

For $x > 0$

$\overline{C} = 1$

$\theta = 0$

and for $x < 0$,

$\overline{C} = 0$

$\theta = 0$

The boundary conditions

$x \longrightarrow 0$

$$\left(\frac{\partial \overline{C}}{\partial x}\right) - B_0 \overline{C} = 0$$

And

$x \longrightarrow 0$

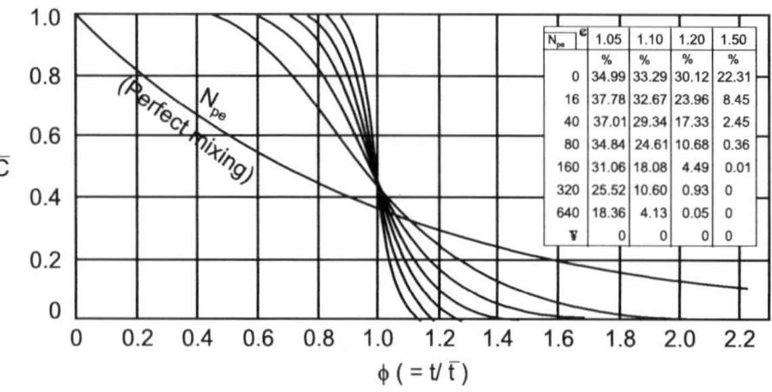

N_{pe} \ e	1.05	1.10	1.20	1.50
	%	%	%	%
0	34.99	33.29	30.12	22.31
16	37.78	32.67	23.96	8.45
40	37.01	29.34	17.33	2.45
80	34.84	24.61	10.68	0.36
160	31.06	18.08	4.49	0.01
320	25.52	10.60	0.93	0
640	18.36	4.13	0.05	0
¥	0	0	0	0

Fig. 4.14 Effect of different types of flow (as shown by different N_{pe} values and different ratios of the holding time, t, to the nominal holding time, t), in continuous sterilization of media

$$\left(\frac{\partial \overline{C}}{\partial x}\right) = 0$$

Provide solution of Equation (4.65)

$$\overline{C} = \int_{32=1}^{\infty} \frac{B_0 \lambda (4\lambda^2 \cos 2\lambda x + B_0 \sin 2\lambda x}{(16\lambda^2 + 4B_0)(16\lambda^2 + B_0^2)} \exp\left(\frac{B_0 x}{2} - \frac{B_0^2 + 16\lambda^2}{4 B_0} \cdot \phi\right) \quad (4.65)$$

Now, when

$$B_0 = 0 \qquad \overline{C} = \exp\left(-\frac{16\lambda^2}{4}\phi\right) \quad \ldots (4.66)$$

$$= \exp(-4\lambda^2\phi)$$

and when $B_0 = \infty$

$$\overline{C} = 0$$

So it implies that for, $B_0 = \infty$ (ideal), percent overheat is negligible and for $B_0 = 0$, the percent overheat is maximum (Fig. 4.14).

Case 2 : Considering steady state destruction of micro organisms to follow first order kinetics.

$$D\frac{d^2\overline{C}}{dx^2} - U\frac{dc}{dz} - kC = 0 \quad \ldots (4.67)$$

One may get in dimensionless form as

$$\frac{d^2\overline{C}}{dx^2} - B_0\frac{d\overline{C}}{dx} - B_0\frac{KL}{U}\overline{C} = 0 \quad \ldots (4.68)$$

Using boundary conditions

$$x \longrightarrow 0, \qquad \frac{d\overline{C}}{dx} + B_0(1 - \overline{C}) = 0$$

$$x \longrightarrow 1, \qquad \frac{d\overline{C}}{dx} = 0$$

gives

$$\overline{C}_{x=1} = \left(\frac{C}{C_0}\right)_{z=L}$$

Or

$$\left(\frac{C}{C_0}\right)_{x=1} = \frac{4\alpha \exp.\left(\frac{B_0}{2}\right)}{(1+\alpha^2)\exp.\left(\frac{\alpha B_0}{2}\right) - (1-\alpha^2)\left(\frac{-\alpha B_0}{2}\right)} \quad (4.69)$$

where

$$\alpha = \sqrt{1 + 4\left(\frac{Nr}{B_0}\right)}$$

and $$N_r = \frac{KL}{U} = \text{Reaction number}$$

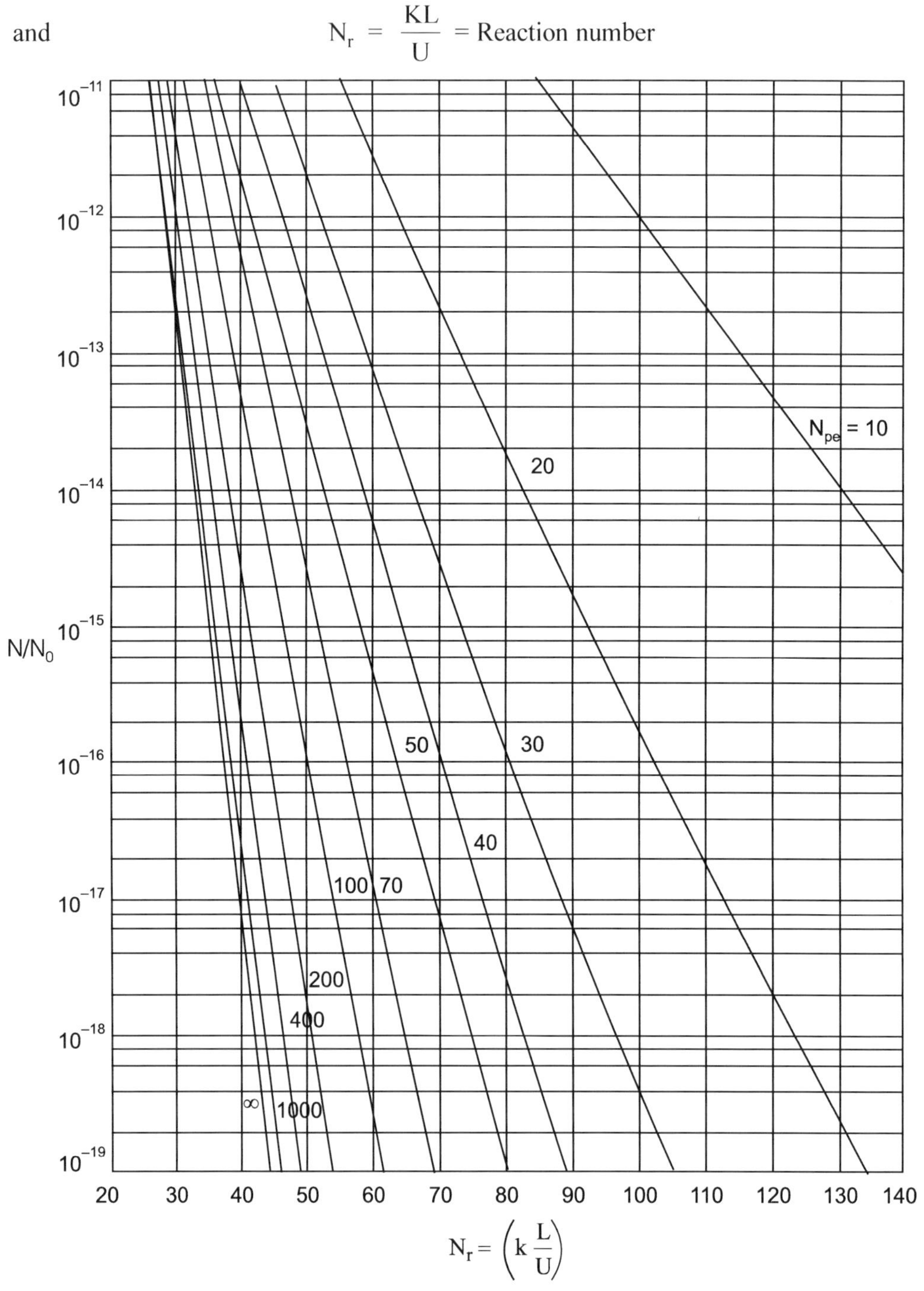

Fig 4.15 Effect of different types of flow (as shown by different N_{Pc} values) on the destruction of organisms (N/N_0) at different rates of destruction (measured as $N_r = kL/U$)

Effect of residence time distribution of continuous sterilizer

k *(min^{-1})*	*Av.Rt* *(sec)*	N_{pe}	*Reduction of Containment Level (N/N_0)* *Plug Flow*	*Actual*
10	5	200	1.8×10^{-22}	10^{-18}
10	5	100	1.8×10^{-22}	1.5×10^{-16}
10	5	70	1.8×10^{-22}	3×10^{-15}
10	5	50	1.8×10^{-22}	2×10^{-23}

Case 3 : Ideal Case

When $B_0 = \propto$ (ideal)

$$\left(\frac{C}{C_0}\right)_{X=L} = \exp.\left(-\frac{kL}{U}\right)$$

In reality the flow of real fluid will have B_0 or N_{pe} between zero and infinity. (Fig. 4.15)

4.4.6 Sterilization of non-Newtonian liquids

Non-Newtonian liquids without initial yield stress follow the relation between shear stress and radial velocity distribution as

$$R = K\left(\frac{du}{dr}\right)^n \tag{4.70}$$

(shear stress) (radial velocity distributions)

in which K = consistency factor and n = the power law index

For laminar flow of non-Newtonian liquids

$$U = \left(\frac{n}{n+1}\right)\cdot\left(\frac{\Delta P}{2LK}\right)^{\frac{1}{n}}\cdot\left(a^{\left(\frac{1}{n}+1\right)} - r^{\left(\frac{1}{n}+1\right)}\right) \tag{4.71}$$

$$U_{mean} = \frac{a.n}{3n+1}\left(\frac{a.\Delta P}{2LK}\right)^{\frac{1}{n}}$$

$$U_{max} = \left(\frac{n}{n+1}\right)\cdot\left(\frac{\Delta P}{2LK}\right)^{\frac{1}{n}}\cdot a^{\left(\frac{1}{n}\right)}$$

or
$$\left(\frac{a\Delta P}{2LK}\right)^{\frac{1}{n}} = \left(\frac{n+1}{an}\right)U_{max}$$

So,
$$U_{mean} = \left(\frac{an}{3n+1}\right)\cdot\left(\frac{n+1}{an}\right)\cdot U_{max}$$

or
$$U_{mean} = \left(\frac{n+1}{3n+1}\right)U_{max} \tag{4.72}$$

It expresses the behaviour of the non-Newtonian fluids of different n values in graphical form in general as shown in the Fig. 4.16.

$$\text{So}\quad \frac{U}{U_{mean}} = \frac{\frac{n}{n+1}}{\frac{an}{3n+1}} \cdot \frac{\left(\frac{\Delta P}{2LK}\right)^{\frac{1}{n}}}{\left(\frac{a\Delta P}{2LK}\right)^{\frac{1}{n}}} \cdot \left(a^{\left(\frac{1}{n}+1\right)} - r^{\left(\frac{1}{n}+1\right)}\right)$$

$$= \frac{3n+1}{n+1} \cdot \frac{1}{a} \cdot \frac{1}{a} m \left(a^{\left(\frac{1}{n}+1\right)} - r^{\left(\frac{1}{n}+1\right)}\right)$$

$$= \frac{3n+1}{n+1} \cdot \left(1 - \left(\frac{r}{a}\right)^{\frac{1}{n}+1}\right) \quad (4.73)$$

For $n = 0$

$$\frac{U}{U_{mean}} = \frac{3 \times 0 + 1}{0+1} [1 - 0] = 1$$

For $n = \infty$

$$\frac{U}{U_{mean}} = \frac{3\infty}{\infty} = 3$$

For $n = 1$

$$\frac{U}{U_{mean}} = \frac{3 \times 1 + 1}{1+1} \cdot \left(1 - \left(\frac{-r}{2}\right)^2\right)$$

$$= \frac{4}{2}\left[1 - \left(\frac{r}{a}\right)^2\right] = 2\left[1 - \left(\frac{r}{a}\right)^2\right]$$

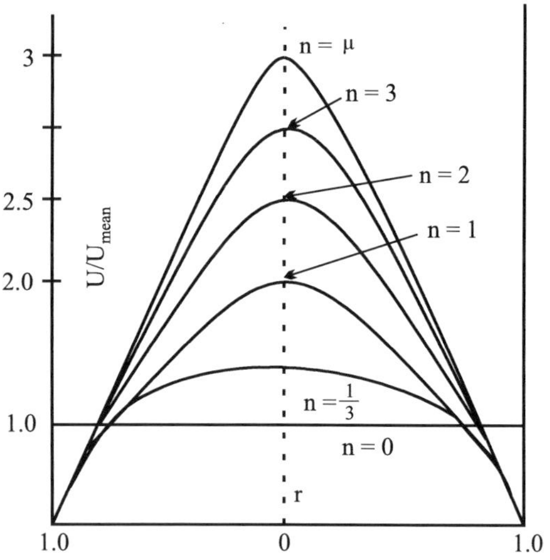

Fig. 4.16 Relation of U/U_{mean} as a function of *r* with n as parameter (Equation 4.73)

For non-Newtonian fluid/liquid sterilization

$$U = \frac{3n+1}{n+1} \cdot \pi a^2 \cdot \left(1 - \left(\frac{r}{a}\right)^{\frac{n+1}{n}}\right) \cdot Q_r$$

$$\therefore \quad \frac{C}{C_0} = 2n \frac{(3n+1)}{(n+1)^2} A^2 \int_A^\infty \left(1 - \frac{A}{x}\right)^{\frac{n-1}{n+1}} \exp(-x)\, x^{-3}\, dx \quad (4.74)$$

in which $$A = \frac{n+1}{(3n+1)} \cdot \frac{\pi L a^2}{Q_0 D''}$$

$$x = A\left(1-\left(\frac{r}{a}\right)^{\frac{n+1}{n}}\right)^{-1}$$

Special Case :

For $n = 1$, the above equation becomes

$$\frac{C}{C_0} = 2\frac{3.1+1}{(1+1)^2} \cdot 1 \cdot \left(\frac{1}{2}\frac{\pi L a^2}{Q_0\, D''}\right)^2$$

$$= 2 \cdot \frac{4}{4} \cdot 1 \cdot \left[\frac{1}{2}\frac{\pi L \cdot a^2}{Q_0 D''}\right]^2$$

$$= 2\left[\frac{1}{2}\frac{\pi}{Q_0}\frac{L \cdot a^2}{D''}\right]^2$$

$$= \frac{1}{2}\left[\frac{\pi}{Q_0}\frac{L.a^2}{D''}\right]^2$$

4.5 REFERENCES

1. S. Aiba, A. E. Humphrey and N.F.Mills, *Biochemical Engineering* 2nd edn., Chapter 10,Univ. of Tokyo Press, 1973
2. H.T. Kim, S. B. Kwon, Y.O. Park and K.W. Lee, "Diffusional Filtration of Polydispersed Aerosol Particles by Fibrous and Packed-bed Filters", *Filtration and Separation*, pp 37-40, 2000.
3. C. Y. Chen, "Filtration of Aerosols by Fibrous Media", *Chem., Review*, pp 55, 595, 1955
4. W. H. Stark and G.M. Pohler, Sterile Air for Industrial Fermentation, *Ind. Eng. Chem*, pp 42, 1789, 1950
5. J. Heintzenberg, "Property of the Log-Normal Particle Size Distribution", *Aerosol Sci Technol* pp 21, 46-48, 1994
6. J.E. Bailey and D. F. Ollis, *Biochemical Engineering Fundamentals*, 2nd edn., McGraw Hill Book Co. New York, 1986
7. R. Lee and J.Waltz, "Consider Continuous Sterilization of Bioprocess Wastes", *Chem. Eng. Prog.* pp 44-48, 1990
8. T.G. Mezger, The Rheology HandBook, Vincentz Verlag, Hannover, Germany, 2002
9. N.J. Alderman and N.I. Heywood, Improving Slurry Viscosity and Flow Curve Measurements, CEP, April 2004, pp 27-32
10. Aspen Technology, "Applied Rheology" Technical Area of Process Mannual, Didcot, Oxfordshire, U.K. 2004

Chapter

5

CONCERNS OF AERATION AND MIXING/AGITATION IN BIOPROCESSING

5.1 INTRODUCTION

Various types of oxygenation hardware designs have been developed to suit specific purposes in biosystems.[1–6] For example, oxygenation required in cell culture uses bioreactor hardware of various designs to take care of biosystem characteristics. For this purpose, conventional stirred tank bioreactor (STBR) designs have been used for a long time to oxygenate or aerate the bioreaction liquid. Many bacteria and yeasts, as well as a few other microorganisms, can grow well when floating free in a liquid culture medium in vessels with a capacity as high as several thousand liters, resisting damage even when they have proliferated to form a thick suspension, and even when the suspension is oxygenated and agitated vigorously with a mechanical sparger and agitator. Many microbial, mammalian, and plant cells are different. They are either highly shear sensitive, flocculating or pellet forming, or larger than most microorganisms, more fragile and more complex. Moreover, the delicate plasma membrane that encloses mammalian cells is not encased in a tough cell wall, similar to many plant cells. Mammalian and plant cells that multiply in suspension can usually be cultivated by oxic techniques, similar to those used in microbial fermentation.[7,8] However, most animal or mammalian cells do not grow at all in suspension, but grow only when they can attach themselves to a surface. They are called anchorage-dependent mammalian cells. Anchorage-dependent cells have traditionally been grown on a large scale on the inner surface of a roller bottle reactor. As the bottles roll, the cells are exposed to oxygen in the air space and to the growth medium. The design of rotary oxygenators has been used also in microbial bioprocessing for product formations[9-12] as well as in effluent treatment for pollution control (rotary biological contactors).[13]

In the human body, the need for oxygenation requires no emphasis. With respect to oxygenation, apparently the function of an artificial lung is to oxygenate at least 4.5 ml of O_2/100 ml of blood at the maximum rated blood flow.[14] Many manufacturers design and produce membrane oxygenators that utilize microporous polypropylene membrane for gas exchange. Designs of these oxygenators include submerged bioreactor oxygenator, hollow fibers, a flat-plate type, or sometimes other types of configurations. Hollow-fiber membrane oxygenator designs have been greatly improved in the past few years.[15-18] In the perfusion mode of the mammalian cell culture system, the use of tubular spiral film oxygen-permeable membrane oxygenator has become a common technique.[19] This type of cell culture technique using perfusion oxygenation has been developed mostly to avoid fluid mechanical damage of animal cells in conventional oxygenated bioreactors.[20] Likewise, it has been discussed in the literature that in the plant cell culture system, the oxygenation situation may become very critical in terms of cell growth and cell division. Whatever the oxygenator used, the biomass yield usually serves as a valuable parameter in bioprocessing. For prediction of biomass yield, oxygen efficiency (η_0) has been used by

some investigators.[21–23] Minkevich and Eroshin[22] proposed oxygen efficiency by defining it as the ratio of the amount of electrons conserved in biomass over the amount of electrons available in organic substrate by aerobic cumbustion to HCO_3^-.

It has been shown[23] that η_0 follows from Y_{DX} (biomass yield on electron donor, per mol, or per C-mol for carbon compounds (C-mol/mol) using only the black box conservation relationship. Hence, η_0 being a true black box, it can only be applied to aerobic systems and, therefore, lacks general applicability. A simple example of black box information for aerobic growth of *Pseudomonas oxalaticus* on oxalate with a yield of 0.586 C-mol/mol, as given above, provides the corresponding macrochemical mass balance relationship as follows:

$$- 5.815\ C_2O_4^{2-} - 0.2\ NH_4^+ - 1.857\ O_2 - 0.8\ H^+ - 5.414\ H_2O$$
$$+ 1.0\ CH_{1.8}\ O_5\ N_{0.2} + 10.63\ HCO_3^- = O$$

Here, there is no intrinsic limit based on the second law of thermodynamics.

5.2 OXYGEN PATHWAYS IN CELL CULTIVATIONS

In all cell culture media, the aqueous solution of the substrate has two major components, water and substrate. During cultivation of cells in the medium, surface active material may be produced or need to be added for certain purposes. If oxygen or air is passed in the medium during cultivation, it has to be transferred to cells properly for its participation in the cellular pathway. Figure 5.1 depicts the oxygen transfer pathway in a typical aerobic microbial cell reaction system to reach oxygen from the gas phase to the cell surface through the liquid pathway.[24]

5.2.1 Extracellular Pathways in Liquid

It has been clearly shown by Finn[25] that in a cell culture system, the rate-controlling step for oxygen transfer is that from gaseous bubble interface to the bulk of the liquid. Therefore, it is

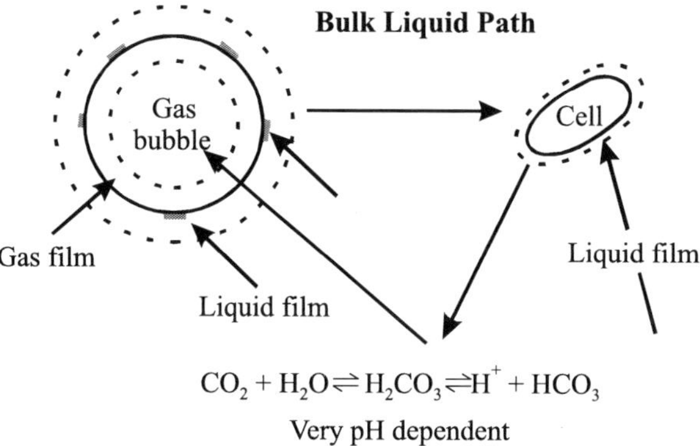

Fig. 5.1 Oxygen and CO_2 pathways in a typical fermentation bioprocessing liquid

primarily an engineering task to provide the microorganism with adequate oxygen for various end results. In aerobic submerged cultures, cells remain immersed throughout the liquid broth. Oxygen or air is purged and aerated for absorption by its passage from the gas phase in bubbles to culture liquid and then to cells. As shown by Finn, this transfer of oxygen from the gas phase to liquid and then to cell frequently becomes a critical factor in fermentation, the reason being the low solubility of oxygen in culture medium. This depends on several steps, each of which encounters certain resistance. In order to assess the efficiency of this aeration process, engineers have defined the rate of transfer equal to the product of the mass conduction (*diffusivity*) times the concentration driving force. For an aerobic fermentation, this rate of oxygen transfer has been expressed as:

$$\text{Rate of oxygen transfer or demand} = \text{Diffusivity of oxygen in liquid} \times \text{Oxygen concentration gradient (driving force)} \quad (5.1)$$

Following the dissolution of oxygen from bubbles in the local liquid, the oxygen has to pass through the bulk liquid path to reach equilibrium concentration. Therefore, it has been possible to represent the local transfer or rate per unit area by the following equation:

$$\left(\frac{dC_L}{dt}\right) = \frac{D}{h}\ (C^* - C_L) = K_L\ (C^* - C_L) \tag{5.2}$$

In this equation, K_L = D/h is the mass transfer coefficient for oxygen transport from the gas bubble interface to the liquid interface with gas. C_L is the oxygen concentration in the bulk liquid, C* is the oxygen concentration in equilibrium with the oxygen partial pressure at the bubble interface, D is the molecular diffusivity of oxygen in the liquid (cm^2/h), and h is the assumed liquid film thickness around the bubble transfer surface area (cm). In fermentation bioreactor the mass transfer concern in fermentations is that of oxygen transfer. CO_2 ventilation could be important. However, definitive studies to show the importance of the latter have not been undertaken.

The data of Fiechter and von Meyenburg (*Biotech. Bioeng.* 10, 535, 1968) for the batch growth of *S. cerevisiae* on glucose medium is reasonably typical of the events that can occur in a fermentation. It is to be noted that in this particular case the maximum CO_2 ventilation rate (29 millimoles/liter-hr.) is much larger than the maximum O_2 uptake (4.2 millimoles/liter-hr.) and is not coincidental with it. Also it is to note that neither transfer rate is very high as a well designed fermenter should have the capability of transferring up to 250 millimoles O_2/liter-hr.

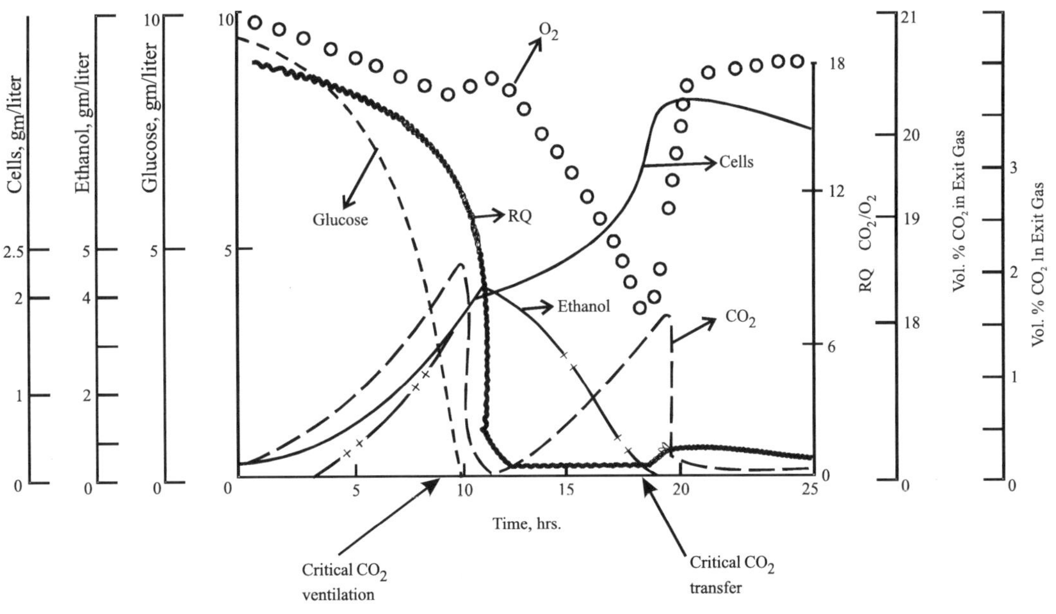

r_{O_2} = 2.0 millimoles/liter-hr.
r_{CO_2} = 29 millimoles/liter-hr.

r_{O_2} = 4.2 millimoles/liter-hr.
r_{CO_2} = 2.0 millimoles/liter-hr.

Fig. 5.2 Batch growth of *S. cerevisiae* on glucose

5.2.2 Why the Concern Over O_2 Transfer?

Most fermentations, but not all, are run under conditions of O_2 limitation.

A typical carbohydrate utilization can be represented (for 200 grams of carbohydrate) by

$$\underset{(200\text{ gm})}{6.67\ CH_2O} + \underset{(67.2\text{ gm})}{2.1\ O_2} \longrightarrow \underset{(74.6\text{ gm})}{\text{Yeast}\ (C_{3.92}H_{6.5}O_{1.94})} + \underset{(121.0\text{ gm})}{2.75\ CO_2 + 3.42\ H_2O}$$

from which there can be obtained

$$Y = \text{Yield} = \frac{74.6}{200} = 0.373 \text{ gm yeast/gm sugar}$$

$$RQ = \text{Respiratory quotient} = \frac{CO_2 \text{ evolution}}{O_2 \text{ uptake}} = \frac{2.75}{2.1} = 1.3.$$

Usually RQ is nearly 1. Hence, because at room temperature and at pH 7 water saturated with air gives a dissolved O_2 concentration (7.8 ppm O_2) which is much less than that for air containing 1% CO_2 (200 ppm CO_2). Most researchers believe oxygen is the crucial mass transfer component.

5.2.3 Comparison of Concentration Driving Forces for Glucose, O_2 and CO_2

	1% Sugar solution	Broth sat. with air @ S.C	Broth sat. with 1% CO_2 air
Concentration in fermentation broth	10,000 ppm	7ppm	15ppm
Critical Concentration which affects growth rate	100 ppm	0.8 ppm	1500 ppm
Rate of uptake or evolution (millimoles/gm cell/hr.)	2.8	7.7	7.7
Diffusion coefficient (cm^2/sec)	0.6×10^{-5}	1.8×10^{-5}	1.4×10^{-5}

Since

(Rate of demand) = (Conduction) (Concentration driving force)

Uptake or evolution i.e. I = (1/R) (E),

It seems obvious that the conduction of oxygen may well be the critical or limiting one.

5.3 VOLUMETRIC OXYGEN TRANSFER COEFFICIENT (K_La)

Since it is extremely difficult, if not impossible, to measure K_L and the amount of bubble transfer area in a bioreactor or fermenter, an engineering parameter known as volumetric oxygen transfer coefficient, expressed by K_La, has been used to represent volumetric oxygen transfer coefficient as:

$$\left(\frac{dC_L}{dt}\right) = K_La\ (C^* - C_L)_{mean} \tag{5.3}$$

where a is the amount of surface area per unit volume. In this relation, the volumetric oxygen transfer coefficient, K_La, has the units of m mol, of O_2/ml. h. unit concentration gradient. Using the proper concentration units, K_La has the unit of reciprocal of time (i.e., time^{-1}). In equation 5.2, the term ($C^* - C_L$) represented a "local" concentration difference. However, in equation 5.3 it represents a mean driving force in the whole reaction volume in the fermenter. For the system where the liquid is very well mixed but when the bubbles rise through the broth in a tall bioreactor without adequate mixing, then the proper driving force should be a log mean driving force, i.e.,

$$(C^* - C_L)_{mean} = \frac{C^*_{inlet} - C^*_{outlet}}{2.303 \log \left[\frac{C^*_{inlet} - C_L}{C^*_{outlet} - C_L} \right]} \quad (5.4)$$

When both the liquid and gas bubbles are perfectly mixed, then the outlet gas bubble concentration represents the average gas bubble concentration in the fermenter. Therefore,

$$(C^* - C_L) = C^*_{outlet} - C_L \quad (5.5)$$

Hanhart *et al.*[26] have recommended this form. In most fermenters the actual operating condition is somewhere between these two (i.e., neither the gas bubbles nor the liquid phase are perfectly mixed in the true sense). Probably the later mean is to be preferred, although it is highly sensitive to experimental error when the uptake rate by cells is very low and $C^*_{outlet} - C_L$ is high. For this reason, some industrial engineers have preferred to use the K_La value computed from:

$$K_La = \frac{\text{Uptake rate by cells}}{C^*_{inlet} - C_L} \quad (5.6)$$

It appears that engineering problems of oxygen transfer in culture liquid in the bioreactor arise because of (1) the resistance encountered in the transfer process, thereby influencing mainly the K_L value, and (2) the hindrance to increase interfacial transfer area "*a*".

5.4 OXYGEN TRANSFER MECHANISM AND PARAMETERS

The oxygen transfer concept as discussed above has been explained by various theories. The simplest theory is the stationary film theory as proposed by Whitman and depicted in Fig. 5.2.

Bulk gas	
	C^* p^*
Stationary liquid film	
	C_i p_i
Bulk liquid	

(a)

Bulk gas	
	p^*
Stationary gas film	
	p_i C^*
Stationary liquid film	
	p_i, C_L
Bulk liquid	

(b)

Bulk liquid	
	C_L
Stationary liquid film	
	C_b
Biomass	

Fig. 5.2 Mechanism showing oxygen transfer from gas to liquid to cell

It assumes that in the interface proper, the liquid is saturated with oxygen gas (symbolized as C*). In the bulk dissolved oxygen (DO), concentration is C_L

$$R = \frac{dC_L}{dt} = \frac{K_L a}{h}(C^* - C_L) \tag{5.7}$$

where h is the stationary film thickness, and k_L is a constant dependent on diffusivity coefficient of the gas. In general, h is not known, that is why it is combined with k_L to give K_L. Therefore,

$$\frac{dC_L}{dt} = K_L a\,(C^* - C_L) \tag{5.8}$$

In Equation 5.7, $(C^* - C_L)$ is the concentration gradient or driving force in overcoming the barrier in diffusion. The oxygen absorption rate in terms of partial pressure can be expressed by:

$$\frac{dC_L}{dt} = K_L a\,H\,(p^* - p_i) \tag{5.9}$$

because, from Henry's law (H = Henry's constant)

$$C^* = Hp^* \tag{5.10}$$

and $$C_i = Hp_i$$

Aeration efficiency or oxygenation efficiency is expressed by $K_L a$ or $K_L a$ H. For maximum oxygen absorption rate,

$$C_L = 0$$

and then $$\left(\frac{dC_L}{dt}\right) = K_L aC^* = K_L aHp^* \tag{5.11}$$

Stationary film theory has been elaborated in many ways.[27–29] One of them is the two-film theory, which presupposes a stationary gas film in addition to the stationary liquid film, as shown in Fig. 5.2. At a steady state, it is possible to write,

$$\frac{dC_L}{dt} = K_g aH(p^* - p_i) = K_L aH(p^* - p_i) = K_L aH(p^* - p_i) \tag{5.12}$$

where $1/K_g$ is the gas film resistance, $1/K_L$ the liquid film resistance, and $1/K_t$ the overall resistance. Therefore,

$$1/K_t = 1/K_g + 1/K_L \tag{5.13}$$

For a highly agitated Newtonian system, K_g is negligible[27 – 29] and then $K_t = K_L$. It may thus be stated that

$$\frac{dC_L}{dt} \begin{array}{l} \propto a \\ \propto \text{partial pressure} \\ \propto 1/K_L \end{array} \tag{5.14}$$

A stationary liquid film is supposed to remain surrounding the cell, and it offers an additional resistance to oxygen uptake by the cells. The magnitude of this resistance can be conceived from the data on the respiration in yeast cells provided by Finn.[30] A maximum concentration difference of 2×10^{-7} molar (M) is required to overcome this resistance. In agitated liquid suspension, stationary liquid film thickness and, consequently, concentration difference across it would be smaller. The concentration difference is considered negligible compared to DOT (Dissolved Oxygen Tension) value of about 10^{-6} to 10^{-5} M, at which respiration rate starts to be oxygen limited.

The possibility of penetration of stationary liquid film at the gas-liquid interface by cells is reported,[31] which suggested further that cells may concentrate on the interface owing to the surface activity of the cells. The overall effect of such concentrations of cells on the interface is to decrease the film thickness, thereby increasing K_La. The validity of such an approach, however, still awaits experimental verification.

The following resistances counteract to improve the K_L value in the gas-liquid transfer.[32]

5.5 RESISTANCES TO GAS-LIQUID INTERFACE AND BULK MIXING

Three distinct resistances at the gas-liquid interface have been visualized. The first is concerned with gas film resistance. This encompasses the resistance between the bulk of the gas and the gas-liquid interface, and it gives a measure of stagnation that may occur inside the air bubbles. The second manifests as internal resistance in the form of an energy barrier which excludes oxygen molecules below a threshold velocity. The third includes liquid film resistance. It extends from the gas-liquid interface into the bulk of the liquid, and naturewise it provides a measure of stagnation in the liquid around the bubbles. This resistance is a measure of the mean separation distance between the bubble and organism, but it is not generally assumed to be constant within the liquid in any zone. However, for a fermentation broth having high rheological property, this resistance might have a significant contribution. In that case, DO concentration may vary from region to region in the fermenter.

The intraclump resistance has four counterparts.[30] The first is liquid film resistance that exists around the cell or clump of cells—again, a stagnation effect. The second manifests as clump resistance. It is a measure of the diffusion barrier between organism surface and metabolic site. Eventually, it may become significant in a large single cell or in clumped cells. The third one indicates cell membrane resistance to transport. It extends from the exterior surface of the cell membrane to its interior surface, and it is associated perhaps with an endergonic reaction. The fourth one is reaction resistance, perhaps also related to an energy barrier for the reaction of oxygen molecules with terminal electron carriers.

5.5.1 Problems to Increase "a"

The problems of increasing the gas-liquid interfacial area "a" are not so acute in Newtonian broth. However very often it becomes a serious problem in many non-Newtonian broths, where large agitation power input is needed to increase the gas-liquid interfacial area. Although increased power input produces a large value of a with marginal effect on K_L[33], in large-scale systems it increases the overall cost, thus becoming a problem with increasing a with minimum power expenditure. This becomes especially crucial for some high oxygen-demanding microbial systems that are shear sensitive. Problems with such systems arise because of the tendency of the cells to be ruptured by the shear force exerted in agitation. Transport of oxygen across cell membranes has been described in many reports to be an active transport.[34] For pellet, aggregates, and floc-forming mold as well as actinomycetes and yeast fermentations, oxygen diffusion from bulk to the mycelial pellets, aggregates, or flocs frequently becomes controlling. This means that the rate of transport of oxygen across the cell membrane rather than the rate of oxygen dissolution in the bulk becomes a controlling step, as shown in Fig. 5.3. Another important problem encountered in many mycelial fermentations is that the broth viscosity in the region of the impeller may be low, while that in the distant part of the fermenter is very high. In effect, bulk mixing becomes poor and channeling of the air bubbles is most likely to take place, the net result being that a large part of the culture in the vessel remains under oxygen-starved conditions, thereby hampering the overall process. In such cases, DO distribution at low power expenditure becomes a problem.

5.5.2 Beneficial Effects of Agitation

Many of the engineering problems described above have been overcome by providing agitation arrangement during fermentation.[35] This greatly reduces the resistances by imparting its fourfold functions, namely, (1) creating a large air-liquid interfacial area by bubble disruption; (2) reducing the thickness of the liquid film around the air bubble, thus enhancing oxygen diffusion and increasing the K_L value; (3) maintaining the homogeneity of DO in the liquid by reducing

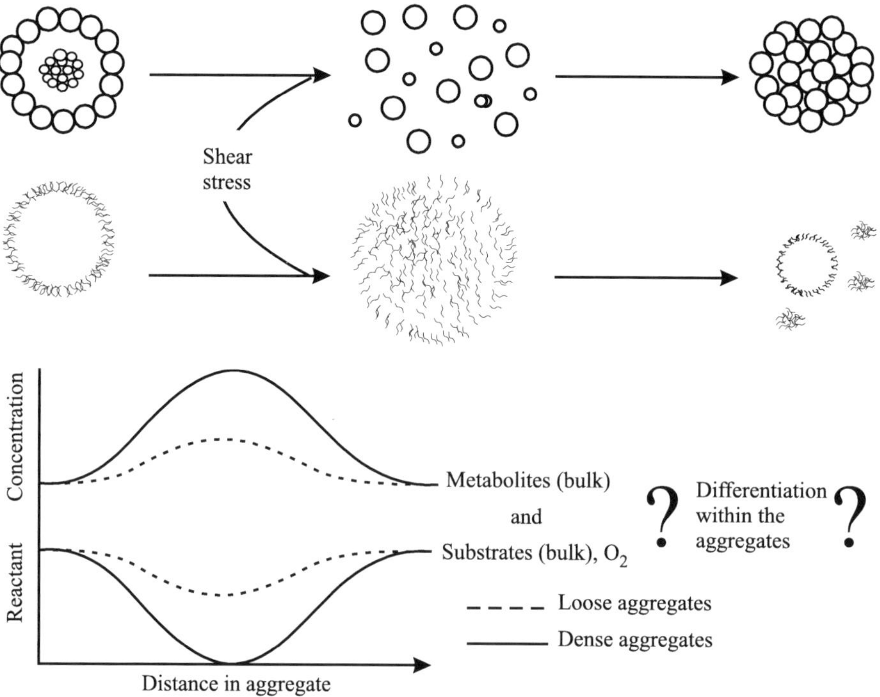

Fig. 5.3 Problems resulting from aggregation

resistance to bulk mixing; and (4) controlling clump size, a phenomenon common with mold and actinomycetes, by reducing the chances of agglomeration of cells, thereby decreasing intraclump resistance.

5.6 RECENT CONCEPT IN OXYGEN TRANSFER PATHWAY

A concept of emulsified oxygen vector pathway for enhanced oxygen mass transfer in bioprocessing liquid has been proposed. According to this concept, the presence of a nonaqueous liquid phase may provoke a significant increase in the oxygen transfer rate from the gas phase to the biocells without necessitating an increased energy input. The principle of oxygen vectors consists of adding to the growth medium a liquid phase in which oxygen has a higher solubility than in water (Fig. 5.4).[36] Examples of oxygen vectors used in bioconversions are hydrocarbonsand perfluorocarbons.[37] Biotechnological efforts to develop and achieve optimal use of oxygen vectors in oxygenators have been reported.[38] In order to explain the role of oxygen vectors in

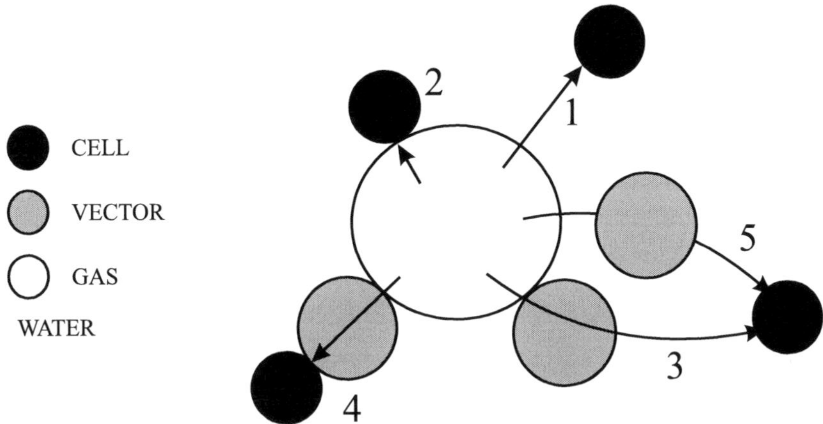

Fig. 5.4 Possible pathway of oxygen transfer from gas bubbles to microorganisms in the presence of oxygen vectors

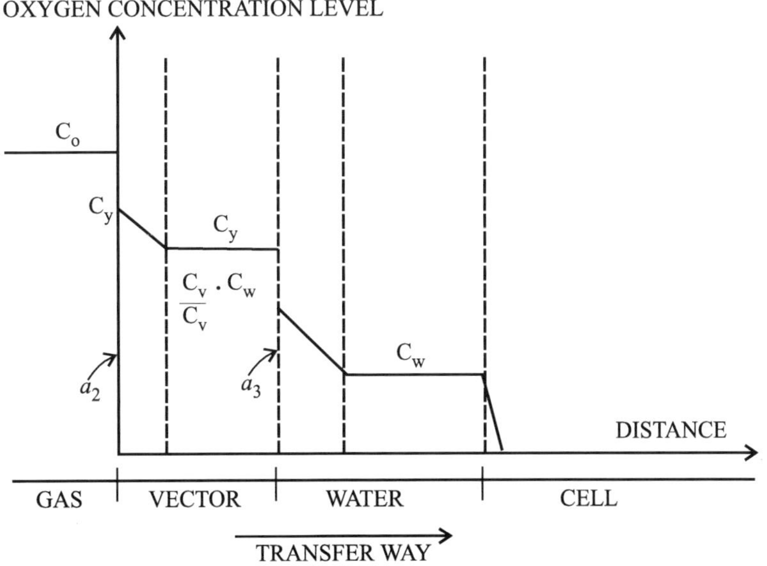

Fig. 5.5 Oxygen transfer from gas bubbles to cells via the oxygen vector

processing systems, some mechanisms have been proposed which need to be experimentally verified. In an oxygen vector-mediated biosystem, four phases exist. These are: gaseous phase (e.g., air), liquid organic phase (the vector), aqueous phase (nutrient water solution), and solid microbial cells. As shown in the figure, the oxygen transfer profile from gas bubbles to cells may take five routes incorporating the fifth vector pathway to propose a mechanism explaining the enhancement of oxygen transfer rates (Fig. 5.5).

From the above discussions, assuming that air at or near atmospheric pressure is used to supply oxygen to cellular systems in aqueous biomedia (thus fixing the maximum value of the driving force), the only variables that may be changed to effect an increase in oxygen mass transfer rate are K_L and a. Besides the Whitman film theory, as discussed above, several other theories are also available based on Fick's law of diffusion. They have been proposed in an attempt to provide a physical developmental explanation of K_L and its components.

5.7 MIXING/AGITATION IN BIOFLUIDS

As discussed in previous section in aeration in form of bubbling or sparging imparts some mixing action in the liquid. Mixing and agitation are used for blending of liquid. Mixing, actually, describes more precisely an operation in which two or more materials are intermingled to attain a desired degree of uniformity. Agitation on the other hand describes those operations by which turbulence in a liquid is promoted. Mixing and agitation find wide applications in microbial engineering processes. Depending on the nature of fluid and the mixing vessel different types of impellers are used to achieve the required degree of blending (Fig. 5.6).

Impeller Types

Propellers: The marine propeller is a relatively small, high speed impeller widely used in low viscosity liquid systems. It has a high rate of flow displacement and generates strong currents in an axial direction. Speed of rotation will vary from 400 rpm for large diameter propellers to 1750 rpm for those having smaller diameters.

Turbines: A flat blade turbine (FBT) impeller is widely used in many submerged microbial/ biochemical reactions. A FBT consists of several straight blades mounted vertically on a flat plate. The blades of some turbine impellers are curved or tilted from the vertical. Fish fin impeller is another example of this type. In this type of impellers rotation is at moderate speeds and fluid flow is generated in a radial and tangential directions.

Paddles: Paddle impellers range in design from a single, flat paddle on a vertical shaft to a battery of multi-blade flocculators mounted on a long, horizontal shaft. These impellers run at a slow to moderate speed (2 to 150 rpm) and are used to mix high viscosity liquids. Radial and tangential currents are generated during rotation of paddles. In selection in most cases it is basically the same as that of a turbine with large D_i/D_t ratio—for such applications as blending of viscous non-Newtonian fluids.

Hydrofoil Impellers: These are a class of axial flow impellers[107, 108] with low power numbers than pitched blade turbines. They have been designed to produce high flow with low turbulence.

Impeller Selection: Each of the impellers discussed above has its own characteristics and suited for particular services. Although in some cases two impeller types may perform equally good, but, in general, a given service will be satisfied best by only one. In microbial reaction system impeller shear forces and conversion of impeller power input into heat are important factors. For filamentous and mycelial systems high impeller shear stress may cause disruption of the cells leading to less product yield. Also, all the power input into the biological fluids where the microbial cell cize increases, is eventually converted into heat at the rate nearly 2545 BTU/hr/HP. It needs adequate control of temperature in the biological systems which are thermosensitive. Therefore heat transfer phenomenon has a great significance to regulate microbial reactions and accordingly impeller type should be selected. Types include flat blade turbine (FBT), pitched blade and curved blade. In mycetial fermentations fish fin impellers have been found to be suitable as it suited in many other biological sustem.

As the K_L term in K_La is relatively insensitive to agitation intensity, the area per unit volume is the primary cause of change of K_La. In effect, a better dispersion of the gas to finer bubbles causes an improvement in the measured K_La. One of the important features of agitator drive selection procedure considered for various levels of gas dispersion, superficial gas velocity, and equivalent volume—enables the selection of commercially available turbine agitators. Turbine agitators are identified in terms of prime-mover power, H_P and shaft speed, N. Tables are available in condensed versions listing turbine agitators capable of producing gas dispersion levels ranging from 1 to 10 in equivalent—volume sizes ranging from 750 to 75,000 gal for gas velocities of 0.07 and 0.20 ft/sec.

At higher levels of gas dispersion, agitator selections become independent of superficial gas velocity and are a function only of equivalent volume, defined as Veq = SgV where Sg is specific gravity of the liquid and V is volume of the ungassed liquid. At lower levels, where proximity to flooding affects the degree of gas dispersion, the selection are functions of both superficial gas velocity and Veq.

High Shear Impellers: High shear agitation includes applications generally known as emulsification, dispersion or homogenization. It is the relatively narrow processing area lying between the agitation intensity of conventional impellers at high P/V and the shear forces generated by homogenizers or colloid mills. Proper selection of impellers for this service involves maximizing the impeller head $N^2D_i^2$ and minimizing the flow ND_2^3. This is done by using a relatively small D_i/D_t ratio, a high speed and small blade area. For a quantitative evaluation of the performance of various impeller types a paper by Fondy and Bates (AHChE J, 9, 338, 1963) provides good reference.

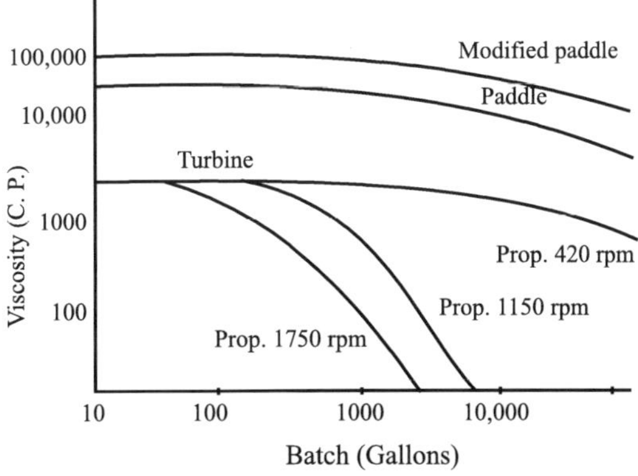

Fig. 5.6 Agitator selection — Effect of viscosity and volume

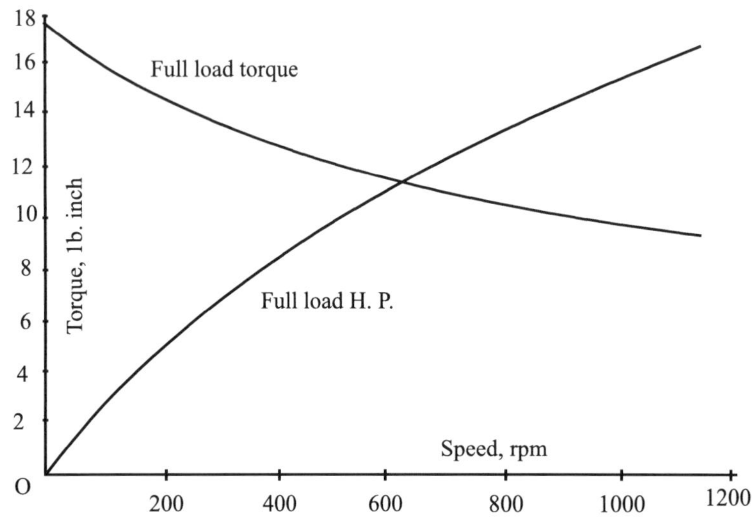

Fig. 5.7 Torque, speed characteristics of FBT (Bench Scale Equip. Co. Dayton, Ohio)

Based on predominant flow pattern impellers are grouped under three heads as below (Fig. 5.8)

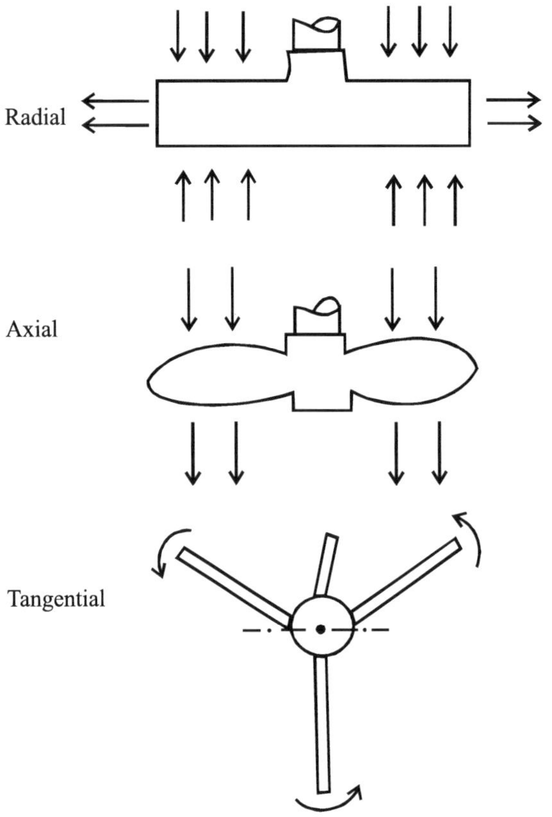

Radial

FBT is a non-swirling, low viscosity system is an ideal example.

Axial

Ex. Marine propeller, Hydrofoil impeller.

Tangential

Any impeller at a low apparent viscosity if swirl exist, occurs usually with paddle at high viscosities.

Fig. 5.8 Flow pattern classification of impellers

Impeller Design Factors : In submerged microbial reactions FBT is widely used. In designing an impeller for a stirred tank bioreactor its geometry should bear proper dimensional ratio with tank geometry. Conventional ratios of the dimensions in a FBT are as below.

(i) $\frac{\text{Impeller diameter}}{\text{Bioreactor diameter}} = \frac{D_i}{D_i} = 0.3 \text{ to } 0.5$

(ii) $\frac{\text{Sparger to impeller spacing}}{\text{Bioreactor diameter}} = \frac{H_r}{D_t} = 0.33$

(iii) $\frac{\text{Impeller pitch length}}{\text{Impeller diameter}} = \frac{B}{D_t} = 1.0 - 1.2$

(iv) $\frac{\text{Impeller blade width}}{\text{Impeller diameter}} = \frac{W_i}{D_i} = 0.20$

(v) $\frac{\text{Impeller blade length}}{\text{Impeller diameter}} = \frac{L_i}{D_i} = 0.25$

(vi) Sparger to impeller spacing Hr = 1/3 D_t

(vii) Blade weight of the impeller
(4 blade turbine) weight = $(0.35\ D_i\ Hp/N)^{1/2}$

(viii) Baffle ratio = $\frac{N_b W_b}{D_t}$

N_b = Number of baffles,
W_b = Width of baffles
D_t = Tank diameter

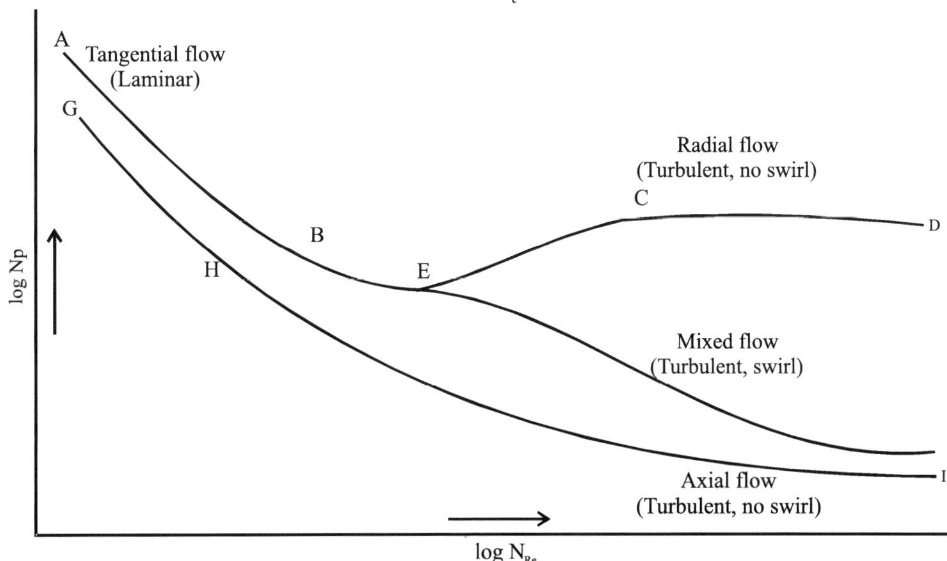

Fig. 5.9 Characteristic impeller power curves

Power Theory : Power theory has been discussed for many years. Impeller power data available are mostly based on a simplification of the full correlation. Assuming full geometric similarity of impeller system and considering gravitational effects, the relationship is

$$N_p = K\,(N_{Re})^a\,(N_{Fr})^b$$

Where N_p and N_{Re} are power and Reynolds numbers respectively and are dimensionless. Here N_{Fr} is also a dimensionless number, known as Froude number and a and b are exponents where as K is a constant. Gravitational force represented by N_{Fr} is effective only when flow is turbulent and vortex is formed around the axis of the impeller. Characteristic impeller power curves in the figure 5.9 is the typical representation of the simplified relations.

Power Input : The productivity of most aerobic fermentations depends greatly on the aeration capacity and blending efficiency in the liquid. Aeration capacity and blending efficiency in turn are related to energy consumption. Power input defined as the rate of doing work or the rate of flow of energy provides a measure of energy consumption. In SI units power is measured in watts (W). The traditional units of power is hp (550 ft lbf/s) which is related to watt as 1hp = 745.7 W.

Electrical energy is determined as the quantity of power supplied over a period of time (t). Thus energy = Pt with the units of KWh [Electrical power P = current flow (A) × electrical potential (v)]. The power input is conventionally expressed as hp/100 gal which in SI units is equivalent to 1.64 KW/m^3. It is difficult to correlate the impeller power input in gassed and non-gassed system to operating and geometric parameters of the bioreactor by analytical approach. When the analytical approach does not yield a solution, the technique of dimensional analysis may be used in the rational treatment of a problem.

Here

$$N_P = \frac{P g_c}{\rho N^3 D_i^5}$$

P = Power, g_c = Gravitational conversion constant
ρ = Density, N = Impeller speed, D_i = Impeller diameter

$$N_{Re} = \frac{\rho N D_i^2}{\mu}$$

μ = Viscosity

In the laminar range, the slope shown (A-B and G-H) are typical for all types of impellers. In this range the slope is -1 and the relationship is (Fig 5.9)

$$P \propto \mu N^2 D_i^3$$

In the turbulent range (C-D and point I) where the slope is zero, viscosity has no effect and

$$P \propto \rho N^3 D_i^5$$

In the transition range the change from laminar to fully turbulent flow is gradual, but the curves for various impeller types differ in shape and extent. Both μ and ρ have an effect on power.

5.8 DEVELOPMENTS IN PHYSICAL CONCEPTS IN LIQUID PHASE OXYGEN TRANSFER COEFFICIENT (K_L)

5.8.1 Stagnant Film Concept

Whitman[27] based his film theory on Fick's first law. In this concept, oxygen mass transfer occurred by molecular diffusion through a thin film in stagnant fluid underlying the surface of the bulk liquid phase. His theory is shown as,

$$(K_L)_W = \frac{D}{h} \tag{5.15}$$

D is the diffusivity of oxygen in the fluid/liquid.

5.8.2 Penetration Concept

The assumptions made by Whitman in proposing his theory were modified by Higbie in his penetration theory.[39] He assumed that contact between gas and liquid occurs in a series of intermittent steps, and the length of time (t_c) that each element remains in contact with the gas is constant. On the basis of these assumptions, Higbie showed that

$$(K_L)_H = 2 \cdot \sqrt{\frac{D}{\pi t_c}} \tag{5.16}$$

where t_c is the time of contact between gas and liquid in hours.

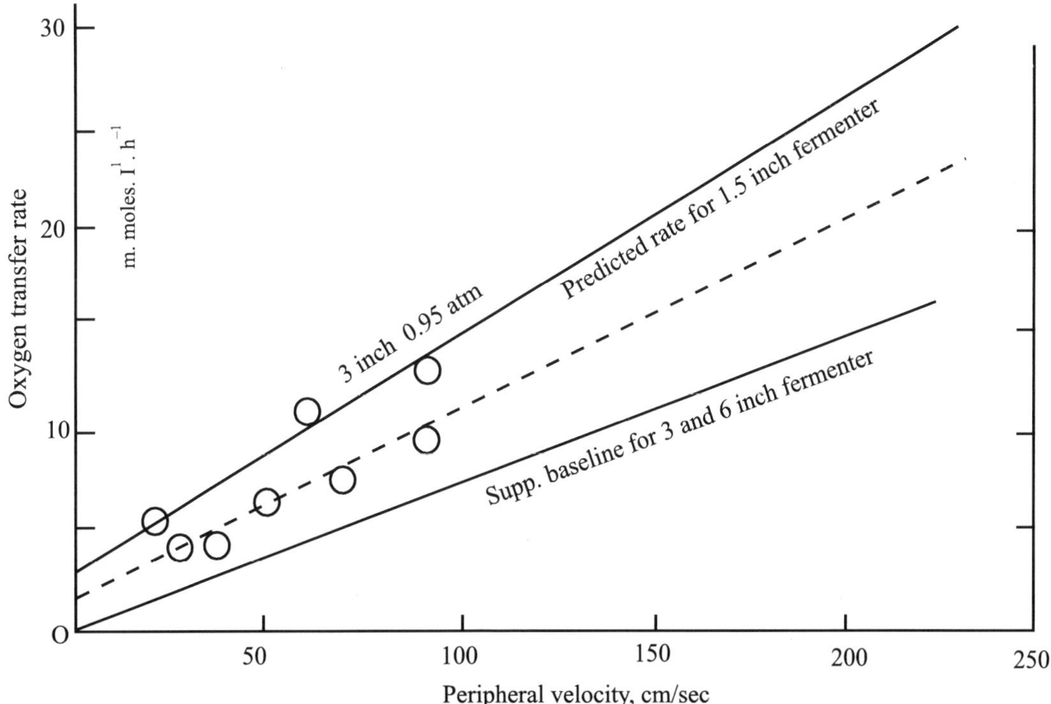

Fig. 5.10 Oxygen transfer rates in the 3.8-cm diameter fermentor at 0.95 atmospheric pressure

5.8.3 Surface Renewal Concept

Danckwerts [40] proposed a modification to the penetration theory of Higbie. It did not require the assumption of constant time of contact betweeen the gas and elements of the liquid surface, and it considered continuous surface renewal of gas in the liquid. According to his surface renewal theory,

$$(K_L)_{/D} = \sqrt{DS} \tag{5.17}$$

where S is the fractional rate of surface renewal per hour.

Kishenevsky,[41] in a critical appraisal of the theoretical work of Danckwerts in the field of gas–liquid absorption, noted several inconsistencies in the surface renewal theory. Therefore, he concluded that Danckwert's quantitative theory, based on the concept of molecular diffusion mechanism of mass transfer during the period of surface layer renewal, was contrary to the experimental data. This divergence of opinion concerning the physical meaning of K_L led to extensive studies on the oxygen mass transfer coefficient in gas–liquid absorbers. In a conventional air sparged and stirred bioreaction system, it is difficult to study K_L independent of the area term a, because the gas–liquid interfacial area available for oxygen mass transfer can not be determined with any degree of accuracy. Because of this difficulty, it was necessary to design a bioreactor system with a defined total surface area, through which gas–liquid transfer could occur and in which the dependence of K_L on hydrodynamic conditions could be studied by varying liquid flow or stirring intensity in absorption by the liquid film having a large surface area.

5.8.4 Simultaneous Adsorption-Absorption Concept

In discussing controlling factors in liquid film absorption, a hypothetical case[42] has been propsed in which the gas was completely insoluble in the liquid and could be adsorbed only on the surface. For such a case, the transfer rate of the gas would depend only on the rate of new surface generation instead of diffusion through a liquid film. It was proposition by Hartman[43] that, in all probability, without adsorption, no absorption would occur, although adsorption might occur without absorption. It was also stated that before absorption can take place, the surface must be wetted by the substance to be absorbed. In order to wet the surface by the substance, it must be adsorbed first on the surface. To verify this, Phillips[44] conducted experiments in the horizontal rotary thin-film bioreactor (HRTFB) of 3.8 cm diameter and 92 cm long using *Candida utilis* fermentation at 0.95 and 1.95 atm pressures. The results are shown in Figure 5.10. Analysis of these results showed that the theoretically calculated amount of air that could be accommodated on 1 cm^2 surface was 9.7×10^{-7} mmol, which is in close conformity with the reported values with other gases. Considering that air contains 21% oxygen, the amount of oxygen that would be carried into the liquid when rotating surface liquid film was submerged would be theoretically 2.04×10^{-7} mmol/cm^2. This value compares most favorably with the value 2.0×10^{-7} mmol/cm^2 determined from the experimental results of Phillips (Fig. 5.10) as mentioned above. Based on these reports and his findings, Phillips proposed a modified oxygen transfer rate equation in the liquid as

$$\frac{dC_L}{dt} = K_La\,(C^* - C_L) + 9.7 \times 10^{-7} \cdot A_f \cdot Y \tag{5.18}$$

Here, the first term contributes for absorption and the second term for adsorption of oxygen in the liquid medium. A_f and Y are indicating the rate of surface formation or submergence

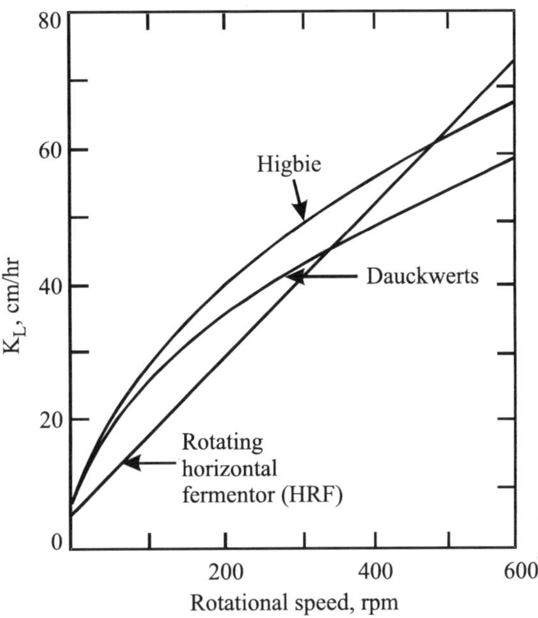

Fig. 5.11 Comparison of values for K_L determined in the 3-in. diameter HRTFB with those calculated from different theories

($cm^2\,h^{-1}$) and volumetric or mole fraction in the gaseous phase of gas being absorbed. Thus, the above equation may be referred to in defining the simultaneous adsorption–absorption concept.

5.8.5 Comparison of Concepts

If it is assumed that the rate of fraction of surface renewal is equivalent to the reciprocal of contact time K_L in Higbie's concept, then the ratio

$$\frac{(K_L)_H}{(K_L)_D} = \frac{2}{\sqrt{\pi}} = 1.13 \tag{5.19}$$

applies. Thus, the value of Danckwerts $(K_L)_D$ is 1.13 times as large as Higbie's $(K_L)_H$. A comparison of values of K_L in different concepts is shown in Fig. 5.11. It should be noted that both the Higbie and the Danckwerts theories predicted that K_L should vary nonlinearly with the time of contact or fractional rate of surface renewal. The validity of the same could be checked by Phillips, as shown in Fig. 5.11. However, in the case of HRTFB, the relation was linear for surface renewal over a wide range of values. Shake flasks and unbaffled stirred vessels with surface aeration were not suitable for such a study, since the surface area in either system was difficult to define and varied as the shaker or stirrer/agitator speed was changed. In addition, the surface-to-volume ratio was unfavorable for obtaining high oxygen transfer rates. Wetted-wall columns have been used for gas-liquid transfer studies. However, the rate of flow down or up the wetted wall is limited by gravitational force, and the requirement for recirculation of the fermentation liquid dictated an aseptic pumping operation.

Heaviside Theory (HST) based Concept:

In oxic bioprocess engineering system in liquid culture transfer of oxygen from air to liquid has been measured by fast response steam sterilizable dissolved oxygen probe on line. In the measurement, the concept of flow of oxygen from higher concentration (heaviside) to lower concentration has been conceived. Thus, heaviside theory (HT) in oxygen transfer is of significance. The first aim of the present work is to make a mathematical foundation of HT pertaining to simple air-liquid contacting system that prevails in bio-liquids. With this primary objective we have considered unsteady state mass transfer of oxygen into aqueous water. Thus, our starting point was the second law of diffusion equation,

$$\frac{\partial C_L}{\partial t} = D\frac{\partial^2 C_L}{\partial z^2} \tag{5.20}$$

Its transformed dimensionless relation is

$$\frac{\partial \pi}{\partial \tau} = \frac{\partial^2 \pi}{\partial \xi^2} \tag{5.21}$$

in which $\pi = \frac{(C_L - C_O)}{(C^* - C_0)}$, $\tau = \frac{Dt}{l^2}$ and $\xi = \frac{z}{l}$

Its Laplace transform gives

$$F(\xi,s) = L(\pi(\xi,\tau)) = \int_0^\infty \pi(\xi,\tau)e^{-s\tau}d\tau \tag{5.22}$$

From this one may arrive at

$$L\left(\frac{\partial^2 \pi}{\partial \xi^2}\right) = \frac{d^2F}{d\xi^2} \tag{5.23}$$

which by proper substitution results in

$$\frac{d^2F}{d\xi^2} = sF \tag{5.24}$$

On solving equation 5.24 one gets

$$F(\xi,s) = \frac{1}{s}\cosh\sqrt{s}\xi - \frac{1\cosh\sqrt{s}}{s\sinh\sqrt{s}}\sinh\sqrt{s}\xi \tag{5.25}$$

or

$$F(\xi,s) = \frac{1}{s}\left[\frac{1\sinh(1-\xi)\sqrt{s}}{\sinh\sqrt{s}}\right] \tag{5.26}$$

which has two poles. Considering these poles, from HT one gets

$$H(\xi,\tau) = L^{-1}(F(\xi,s)) \tag{5.27}$$

or

$$H(\xi,\tau) = E(t) = 1 - \xi - \frac{2}{\pi}\sum_{n=1}^{\infty}\frac{e^{-n^2\pi^2\tau}}{n}\sin n\pi\xi \tag{5.28}$$

or

$$1 - E(t) = \xi + \frac{2}{\pi}\sum_{n=1}^{\infty}\frac{e^{-n^2\pi^2\tau}}{n}\sin n\pi\xi \tag{5.29}$$

or

$$1 - E(t) = \frac{z}{l} + \frac{2}{\pi}\sum_{n=1}^{\infty}\frac{e^{-n^2\left(\frac{C_L - C_o}{C^* - C_o}\right)^2\frac{Dt}{l}}}{n}\sin n\left(\frac{C_L - C_o}{C^* - C_o}\right)\frac{z}{l} \tag{5.30}$$

In this relation, E(t) denotes millivolt probe reading. Significance of the equation and symbols in terms of fastness of the probe response was explained earlier.

Further reading

1. S. Aiba, J.I. Koizumi, J. ShiRu and S.N. Mukhopadhyay, *Biotechnology and Bioengineering*, Vol. 26, 1984 pp 1136-1138
2. S.N. Mukhopadhyay, *Indian Chemical Engineer,* Section A 43(3), 2001, pp 147-151.
3. J.E. Bailey and D.F. Ollis, *Biochemical Engineering Fundamentals*, McGraw-Hill Book Company, 2nd edition, New York, 1986, pp 524-532.
4. N. Piskunov, *Differential & Integral Calculus*, Mir Publishers, Moscow, 1969, pp 854-857.
5. V. Matta, S.N. Mukhopadhyay, *In Biohorizon 2003,* Abstr.BE 28, Organized by B.E.T.A, I.I.T. Delhi, March 7-8, 2003.

5.8.6 Additional Information

Revolving drums equipped with internal baffles and buckets or concentric horizontal rotary cylinders with spargers were used in the microbial production of gluconic acid.[9,10] Various types of horizontal thin-film rotary bioreactors/fermentors have been used with diverse objectives (Fig. 5.12 and 5.13). The rotational speed of these drums/cylinders was limited to only 13-20 rpm because of foam formation caused when the liquid was aerated. It was reported that at very low rotational speeds of this type of gas-liquid contactor, K_La was found to decrease appreciably. At lower speeds, surface renewal rates of the liquid film around the inner periphery of HRTFB are slow, so a low K_La results (Fig. 5.14). At high rotation speeds, oscillation of the bulk liquid inside the vessel may occur because of liquid drag. However, in the fermentations thus far investigated in HRTFB, low rotational speeds have been used. At such speeds, oscillation of bulk liquid does not appear because of low drag force. When air is allowed to flow through an HRTFB, oxygen is mainly absorbed in the thin film of liquid formed on the peripheral surface when the rotational speed is low with no oscillation in bulk liquid. Oxygen transfer behavior of the system can be analyzed with the assumptions that (1) there is negligible change in the specific surface area of oxygen transfer due to an increase in rotation speed; (2) liquid film thickness is uniform and small, so that the distance from the center of the vessel to the film surface is approximately equal to the radius of the vessel; and (3) the angle formed by the film surface edges with the center of the vessel is constant under nonoscillating conditions of the bulk liquid. Under these conditions, the specific liquid film surface renewal per unit contact time with the gas can be written as[45]

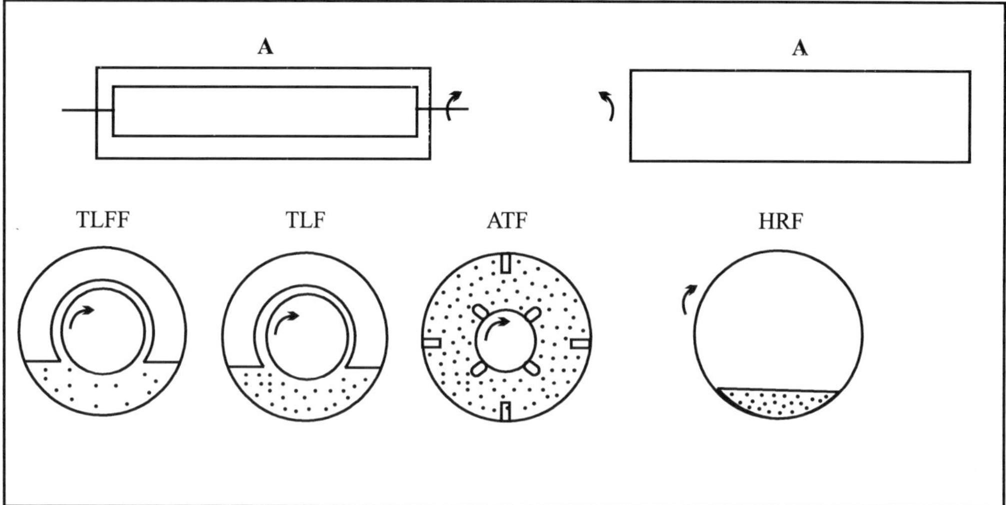

Fig. 5.12 Bioreactors with thin-layer characteristics

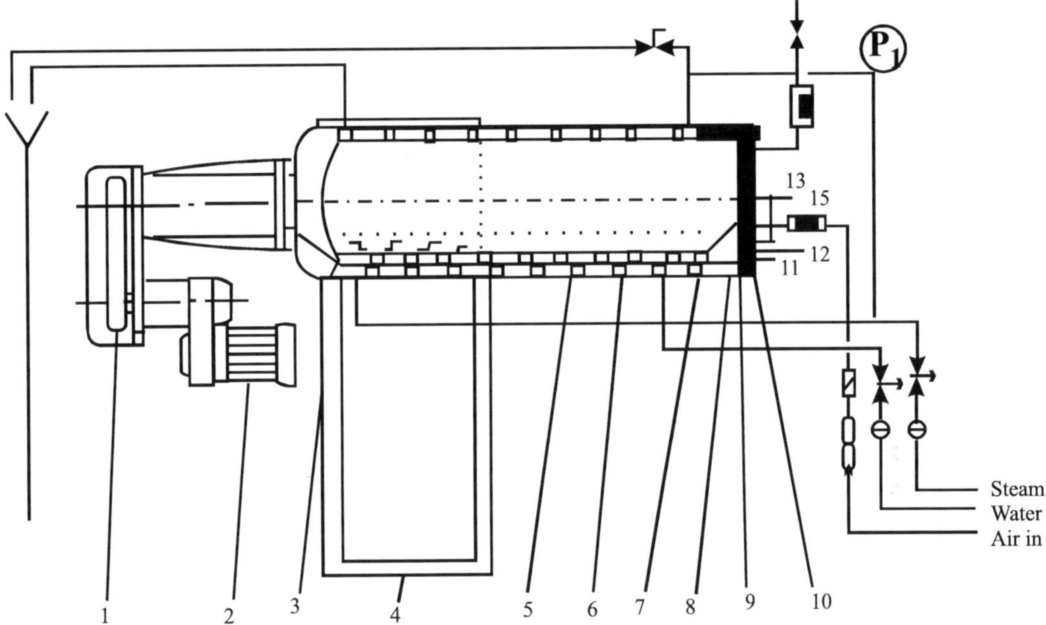

Fig. 5.13 A typical HRTFB (BERC, IIT. Delhi, Design). (1) chain drive; (2) variable-speed drive; (3) mechanical shaft seal; (4) switch and speed control board; (5) chamber for condensate; (6) cooling tube; (7) sliding bearing; (8) packing rings (9) gland; (10) cover; (11) temperature probe; (12) DO probe; (13) pH probe; (14) spindle shaft; (15) air filter

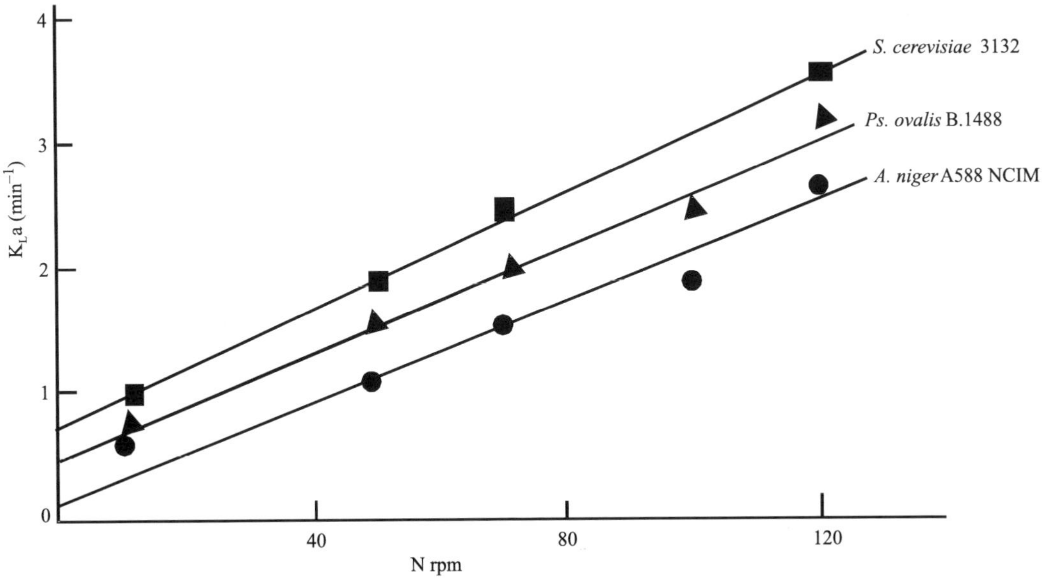

Fig. 5.14 K_La as a function of rotation speed of the HRF

$$\frac{a'}{t_c} = \left(\frac{2\pi rl}{V}\right) \cdot \left(\frac{\theta}{360}\right) \cdot N \tag{5.31}$$

where

a' is specific liquid film surface renewal (cm^2/cc);
t_c is contact time between liquid film surface and gas (min);
r is distance of the liquid film from the center of the vessel = radius of the vessel (cm);
l is longitudinal length of the liquid film (cm);
v is volume of the culture liquid in the fermenter, (cc);
θ is angle formed by the film surface and the center of the vessel, (deg); and
N is rotational speed of the fermenter (min^{-1}).

Therefore, from the equation above, the fraction surface renewal rate is

$$S = \frac{1}{t_c} \equiv \frac{\theta N}{360} \tag{5.32}$$

Since the renewal of the liquid film surface exposed to gas is continuous, Danckwerts' surface renewal theory is applied to obtain the liquid film transfer coefficient K_L as :

$$K_L = \sqrt{D \cdot S}$$

or

$$K_L = \sqrt{D \cdot (\theta \cdot N/360)} \tag{5.33}$$

Since during fermentation the physical environment remains unchanged, D may be assumed constant, thus,

$$K_L \propto N^{1/2} \tag{5.34}$$

This means that with a given surface area in the HRTFB, K_L is directly proportional to the square root of the rotation speed of the vessel.

For verification of these relations, studies (Figs. 5.12 and 5.13) were carried out with different microbial systems at five rotational speeds of HRTFB. The values of K_La were determined at each speed. No oscillation of the bulk liquid was observed in the range of rpm employed. A plot of K_La as a function of rotation speed is shown in Fig. 5.14. The value of the liquid film surface area of oxygen transfer a and the angle θ formed by the liquid film surface edges with the center of the vessel were computed from the vessel's geometry. From the known values of θ, the contact time t_c between the gas and the liquid film surface areas, and fractional surface renewal rates, *S* could be determined from the above equations easily for each rotation speed, N. The variation of t_c and S as functions of N is shown in Fig. 5.15. From the measured value of K_La and the known value of a versus N plot (Fig. 5.15) indicated a linear relationship according to equation 5.34. It follows that the rotational speed of an HRTFB changes only as a square of K_L, provided the hydrodynamic conditions remain unaltered. The positive intercept on the ordinate as noticed at zero rotation speed (Fig. 5.16) represents the net transfer of oxygen through a still surface having a total area equivalent to the wetted surface exposed to air when the fermenter/bioreactor was not rotated.

In a horizontal rotary thin-film bioreactor, transport of oxygen from gas phase to liquid depends on rotation speed or peripheral velocity (V_P), thickness of the liquid film (h_f) on the rotating surface, and hydrodynamics of physical properties of liquid containing respiring microbial cells. After sparging of air in the liquid pool in the HRTFB through a longitudinal sparger, the transport of oxygen from air into the liquid takes place mostly through the rotating

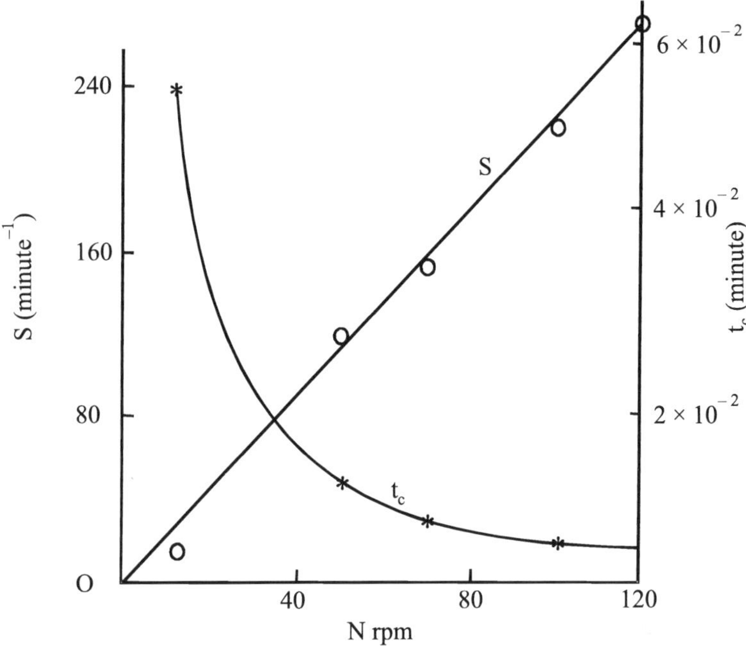

Fig. 5.15 Fractional surface renewal rate and contact time as functions of rotation speed of the HRF

liquid film having a large surface area, and a small fraction of it is absorbed due to sparging. Thus, equation 5.34 can be written in rate equation form as :

$$\frac{dC_l}{dt} = K_L a_0 (C^* - C_L) - rX \tag{5.35}$$

where $K_L a_0$ is is overall volumetric oxygen mass transfer coefficient during sparging, rX is the oxygen uptake rate in which r is the specific oxygen uptake rate and X is the cell mass concentration. In HRTFB actually,[46]

$$K_L a_0 = K_L a_f + K_L a_s \tag{5.36}$$

where $K_L a_f$ and $K_L a_s$ are the values of volumetric oxygen transfer coefficient in the rotating liquid film, and due to sparging in the liquid pool without rotation, respectively. $K_L a_o$ and $K_L a_s$ are determined by the standard method. From the difference of the known values of $K_L a_o$ and $K_L a_s$, the value of $K_L a_f$ can be obtained. The value of $K_L a_f$ is also computable as below.

$$K_L a_f = \frac{\sqrt{DS}}{h_f} \tag{5.37}$$

where S is given by equation 5.32. Combining these relations,

$$K_L a_f = K \cdot \frac{\sqrt{N}}{h_f} \tag{5.38}$$

To check this relation, the film thickness of liquid (h_f) on the rotating surface is computed from the following correlation:

$$h_f = \frac{(\mu_{am} \cdot V_p)^{2/3}}{\sigma_a^{1/6}} (\rho_a \cdot g)^{1/2} \tag{5.39}$$

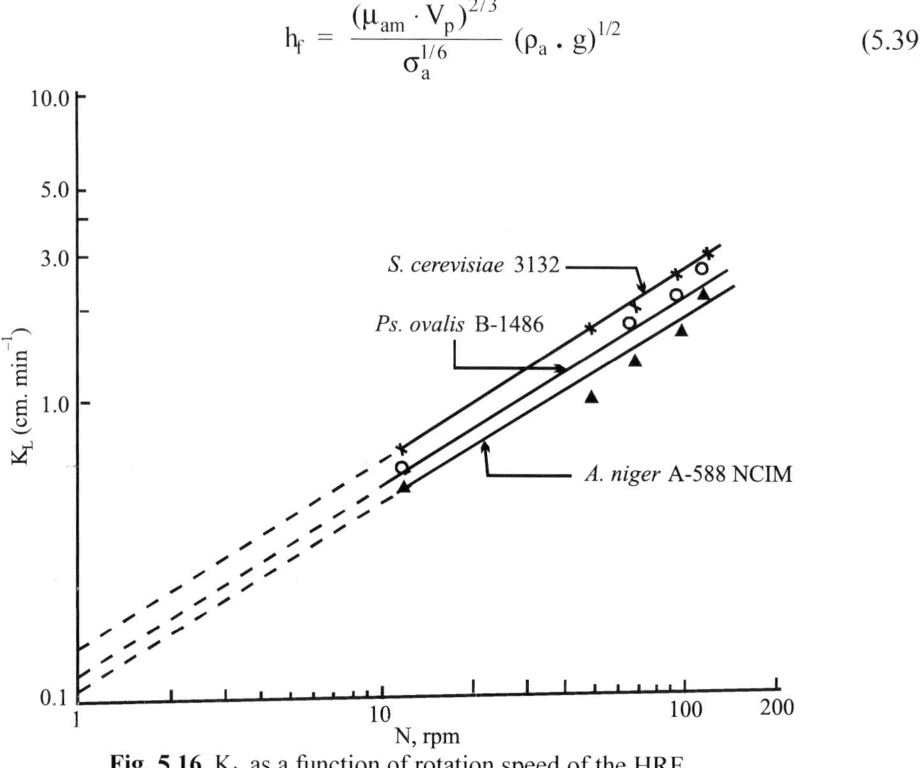

Fig. 5.16 K_L as a function of rotation speed of the HRF

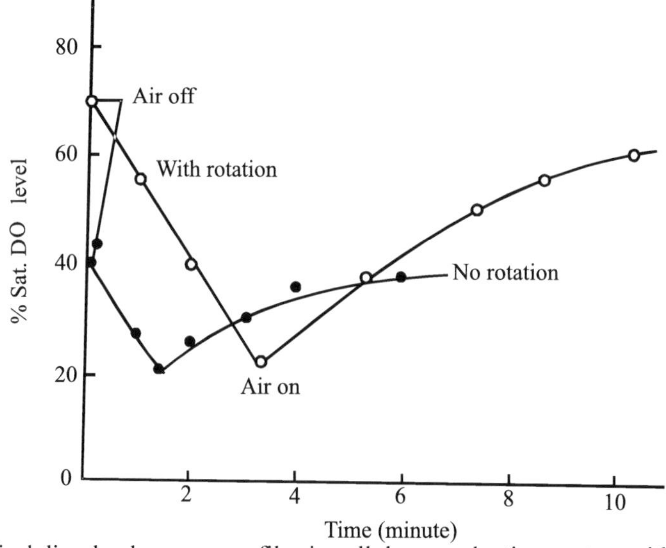

Fig. 5.17 Typical dissolved oxygen profiles in cellulase production system with and without rotation of HRF

Here μ_{am} is the value of maximum apparent viscosity, ρ_a is apparent density, and σ_a is value of surface tension, K is a constant, and g is acceleration due to gravity. In order to check the validity of the correlation experiments with *Trichoderma reesei*, QM9414 cell cultivations were conducted at different rotation speeds in a 60-liter HRTFB at 30°C for 160h. In the cultivation broth, typical dissolved oxygen traces obtained by the gassing out method with/without rotation of the HRTFB were as given in Fig. 5.17.

Evaluation of K_La_0 and K_La_s from these profiles at different rotation speeds of HRTFB showed values listed in Table 5.1, which indicated that with no rotation the value of K_La_s is very small. In the used rotation speed range, K_La_0 and K_La_f increased with the increase in reactor rotation speed. At a given V_p, when the maximum respiration of cell culture was observed, maximum cell growth rate occurred. At this state, the values of μ_{am}, ρ_a, and σ_a were measured in the cell culture liquid. Values of h_f were computed and are shown in Table 5.1, from which it was seen that the computed values of $\frac{\sqrt{N}}{h_f}$ had a correlation with K_La_f as shown in Fig. 5.18, indicating inverse proportionality. The proportionality constant was $\sqrt{D\theta / 360}$ whose value was obtained from the slope of Fig. 5.18. From this slope, the value of D was found to be

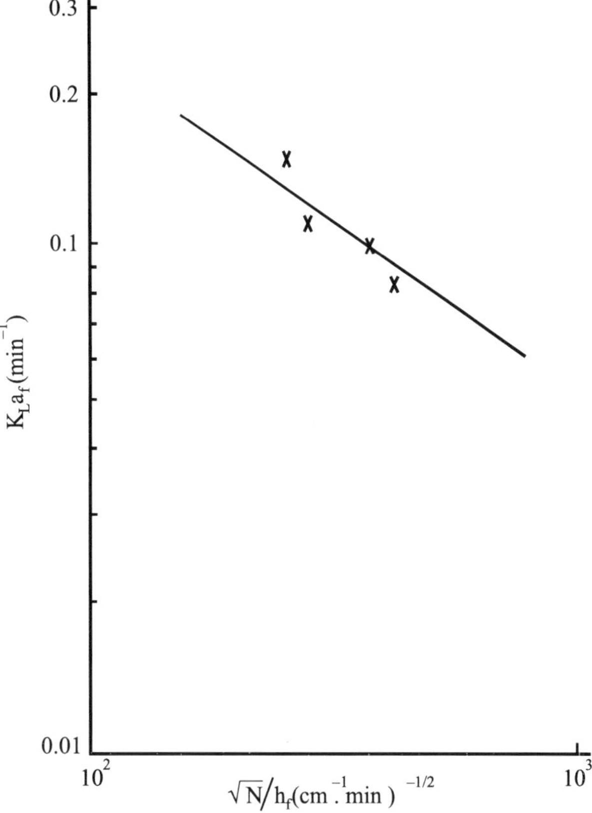

Fig. 5.18 Plot of K_La_f as a function of $\frac{\sqrt{N}}{h_f}$

Table 5.1 Values of K_La_0, K_La_f, and h_f with the variation of rotation speed (N) of HRTFB or V_p, $(K_La_s) = 0.01$ min^{-1}

N (rpm)	V_p (min s^{-1})	K_La_0 (min^{-1})	K_La_f (min^{-1})	h_f (cm)
8	8.50	0.09	0.08	0.007
15	16.00	0.11	0.10	0.011
45	48.00	0.12	0.11	0.025
80	85.60	0.16	0.15	0.036

0.20×10^{-5} cm^2 s^{-1}. This value of D is of the same order of diffusivity of oxygen in water (20°C), but the value is about 8-10 times less. The low value of D was perhaps due to the presence of solute content in the liquid.

From these results, it was concluded that in the transport of oxygen in the gas-liquid microbial system in HRTFB, liquid film thickness on the rotating surface has a great influence on the overall volumetric oxygen transfer coefficient. A large fraction of oxygen is absorbed in the liquid film having a large surface area. In stirred tank reactor mixing/agitation become advantageous by:

1. creating large air-liquid interfacial area by bubble disruption,
2. reducing the thickness of the liquid film around the air bubble thus enhancing oxygen diffusion,
3. maintaining homogenity of dissolved oxygen (DO) in the liquid by reducing resistance to bulk mixing and
4. controlling clump size, a phenomenon common with mould and actinomycetes, by reducing chances of agglomeration of cells thereby decreasing intraclump resistance.

5.9 ADVANCES IN OXYGEN ABSORPTION MECHANISM AND INFLUENCIAL FACTORS

The basic mechanism in oxygen transfer in a gas-liquid-cell dispersion has been described earlier. Dissolved oxygen in the liquid is picked up by microbial cells and consumed in metabolic processes. However, many other possible pathways of oxygen transfer in fermentation systems have been described (Tsao & Kemp, 1960, Bennet and Kempe, 1967, Muchmore, 1971; Tsao, 1970). Some of them have depicted the possibility of direct oxygen uptake from gas phase to the microbial cell, (Muchmore, 1971). Tsao (1970, 1972) has established that in oxygen absorption process the presence of microbial cells in the liquid enhances the rate of oxygen absorption. This enhancement mechanism by demarketing physical, chemical and gas-liquid-cell absorption has been illustrated in Figs. 5.19 and 5.20. It can be visualised a situation with cells totally or partially submerged in the liquid film. Foam fractionation technique of bacterial cell concentration prove that cells, infact, have a tendency to crowd themselves into the liquid film due to surface absorption. In other words, cell concentration at the bubble surface is usually higher than that in the bulk liquid.

Since cells consume oxygen molecules being absorbed right at the gas-liquid interface it is believable that cells will effect and enhance the oxygen abosorption rate. Illustration of this idea is depicted in Fig. 5.19. This enhancement factor was quantified to be

$$E = \frac{\overline{R}}{R^{o}} = \sqrt{1+M} \qquad (5.40)$$

where $M = Dk_1/K_L^{o2}$. k_1 being first order rate constant, R° is the rate per unit interface in physical absorption and $\overline{R}$ is the rate of gas-liquid interface mass transfer per unit interface.

Yagi and Yoshida (1975) has also tried to analyse the character of enhancement-factor for oxygen absorption into fermentation broth using *Candida tropicalis* in STF. Defining time avarage mass flux without viable cells as

$$N = \frac{\int_0^1 \left[C(x, T_\theta) - \bar{C}\right] dx}{T_\theta} \tag{5.41}$$

and that with viable cells by

$$N^* = \frac{\int_0^1 \left[C(x, T_\theta) - \bar{C}\right] dx}{T_\theta} + R \tag{5.42}$$

The enhancement factor, E, was given by the relation

$$E = \frac{N^*}{N} \tag{5.43}$$

In equation (5.42) R is a dimensionless oxygen uptake rate ($r_1 C_k . l^2/D_L . C_1$), which is proportional to the respiration rate r_1, and/or the cell concentration C_x for a given value of l, x, T_θ, $\bar{C}$ and *l* designates dimensionless liquid depth from gas-liquid interface (x/l), dimensionless time (D_L/l^2), the dimensionless DO concentration (C/C_1) for x > O and T = O (initial conditions) and liquid depth corresponding to half the distance between adjacent bubbles respectivily. X and t being liquid depth from gas-liquid interface (cm) and time (secs). Assuming three models as shown in Fig. 5.19 to 5.21 theoretical analysis indicated that in the usual case E has a value negligibly larger than unity, even when accumulation of microorganisms at or near the gas-liquid interface is assumed. Results of experiments with *C. tropicalis* also confirmed the theoretical prediction and thus it was concluded that except for extreme cases, the effect of respiration of microorganisms on K_La values can practically be ignored.

The above mechanisms, however, do not provide any information on the effect of air bubbles distribution and bubble coalescence and redistribution on the oxygen absorption rates in aerated mixing vessels. An integrated mechanism of oxygen absorption in fermentation systems considering distribution of air bubble sizes, concentration of DO, partial pressure of oxygen in bubbles, residence time of bubbles, the volumetric oxygen transfer coefficient, the interaction of liquid flow and moving bubbles and the rate of bubble coalescence and redispersion has been forwarded by Taguchi *et al.* (1972). Dynamic characteristics of bubble flow and mixing has been demarcated into four zones (Fig. 5.22) each with properties as described in Table 5.2. Although it is a complicated mechanism but its expertised appliance in practical system will lead to its better understanding and control.

5.10 ABSORPTION MODELS

In explaining oxygen transfer mechanisms various quantitative mathematical models have been put forwarded (Table 5.3). Need of such models are (i) as an aid to thoughts of oxygen absorption mechanism, (ii) organisation of scientific informations; (iii) quantification of concepts; (iv) system analysis, (v) parameter determination (vi) aid to control studies, (vii) explanation of ideas and (viii) data logging for optimization studies. These models are primarily a set of relationships between variables of interest in explaining the mechanism of system. System referred to here is a bioreactor or fermenter containing microbial cell suspension into which air is sparged. The absorption reaction is aimed to produce more cell mass, industrially important biochemicals or disposal of waste materials. Thus every model relates to various engineering activities.

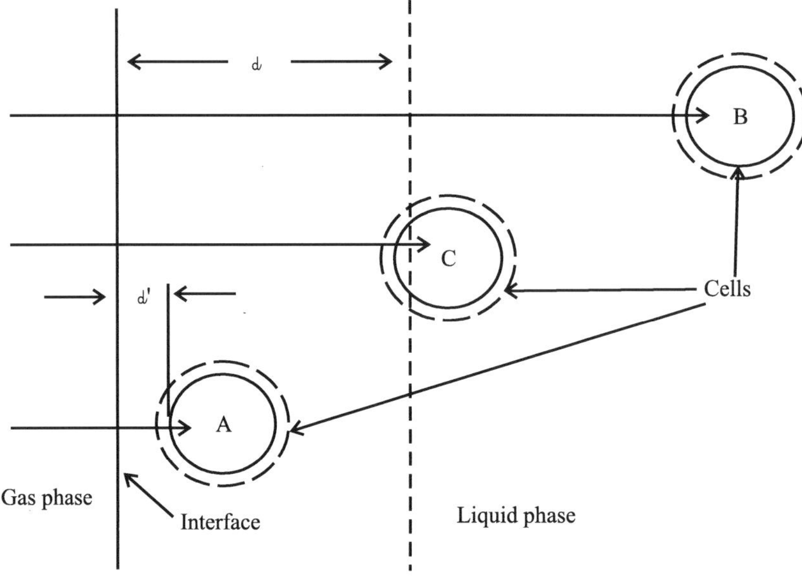

Fig. 5.19 Cells at interface and in bulk. Dotted lines show films at various interfaces

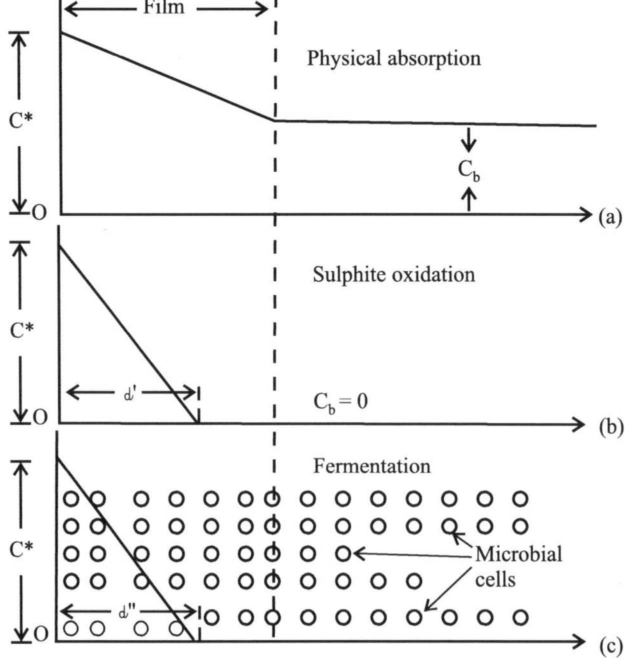

Fig. 5.20 Physical, chemical and gas-liquid-cell absorptions

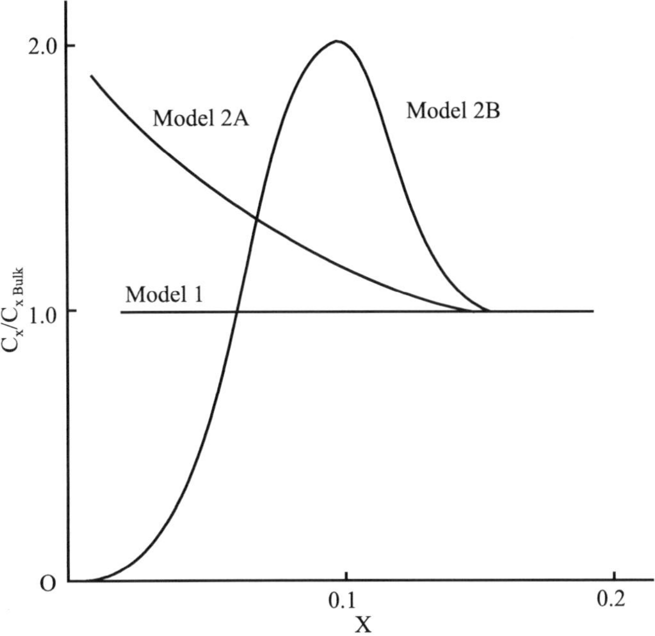

Fig. 5.21 Models for cell concentration distribution

Model 1 : Assumes the microorganisms distribute uniformly in the fermentation broth.

Model 2A : Assumes that microorganisms adhere to the gas-liquid interface and the cell concentration is maximum at the interface.

Model 2B : Assumes microorganisms accumulate near the gas-liquid interface, but the cell concentration is maximal at some distance from the interface and almost zero at the interface.

(*Yagi and Yoshida; Biotechnol Bioeng,* 1975)

5.10.1 Factors Affecting Oxygen Transfer

Volumetric oxygen transfer coefficient (K_La) serves as a determinant of aeration efficiency of a bioreactor. Maintenance of uniform K_La throughout the liquid is most important in aerobic submerged fermentation. In fact K_La is influenced by several factors as described in the following sections.

1. Broth viscosity

A relation between apparent viscosity (η_{app}) and K_La for penicillin fermentation broth was provided by Deindoerfer and West (1960). Other available informations also described the influence of broth consistency on oxygen absorption (Jarai *et al.*, 1969 and Taguchi, 1971). For same volume and similar geometry of the vessel change in rheological property of the broth changes K_La value during fermentation. Fermentation broths of penicillin, nystatin, cycloserine and some other antibiotics confer this property. They are highly non-Newtonian and contain mold myceleum in pellet or dispersed forms in the broth. A relation of change of K_La with broth consistency index (K) along with other parameters like surface tension, flow behavior index (n) and culture age of cycloserine fermentation has been provided by Jarai *et al.* (1969). A continuous decrease of K_La with fermentation age was observed. The increasing value of K and slowly decreasing value of n might be the cause of such a decrease of K_La.

A logarithmic relation between decrease of K_La and η_{app}. was shown in penicillin broth (Deindoerfer and West, 1960). Besides η_{app} other engineering parameters like power input per unit volume (P/V), impeller spacing to its diameter (S/D_i), linear air velocity (V_s), impeller speed (N) also exercise their effects on oxygen absorption capacity of the system. Mathematically, therefore,

$$K_La = f\left[\left(\frac{P}{V}\right)^{\propto}\left(\frac{S}{D_i}\right)^{\beta}(V_s)^{\chi}\,N^{\delta}\,\eta_{app}^{-\theta}\right] \tag{5.44}$$

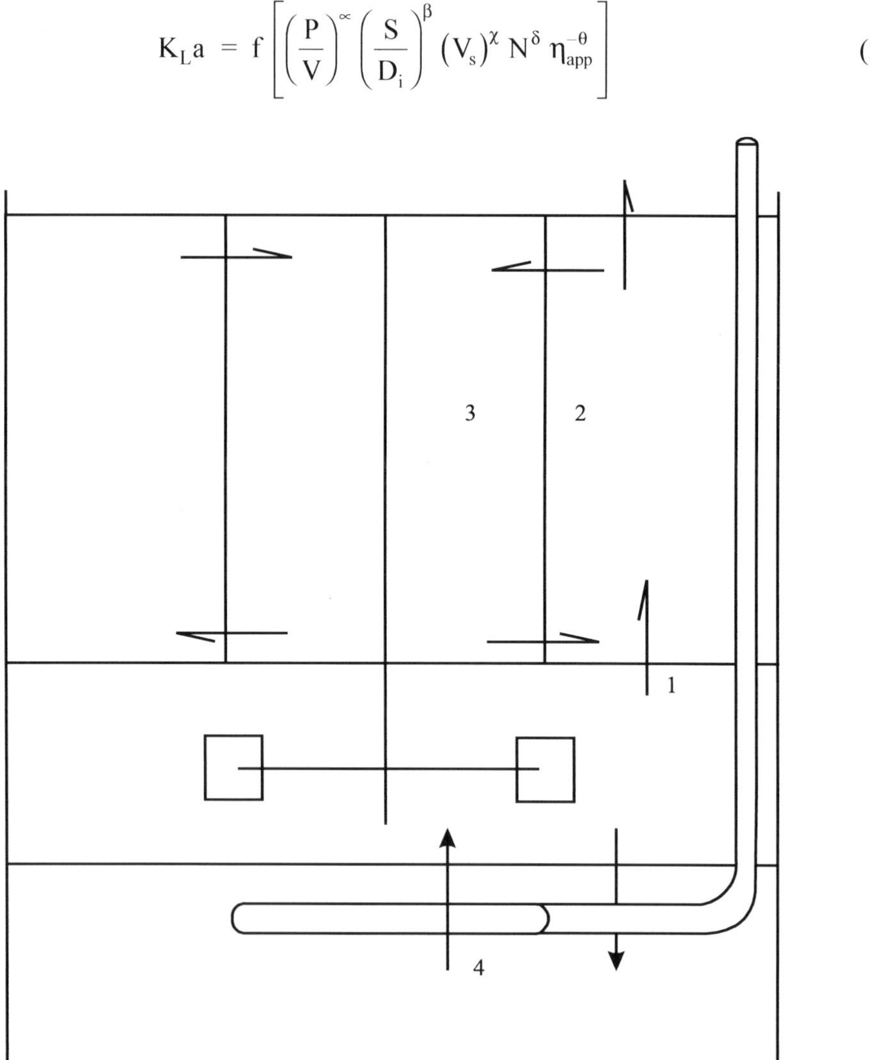

Fig. 5.22 Bubble flow pattern in gas-liquid contactor with four demarcated zones[1-4]

Table 5.3 Various oxygen transfer models useful in fermentation systems.

Sl. No.	*Proposer / Reference*	*Model*	*System Used*	*Purpose of the Model*
1	Whitman (1923) (Chem. & Met. Engg., 29, 146)	**Film model :** $DC_L/dt = K_L a (C^* - C_L)$ where $K_L = D/\sigma$, σ = film thickness	Air–water	To explain the mechanism of oxygen absorption in water.
2.	Higbie (1935) (Am. Inst. Chem. Engrs., 31, 365)	**Penetration model :** $DC_L/dt = K_L a (C^* - C_L)$ where $K_L = 2\sqrt{D/\pi t}$ t = exposure time	Air-water	To explain the mechanism of oxygen transfer modifying the limitation of non-prediction or prediction of dependence of concentration profile on time in the film model.
3.	Danckwerts, (1951) (Ind. Eng. Chem. 43, 1480)	**Surface renewal :** $dC_L/dt = K_L a (C^* - C_L)$ where $K_L = \sqrt{D \cdot S}$	Air-water	Improvement of the unrealistic consideration of specifying the same time of exposure of all elements of surface of the film as proposed in Higbie's model.
4.	Kishinevskii (1954) (J. Appl. Chem. USSR Eng. Trans. 27, 359)	**Surface breach model :** $dC_L/dt = K_L a (C^* - C_L)$ where $K_L = \sqrt{D/\Delta\tau}$	Air-water	To account for the discripancies between other models and the experimental results obtained.
5.	Bird *et al* (1962/Transport Phenomena, John Wiley, New York)	**Boundary layer model :** $dC_L/dt = K_L a (C^* - C_L)$ where $K_L = f(N_{Re}, N_{SC})$	Air-Water	To account how N_{Re}, and N_{sc} are responsible in oxygen transfer.
6.	Phillips (1961) *et al* (Ind. Eng. Chem. 53, 799)	**Simultaneous adsorption-absorption model (HRF)** $dC_L/dt = \frac{K_L a (C^* - C_L)}{\text{absorption}} + \frac{9.7 \times 10^{-7} A_f . Y}{\text{adsorption}}$	Air-fermentation liquid-cells	To account for the results obtained in HRF

Contd.

Sl. No.	Proposer / Reference	Model	System Used	Purpose of the Model
		where $K_L = 3.3 \times 10^{-5} vp + 6$ v_p = peripheral velocity of HRF		
7.	Tsao (1968) (Biotechnol. Bioeng., 10, 765)	**Model involving effect of surface active agent:** $dC_L/dt = KA_e (C^* - C_L)$ where $KA_e = (KA)_I (1-S) + (KA)_{II} S' . \left[\frac{f(C_i)}{C^* - C_L}\right]$	Air-fermentation liquid-surface active agent-cells	Explanation of the effect of surface active agents on oxygen transfer rate in fermentations considering two mechanisms (I & II)
8.	Tsao (1970) (Biotechnol. Bioeng., 12)	**Zero-order microbial reaction model :** $dC_L/dt = K_L a (C^* - C_L) . E$ where $E = K_L/K_L{}^\circ$ $= \frac{1/2 \cdot \sqrt{\pi t^* / D}}{1/2 \cdot \sqrt{\pi t^* / D} - 2/3\, t^* A}$	Air-fermentation liquid-cells.	Theoretical prediction of enhancement of oxygen transfer rate in presence of microbial cells.
9.	Tsao (1972) *et al.* (Proc. IV. IFS. : Ferment, Technol. Today 65-71)	**First order microbial reaction model :** $dC_L/dt = \overset{\circ}{K_L} a . E' (C^* - C_L)$ Where $E' = \overline{R}/\overline{R}^0 = \sqrt{1+M}$ $M = Dk_1/K_L^{02}$, K_1 = first order rate constant	(i) Air-liquids catalyst	To describe theoretical explanation of oxygen transfer with simple diagrams to present experimental evidence and there by predict mathemetical model.
10.	Bungay *et al.* (1969) (Biotech. Bioeng. 11)	**Oxygen diffusion model:** $\delta C_L/\delta t = -(R_1/D) . X + K$	Air-liquid-slime forming organism	To describe mathematically oxygen uptake in microbial slime system.
11.	Topiwala (1972) (J. Ferment, Technol. 50, 668)	**Surface absorption model:** $d(C_2V_2/dt) = Q_6C_3 + Q_1C_1 - Q_5C_2$ $d(C_3V_1/dt) = Q_5C_2 - (Q_3 + Q_6) C_3$ (dividing the system into two regions)	Air-liquid	To explain the mechanism of oxygen absorption of air from the head space of the gas-liquid contactor.

Contd.

Sl. No.	*Proposer / Reference*	*Model*	*System Used*	*Purpose of the Model*
12.	Muchmore *et al.* (1971) (Biotechnol. Bioeng. 13, 271)	**Mechanistic model of gas-cell transfer :** $dC/dt = -(XK_LA + XK_SA)C_L + XK_LAC^*$	Air-liquid-cell	Theoretical prediction of the possibility of direct gas-cell oxygen transfer.
13.	Mimura *et al.* (1971) (J. Ferment, Technol. 49)	**Gas-oil oxygen absorption model :** $dP_o/dt = (V/v)\,R\,.\,K_La\,(C_G - C_L)$	Air-oil-water	Explanation of oxygen absorption in gas-oil-water dispersion
14.	Aiba and Kobayashi (1969) (Biotechnol. Bioeng., **11**, 605)	**Oxygen transfer model in pellets** $\delta C/\delta t = D\,(\delta^2C/\delta r^2) + \frac{2}{r}(\delta C/\delta r) - \rho mQO_2$	Air-liquid-mold	Prediction of oxygen diffusion rate in mold aggregates or pellets.
15.	Taguchi *et al.* (1972) (Proc. IV IFS : Ferment Technol. Today. 83, 89)	(*i*) **With bubble coaliscence and redispersion :** $dC_L/dt = S_1\,.\,K_La/V\,(\overline{P}/H - C_G)$ (*ii*) **Without bubble coalescence and redispersion** $dC_G/dt = \frac{RT}{H}\cdot\frac{K_La}{V}\int_0^{P_0}\int_0^{\infty} A\,(p/H - C_G)\,f(v_1p)\,dv\,dp$	Air-liquid system (*i*) Air-water	To define a model integrating distribution of gas bubble sizes, DO concentration, O_2 p.p. in bubbles, the residence time, the mass transfer coefficient, the interaction of liquid flow and bubble movement and rates of bubble coalescence and redispersion.

Table 5.2: Dynamic characteristics of the bubbles in each of the four zones

Zone	*Pattern of Bubble Flow*	*Coalescence and Redispersion*	*Residence Lime*
1	Backmix flow	Vigorous	Very short
2	Plug flow	Slight	Short
3	Backmix flow	Moderate	Long
4	Plug flow	Slight	Long

where f represents a function of the variables indicated in the bracket and α, β, γ, δ and θ are exponents. Maximum oxygen transfer rate (OTR_{max}) in the broth can be computed from

$$OTR_{max} = K_L a_m (C^* - C_L) \tag{5.45}$$

where $K_L a_m$ is the maximum value of $K_L a$ under optimum operating conditions of the engineering parameters. Maximum oxygen demand over OTR_{max} can then be assessed easily. Under steady state oxygen uptake rate (OUR) would be such that

$$OUR \le OTR_{max} \tag{5.46}$$

where

$$OUR = r\, C_X \tag{5.47}$$

r being specific oxygen uptake rate, m mole O_2 consumed g^{-1} hr^{-1} and C_x is cell concentration gl^{-1}. Change in broth rheology during fermentation can affect OTR as well as OUR by increasing resistances to oxygen transfer pathways and rendering poor flow condition in the fermenter.

2. Power expenditure

With the variation of power expenditure for aeration and agitation in fermentation oxygen transfer rates vary appreciably. Quantitative relationship between power expenditure in aeration and agitation in fermentation oxygen transfer rates vary appreciably. Quantitative relationship between power expenditure in aeration and agitation has been developed by many workers (Mitchell & Miller, 1962, Kanzaki et al, 1968). Analysis of the data provided by Taguchi (1968) as shown in Table 5.4 indicates the significance of power expenditure on aeration. It shows that the agitational power (KWH/Kg broth) is increased by about two times when fermenter volume increases ten folds while air compression energy increased by about three times. At this condition total energy expenditure per kilogram of oxygen transfered is just a little over double. Data of Kanzaki *et al.*, (1968) obtained with Na_2SO_3 solution in 4200 *l* fermenter (Table 5.5) further show that for the same liquid volume a three fold increase in agitational power increases total energy requirement by two fold when OTR increased from 20 to 100 m mole l^{-1} hr^{-1}. The corresponding increase in energy requirement for air compression is five fold. Bylinkina *et al.*, (1972) observed in oxytetracyclin fermentation that OUR changes depending on the energy expended in impeller rotation with reference to various periods of its production.

Table 5.4 : Oxygen transfer rate (OTR) as a function of power expenditure in non-Newtonian broth (calculated from the data of Taguchi et al (1968))

Liquid Volume in Fermenter (liters)	*OTR m.mole l^{-1} hr^{-1}*	*Power Per Unit Vol. HP/1000.1*	*Gas Velocity in cm min^{-1}*	*Agitation Energy KWH. Kg^{-1}*	*Air Energy KWH. Kg^{-1}*	*Total Energy KWH. Kg^{-1}*
3000	23.2	0.49	95	0.49	0.102	0.592
3000	30.6	1.44	95	1.10	0.153	1.26
30000	15.5	0.35	133	0.53	0.410	0.94
30000	21.3	0.92	133	1.00	0.294	1.29

Table 5.5 : Variation of OTR with Power expenditure (Calculated from Kanzaki *et al's* data (1968)) (Fermenter Vol. 42001, Superficial air Vel. 32 cm min^{-1})

Total Energy Expanded KWH. KgO_2^{-1}	*Energy Expanded for Air Compression KWH. KgO_2^{-1}*	*Power Input Per Unit Volume HP/10001*	*Agitation Energy KWH. KgO_2^{-1}*	*OTR m. mole O_2 l^{-1} hr^{-1}*
0.359	0.102	0.22	0.257	20
0.447	0.051	0.68	0.396	40
0.547	0.034	1.32	0.513	60
0.643	0.026	2.12	0.617	80
0.720	0.020	3.00	0.700	100

3. Vessel geometry and liquid depth

Geometric parameters of the vessel have a marked effect on oxygen absorption. Influence of the ratio of impeller diameter to fermenter diameter (D_i/D_t) on oxygen absorption has been reported by some workers. The flow component of power consumption is greater and turbulence component is less with larger D_i/D_t ratio. Larger impeller with higher flow component would effect a more uniform distribution of oxygen transfer throughout the fermenter. The smaller impeller causes a high local turbulence and increased OTR in viscous fermentation fluids. However, with sulfite and non-viscous fluids all impeller diameters produce almost same oxygen absorption rate. Different conditions showing oxygen transfer coefficient as function of fermenter geometric parameters has been presented in Table 5.6.

Influence of liquid depth and fermenter geometry on oxygen absorption can be visualized from the report of Lister and Boon (1973). In deep tank agitation vessel (like batch air lift fermenter) the conventional oxygen absorption equation (5.7) requires modification as C*, which is usually assumed constant, will actually depend on liquid depth since partial pressure of oxygen in bubbles and OTR from the same depends on their position under hydrostatic head. The compositon of the air bubble flowing through out the liquid will vary from bottom to the top of the tank and with time during the experiment. The modified oxygen absorption equation will then be given by

$$\frac{dC_L}{dt} = K_La\ (C_{sm} - C_L) \tag{5.48}$$

where C_{sm} represents the average saturation concentration. Its value can be computed from

$$C_{sm} = \frac{1}{2}\ C_{si}\left[\left\{\frac{X_0}{X_i}\right\} + 1\right] \tag{5.49}$$

Here C_{si} is the saturation concentration of oxygen when water is in equillibrium with inflowing air in which the proportion of oxygen is X_i, X_0 is the proportion of oxygen in out flow air from the vessel.

Downing (1960) observed in a furrow bottomed tank that K_La and oxygenation efficiency decreased with increase in liquid depth. In a square section tank fitted with dome diffuser Lister and Boon (1973) measured DO concentration at different liquid depth and could not notice appreciable change in K_La and oxygenation efficiency at different depths. It was, therefore, contradictory to Downing's report. However, when they conducted the experiments with flat bottomed tank modified to a furrow similar to that used by Downing they could observe comparable results. It was concluded that the differences in the results obtained between furrow and square bottomed tanks was due to difference in their geometry. The vessel shape determines the hydraulic mixing pattern in the tank under different conditions of aeration. Improved mixing in furrow vessel resulted higher relative velocities of air bubbles and the liquid ultimating increased oxygen transfer coefficient. So considerations of fermenter vessel geometry and liquid depth in it are important in oxygen transfer studies.

It is clear from the above discussions in aerated well mixed STBR one may conceive the existence of distributed tiny and large air bubbles throughout the liquid in a given bioreactor/ fermenter vessel geometry and liquid depth. So, in computation/ measurement of overall volumetric oxygen mass transfer coefficient (VOMC, K_La) there will be contributions from both tiny and large air bubbles in the system. Tiny bubbles fraction receives a supply of oxygen continuously through the fraction of sparged air flowing (FQ_G) through the liquid. Considering the whole system of tiny bubbles one may write an oxygen balance equation covering this fraction as below (5.50).

$$\frac{FQ_GP^of^o}{RT} - \frac{FQ_GP^of}{RT} - (K_La)_t\left(C_2^* - C_L\right)V = 0 \tag{5.50}$$

In this equation P^o is the atmospheric pressure, f^o is the mole fraction of oxygen in the inlet, f is the mole fraction of oxygen in the tiny air bubble fraction, R is the universal gas constant, T is the experimental temperature in absolute scale, $(K_La)_t$ is the VOMC due to tiny bubbles, C_2^* is the solubility of O_2 corresponding to the tiny bubble fraction and C_L is the concentration of dissolved oxygen in the feed of the bioreactor and V is the liquid volume. In the above equation the first and second terms on the left hand side represent the rates at which oxygen flows in and out of the tiny bubble fraction, respectively. Third term in this equation represents the rate of oxygen transfer to the liquid through this fraction. The solubility of O_2 corresponding to its partial pressure in the tiny bubble fraction is computable from $C_2 = \frac{P^oY}{H^*}$, here H* being the Henry's constant. Further, also following assumption that a large bubble fraction flowing through the liquid in a plug flow manner with oxygen partial pressure (P.P.) comparable to that of the inlet air, the solubility of oxygen corresponding to its partial pressure in the large bubble fraction is given by

$$C_t^* = \frac{P^oY^o}{H^*} \tag{5.51}$$

considering that

$$C_1^* - C_2^* - N_D\left(C_2^* - C_L\right) = O \tag{5.52}$$

where C_t^* is the solubility of oxygen corresponding to large bubble fraction.

It follows from Eqn. (5.52) that

$$C_2^* = \frac{C_1^* + N_D C_L}{1 + N_D} \tag{5.53}$$

In Eqn. (5.53) N_D is a dimensionless number and its value is

$$N_D = \frac{(K_LQ)_t VRT}{FQ_GH^*} = \frac{V/FQ_G}{H/(K_La)_t RT} \tag{5.54}$$

From this relation the significance of N_D is given by

$$N_D = \frac{\text{Mean residence time for tiny bubbles to traverse through the liquid}}{\text{Characteristic time for oxygen transfer from these bubbles}} \tag{5.55}$$

From measurements, low value of N_D will indicate that the tiny bubble fraction is actively transferring oxygen. For extreme case when $N_D \to O$ equation 5.42 gives $C_2^* = C_1^*$ indicating that solubilities and oxygen partial pressure of the large and tiny bubble fractions are similar. In contrast, a high value of N_D indicates greater mean residence time of the tiny bubbles in relation to the characteristic time for oxygen transfer, which enables tiny bubbles to equillibriate with the liquid. For the case where N_D >>1 equation 5.54 simplifies to $C_2^* = C_L$. It is now possible to estimate the ratio of the rates of oxygen transfer between large bubbles (γ_l) and tiny bubbles (γ_t) that can be expressed by

$$\frac{\gamma_t}{\gamma_L} = \frac{(K_La)_t\left(C_2^* - C_L\right)}{(K_La)_l\left(C_2^* - C_L\right)} \tag{5.56}$$

substituting or C_2^* from equation 5.53 equation 5.56 becomes

$$\frac{\gamma_t}{\gamma_l} = \frac{1}{1+N_D} \cdot \frac{(K_La)_t}{(K_La)_\ell} \tag{5.57}$$

Taking a conservative estimate of $(K_La)_t$ $(K_La)_\ell = 1$and $N_D = 1$ equation 5.57 reduces to

$$\frac{\gamma_t}{\gamma_l} = \frac{1}{2} \tag{5.58}$$

This implies that in a continuously stirred tank aerobic/oxic bioreactor half of the oxygen mass transfer might be considered to take place through tiny bubbles. Also, this analysis reveals that tiny bubbles in viscous liquid cannot be assumed to equilibriate with the liquid phase.

4. Antifoam and impurities

Several reports concerning the effect of antifoam agents on oxygen transfer are available (Evans and Hall, 1971; Mimura *et al.,* 1973; Bell and Gallo, 1971). Since fermentation is usually conducted at constant temperature and pressure so thermodynamically antifoam agents make the foam unstable causing $\Delta G < v_a \Delta A$ (where ΔG is the free energy change, v_a is the surface tension and ΔA is the change in area). At this condition it destroys the surface elasticity and viscosity of the air bubble and spreads quickly over the bubble lamellae. On the basis of the above reports it appears that as the antifoam agents spread over the bubble depending on their concentration they can influence on K_La in different ways as classified below.

Decreasing Effect : It might (i) be due to formation of larger bubbles with smaller surface to volume ratio, (ii) decrease in residence time of the bubbles and hold up volume when foaming is restricted and (iii) cause additional gas liquid interfacial resistance resulting from the barrier imposed by the agent forming a film around the bubbles. Thus in bubble dispersion systems K_La decrease by antifoam can be due to the decrease of K_L or a or both.

Increasing Effect : It is due to the release of bubbles from adsorbed cells there by making it unstable and rendering larger interfacial area between air and liquid thereby increasing K_La. Bell and Gallo (1971) showed (Table 5.7) that minute amount of adventuties surface active impurities improved oxygen transfer in the liquid. The action of these contaminants was greater in the alkaline range.

Table 5.6 Correlations of mass transfer coefficient with geometric parameter obtained by various investigators.

Investigator /Reference	*Specification of the Equipment Used*	*Type and Number of Impellers/ Blades Used (n_b)*	*Values of Impeller Rotation (D_i) Used*	*K_La Correlation*
Cooper *et al.*,	$V = 27 - 67l$	Varid disc	$N^{2.85}, D_i^{2.57}$	$K_La = C\left(\frac{P_g}{V}\right)^{0.96} (V_s)^{0.67}$
(Ind. Eng. chem. 36, 504, 1994)	$D_t = 15, 21, 24, 43$ cm $D_i/D_t = 0.4$	$n_b = 16$		
Maxon and Johnson (IEC 45, 2554, (1953))	$V = 1.5l$	Propeller	$N^{1.7}, D_i^{1.2}$	
Oldshue (IEC 48,	$V = 10{,}000\,l$	Turbine	$N^{1.5}, D_i^{1.4}$	$K_La = C\left(\frac{P_g}{V}\right)(V_s)^{0.4}$
2194, 1956)	$D_t = 6.1$ m $D_i/d_t = 0.2$	$n_b = 8$		
Yamamoto (Chem.	$V = 4.6 - 5.2\,l$	Paddle	$N^{3.0}, D_i^{2.5}$	$K_La = C\left(\frac{P_g}{V}\right)(V_s)^{0.5}$
Eng. Japan, 597, 1969)	$D_t = 21.2$ cm Di = 7.0 cm	$n_b = 2$		
Friedman and Lightfoot (IEC 49, 1227, 57)	Dt = 15.1 cm Di = 3, 7.6 cm	Paddle $n_b = 4$	$N^{3.08}, D_i^{4.94}$	$K_La = C \cdot V_s \cdot N^{3.08} D_i^{4.94}$
Yoshida *et al.*, (IEC 50, 435, 1960)	Vessel Dt (cm) Di cm A 15 6 B 25 10 C 37.5 15	Vanied Disc $n_b = 16$ Turbine $n_b = 12$	$N^{1.68}, D_i^{1.73}$	$K_La = C \cdot V_s^{0.4-0.84} \times (N_3D_i^2)^{0.43-0.68}$

Contd.

Table 5.6 Correlations of mass transfer coefficient with geometric parameter obtained by various investigators.

Investigator/ Reference	*Specification of the Equipment Used*	*Type and Number of Impellers/ Blade Used (n_b)*	*Values of Impeller Rotation (D_i) Used*	*K_La Correlation*
Richards (Prog. Ind. Microbiol. 3, 141, 1961)	—	—	$N^{1.7}$, $D_i^{1.3}$	$K_La = C\left(\frac{P_g}{V}\right)^{0.4} . V_s^{0.5} N^{0.5}$
Westerterp *et al.* (Chem Eng. Sci. 18, 157, 1963)	$V = 2.2 - 570\,l$ $D_i = 14 - 90$ cm $D_i/D_t = 0.2 - 0.7$	Turbine Paddle	$N, D_i^{-0.5}$	$K_La = H_L^{-1} N D_i C_s D_t^{0.5}$
Kanzaki *et al* (J Ferment-tech. 46, 338, 1968)	V D_i/D_t 100 0.55 700 0.45 1500 0.50	Turbine	$N^{2.38}$, $D_i^{1.82}$	$K_La = C\left(\frac{P_g}{V}\right)^{0.50} V_s^{0.7} N^{0.7}$

Mimura *et al.* (1973) observed in hydrocarbon fermentation by yeast cells that air bubbles which are completely covered with yeast cells become very stable. Addition of silicone oil, however, makes such bubbles unstable and release yeast cells from their surface. It causes higher oxygen consumption rate by the cells and aids in higher oxygen absorption in the culture liquid. K_La value also becomes three times higher than K_La measured without the antifoam in the liquid. Antifoams which cause bubble coalescence and shortend residence time, reduce oxygen transfer rate by effecting mainly on gas-liquid interfacial resistance. Those lowering surface tension increase oxygen transfer rate which might be due to decreased bubble size rather than any direct-interfacial film effect.

5. CO_2 accumulation

In cases of secondary metabolism of microorganisms CO_2 plays a role, both in dissolved and in gaseous phase, on oxygen transfer in the liquid. Our present knowledge regarding the extent of this factor as a controlling one is rather limited. Inhibitory effect of CO_2 accumulation on fermentations like glutamic acid (Hirose *et al.,* 1973 & Okada and Sonoda, 1965), inosine (Shibai *et al.,* 1973) and in some other microbial fermentations are reported. Okada demonstrated that removal of CO_2 from the environment by increasing air flow rate from 0.31 to 0.50 vvm gradually increased glutamic acid yield. Observing remarkable inhibitory effect of CO_2 generated during fermentation some investigators (Richards, 1961 and Nyiri and Lengyal, 1965) have recommended for provision of ventilation in the unit operation of aeration and agitation. Aeration- agitation condition should therefore be estimated properly for scale up of submerged fermentations in which CO_2 was inhibitory. The rate of aeration is to be established to make sufficient ventilation and overcome this inhibition. A procedure of estimating aeration-agitation condition in fermentation considering both oxygen supply and ventilation is provided by Ishizaki and his associates (1973). This procedure was used in inosine fermentation. Inhibition of product formation and resistance to oxygen transfer pathway by CO_2 is not clearly understood. However, the pathways of oxygen and CO_2 as shown by Humphrey (1968) indicates that product inhibition by CO_2 might be due to (i) its action as a metabolic poison or (ii) the reduction of partial pressure of oxygen in the system thereby reducing its availability.

6. Suspended solids

Presence of suspended cells or insoluble substrates might influence on oxygen transfer property in the liquid. In order to relate the rate of oxygen transfer measured in a mixed liquor (in activated sludge) to that in a clean water Lister and Boon recommended a factor of proportionality given by

$$a' = \frac{K_L\ a \text{ in mixed liquor}}{K_L\ a \text{ in clean water}}$$

Table 5.7 : Effect of trace contaminants on OTR

Water Used	*pH of the Liquid*	*OTR m mole O_2 l^{-1} hr^{-1}*		*Foam Formation*
		Determined Values	*Mean Values*	
(i) Normal distilled water	4.0	49.2, 52	51	None
	7.5	120	120	Yes
	8.5 – 9.0	129, 119, 132	126	Yes
(ii) Double distilled water with no cleaning of reactor	7.5	105	105	Slight
(iii) Double distilled water in reactor, cleaned by chromic acid	4.0	43.5, 45	44	None
	7.5	52, 75	54	Trace

A decreasing ratio of K_La with increasing cell concentration at different agitational intensity was noticed in a n-parafin hydrocarbon fermentation (Mimura, 1973). It was believed that air bubbles covered with large number of cells resulted in a lower K_L than with normal bubbles. Also available interface area (a') between air and liquid where

$$a' = 1 - \beta' \left(\frac{D_b \cdot C_x}{V_b} \right) \tag{5.59}$$

in which $\beta' = (\frac{1}{4}\ \rho_c\ f_c D_c$ = constant) indicates that the bubble size (D_b), cell concentration C_X and air bubble hold up volume (V_b) in the liquid are important in computation of a'. Also, Mukhopadhyay and Ghose (1976) observed a decrease of K_La with increase in *Ps. ovalis* B 1486 cell concentration beyound 4.0 g l^{-1} in their studies in HRF. It was believed that this decreasing effect was probably due to over crowding of cells in the film of liquid.

7. Bubble size and ionic strength

Decrease in bubble diameter exposes greater surface area for transfer of gas from the bubble into liquid thus increasing K_La value. Benedeck and Heideger (1971) in the range of bubble size of 0.1 cm < d_{sm} < 0.4 cm observed a linear relation between K_L and d_{sm} (souter-mean bubble diameter) as given below :

$$K_L = 0.171\ d_{sm} - 0.0043 \tag{5.60}$$

This equation predicts the influence of d_{sm} or K_L within limited range of d_{sm} and indicates that in computation of K_La factors influencing bubble size distribution should be given importance. Ionic strength in the liquid is such a factor that can appreciably decrease bubble size (Calderbank, 1967; Marruci & Nicodeino, 1967 and Robinson & Wilke, 1973) even though the physico-chemical properties of the liquid remains essentially same. Fermentation liquid usually contains many ionic mineral components. The ionic strength, Γ in the liquid is defined as (Robinson & Wilke, 1973)

$$\Gamma = \frac{1}{2}\,\Sigma\, Z_i^2\, C_i \tag{5.61}$$

where Z_i is the charge on an ionic species and C_i is its concentration. In actual soluble substrate fermentation containing electrolytes a generalized correlation of $K_L a$ was obtained by Robinson and Wilke (1973) as below

$$\varepsilon = \lambda\,(P_G / V_L)^n \,.\, (V_s)^m \,.\xi \tag{5.62}$$

in which ξ is a physical property group and is given by

$$\xi = \frac{\rho_L^{0.533}\, D_L^{2/3}}{\sigma^{0.6}\, \mu L^{1/3}} \tag{5.63}$$

In these equations ε denotes $K_L a$ or $K_L^r\, a/Ø$ where K_L^r a is effective over all volumetirc mass transfer coefficient with reaction and $Ø = (K_L^r/K_L)$ is dimensionless absorption factor for mass transfer with chemical reaction, λ is a proportionality constant, m and n are exponents dependent on ionic strength of the liquid. Equation (5.62) expresses the dependency of $K_L a$ on ionic strength along with other physico-chemical parameters as ξ is dependent on density (ρ_L), viscosity (μ_L), surface tension (σ) and D_L of the liquid.

Ionic solutes in the liquid decrease average bubble size and increase dispersed gas fractional hold up. The gas hold up influences on $K_L a$ in the way as explained by Topiwala (1974).

8. Evaporation

Water evaporation during fermentation that prolongs several days can effect on oxygen transfer coefficient (Aiba *et al.*, 1973). Available information for elucidation of evaporation effect on $K_L a$ is scanty. The graphical correlation between oxygen transfer coefficient and water evaporation through the closure in shake flask is given in the book by Aiba *et al.* (1973). From this relation two possibilities might be assumed. First, evaporation might decrease oxygen absorption rate by increasing the solute concentration in the liquid. Second it might increase OTR due to greater partial pressure of oxygen inside the enclosure. However, which one of the two facts will be predominant depends on the system charateristics. Now a days in bench scale bioreactors asceptic cold finger has been installed to prevent evaporation loss.

9. Surface aeration

Fuch *et al.* (1971) determined the effect of surface aeration on $K_L a$ with air-water systems in different size of fermenters (Table 5.8) in order to include surface aeration in scale up. Power factor, N_P, defined as

$$N_P = \quad (N^3\, D_i^5/V) \tag{5.64}$$

has great relevance to surface aeration. Here denotes a function. Other symbols has the same significance as used earlier. Variation of K_La as a function of N_P showed a general trend towards decreasing K_La of surface aeration for smaller values of N_P as the fermenter size increases. It showed that a contribution of surface aeration on K_La generally increases as fermenter size

Table 5.8 : Effect of surface aeration on K_La (Fuch *et al*, Ind. Engg. Chem., Proc. Design Dev. 10, 190, 1971)

Fermenter Size (Liters)	*Surface Aeration K_La at 2 Watts / l*	*Surface Aeration K_La Per Unit Vol. $1/hr - m^3$*	*Surface Aeration K_La Per Unit Cross Sectional Area, $1/hr - m^2$*
51000	3.6	0.071	0.41
3000	15.0	5.0	8.2
550	20.0	36.0	45.0
200	110.0	550.0	390.0
10	21.0	2100.0	610.0

decrease (Table 5.8). Surface aeration K_La is shown to be related to (P/V) ratio as

$$(K_La)_{sj} = (P/V)_j^{\sigma_j} \tag{5.65}$$

in which σ_j is dependent of N_P. Oxygen transfer on the basis of unit volume of liquid and per unit cross sectional area also shows the increasing trend of surface aeration K_La with decreasing fermenter size.

5.10.2 Intracellular Oxygen Pathways

When the dissolved oxygen reaches the microbial cell surface through the bulk liquid pathway, the molecular oxygen may be transported to the interior of the cell through cell wall and cell membrane by mechanisms like diffusion, active transport, and others.[47] A typical active transport mechanism scheme of oxygen transfer inside the cell has been depicted in literature. After getting inside the cells, oxygen may participate in intercellular reaction in several pathways as depicted mechanistically in Fig. 5.23. Many microorganisms are provided with a mechanism whereby the hydrogen removed by dehydrogenation may be passed to gaseous oxygen. In this process (called cell respiration), oxygen gas serves as the terminal electron acceptor. This mechanism is also shown in the literature. The available electrons in these reactions may yield energy in a form available to the cell. In bacterial physiology in this pathway to oxygen, the removal of low hydrogen atom does not generally take place by reacting with molecular oxygen without the participation of enzymes and coenzymes. Several pathways exist in cells from substrate 2H to oxygen, namely, direct oxidation, the direct cytochrome pathway, and the indirect cytochrome pathway.

In certain oxidase enzymes, for example, the *d*- or *l*-amino acid oxidases, the involved enzyme construction can directly react with oxygen. In this pathway (Fig. 5.23), these enzymes are known to be capable of combining the 2H from the substrates. This pathway may be vital for generation of intermediates that are required by the cell. In some organisms, a few dehydrogenases (e.g., succinic dehydrogenase, Fig. 5.23A) are capable of directly reducing a series of cytochrome pigments. The latter are capable of reacting with oxygen to form water. This pathway comprises the only path out to oxygen, but it is generally of much smaller significance. An example of a cytochrome pathway is shown in Fig. 5.23B. This oxygen pathway may yield energy to the cell. The indirect cytochrome pathway to oxygen as shown in Fig. 5.23C is probably the most important. In many microorganisms, dehydrogenases reduce the nicotinamide coenzymes. In the reduced state, these coenzymes neither react with molecular oxygen nor reduce the cytochrome pigments, but they are able to reduce certain flavoproteins. Many such flavoproteins can react with the cytochrome pigments producing oxygen. Oxidation along this pathway (as shown in Fig. 5.23C) may yield energy in a form available to the cell.[48]

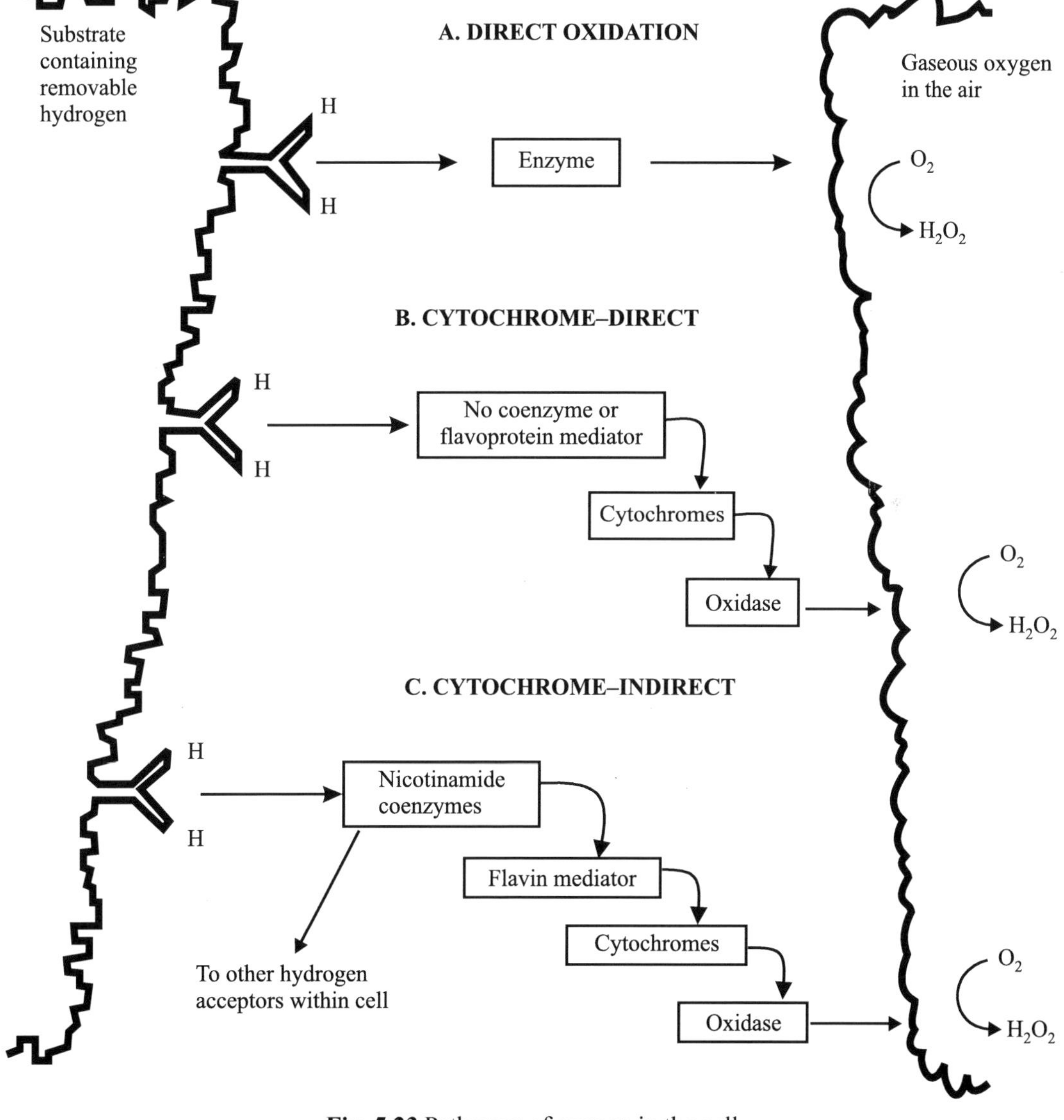

Fig. 5.23 Pathways of oxygen in the cell

5.11 MEASUREMENT OF DISSOLVED OXYGEN (DO), K_La, AND ACTIVE OXYGEN SPECIES

5.11.1 Measurement of DO

In the book, the interrelation between ionization and redox potential of oxygen has been illustrated.[102] It showed the importance of accurate measurement and monitoring of dissolved oxygen, as its solubility depends on the nature of the biomedia and operating conditions. Prior to the development of the DO electrode probe, the titrimetric method was in vogue. However, in bioprocessing this method did not simulate an actual reaction system and was prone to analytical error. Thus, its use in monitoring oxygen participation in biosystems was discarded. In essence, this chemical method of monitoring DO in biomedia is as described in the following section.

1. Chemical method

The determination of DO concentration in pure water or in waste water involves the addition of known excess quantities of a standard solution of reduced ion (such as ferrous or manganous), followed by a back titration of the excess with a known standard oxidizing agent. Among these methods, Winkler's method [49] was widely used until the development of the DO probe. In principle, this method involves the formation of a precipitate of manganous hydroxide. This is oxidized to $MnO(OH)_2$ by oxygen in the solution, which in turn oxidizes iodine. This liberated iodine is estimated by back titration with standard $Na_2S_2O_3$ solution. From these results, DO concentration in ppm can be determined using the following relation:

$$\text{DO concentration (ppm)} = \frac{\text{Normality of thiosulphate} \times \text{Vol. of thiosulphate used}}{\text{Vol. of sample taken}} \times 200 \tag{5.66}$$

2. Physical method

This method makes use of the oxygen probe which measures DO concentration in the solution directly.[50] The partial pressure of oxygen in a mixture of gases or in an aqueous liquid in dissolved form can be monitored by use of specially designed galvanic or amperometric electrodes or probes. An oxygen electrode, in principle, is a device that produces an electric current which is proportional to the DO in the liquid medium in which the probe (electrode) is placed. Various types of DO electrodes are in use to determine DO concentration in fermentation broths and other biochemical reactions. On the basis of their operational characteristics, these oxygen electrodes may be classified as in Table 5.9.

Some of these electrodes are steam sterilizable, while many are not. The most popular oxygen electrodes used for the respiratory measurements and DO concentration measurements in microbial and medical engineering systems are membrane-covered electrodes.[51] In determining DO concentration, the DO probe is placed in an electrical circuit which functions in the following most widely used way.

a. It imposes a potential difference between the oxygen electrode and some reference anode, which is ususally a calomel half-cell or Silver-Silver chloride half-cell.

b. It measures the current passing through the electrode.

Typical examples of membrane-covered polarographic and galvanic type of DO probes are shown in the literature. Basically, the current output of the probe depends on the tension of oxygen that participates in the electrochemical reaction. It is obvious that the response time of the electrode depends on the membrane type and its thickness. It is determined by the time required for an equilibrium. Oxygen gradient will be established in the captive electrolyte film and the membrane following a change in oxygen level. The average 97.5% response time for a 1-mil Teflon membrane electrode is 10 s, which for a 1-mil polypropylene is closer to 40s. Table 5.9 provides the typical 97.5% response times obtained with several oxygen electrodes having membranes of differing composition and thickness. Electrode output and response time as a function of cathode membrane and membrane thickness are given. It was shown earlier that the magnitude of the current produced by the electrode is

Table 5.9 Time of 97.5% resoponse in different DO electrodes

Electrode Type	*Membrane Type*	*Membrane Thickness (mil)*	*Output*	*97.5% Response Time (s) Air → N_2*
Galvanic (55-mil cathode)	Teflon	0.5	4.4 μA	2.0
	Teflon	1	1.63 μA	8.0
	Polypropylene	0.5	0.80 μA	10
	Polypropylene	1.0	0.222	30
Polarographic (1-mil cathode)	Polypropylene	0.5	0.80 nA	18
	Polypropylene	1.0	0.41 nA	45
	Teflon	0.125	8.3 nA	0.30
	Teflon	0.25	4.2 nA	0.60
	Teflon	0.375	3.75 nA	1.00
	Teflon	0.50	2.70 nA	2.0
	Teflon	0.75	2.34 nA	7.0
	Teflon	1.0	1.78 nA	17.0
For fermentation Polarographic (10-mil cathode)	Special Silicone Composite	—	0.110nA	44.0

1 mil = 0.00254 inch

directly proportional to the oxygen concentration, provided D remains constant.[52] The current produced when the electrode is exposed to oxygen is actually a function of the individual electrode and its functional state and environmental conditions (e.g., temperature, ionic strength of the liquid, etc.). Consequently, it is essential to calibrate the ammeter or recorder response by exposure to known concentrations of dissolved oxygen.

Two conventional reference concentrations of oxygen are selected to calibrate a DO electrode, since the current output by the electrode is usually linear with oxygen concentration.[53] The most convenient oxygen concentrations to use are those of air-saturated solution and a solution with zero oxygen content. The former is easily prepared by the continuous gentle bubbling of air through the buffer in use at the desired working temperature. Solutions with zero oxygen-content may be prepared by the following methods:

1. *Dithionite method,*[54] which includes the following steps: Span control of the amplifier/recorder is adjusted to 95-100% of full-scale deflection for the electrode immersed in an air-saturated solultion. Next, sodium dithionite solution prepared by injecting saturated solution of $Na_2S_4O_6$ (freshly prepared, pH 7.5-8, in absence of oxygen) is added to the reaction liquid in 1 : 30 v/v ratio, and a new value in the recorder is noted (usually 0-1% of the full-scale deflection). It is due to a residual current output of the electrode in the absence of oxygen. The addition of more dithionite should produce no further change, and thus it is calibrated. The demerit of this method is that prolonged exposure to dithionite causes poisoning of the electrode. Therefore, the electrode must be removed from the dithionite solution immediately after the measurement.
2. *Nitrogen discharging method,*[55] in which a standard buffer solution is equilibrated with nitrogen by discharging the gas in it. Nitrogen discharge drives out any oxygen present in the buffer, leading to a buffer with zero oxygen content.

Therefore, by measuring the current output by placing the oxygen electrode into solutions of zero oxygen content and in solutions saturated with oxygen, respectively, a standard curve is plotted which gives the relation between current/voltage output of the electrode and DO concentration in the liquid. By measuring the current/voltage output of the calibrated electrode in an unknown solution, its DO concentration can be known from this standard curve. After calibration, the probe is sterilized (if required) and is put into the bioreaction liquid asceptically or gas mixture in which oxygen is to be measured.

In medical engineering, a probe that was used to monitor oxygen tension in anaesthetic circuits (modification of Meckereth electrode)[56] utilizes a silver cathode, lead anode, and potassium hydroxide electrolyte. Oxygen used to be admitted to the electrode through a teflon membrane, which is pervious to gas, but not to the electrolyte. Oxygen is reduced at the cathode to form a hydroxyl ion in a reaction catalyzed by the silver. These ions combine with lead at the anode to form lead hydroxide. The electron flow from the lead to the silver cathode through a microammeter is a measure of the rate at which the reaction proceeds. Hence, the meter reading depends on the rate at which the external tension forces oxygen to diffuse through the membrane and contact the silver electrode. These probes are rugged, operable in any position, unaffected by humidity, and self-contained (requiring no amplifier, pump, or heat source). They are compact—a probe of this type has been used by mounting it on the tip of a cardiac catheter for *in vivo* recording of blood oxygen tensions. Their readout can be made linear and accurate to within 5% of full scale. The reading is not altered by the addition of compounds like halothane, methoxyflurane, or ether to an atmosphere of 20% oxygen and 80% helium. On the other hand, the probes are relatively expensive and short-lived. A commercial model, however, is warranted for 80,000 hours. At 21% oxygen, this would give a life expectancy of 80,000/21 = 3810 h, or approximately 23 weeks. Their response is slow, varying from one to several seconds. Carbon dioxide shows response time and in continuous exposure shortens probe life.

An oxygen probe employing a zirconium oxide galvanic electrode (similar to that described by Elliot and his associates)[57] is commercially available. Its response time is so rapid (less than 100 ms) that the effect of pulsatile blood flow is detectable in the recording of oxygen tensions during a single expiration. CO_2 has no effect on the probe output, but the presence of gaseous anaesthetic agents causes gross inaccuracy. This monitor has a built-in heater, because the probe must be operated at 8.50°C. It also incorporates a vacuum pump and an amplifier.

3. Biological method

In this method, a highly selective flow system has been used by coupling immobilized whole biocells or enzymes with electrochemical sensors. In principle, two types of biosensors have been reported.[58, 59] The first type consists of enzyme or biocell electrodes in which immobilized whole biocell or enzyme is in direct contact with the potentiometric or amperometric sensor. In the second type, the enzyme, or whole cell, immobilized on a solid support (bioreactor) is incorporated in the flow line into which the analyte is injected. The product generated is detected and measured with an electrochemical sensor downstream. A bioelectrochemical system with immobilized whole biocell or enzyme has been applied to flow injection analysis to monitor oxygen.

For glucose determination in flow systems, glucose oxidase has been frequently employed because of its high selectivity for β-D-glucose, which is oxidized producing H_2O_2.[60] The H_2O_2 produced enzymatically can be monitored electrochemically. As anoxic oxidation of the hydrogen peroxide is irreversible, calibration curves for glucose with glucose electrodes are shown in Table 5.10.

Table 5.10 Calibration curves for glucose with both glucose eletrodes

		Calibration Curve		
Electrode	*Sample Size (μl)*	*Linear Range (mg dl^{-1})*	*Correlation Coefficient*	*Time to Return to Baseline (s)*
GOD-CT	5	20–800	0.9998	6.4
GOD-POD	1	30–400	0.9997	6.0

5.12 GASEOUS OXYGEN MEASUREMENT

Oxygen is unique among common gases. It is strongly paramagnetic by virtue of its magnetic susceptibility, and this property has been utilized in gaseous oxygen monitoring.[61, 62] A lightweight, dumbbell-shaped, glass rotor is suspended by a torsion spring in a nonuniform magnetic field. Oxygen tends to accumulate in this field to displace the nonmagnetic rotor. This rotation is opposed by the torsion spring and occurs to a degree proportional to the oxygen tension. Readout depends on the position on a translucent scale of a slit of light reflected from a mirror that turns with the rotor. This meter is accurate, requires no external power, and will function indefinitely if not abused. However, the gas to be analyzed must be pumped through the chamber, and the response to changes in oxygen concentration is slow.

An analog signal could be obtained from this type of analyzer by arranging for the light reflected from the motor mirror to strike a photocell. A mask with a triangular aperture overlies the light-sensitive area of the cell. As the mirror rotates, an increasing amount of the reflected slit of light passes through the widening aperture, and the electrical output of the photocell rises. Accuracy can be increased by the use of a null balance method. Wound on the rotor is a coil so oriented that current flows through it, producing a magnetic torque opposed to torque resulting from the presence of oxygen. A photocell detects the rotor movement. The amplified output of this cell adjusts coil current to a level just sufficient to balance the initial torque and prevent rotation. The magnitude of balancing current required is proportional to the oxygen tension.

5.12.1 Oxygen Analyzer

One of the paramagnetic oxygen analyzers that has been used in investigations for a long time is DCL Servomex Oxygen Analyzer, type 83, from the United Kingdom. This is strictly a linear measuring device and is a dumbbell-type paramagnetic oxygen analyzer.[63]

5.12.2 Standardization of Oxygen Analyzer

Since it is a strictly linear measuring device, it can therefore be standardized for all scales by checking at two points only. For convenience, 0% oxygen (pure nitrogen) and 21% oxygen (air) are used. After switch-on, the instrument is allowed to warm up at a temperature of 35°C. It is held at this temperature for 2 hr. The following steps are observed. Pure nitrogen (oxygen free) is passed through the instrument at a set flow rate. With the help of control switches provided on the instrument, the meter indicator is adjusted accurately at zero following the standard set procedure. Next, drier air at 29°C (room temperature) is passed through the instrument at the selected flow rate. When the indicator needle shows a steady reading, the standardized control switch on the instrument is adjusted until the meter reads exactly 21 %. The instrument is now standardized. It is connected through a sterile rotameter and $CaCl_2$ absorber to the bioreactor exit gas line. Percentage oxygen in the gas stream is measured periodically during bioreaction.

5.13 ASSESSMENT OF K_La

5.13.1 Chemical Method

The chemical method is known as the sulfite oxidation method.[64] It involves the determination of the maximum rate of oxidation of sodium sulfite to sodium sulfate in the presence of $CoSO_4$ or $CuSO_4$ catalyst, in which there is no back pressure of dissolved oxygen. The reaction is independent of sulfite concentration in the range of 0.8 M to 0.02 M. Usually, 0.5-0.8 M sodium sulfite solution at pH 7.5-7.8 is used in K_La determination. The course of oxidation is followed by analyzing the unreacted sulfite concentration, using the excess of standard iodine, and back-titrating the unreacted iodine with sodium thiosulfate solution. The reactions involved are :

Absorption reaction in reactor: $O_2 + 2Na_2SO_3 = 2Na_2SO_4$

Detection of sulfite: $2Na_2SO_3 + 2I + 2H_2O = 2Na_2SO_4 + 4HI$

Back titration (unreacted I_2): $4Na_2S_2O_3 + 2I_2 = 2Na_2S_4O_6 + 4NaI$

Thus,

$$\frac{O_2}{4} = \frac{Na_2SO_3}{2} = Na_2S_2O_3 \tag{5.67}$$

or, l mol of O_2 = 4 liters of (N) $Na_2S_2O_3$ solution.

Based on liquid film overall coefficient, the absorption rate is :

$$\frac{\text{m.mol } O_2 \text{ absorbed}}{\text{liter} - \text{hour}} = K_La \text{ (Driving force)} \tag{5.68}$$

Since oxygen absorption is very rapid with sulfite, the concentration of oxygen in the bulk of the liquid is zero (i.e. $C_L = 0$). The driving force, therefore, is just the solubility of oxygen in 0.5 M sulfite solution (0.20 mM per liter at 25°–30°C). Thus,

$$K_La = \frac{1}{4}\,\frac{\text{mmol Thiosulfate used}}{\text{liter} - \text{hour}} \times \frac{1}{0.20\ \text{mMl}^{-1}} \tag{5.69}$$

or

$$K_La = \frac{\text{(Normality of thiosulfate used).(ml used)}}{\text{(ml sample) (minute in test)}} \times \frac{1000 \times 60}{4 \times 0.20}\ h^{-1} \tag{5.70}$$

The experimental procedure of this method as described by Cooper *et al.* [64] has certain limitations of cell concentration.[65] In nonrespiring[66] system in a well-agitated fermenter, it is assumed that the DO concentration is uniform throughout the bulk liquid. Transfer of oxygen to a respiring culture is given by:

$$\frac{dC_L}{dt} = K_La\,(C^* - C_L) - rC_x \tag{5.71}$$

Since nonrespiring culture is used in this method, $rC_x = 0$. Therefore, integration of equation 5.71 gives:

$$\int_0^{C_L} \frac{dC_L}{C^* - C_L} = K_La \int_0^t dt$$

or

$$\ln\,(C^* - C_L) = -\,K_Lat + \ln C^* \tag{5.72}$$

This equation shows that the plot of $(C^* - C_L)$ against time on a semilog graph will give a straight line having a negative slope of $-K_La$ and intercepting $\ln C^*$. Therefore, from the slope and intercept, K_La and C^* can be determined.

5.13.2 Dynamic Differential Gassing-Out (DDGO) Method

This method, developed by Bandyopadhyay *et al.*,[67] is based on following the DO trace during a brief interruption of aeration in the fermentation system. Only a fast-response, sterilizable DO probe is needed to obtain the necessary data.

The experimental procedure involves degassing (air turn-off) of an actively respiring fermentation mash to record the decrease in DO concentration due to respiration and to obtain the rate of oxygen uptake by the total cell mass. Before critical DO concentration of the organism is reached, aeration is resumed and the increase in DO concentration is recorded as a function of time. The rate of change of DO concentration is measured from this trace. When air is turned off,

$$\text{Rate of oxygen uptake} = \frac{dC_L}{dt} = -r\,C_x \tag{5.73}$$

When aeration is resumed following degassing, the rate of change of DO concentration would be given by equation 5.71. Assuming that probe measures the bulk DO concentration and C* can be represented by some mean value, equation 5.71 can be rearranged as follows :

$$C_L = -\frac{1}{K_La}\left[\frac{dC_L}{dt} + rC_x\right] + C^* \tag{5.74}$$

This equation shows that the plot of C_L against $\left(\frac{dC_L}{dt} + rC_x\right)$ on the arithmetic coordinate would result in a straight-line relation with a slope of $-1/K_La$ from which K_La can be determined easily. The value of C* can be obtained from the extrapolated intercept of this line on the ordinate, and rC_x can be known from the slope of the dissolved oxygen trace in the degassing period.

5.13.3 Dynamic Integral Gassing-Out (DIGO) Method

The differential gassing-out method has been widely used, but it may incorporate several weak points (as discussed in a later section). For improving some of these weak points, Fujio *et al.*[68] developed a dynamic integral gassing-out technique based on the differential gassing-out method. Basically, the experimental procedure is the same as that in the previous method. However, in the case of low DO concentration in equilibrium in microbial cultivation, if one takes the integral form of equation. 5.71, more accurate values will be provided for rC_x and dC_L/dt, and hence for K_La. The value of rC_x in equation 5.71 may be regarded as having a constant value during a short period of time. By rearranging the equation, one can write

$$\frac{1}{K_La}\cdot\frac{dC_L}{dt} = B' - C_L \tag{5.75}$$

where

$$B' = C^* - \frac{A}{K_La} \tag{5.76}$$

and

$$A = rC_x \tag{5.77}$$

From equation 5.75, we get

$$\frac{1}{B}\frac{dC_L}{\left(1-\frac{C_L}{B'}\right)} = K_La\,dt \tag{5.78}$$

Integrating this equation with initial conditions, $C_L = 0$, at $t = 0$, and $C_L = C_{L1}$ at $t = t_1$, one may obtain

$$\ln\left(1 - \frac{C_L}{B'}\right) = K_L at \tag{5.79}$$

and

$$\ln\left(\frac{C_{L_t} - B'}{C_{L_t} - B'}\right) = K_L a\,(t_1 - t) \tag{5.80}$$

Equations 5.79 and 5.80 show that the plot of $\ln\left(1 - \frac{C_L}{B'}\right)$ against t or $\ln\left(\frac{C_{L_t} - B'}{C_{L_{t_1}} - B'}\right)$ against $(t_1 - t)$ gives a straight line, the slope of which directly predicts K_La. The numerical value of B' will be equal to the equilibrium concentration of DO in the broth under aerated cultivation. Values of rC_x and B' can be obtained from DO trace by performing the experiment as in the method of Bandyopadhyay *et al.*[67]

5.13.4 Oxygen Balance (OB) Method

Some investigators[69] are of the opinion that oxygen balance over the whole system is the best method for evaluation of K_La in fermenters, because no assumption need be made on the effects of cell, surface active agents, viscosity, and forth. Based on the oxygen balance concept, Mukhopadhyay and Ghose[70] developed a linear mathematical correlation between DO concentration and the proportion of oxygen in inlet and exit air of laboratory fermenter from which K_La can be determined very easily and rapidly, as described below.

When air is blown to a fermentation mash, a fraction of oxygen present in incoming air is dissolved in the liquid, from which the microorganisms absorb oxygen for their respiration and metabolic activities and unabsorbed oxygen goes out with the exit gas. Assuming that during fermentation air density in inlet and exit air does not change appreciably, the incoming air flow rate is equal to the outgoing flow rate (i.e., the pressure drop in the vessel is very low and evaporation loss of the medium is negligible), one can make an oxygen balance in the aerobic bioprocessing system at any time and can write:

Mathematically

$$O_{2inlet} = O_{2med} + O_{2cell} + O_{2exit} \tag{5.81}$$

$$\rho_a Qfi = V \,.\, \frac{dC_L}{dt} + VrC_x + \rho_a Qfo \tag{5.82}$$

where ρ_a is the density of air at experimental temperature (gl^{-1}); Q is volumetric air flow rate (hr^{-1}); V is working volume of the fermenter (1); and f_i, f_o are the proportion of oxygen in inlet and exit air, respectively.

From equation 5.82,

$$\frac{dC_L}{dt} = \frac{\rho_a Q}{V}(f_i - f_o) - r\,C_x \tag{5.83}$$

The oxygen absorption rate in the broth is given by equation 5.83. By combining equation 5.82 and equation 5.83, one can write,

$$K_La\ (C^* - C_L) - rC_x = \frac{\rho_a Q}{V}\ (f_i - f_o) - rC_x \tag{5.84}$$

from which

$$C_L = \frac{-\rho_a Q}{K_L aV}\ (f_i - f_o) - C^* \tag{5.85}$$

For a particular fermentation condition in this equation, K_La, V, ρ_a, Q, C*, and fi may be assumed to have constant values, with the only variables being C_L and f_o. Thus, a plot of C_L versus $(f_i - f_o)$ in arithmetic coordinates will produce a straight line with a slope of $\frac{-\rho_a Q}{K_L aV}$ and intercept C*. From the slope, K_La can be obtained easily knowing ρ_a, Q and V from the experimental conditions.

The value of rC_x can be determined from Equation 5.80, which can be written as :

$$rC_x = \frac{\rho_a Q}{V}\ (f_i - f_o) - \frac{dC_L}{dt} \tag{5.86}$$

Since the second term on the right side of this equation is negligible compared to the first term, we can write,

$$rC_x = \frac{\rho_a Q}{V}\ (f_i - f_o) \tag{5.87}$$

which gives the value of rC_x at any time. By plotting rC_x against $(f_i - f_o)$ values, the maximum value of rC_x can be determined.

5.13.5 Enzymic Method (GGO)

Based on the Heineken theory,[71] Linek and his associates[72,73] developed a dynamic method to determine K_La in a fermenter using the glucose-glucose oxidase (GGO) system. Assuming absorption of oxygen in the liquid phase as the first-order reaction as well as perfect mixing conditions, the rate of oxygen absorption in the GGO system in a mechanically agitated dispersion (MAD) of gas is given by :

$$\frac{dC}{dt} = K_La\ (C_2^+ - C) - K_1C \tag{5.88}$$

where C_2^+ represents equilibrium oxygen concentration with respect to gas leaving the dispersion, C is oxygen concentration, and K_1 is constant. Integrating equation 5.88 with the initial condition

$$C = 0, \quad t = 0 \tag{5.89}$$

One gets

$$C = \frac{C_2^+}{(1 + K_1 K_L a)} [1 - \exp(-Kt)] \tag{5.90}$$

where

$$K = K_L a (1 + K_1 K_L a) \tag{5.91}$$

In the dynamic method, $K_L a$ estimation is based on the tracing of DO concentration by DO probe in MAD caused by sudden interruption and subsequent resumption of aeration. Under air turn-off condition, oxygen concentration in GGO decreases to zero value (condition 5.79) as a result of the reaction between DO and glucose. On resumption of air, the DO trace is given by equation 5.92. The normalized response (Γ') of the DO probe after air resumption is given by :

$$\Gamma' = 1 - A \exp(B_2 \kappa t) + F \tag{5.92}$$

where

$$A = \pi \sqrt{B_2} / \sin \pi \sqrt{B_2} \tag{5.93}$$

$$B_2 = K/\kappa \tag{5.94}$$

and F is a function of B_2, and κt and K are defined in equation 5.94.
At steady state, oxygen concentration in GGO is obtained from the equation as :

$$C_0 = \frac{K_L a C_2^+}{K_1 + K_L a} \tag{5.95}$$

in which C_0 is steady-state oxygen concentration.
Putting

$$Z = \frac{C_2^+}{C_0} \tag{5.96}$$

at steady state

$$Z = \frac{C_2^+}{C_0} - 1 + (K_1/K_L a) \tag{5.97}$$

From equation 5.94 $B_2\kappa = K = K_L a + K_1$. Putting this value of $(K_L a + K_1)$ in equation 5.97, we get

$$K_L a = \frac{K_L a + K_1}{Z} \tag{5.98}$$

$$K_L a = \frac{B_2 \kappa}{Z} \tag{5.99}$$

The values of B_2 and κ can be obtained from the plot of $(1 - \Gamma')$ against κt values, with B_2 as the parameter. The value of Z is obtained from the enzyme probe readings by placing the probe in the gas stream from fermenter and in the GGO system under steady state. For illustration, the plot of the actual concentration in the GGO system and the oxygen probe reading is given in the literature.[72, 73]

5.13.6 Merits and Demerits of the Methods

1. Limitations of the chemical method

The chemical method suffers from serious limitations which restrict its use in determining K_La in many chemical and microbial systems. The primary limitation is that aqueous sulfite solution does not adequately simulate fermentation mashes in many properties, which can strongly affect the mass transfer coefficient e.g. viscosity, the presence of surface active agents, the solute concentration, and the presence of microbial cells. It is common for highly viscous mycelial fermentations to exhibit K_La substantially lower than predicted by this method.

Investigations in sparged systems with/without mechanical agitation as well as in a stirred transfer cell without sparging indicate that physical absorption is the rate-controlling process in copper-catalyzed systems if K_L is greater than 3×10^{-4}m S^{-1}. This can be used to determine the types of equipment and the conditions for which the method can give valid assessments of mass transfer characteristics applicable to fermentation processes and other systems in which the rate of absorption is physically controlled. It has also been possible to compare coefficients determined in this way with those determined in cultures of *E. coli* growing in an unstirred, sparged column. These results indicate that K_La increases with expansion of cell concentration, probably because of the effects of the suspended solids on the hydrodynamic conditions near the gas/liquid interface.

This method has also been applied to determine interfacial areas, and this application depends on the rate being reaction controlled. Between the two extremes of diffusion and reaction control regimes, there is a transition zone in which the sulfite method cannot be applied for either purpose. The results of this method frequently are reported to depend on the choice of catalyst.

The demerit of this method for application in biosystem also relates to difficulties in its use for colored biomedia.

2. DDGO method

The merits of the DDGO method are the following: (1) it avoids the restrictions of nonrespiring mash; (2) it measures K_La in the actual fermentation system so that the number of assumptions required are less; (3) results of this method are internally consistent, since only a single measuring device (i.e:, DO probe) is used; and (4) the method is very simple.

However, many disadvantages of the method have been pointed out,[69] including: (1) its applicability to viscous mycelial fermentations is questionable; (2) it assumes a rapid disengagement of air bubbles from the mash upon termination of aeration (which is not usually the case with highly viscous non-Newtonian mashes); (3) for some systems (non-Newtonian), it gives appreciably low oxygen uptake values; (4) in the case of low DO concentration in equilibrium in microbial cultivation, this method gives inaccurate values of rC_x and dC_L/dt;[68] (5) the time derivative of DO concentration must be calculated from the DO trace (which might incorporate error during calculations), (6) at higher broth respiration, accurate measurement itself is difficult; and (7) for genetically redesigned cell cultivation, transient degassing may be detrimental.

3. DIGO method

This method also has its limitations, due to the fact that it also interrupts the process for a while. For highly responsive biosystems like genetically engineered or redesigned biocell processing, this may be undesirable.

4. OB method

As this method does not interrupt the bioprocessing in any manner, traces of DO concentration and percent of oxygen in inlet air and exit gas need to be determined only up to the end of the logarithmic phase of growth. The calculation does not have the scope to incorporate errors, it is easy, and the value is more realistic. It also gives a better result for the recombinant cell biosystem.

5. GGO method

This method does not need any knowledge of oxygen solubility data in the bioprocessing liquid during estimation. However, calculation is prone to incorporate errors. This method suffers from the fact that it considers a nonrespiring system which can not be simulated with actual fermentation. The requirement that there be no respiration demand during K_La determination mandates that either noninoculated mash be used, or that respiration be terminated at a particular time by either pasteurization or a respiratory poison. Thus, K_La is measured under artificial conditions.

5.13.7 Role of Reactive Oxygen Species (ROS) [102-111]

1. In BamH1 bioprocessing

In nature and natural systems oxygen and oxygen species do exist in free and combined states. In nature's biosphere four major natural systems of biochemical engineering and biotechnological importances include microbe, animal, plant and environment. In all these systems oxygen play a key role. Depending on the nature and processing of the biosystem the participation of dioxygen species such as free and dissolved molecular oxygen, (like O_2, O_2^-, HOO^- etc) and monooxygen species (O, O^-, OH^-, OH) in biomedia is important.[102-105] Thus oxygenation, oxygen sensing and aerotaxis phenomena bear a great relevance to oxyradical participation in biochemical engineering and process biotechnology. The concerns of oxygenation in microbial bioprocessing are well known. Speculated mechanism of participation of oxygen free radical species in prokaryotic systemic product formation had been proposed in an earlier publication.[104] Further advances of oxygenation property in *Bam* H1 producing system has been proposed in terms of metabolic oxygen concentration coefficient (MOCC).[111] Thus it has been possible to suggest that oxygen or free oxyradicals produced from it, can directly or indirectly affect prokaryotic cells in two pathways in *in vivo* regulation of *Bam* H1 biosynthesis.

In some microbial cell cultivation systems cells adhere on the surface of air bubbles.[32] From the current knowledge of oxygen effects on simple organisms it has been clear that prokaryotes are much more metabolically melleable than eukaryotes. Also, present state of knowledge on the beneficial effects of oxygen in energy conservation and the deterimental effects of oxygen under oxidative/oxygen stress clearly indicated that microbial cells, have evolved and redesigned/modified regulatory networks. It also appeared that cells did develop in respiratory system a mechanism for sensing oxygen concentration in their environment. Important scientific progress on oxygen sensing in living being has discussed how sensing based oxidative stress regulation manifest at the molecular level.[109]

In bacteria aerotaxis has been defined as the movement of a cell or organism toward or away from oxygen/air bubble.[110] Accumulation of cells near air bubbles or other sources of oxygen was observed as mentioned before. Also, oxygen is known for a long time the only substance functioning either as an attractant or repellant in cells like *E. coli* and *S. typhimurium.*[102]

In order to explain this behaviour a signal transducer gene dubbed *aer* has been identified and described for aerotaxis in *E. coli*. *Aer* protein promise to provide a definitive answer to the long standing puzzle to how cells detect oxygen gradients during aerotaxis. Proposed steps and nature of *aer* in the research methodology included the following.

a. Examinig sequence features of the *aer* locus.
b. Construction of an *aer* mutant
c. Air bubble assays for aerotaxis
d. Swarm plate assay for aerotaxis
e. *Aer* is probably a flavoprotein
f. *Aer* may function as a redox sensor.

Also, two major redox systems are involved in maintaining reduced environment in the *E. coli* cytosol; the glutathione – glutaredoxin (GSH/GrX) systems in thioredoxin system which may be involved in controlling defense against oxidative stress[122].

Oxygen being the most important oxidant in the biosphere knowledge of oxygenation and oxygen sensing and aerotaxis indicate that in cell cultivation in bioreactors during the course of aerobic respiration, molecular oxygen is generally reduced by four electrons to give water. A part is reduced to highly reactive intermediate radicals like O_2^- (super oxide), OH^- (hydroxyl), H_2O_2 etc. These partially reduced forms of oxygen, referred to as free radical or reactive oxygen species (ROS) are also produced, independently of respiration, during oxygen uptake reactions in the cytosol of the cells. During cultivation the production of ROS may increase proportionally with partial pressure of oxygen. These unstable reactive compounds may mutate DNA, oxidize cell proteins and damage cell membranes specially in aged cells. In cell cultivation the damages may collectively be referred to as oxygen toxicity or oxidative stress.[104,106] Thus relevance of oxyradicals in aeration, oxygenation, oxygen sensing and aerotaxis is obvious in cell cultivation.

Over aeration for high oxygenation may reduce cellular activity or cause injury to cell culture and stem cell bioprocessing systems. Coping with active functional molecules in cells or tissues of biosystems in presence of stress agents thereby developing its antiinjury capacity to certain extent may be termed as molecular adaptation. When the stress is by over aeration of oxygen its involvement in producing increased level of nascent oxygen radicals or active oxygen species formation may create stressful event which has been termed as oxidative stress. Therefore, coping of functional molecules manifesting adaptive expression in cells or tissues allowing them to recover or survive in presence of oxygen or oxidative stress may be termed as molecular adaptation to oxidative stress (Fig. 5.24). In many cell culture systems this may be very important concern. Attempt has been made to provide a molecular mechanistic explanation of *Bam*H1 production biosystem in relation to oxygenation based on experimental results and available informations (Fig. 5.25).

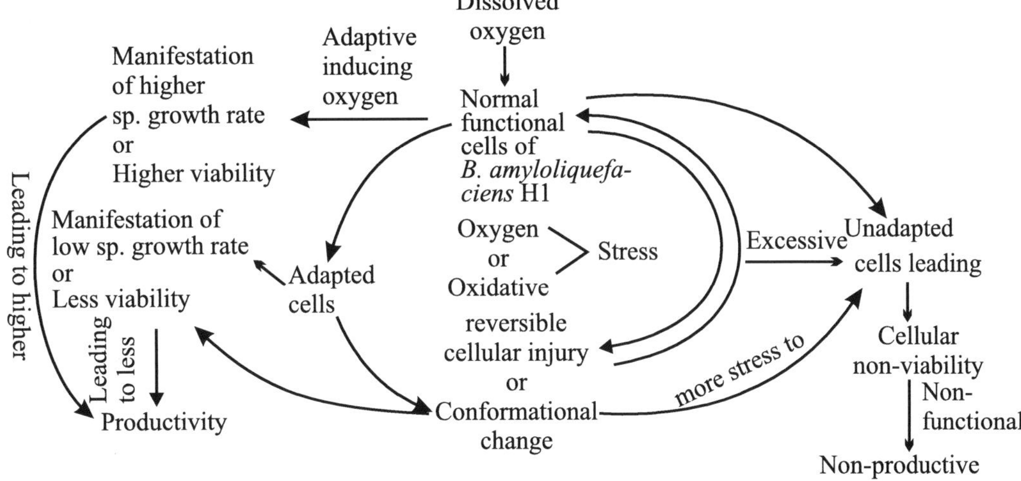

Fig. 5.24 Adaptive and stress inductive manifestation by oxygen in *Bam* H1 cells

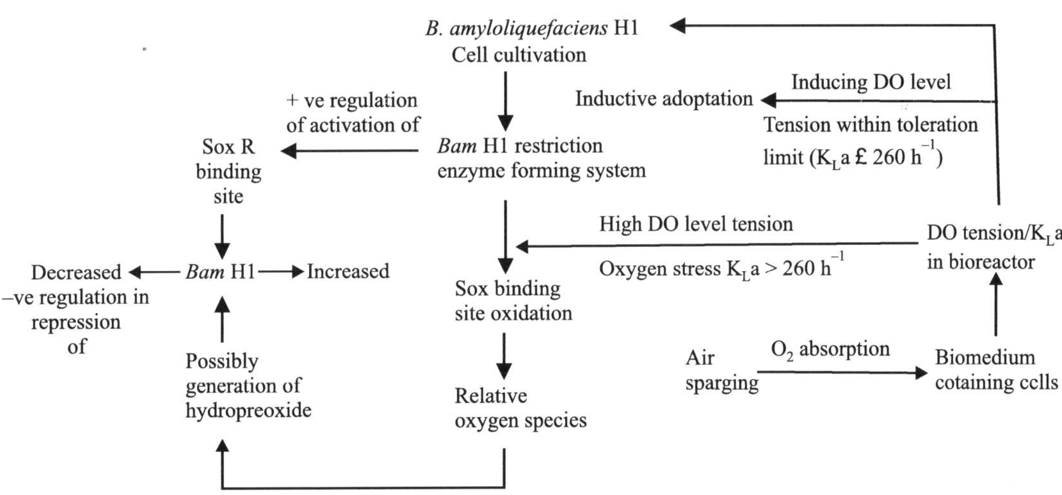

Fig. 5.25 Proposed explanation on the effect of over aeration and under aeration in *Bam* H1 production by *B. amyloliquefaciens* H1

Table 5.11 : Oxygen adaptation and stress in relation to *Bam* H1 productivity (pH = 6.8, T = 35 –37° C)

K_La (h^{-1})	μ (h^{-1})	Max c_x (m. mol O_2 l^{-1} h^{-1})	Production (P) of Bam H1 (units l^{-1})	Observed $C_{L\,me}$ (ppm)
100	0.16	4	5500	3.2
150	0.20	7	7000	4.0
260	0.23	8	10000	4.8
350	0.19	–	6000	4.9
400	0.18	6	3000	5.1

2. *Positive and negative regulation of Bam* H1 *production by* $^1O_2$

In more recent years it was indicated that constitutive restriction enzyme, *Bam*H1 protein biosynthesis in *Bacillus amyloliquefaciens* H1 strains is greatly influenced by oxygen tension in the cell cultivation liquid.[102] The profiles of *Bam* H1 production showed that specific growth rate (μ) and specific restriction enzyme protein yield ($Y_{RE/X}$) of this prokaryotic cell varied as a function of temperature and oxygenation. It can be seen that the value of μ varied largely, but $Y_{RE/X}$ to only a little extent under thermal processing stress. The variations of these bioprocess technology states parameters by oxygenation and shear control parameter was seen to be very pronounced. It appeared that formation *Bam* H1 involved oxygen species reactive stress gene(s) having functional optimality at specific oxygen tension. In prokaryotic system, oxidative stress has been found to induce that heat shock proteins and glucose regulated proteins.[102] This led the scientists to think that such cellular response in eukaryotic cells may be of great significance, since reactive oxygen species have been shown to play a significant role in a variety of disease processes like heat attack, stroke, arthritis and few others.[103] Reactive oxygen species have also been implicated in ischemic and reperfusion injury to a large variety of mammalian tissues. However, information on the prompt response of eukaryotic cells to the oxidative stress is scanty. Prompt molecular adaptation of vascular endothelial cells to oxidative stress as mentioned earlier is an important information. In *Bam* H1 producing prokaryotic cells, the nature of the oxygen species reactive stress genes and corresponding stress factors in the cell is still not identified. Their identification and involvement in thermotolerence and oxygen stress in *Bam* H1 yield increase[102, 104] remains as a future research scope in the area of oxidative stress in prokaryotes. It may also be necessary to know in this organism whether the unknown individual HSPs are under the control of constitutive or inducible promoters.

Oxidative stress developed by exposing bacteria (*Salmonella typhimurium*) to low concentration of H_2O_2 induced several new proteins including HSPs and mRNA of catalase. In the process of oxidative stress adaptation, the bacteria becomes resistant to killing by otherwise lethal doses of H_2O_2 and other strong oxidants. Thus, it may appear in mammalian cells that oxidative stress induction creates a defense action against subsequent cellular injury by expressing a distinct group of proteins such as HSP and GRP, etc. This class of special proteins have been collectively termed as "oxidative stress inducible proteins" (OSIPs). Furthermore, it was shown that among the oxidative stress inducible genes, Sox R-nd OxyR genes are positive regulatory genes for different proteins including catalase, hydroperoxide I, glutathione reductase, and alkyl-hydroperoxide reductase. However, many oxidative stress-inducible proteins are not characterized, and their functions are yet unknown.

3. Possible molecular mechanisms of oxidative stresses

From the influence of dissoved oxygen on constitutive enzymic protein *Bam* H1 formation by *Bacillus amyloliquefaciens* H1 strain as well as prokaryotic systems like *S. typhimurium* and others under oxidative stress, it will be interesting and useful to know about molecular mechanism of participation of oxygen in such situations. The ambivalent mechanism of oxygen in aerobic organisms is really a paradox. A beneficial effect of oxygen in aerobic organisms up-to a certain level has been observed. Above certain level nonbeneficial effect was observed in many cases including *Bam* H1 production. It leads to suggest that below certain level of ($K_La < 260h^{-1}$)[104] oxygen does not activate the regulon of mRNA of the activator protein to react with its SoxR binding site which is responsible for changing oxidation state. It permits *in vivo* Bam H1 synthesis to continue and increase. On the other hand, above certain dissolved oxygen level in other words volumetric oxygen transfer coefficient ($K_La > 260h^{-1}$) it activates the SoxR binding site or the activatior protein. The SoxR protein is, therefore, directly activated by metabolic oxygen stimulus, an oxidant becoming transcriptional inactivator by generating reactive oxygen species. It is generated from high d.o in the medium and interacts with SoxR changing oxidation state of its binding site. This change perhaps causes conformational change that effects the way in which the proteins interact with its corresponding promoters.

So, the SoxR regulon response to high dissolved oxygen stress is one of the few molecular mechanisms for which the translation of an environmental stress into transcriptional control has been defined and some cells were partly resistant to this response to survive harmful metabolic effects of active oxygen species and possibly other oxidants in the medium.

In prokaryotic biosystems molecular oxygen may, therefore, play an ambivalent role.

A substantial oxidative damage rate to DNA can occur as a part of normal metabolism of lipid peroxidation in cells. The oxidative DNA damage rate has been measured by thymidine glycol excretion in mammals. In order to cope with oxidative stress aerobic organisms evolved enzymic and non enzymic molecular level antioxidant defense mechanisms. These molecular mechanisms within the organisms have been evolved to limit the levels of reactive oxidants and the damage they caused. In cells proliferation the molecular mechanism of oxygen stress dependent pathway has been shown to play significant role by regulating uridine phosphate mediated ribonucleotide reductase system.

4. Molecular mechanism types

From various literature informations and above discussions the manifestation of molecular mechanisms of oxidative stress possibly may be of six different types as stated in the first edition of this book (Chapter 11).[104] Among these mechanisms for cell metabolism SOD has been stated to play a key role in molecular adaptation to oxidative stress in many biosystems. For molecular adaptation to prevent or minimize active oxygen species or radical formation a subtle balance is essential between superoxide flux, H_2O_2 generation and intracellular availability of suitable reduced ion. In this balance also SOD plays key role. SOD is found in all microorganisms including archaebacteria. Prokaryotic SODs may be iron and/or manganese SOD. MnSOD is usually found in presence of oxygen whereas FeSOD is found under anaerobiosis. In cell culture control dissolved oxygen (DO) or aeration efficiency (K_La) in the growth media is, therefore, one of the most common approaches for manipulating SOD in cells.

5. Adaptation and control of oxygen stress

Depending on the treatment and/or presence of oxygen in cells or tissues of biosystems H_2O_2 generation vary to a great extent. In cells or tissues if nascent 1μ mol l^{-1} H_2O_2 comes in contact with 1μ mol l^{-1} of Fe it enhances OH radical generation by a second order gene reaction. Its kinetics having a second order

$$H_2O_2 + Fe^{++} \longrightarrow Fe^{+++} + OH^- + OH^0 \tag{5.100}$$

rate constant value K_2 of 76 l mol^{-1} s^{-1}.[23] Moreover, toxic action of nascent H_2O_2 may be exerted by its ability to form hydroxyl free radical via the Fe+++ catalysed Haber-Weiss reaction.[23]

$$O^{-2} + H_2O_2 \xrightarrow{Fe^{+++}} O_2 + OH^- + OH^0 \tag{5.101}$$

In response to the oxidative stress exerted by the presence of oxygen derived free radicals, cells or tissues take up (from the medium), produce and/or secrete antioxidant molecules. So under normal physiological conditions the toxic effects of free radicals are controlled by antioxidants like SOD, catalase, glutathione peroxidase, vitamin E, pyruvate etc. If stressful condition is severe having high oxygen or oxidant level to overwhelm the antioxidants cell injury or even inactivation by conformational change may result.

6. Can DO cause conformation change?

Cells generating H_2O_2 in presence of dissolved oxygen may influence on sites for SoxR or OxyR DNA interactions. The oxidation state of OxyR or SoxR regulon may become determinant in transcription enhancement. In turn protein is directly activated by metabolic stimulus, an oxidant to become transcriptional activator. This activator serves both as a sensor of oxidative stress and the mediator of enhanced transcription of genes. The gene products are part of the adaptive response. In the adaptive response the active oxygen species is generated from dissolved oxygen in triplet dioxygen state in the medium or from oxidant used in the medium. The reactive oxygen in turn interacts with the regulon altering its oxidation states. Alteration of oxidation state has been stated to cause a conformational change affecting protein interactive target promoters. In *Bacillus amyloliquefaciens* H1 strain there may exist systems involving coordinately regulated yet scattered genes which may be regulons. OxyR and SoxR regulons may presumably be functional. The OxyR and/or SoxR regulon response to oxidative stress by disssolved oxygen (DO) and translation of environmental stress into transcription control is presumably manifested. Organisms use this response in part to adapt or survive the injurious metabolic effects of DO or other oxidants in the medium. This implies that DO may cause conformational change by oxidation-reduction state alteration of a molecule. In this alterations operon consisting of regulons may be under negative or positive control depending on redox state. It can be referred to as inductive if the presence of some secondary effector like DO molecule is required to achieve an increased expression of structural genes. Likewise the same operon can be described as repressive if the effector DO molecule must bind to regulatory protein before it will inhibit transcription of the structural genes.

7. Can dissolved triplet dioxygen alter redox state?

It is known that DO has a triplet ground state $^3\Sigma O_{2g}$. This state having the following biradical electronic configuration indicates possibility of its electron $O_2\,(\pi_s)^2\,(*\pi s)^2\,(\pi 2S)^2\,(\sigma 2pz)^2\,(\pi 2px)^2\,(\pi 2px)^2\,(\pi 2Py)^2\,(\pi^*2Px)^1\,(\pi^*2Py)^1\,(\pi^*2Pz)^0$ acceptibility or possibility of its reduction.

For oxygen to be reduced to water four electrons and four protons need to participate as per following reaction

$$O_2 + 4H^+ + 4e^- \longrightarrow 2H_2O \tag{5.102}$$

In biosystems it is known that electrons are transfered from substrates to oxygen. However other alternate reactions step pathways also does exist. These are given in Fig. 5.25. In dissolving oxygen at atmospheric pressure in aqueous biomedia (pH 7.0 25°C) the step's and redox potentials are known. The free energy changes from stepwise reduction of 1 mole of O_2 to two moles of water via nascent H_2O_2 has been related as a function of number of electron transfer as shown in the Fig. 5.26 below.

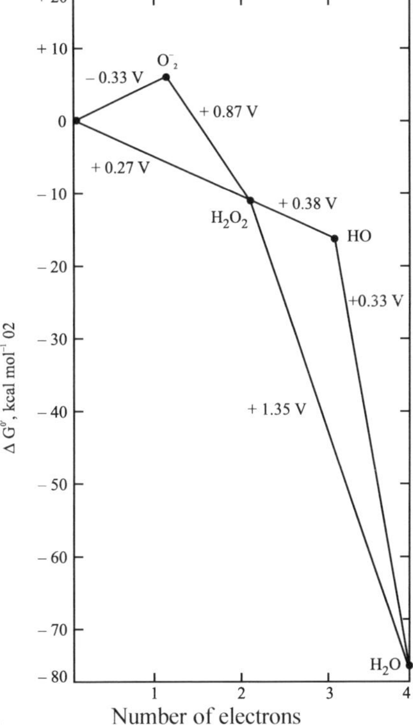

Fig. 5.26 Free energy diagram for the reduction of molecular oxygen to water at pH7 and 25°C. The corresponding oxidation-reduction potential are also given along the reaction lines

It showed that dissolved oxygen is a strong oxidizing agent with a total free energy change of – 74.7 kcal mole^{-1} (–312 KJ mol^{-1}) for complete reduction to water.

It can be noted from Fig. 5.26 that addition of the first electron to O_2 in the triplet ground state is an unfavourable uphill limiting step. This is obvious from the shown low potential of

–0.33 V. All other subsequent steps as shown in the Fig. 5.26 being downhill has no thermodynamic barrier. However, to overcome the thermodynamic barrier to the first step the ridge between activation of dioxygen by regulon protein substrate and its own destabilization is very essential. The oxidation-reduction potentials of the reactive oxygen species given in Fig. 5.26 are for the oxyradicals in aqueous solution.The values may be modified when the species are bound to regulon protein molecule as well as when condition varies.

It is apparent, therefore, that triplet state dissolved dioxygen can alter oxidation-reduction state or conformation of a biomolecule depending on how much tolerence or affinity the molecule has towards oxygen. The values of oxygen transfer, adaptation and stress in relation to *Bam* H1 productivity is given in Fig.5.25. It indicates that *Bam* H1 production may be divided into two regimes with respect to oxygenation. The first regime of inductive adaptation (positive regulation) causing increase in *Bam* H1 productivity and μ reaching to a maxima in relation to oxygen tolerence. The second regime of oxygen stress (at high $K_La > 260\ h^{-1}$) resulting decrease in *Bam* H1 productivity, rx as well as μ (negative regulations). The observed attainable maximum equillibrium DO level in the culture liquid showed however a continuos increase with increase in K_La. From these results the functional relation between normal, partially adapted, reversible cellular injury or conformational change possibility in cells by oxygen stress in terms of productivity may be depicted as in Fig 5.25.

8. Index of molecular adapation to oxygen stress

In *Bam* H1 producing cell culture molecular adaptation to oxygen stress may be assesed by the metabolic oxygen control coefficient (MOCC). The MOCC [111] may be defined as the product of the ratio of μ per unit OUR (rx) to that of the ratio of product concentration per unit aeration efficiency (K_La). Quantitatively,

$$\text{MOCC} = \left(\frac{\mu}{rX}\right)\left(\frac{\Delta P}{\Delta K_L a}\right) \tag{5.103}$$

(μ, h^{-1}; rX, m mole O_2/g cell–h units/gm cell h ; Δ K_La, h^{-1})

9. Estimation of MOCC

This index is easily determinable from a simple batch or continuous steady state culture run by following either time profile or steady state values and computing from equation (5.103).

10. Significance of MOCC

As MOCC indicates the adaptive formation of a metabolite in relation to oxygenation if MOCC > 1, higher is the molecular adaptation to oxygen. If on the other hand MOCC < 1, indicates stress is high and molecular adaptation to O_2 is poor.

5.14 ESTIMATION OF REACTIVE OXYGEN SPECIES

The presence of reactive oxygen species can be monitored both directly and indirectly. Several direct methods are available which include electron spin reasonance spectroscopy, chemiluminescence detection, pulse radiolysis, and high-performance liquid chromatography.

Oxygen free radicals once formed in a biological system attack the membrane lipids causing the peroxidation. The products of peroxidation can also be estimated as an indirect method to monitor the presence of free radicals.

5.14.1 Electron Spin Resonance (ESR) Spectroscopy for Oxygen-free Radical Detection

This is the most widely used technique for the direct detection of oxygen free radicals.[74-77] The method depends on coupling between the electric vector of the magnetic component of electromagnetic radiation and electrical charge in the molecule. The success of this technique, also referred to as electron paramagnetic resonance spectroscopy (EPR), depends on the fact that the paramagnetic resonance is only sensitive to transitions involving unpaired electron, which has a spin of either + 1/2 or – 1/2 and behaves as a small magnet. It can align itself parallelly or antiparallelly to the magnetic field of the ESR, thus attaining two different energy levels. Upon the application of electromagnetic radiation of correct energy, the absorped energy is used to move the electron from a lower energy level to an upper energy level, which can be captured as an absorption spectrum. The technique was originally developed to study the paramagnetic transition metal complexes.[78] It was subsequently modified to examine the presence of free radicals. The schematic diagram for a standard ESR spectrometer is shown in Fig. 5.27.

An ESR spectrometer consists of a microwave source, a loop-gap resonator and an amplifier. The sample is inserted in the microwave cavity in the region of high magnetic field. DC magnetic field is gradually increased until resonance occurs. i.e. until the static magnetic field is swept. This is because most of the ESR spectrometers made to date operate at X-band frequencies at nearly 9000 MHz, with the aid of a monochromatic Klystron source which can be tunable only over a small range. The spectrometer is also equipped with a recording system so that absorption band can be recorded on chart paper. Usually, the first derivative of the absorption band is plotted as ESR spectrum reflecting the rate of change of absorbance as shown in Fig. 5.28 which is subsequently analyzed for the presence of free radicals.

The major factors derived from the ESR spectra consist of the hyperfine coupling constants, line widths and intensities, and g values. As shown in Fig. 5.28, line widths are measured as the distances between points of maximum and minimum slope, intensities are the total extent of each line, and g values are defined as the rate of divergence of the levels. Higher g values and low field resonance are reflected by rapid divergence, whereas lower *g* values occur from slow divergence. *g* value becomes 2.0023 when the total magnetism is drived solely from the electron spin, and can be represented by the following equation:

$$h\nu = gm_bB \tag{5.104}$$

where ν is the fixed microwave frequency, m_b is Bohr magneton constant, and B is variable magnetic field. Orbital motion induced from the free radicals generate magnetic moment, adding to or subtracting from that of the electron. This shifts this *g* value to either higher or lower level characterized by a particular free radical (Fig. 5.29)

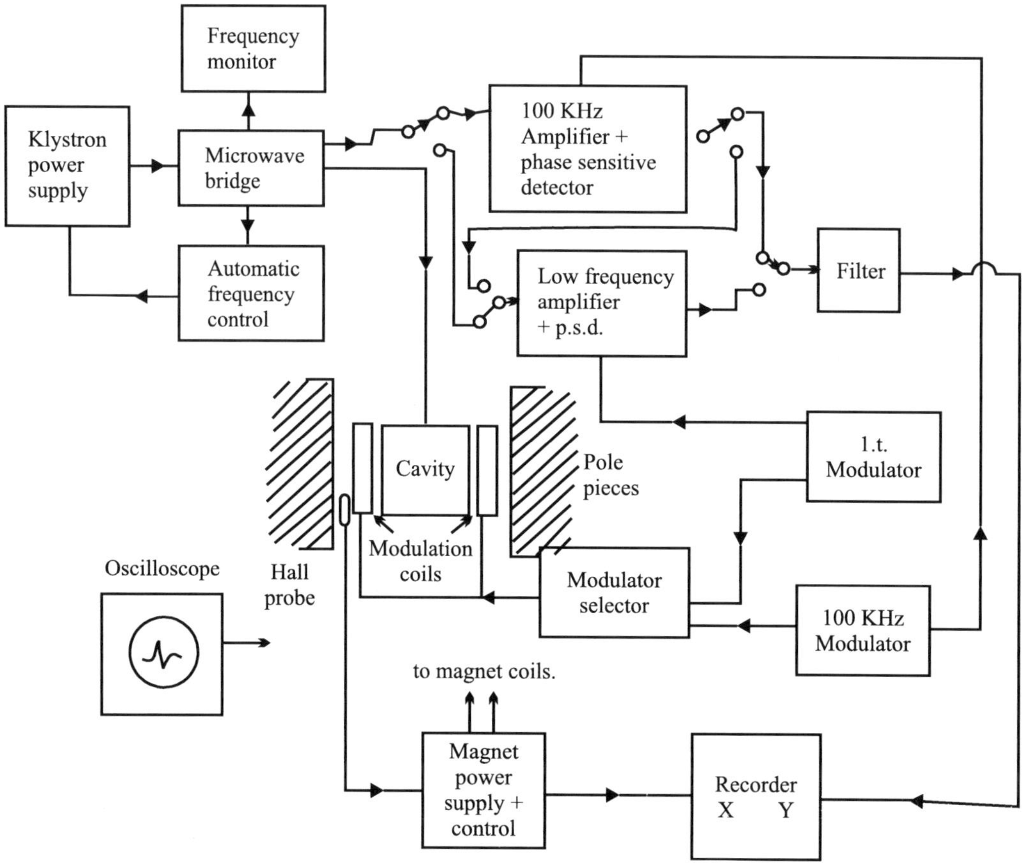

Fig. 5.27 Schematic diagram for a standard C.W.X-band ESR spectrometer. (Reprinted with permission from *Laboratory Techniques in Biochemistry and Molecular Biology*, 22, 52, 1991. Copyright © 1991 Elsevier Science Inc.)

Free radicals also lead to the electron-nuclear hyperfine coupling. The nuclei having net magnetic moments with nuclear spin [*I*] of 1/2 should take up to [± 1/2] orientations, whereas those with *I* of 1 should have three choices (–1, 0 and +1). Thus, a free radical with a single nucleus of $I = 1/2$ should contain two components–half having m_I of +1/2 and the other half having m_I of –1/2, which are reflected in the ESR spectrum producing hyperfine coupling. Similarly, *I* of 1 should produce three ESR transitions from the three possible orientations, again giving rise to hyperfine coupling (Fig. 5.30).

Although ESR is an extremely sensitive method for the detection of oxygen free radicals up to nanomolar range, it is practically impossible to detect them in their native forms. This is because these free radicals are very short-lived, normally in the region of nano seconds. Various techniques are available to prolong the lives of the free radicals, the most practical and widely used technique is by trapping with *spin-trapping* agents.[79,80] Spin-trapping agents can make an

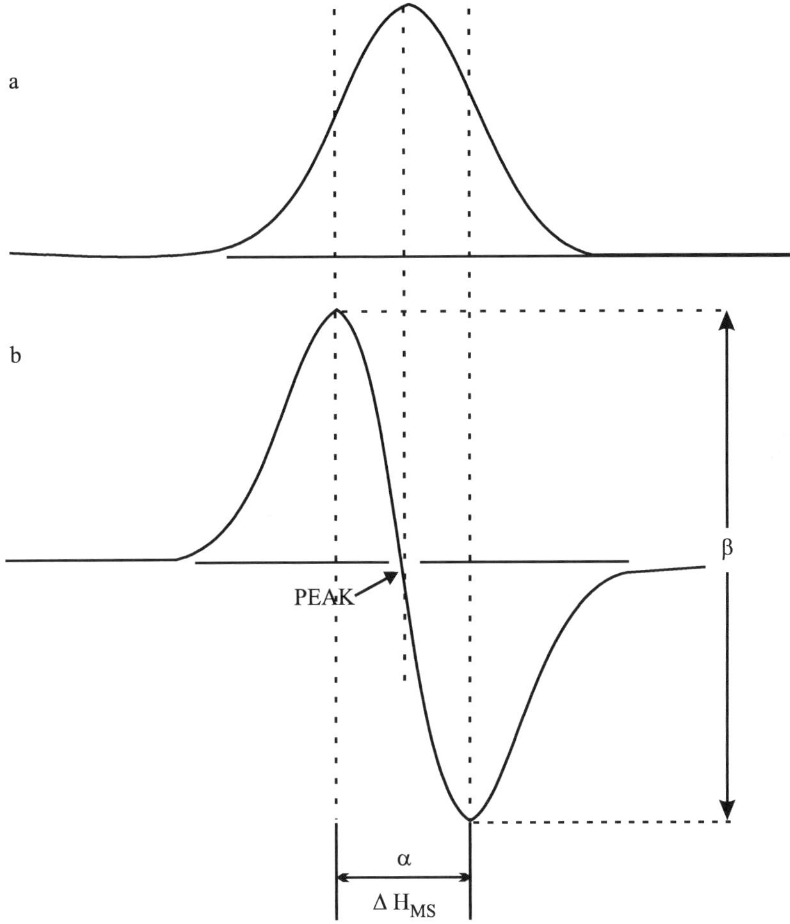

Fig. 5.28 (a) Absorption band; (b) first derivative of the absorption band shown in (a). (Reprinted with permission from *Laboratory Techniques in Biochemistry and Molecular Biology*, 22, 53, 1991. Copyright © 1991 Elsevier Science Inc.)

extremely short-lived radical to live long enough to make the ESR spectroscopic measurement possible. Spin-trapping techniques are widely used in biological systems, and are considered to be the most useful method for the detection of free radicals both *in vivo* and *in vitro* systems.

For *in vitro* trapping of free radicals, a number of trapping agents may be used see Fig. 5.35. Among the trapping agents, the most popular is DMPO. DMPO reacts with superoxide to give the DMPO-OOH adduct. This adduct being very unstable rapidly decomposes into more stable DMPO-OH adduct. The same adduct is formed if DMPO is allowed to react with OH. (Fig. 5.31). DMPO has been successfully used in the author's laboratory to detect OH in the biological system. Thus when OH is generated in the presence of a OH. generating system, DMPO forms a spin adduct with the generated OH.

It is important to remember that a spin-trapping agent must be present at the time of the free radical production. Addition of the spin traps after the completion of free radical production may either detect only a fraction of the total amount of free radicals or may not detect them at all. Addition of a spin trap to the free radical makes the radical inactive. Thus a spin trap functions as a free radical scavenger. Consequently, it often becomes difficult to identify the free radicals from their spin adducts. Generally, the ESR spectra are associated with extra hyperfine coupling characteristics of the trapped species.

DMPO may also be used as *in vivo* spin traps. For the purpose of *in vivo* trapping of free radicals, DMPO must be injected into the biological systems at the time of free radical production (Fig. 5.32).

Although DMPO can trap an oxygen free radical such as OH. when injected into a tissue, the most popular *in vivo* nitrone spin trap is a phenyl N-tert-butylnitrone (PBN), which forms a substituted benzyl *tert*-butylnitroxide spin adduct.

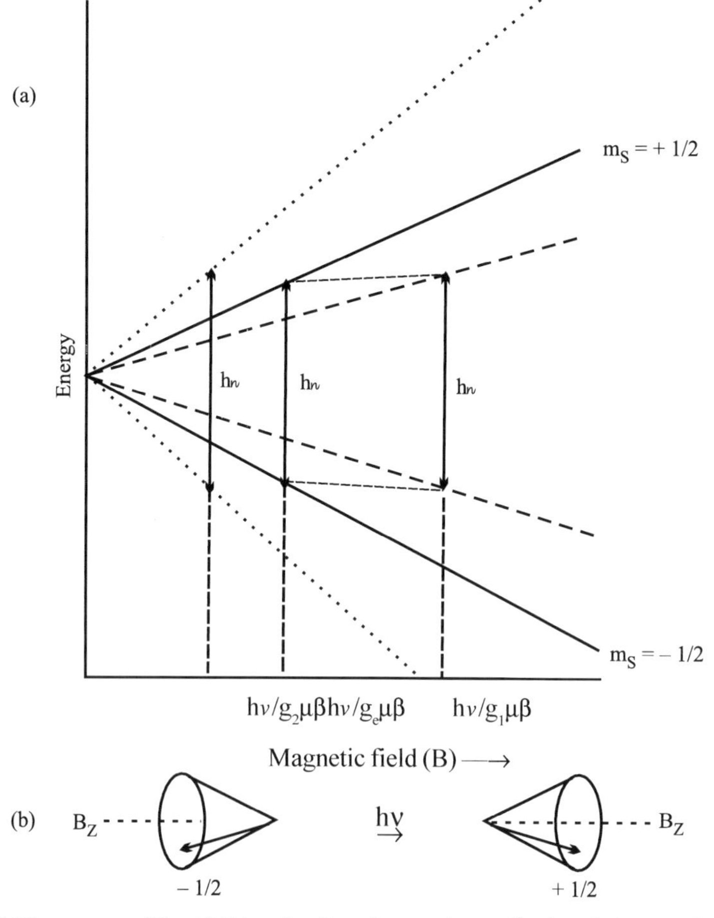

Fig. 5.29 (a) Divergence of the ±1/2 levels of an electron in a radical as the external magnetic field (B) is increased; (b) shows how the processing electron flips its orientation on absorbing *hv* of energy. (Reprinted with permission from *Laboratory Techniques in Biochemistry and Molecular Biology*, 22, 56, 1991. Copyright © 1991 Elsevier Science Inc.)

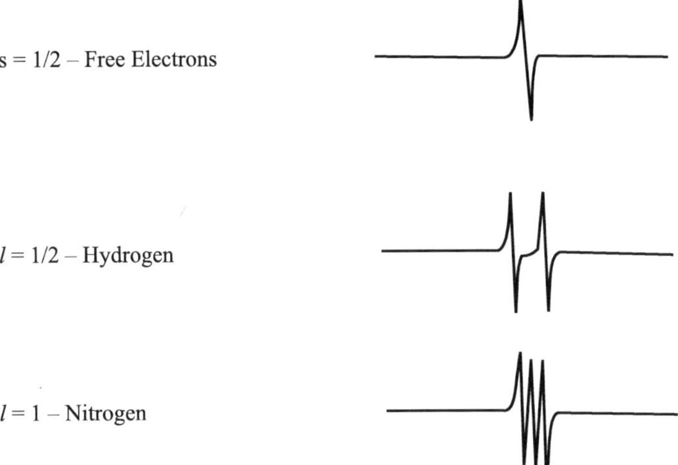

Fig. 5.30 ESR Spectra of free electrons, hydrogen, and nitrogen

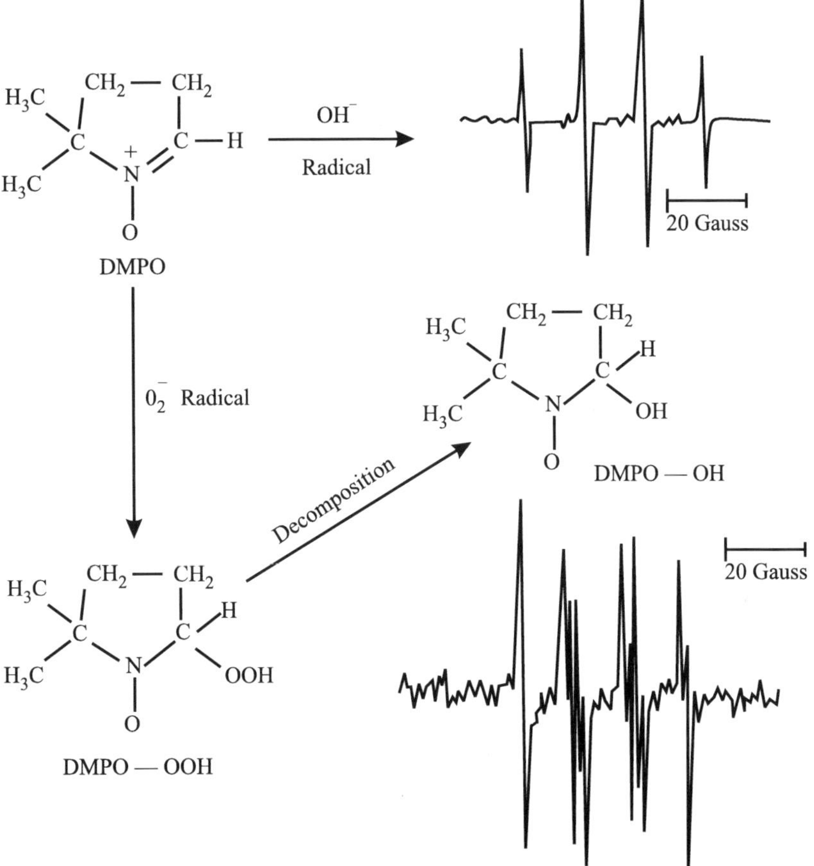

Fig. 5.31 Formation of DMPO-OH· adduct (Reprinted with permission from Hallwell, B., and Gutteridge, J.M.C., *Free Radicals in Biology and Medicine*, Clarendon Press, Oxford, 1989, 53.)

In these nitroxides the unpaired electron occurs in the *p*-orbital on the N_2 and O_2 atoms. Because spin is absent in the O_2 nucleus, the spin will be reflected only for the N_2 nucleus.

5.14.2 High-Performance Liquid Chromatographic (HPLC) Detection of Oxygen Free Radicals

Several HPLC techniques have recently been described to estimate the OH both *in vitro* and *in vivo*.[81,82] The methods utilize either DMPO as spin-trap or salicylic acid as a chemical trap with subsequent analysis of DMPO-OH˙ adduct or hydroxylated benzoic acid formation using electrochemical detection technique. Although both methods have been used in biological systems, the later has been proven to be more successful. The success of the salicylic acid method depends on the formation of two stable compounds, 2, 3-and 2,5-dihydrobenzoic acid, upon the interaction of OH and salicylate.[83] The reaction products also consist of minor amounts of another product, catechol (Fig. 5.33). These hydroxylated products of benzoic acid are very stable and can produce electrical signals when analyzed by HPLC using an electrochemical detector.

Electrochemical detection differs from other methods of detection because it changes the sample. The detection can be performed either amperometrically or coulometrically, the former being the most widely used technique. After the sample is separated on the column, it passes by

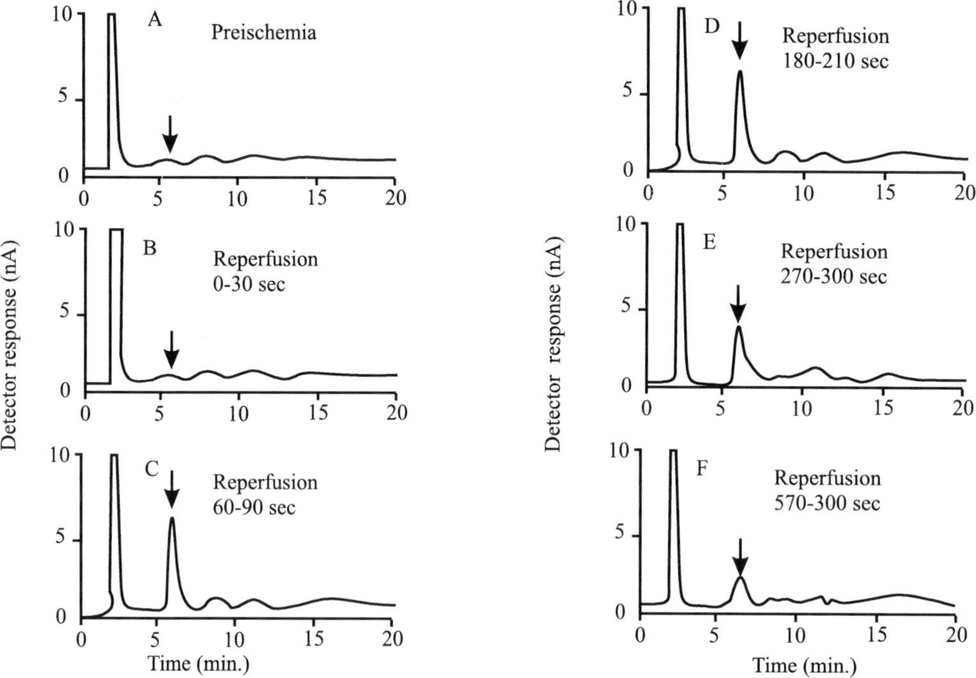

Fig. 5.32 HPLC detection of DMPO-OH. adduct production during reperfusion. Hearts were subjected to 30 minute of global ischemia followed by reperfusion. Effluents were collected; (A) before ischemia; (B) 0-30s; (C) 60-90s; (D) 1801-210s; (E) 270-300 s; and (F) 570-600s after reperfusion. The flow rate of the HPLC mobile phase was 1ml/min, and the chromatographs were recorded at 1 cm/min. The electrochemical detector was set at 10-nA sensitivity. (Data reproduced with permission from *Biochem. Pharmacol.*, 45, 961-969, 1993.)

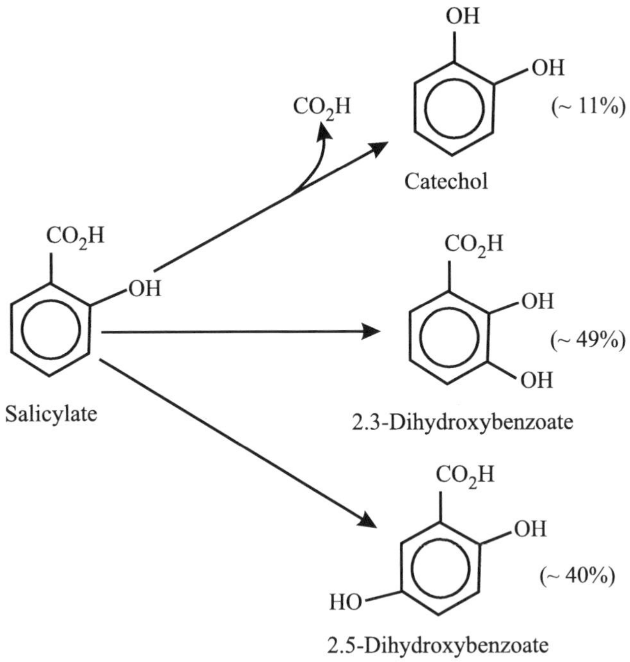

OH

OH

CO_2H (~ 11%)

Catechol

CO_2H CO_2H

OH OH

(~ 49%)

OH

Salicylate 2.3-Dihydroxybenzoate

CO_2H

OH

(~ 40%)

HO

2.5-Dihydroxybenzoate

Fig. 5.33 The products of salicylate-OH- interactions (Reprinted with permission from Hallwell, B., and Gutteridge, J. M. C., *Freee Radicals in Biology and Medicine,* Clarendon Press, Oxford, 1989, 55.)

an electrode (known as the working electrode) in the analytical cell. The working electrode remains at a certain potential with respect to the potential of the electrolyte (as measured by the reference electrode). The electrochemical detector applies a voltage to the working electrode, thus adding energy to the system. The following equation expresses the energy relationship in an electrochemical system:

$$\text{Voltage} = \text{Total energy/Charge}$$

Hence

$$\text{Total energy} = \text{Charge} \times \text{Voltage}$$

where voltage is expressed in electron volts (eV) and the charge is Faraday's constant (96,500 coulombs / mol electrons).

The current produced is proportional to the amount of analyte injected on the column. This equation describes the relationship between the current and the amount injected:

$$I = nKFD^{2/3}C \tag{5.105}$$

where I is the current produced by the electrolysis reaction; n is the number of electrons involved in the reaction; F is Faraday's constant; K is cell constant; D is the diffusion coefficient of the analyte; and, C is the amount of analyte injected onto the column.

An electrochemical reaction occurs in three stages:

1. *Mass transport (diffusion)*: The compound diffuses from the solution in the cell to the electrode surface.
2. *Electrolysis*: At the electrode surface, electrons are either removed from the compound (oxidation) or supplied to it (reduction).
3. *Rediffusion*: The electrolyzed compound passes back into solution.

In principle, an electrochemical detector functions by connecting the working electrode to the electronics. The detector maintains the potential difference between the working and reference electrodes. As the sample flows through the cell, the potential at the working electrode electrolyzes the component(s) of interest, thus producing a current from the electron transfer. The auxiliary electrode remains at ground.

The current flowing through the working electrode is converted to a voltage value. When the sample oxidizes, a positive response results; a reduction reaction produces a negative response. The relationship between current and applied potential is called a *current-voltage curve*, or *hydrodynamic voltammogram*. From the recorded voltage the concentration of the free radicals is calculated.

Both DMPO and salicylate methods have been successfully used in the author's laboratory to detect the formation of $OH^{\cdot}$ in a biological tissue such as heart.[84] Using isolated perfused heart preparation, either DMPO (4.5-5.0 mmol/*l*) or salicylic acid (91mmol/*l*) was infused directly via a side arm of aortic cannula into the heart with an infusion rate of 1 ml/min. The perfusate was sampled, the effluent filtered through a 0.22-mm pore-size Nylon-66 sample filter (Rainin, Woburn, MA) and 20 ml were injected onto a Waters (Milford, MA) HPLC equipped with a model U6K injector, model 510 pump, model 460 electrochemical detector, and a model 740 Data Module. The detector potential was kept at + 0.6 V, employing a glassy carbon working electrode against an Ag / AgCl reference electrode. An Altex Ultrasphere (3 mm ODS, 75 × 4.6 mm) column (Rainin, Wobum, MA) with a Brownlee RP-18 precolumn (Rainin) was used for the detection of the DMPO-$OH^{\cdot}$ adduct at a flow rate of 1 ml/min. The mobile phase consisted of 0.03 mol/*l* of citric acid monohydrate, 0.05 mol/*l* of anhydrous sodium acetate, 0.05 mol/*l* sodium hydroxide, and 8.5% of acetonitrite adjusted to pH 5.1 with glacial acetic acid and was filtered through a 0.22-mm pore-size Nylon-66 solvent filter (Rainin). The DMPO- $OH^{\cdot}$ adduct peak was identified by injecting the DMPO adducts produced from a pure $OH^{\cdot}$ generating system.[84]

To detect the product of salicylic acid–OH- interactions, again the perfusate was filtered through a Rainin 0.22-mm pore-size Nylon-66 sample filter. A 25-ml volume of the sample was injected onto an Altex Ultrasphere (3 mm ODS, 75 × 4.6 mm) column (Rainin) protected by a Brownlee RP-18 precolumn (Rainin). The hydroxylated products of salicylic acid after interaction with hydroxyl radicals, 2,3-dihydroxybenzoic acid (23-DHBA) and 2,5-dihydroxybenzoic acid (2,5-DHBA), were eluted with a buffer containing 0.03 mol/l of sodium acetate and 0.03 mol/l of citric acid (pH 3.6) at a flow rate of 1 ml.min. the detection potential was maintained at +0.6 V, employing a glassy carbon working electrode and an Ag/AgCl reference electrode. Retention times of the peaks of 2,5-DHBA and 2,3-DHBA were varified by injecting authentic standards (Aldrich, Milwaukee, WI) and by injecting the hydroxylated products of salicylic acid from a pure $OH^{\cdot}$ generating system (Fig. 5.34). Examples of a few selected spin traps are shown in Fig. 5.35.

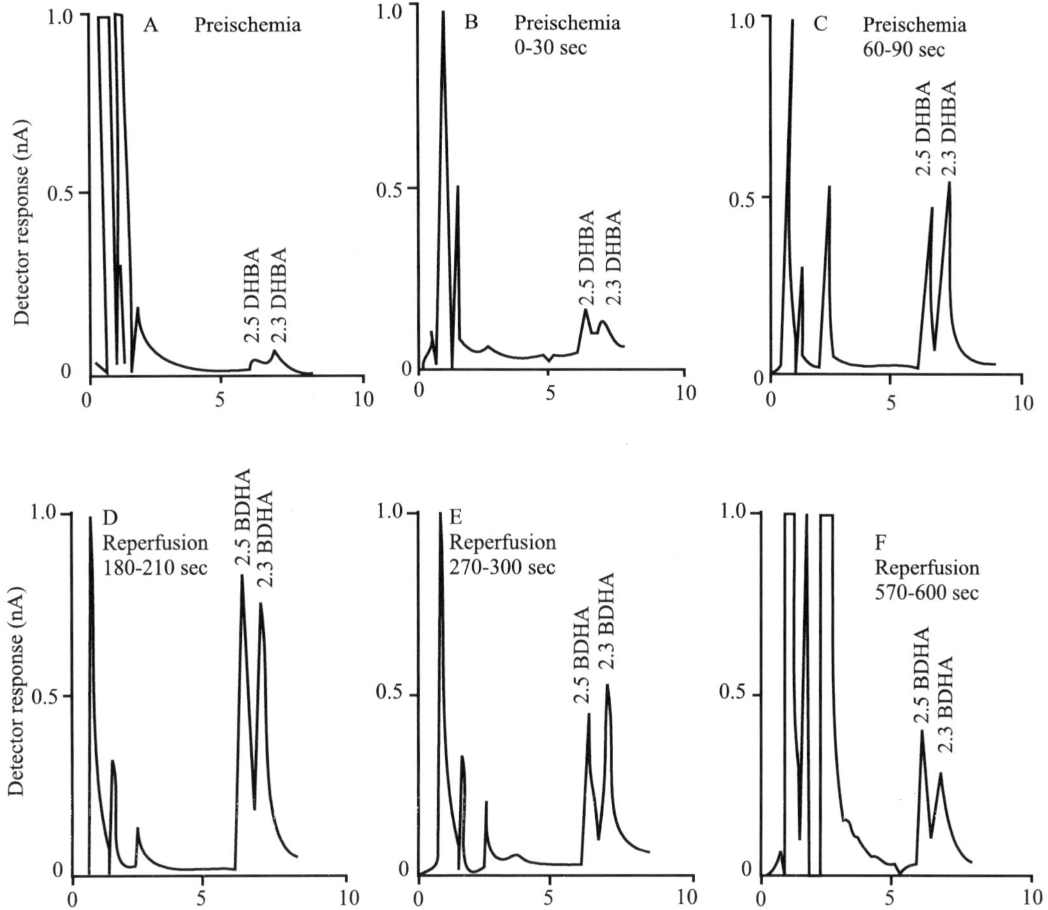

Fig. 5.34 Detection of 2,3- and 2-5-DHBA by HPLC during reperfusion. Hearts were subjected to 30 min of global ischemia followed by reperfusion. Effluents were collected: (A) before ischemia, (B) 0-30s; (C) 60-90s; (D) 180-210s; (E) 270-300s; and (F) 570-600s after reperfusion. The flow rate for HPLC mobile phase was 1 ml/min and the chromatographs were reorded at 1 cm/min. The electrochemical detector was sct at a 1-nA sensitivity. (Data reproduced with permission from *Biochem. Pharmacol.*, 45, 961-969,1983.)

5.14.3 Chemiluminescence Measurement for Oxygen Free Radical Detection

Any free radical species including oxygen free radicals are capable of emitting low-level chemiluminescence. In order to produce luminescence, the energy released from the free radical reactions (viz., oxidation reactions) must be sufficient to produce light. This emitted light can be measured with the help of a luminometer. The reaction rate depends on the concentration of the reacting molecules, thus, chemiluminescence intensity can be recorded as a measure of the concentration of free radicals.

To measure the luminescence in a biological system, the tissue extract or the fluid is mixed with a synthetic compound such as luminol which luminesces during the oxidation by a free radical reaction as shown below[85]:

$$\text{Luminol} + \text{Oxygen free radical} \rightarrow \alpha\text{-aminopthalic acid} + N_2 + \text{Light} \qquad (5.106)$$

As mentioned above, chemiluminescence is measured with the help of a luminometer which consists of an amplifier to convert and amplify the output from the photomultiplier and drive the output device. The output device usually consists of a frequency counter and/or a chart recorder or oscilloscope. The instrument is also equipped with a shutter which allows a continuous operation of the photomultiplier in order to remain dark adapted. The sample is placed inside a chamber which is kept dark all the time.

A luminol stock solution is made by dissolving 1.77 mg of luminol (5-amino-2, 3-dihydrophthalazine 1,4-dione) in 1 ml of demethylsulfoxide (DMSO) to give a concentration of 10^{-2} m. It is diluted before over 10.[85] Although this method is capable of estimating the oxygen free radicals, it cannot distinguish between the individual types, namely, between O_2^-, $OH^{\cdot}$, $^1O_2$, or H_2O_2. The method is still useful for initial screening purposes, and is widely used in free radical detection.

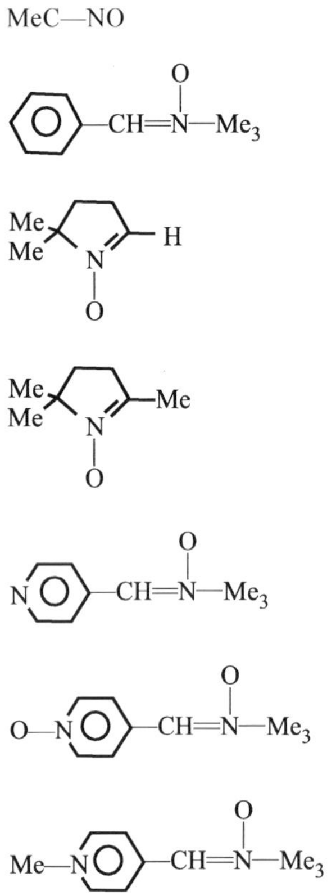

Structure	Agent
MeC—NO	NTB
(benzene ring)—CH=N(→O)—Me$_3$	PBN
Me, Me ring; N—O; H	DMPO
Me, Me ring; N—O; —Me	TMPO
N(pyridine ring)—CH=N(→O)—Me$_3$	4-PyBN
O—N(pyridine ring)—CH=N(→O)—Me$_3$	4-POBN
Me—N(pyridine ring)—CH=N(→O)—Me$_3$	4-MePyBN

Fig. 5.35 Examples of spin-trapping agents

5.14.4 Pulse Radiolysis Method

Pulse radiation is usually generated by linear electron accelerators (Linacs) or by Van de Graaff accelerators, each having certain advantages.[86] The energy carriers are usually accelerated electrons with energies in the MeV range. In aqueous solution, the energy is used for ionization ($H_2O \rightarrow H_2O^+ + e^-$) and excitation ($H_2O \rightarrow H_2O^*$). These reaction products are converted within 10-12 s into hydrated electrons, hydrogen atoms and hydroxyl rddicals:

$$\begin{gathered} H_2O^+ \rightarrow H^+_{aq} + OH^- \\ e^- \rightarrow e^-_{aq} \\ (e^- + H_2O^+) \rightarrow H_2O^* \rightarrow \dot{H}^+ + \dot{O}H^- \end{gathered} \tag{5.107}$$

The equipment for the pulse radiolysis comprises a pulsed accelerator, physical dosimeter, irradiation cell, sample storage and flow system, and detection and signal recording system. Irradiations are performed with pulsed electron beams from a linear or Van de Graaff accelerator as well as with small cyclotrons. Intensity of the electron beam is regulated through a physical dosimeter. The irradiated volume is usually small and irradiation cell is controlled by a flow system with a large sample of unirradiated solution. The resulting signal is monitored by optical or conductivity measurements. For optical measurements, the irradiation cell is penetrated by a beam of intense light rectangularly to the electron beam. Light focusing through the irradiation cell and into a monochromator is achieved by an appropriate lense system. After passing through the monochromator, the light beam is converted into an electrical signal by a photodetector, and finally after amplification the time-resolved signal is displayed on an oscilloscope. For conductivity detection, an electron beam penetrates the area between two electrodes to which a voltage of typically 20-100 V is applied. Any generation or destruction of charged species in the irradiated solution leads to a change in conductance and is recorded as an electrical signal. The major disadvantage of using the pulse radiolysis method is that it is an extremely sophisticated and expensive experimental technique. The instrument is available in only a few selected places. The instrument can be run only with the help of an experienced pulse radiolysist or a physicist.

5.14.5 Biochemical Methods for Oxygen Free Radical Detection

Several biochemical assays are also available to determine oxygen free radicals in biosamples. The two most commonly used methods are the deoxyribose oxidation method to determine $OH^·$ and the cytochrome c oxidation method to estimate O_2^-.

1. Deoxyribose oxidation as a measure for OH^-

The success of the method depends on the fact that deoxyribose reacts with $OH^·$ with a rate constant of $3.1 \times 10^9\ M^{-1}s^{-1}$ producing malonaldehyde.[87] As described previously malonaldehyde can react with thiobarbituric acid to produce a red color which can be measured at 535 nm. The actual assay system consists of (in a total volume of a 1-ml biosample): 28 mM deoxyribose, 20 mM Tris-HCL buffer, pH 7.4, 100 mM $FeCl_3$, 100 mM EDTA, 1 mM H_2O_2 and 100 mM ascorbate. The reaction mixture is incubated at 37°C for 1 h, after which malonaldehyde formation from deoxyribose oxidation is measured using thiobarbituric acid reaction[88] described under malonaldehyde assay.

2. Cytochrome reduction as a measure for O_2^-

The method depends on the ability of superoxide anion to reduce cytochrome c. To determine the amount of cytochrome c reduced by O_2^- the biosample is incubated with 0.75 mM horse-heart ferricytochrome c (type III, Sigma, St Louis, MO).[88] The absorbance is measured at 550 nm using a spectrophotometer. The amount of cytochrome c in the reaction mixture is calculated using an absorbance coefficient of 21.1 $mM^{-1}cm^{-1}$ at 550 nm.

5.14.6 Indirect Methods of Oxygen Free Radical Detection

Several methods are available to detect the presence of oxygen-derived free radicals in the biological systems. The success of the method depends on the interaction between the free radicals and the membrane lipids. Polyunsaturated fatty acids (PUFA) of the membrane phospholipids are extremely susceptible to free radical attack. The reactions generate lipid hydroperoxides and endoperoxides, as well as malonaldehyde. In addition, during the lipid peroxidation after the abstraction of the H atom, carbon molecules rearrange between themselves producing conjugated dienes. Both malonaldehyde and diene formations are considered as powerful tools to measure the extent of lipid peroxidation in biosystems.

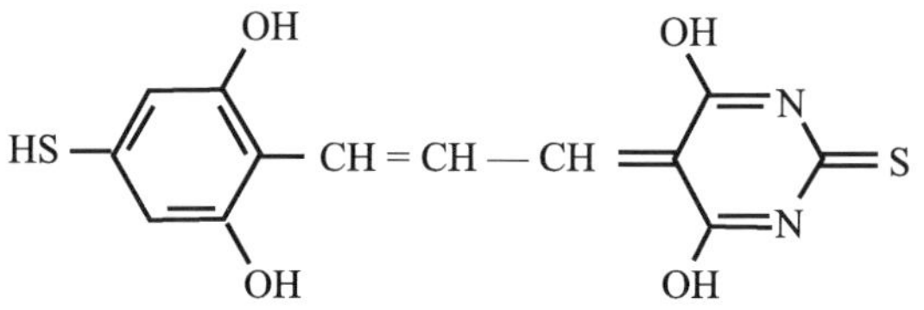

Fig. 5.36 Product of thiobarbituric acid (TBA) and malonaldehyde (MDA) reactions

1. Assay for malonaldehyde formation

The most commonly used method to estimate malonaldehyde formation is the spectrophotometric assay of the malonaldehyde formation following its reaction with thiobarbituric acid (Fig. 5.36). The sample (tissue homogenate or fluid) (91 ml) is mixed with 0.2 ml of 15% trichloroacetic acid and 1 ml of 0.75% thiobarbituric acid in 0.5% sodium acetate, and the mixture is boiled for 15 minute. The red colour of the thiobarbituric acid-malonaldehyde complex is read with a spectrophotometer using a 535-nm wavelength.[89]

Although this method is rapid and relatively simple, the significance of the results is often blunted because of the incorrect interpretation of the results. The thiobarbituric acid-reactive products (often referred to as TBAR) as a measure for malonaldehyde formation is nonspecific, because thiobarbituric acid not only forms a colored complex with malonaldehyde, but it also reacts with many other compounds including ribose, bilirubin, amino acids, pyrimidines, and sialic acid.[90]

Several HPLC methods have been developed to overcome this problem. One such technique depends on measuring malonaldehyde and other lipid metabolic products after derivatizing with 2.4-dinitrophenylhydrazine (DNPH).[91] For derivatization purpose, 310 mg of DNPH is dissolved in 100 ml of 2 M HCl. One-tenth of a milliliter of this DNPH reagent is added to the sample (1.5 ml) in a 20-ml screw-capped Teflon-lined test tube. An aliquot of 0.5 ml is added to the tube, the contents are mixed for 15 min by vortexing, and then 10 ml of pentane are added to the mixture. The tubes are intermittently shaken for 30 min, and reactions are allowed to occur at room temperature. The organic phase is removed, and the aqueous phase is extracted with an additional 20 ml of pentane. The pentane extracts are combined evaporated under a stream N_2 at 30°C, and reconstituted in 200 ml of acetonitrile. In the authors' laboratory, a 25-ml volume of the filtered (0.2-mM Nylon-66 membrane filters in Microfilterfuge tubes from Rainin Instrument Co., Woburm, MA) sample was injected onto a Beckman Ultrasphere ODS C_{18} (3-mm particle size; 7.5 cm × 4.6 mm I.D.) column (Rainin Instrument Co., Wobum,MA) in a Waters chromatograph (Milford, MA) equipped with a model 820 full-control Maxima computer system, satellite Wisp model 700 injector, model 490 programmable multiwavelength UV detector (four channels), two model 510 pumps, and a Bondapak C_{18} Guard-Pak piecolumn. The DNPH derivatives are detected at 307, 325, and 356 nm simultaneously with three channels of the M-490 detector at a flow rate of 1 ml/min with an isocratic gradient of acetonitrile-water-acetic acid (40 : 60 : 0.1 v/v/v) for a total run time of 24 min. The column is washed with acetonitrile-acetic acid (100 : 0.1 v/v) before each day's work to remove any bound reagent.

DNPH derivatives of formaldehyde (FDA). acetaldehyde (ADA), acetone, and malonaldehyde (MDA) are separated using three different wavelengths: 307, 325, and 356 nm. MDA gives absorption maxima at 307 nm whereas the absorption maxima for FDA, ADA, acetone is 356 nm. The retention times of MDA, FDA, ADA, and acetone are 5.3, 6.6, 10.3, and 16.5 min. respectively, making a total run time of 24 min.

In order to confirm the identity of lipid metabolites, GC-MS analyses may be performed.[92] The GCMS system used in the authors' laboratory consisted of a Hewlett-Packard model 5890 gas chromatograph (Fullerton. CA) with a 15 m × 0.32 mm I.D. capillary column 0.25-μm film thickness (Supelco SPB-5, Bellefonte, PA), which was connected directly to the mass spectrometer via a heated transfer line. The transfer line temperature was maintained at 250°C. The carrier gas was helium at an average linear the velocity of 65.8 cm/s, and the injection temperature was 230°C. The injector was operated in the splitless mode. A temperature program was used which consisted of a starting temperature of 75°C which was as increased to 175°C at increments of 25°C/min. Between 175°C and 200°C, the temperature was increased at a rate of 5°C/min and finally to 300°C at increments of 25°C/min. The mass spectrometer was a Finnigan-MAT model 50B quadrupole instrument (Palo Alto, CA) in combination with an INCOS data system. The instrument was set on electron ionization mode. The ion source temperature was 180°C, and the ionization energy was 70 eV. The system was coupled to a Data General model DG 10 computer (Southboro, MA) and a Printronix model MVP printer (Irvine, CA). For GC-MS analysis, the hydrazine derivatives of MDA, FDA, ADA, acetone, and PDA were dissolved in chloroform (50 ng/ml). Similarly, hydrazine-derivatized heart perfusate samples were reconstituted in chloroform. Samples (2 ml) of standard and extracts were injected onto the GCMS system. Following the full-spectrum identification of each of the hydrazones, a selective ion monitoring (SIM) program was developed, and additional spectra were obtained in the SIM mode.

The identity of the peaks may be confirmed by comparing the retention times with those of authentic standards using GC-MS. The HPLC-GC-MS data for the five lipid metabolites are presented in Figs. 5.37, 5.38 and 5.39. The molecular ions (M^+) of the synthetic hydrazones of FDA, MDA, ADA, acetone, and PDA are 210, 234, 224, 238, and 238, respectively.

2. Assay for conjugated diene formation

As mentioned earlier, lipid peroxidation can proceed by hydrogen abstraction or by an addition reaction. The carbon-centered radical formed is then stabilized by spontaneous molecular rearrangement to form conjugated diene (Fig. 5.40). The diene formation can be detected spectrophotometrically.[93] The biosamples are extracted with a methanol-chloroform mixture (1:2, v/v). The mixture is allowed to stand at room temperature for 10 min, and then centrifuged at 260 × G for 10 min. The supernatant fluid is decanted into another centrifuge tube, the volume adjusted to 30 ml with methanol-chloroform (1 : 2, v/v), and then 10 ml of water are added. The contents are mixed gently, centrifuged, and the chloroform layer is transferred to a clean tube. The chloroform is evaporated to dryness under N_2, and the residue is dissolved in spectroscopic grade cyclohexane. The solution is scanned between 220 and 300 nm against a cyclohexane blank.

5.15 CONVENTIONAL AND NOVEL BIOREACTORS FOR CELL CULTURES

In general, a conventional submerged type of bioreactor/oxygenator with agitation system has been used in cell cultivations.[1, 6-8] The same type of oxygenator as used for the homogeneous cultivation of microorganisms may be applied for plant cell cultivation and for microcarrier supported animal cell culture.[94] There are three major types of homogeneous-oxygenator systems used for propagating microbial, plant, and animal cells. These are stirred tank reactors (STRs), thin-film rotary oxygenator and airlift reactors (ALRs).[95, 96] All of these oxygenators are able to exert shear effects on cell cultures. In general, animal cells are much more sensitive to shear stress as compared with microbial and plant cell cultures. In STRs, however, there is conflicting data about this degree of shear sesitivity. Conventional turbine or vibrator-agitated bioreactor oxygenators have been commonly used to produce mammalian cells which can grow independently of a solid support.[97] It has been shown that the growth of specific hybridoma cells decreased at an agitation rate of 240 rpm.[98] This has been stated to be an indication of the sensitivity of hybridoma cells to excessive mechanical agitation. It has been shown that critical shear stress causing progressive loss of viability of insect cells was 1-4 N/m^2. The problem is that it is not an easy task to grow large quantities of mammalian and plant cells in an artificial medium. The well-established technology of industrial microbiology is adapted to the requirements of bacteria, yeasts, and molds. Each single cell of these microorganisms being encased in a tough cell wall serves as an independent metabolic factory with fairly simple nutritional requirements. Microorganisms grow well dispersed and floating free in a liquid cultivation medium in a conventional STR with a capacity as high as 80,000-100,000 liters. In this conventional oxygenator design, microorganisms depending on nature resist damage even when they have proliferated to form a thick suspension and even when the suspension is agitated vigorously with a mechanical agitator. Mammalian and plant cells have different properties. They are larger than those of most microorganisms, more fragile, sensitive to shear and other mechanical forces. and more complex. As can be seen from literature,[102, 103] the delicate plasma membrane that encloses an animal cell is not encased in a tough cell wall. Having these structural characteristics most animal cells will not grow at all in suspensions. They grow only when they can attach themselves to a surface. This requirement led to the development of a novel microcarrier-anchored cell bioreactor. Over the years techniques have

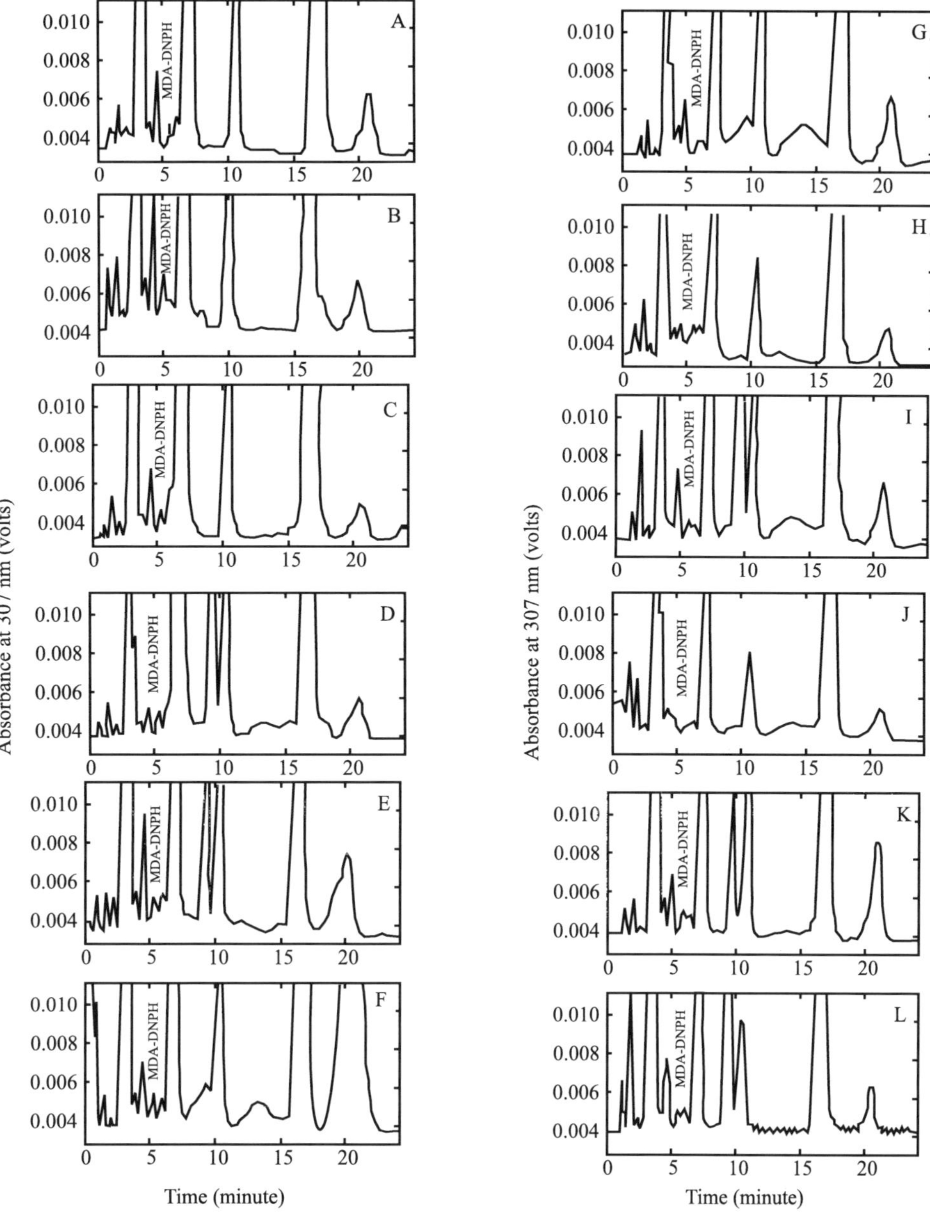

Fig. 5.37 Reverse-phase HPLC separation of MDA-DNPH from perfusates obtained from isolated rat hearts perfused with a OH˙ generating system in the presence and absence of SOD plus catalase. Perfusates were collected, derivatized, and chromatographed. Absorbance was measured at 307 nm. (A) baseline; (B) after 1 min of perfusion with OH˙; (C) after 45 mins. of perfusion with OH˙; (D) after 20 mins. of perfusion with OH˙; (E) after 30 mins. of perfusion with OH˙; (F) after 45 min of perfusion with OH˙; (G) Baseline; (H) after 1 min of perfusion with OH˙plus SOD and catalase; (I) after 20 min of perfusion with OH˙plus SOD and catalase; (J) after 20 mins. of perfusion with OH˙plus SOD and catalase; (L) after 45 mins. of perfusion with OH˙ plus SOD and catalase. (Data reproduced with permission from *J. Chromatographer*., 661, 181-191, 1994.)

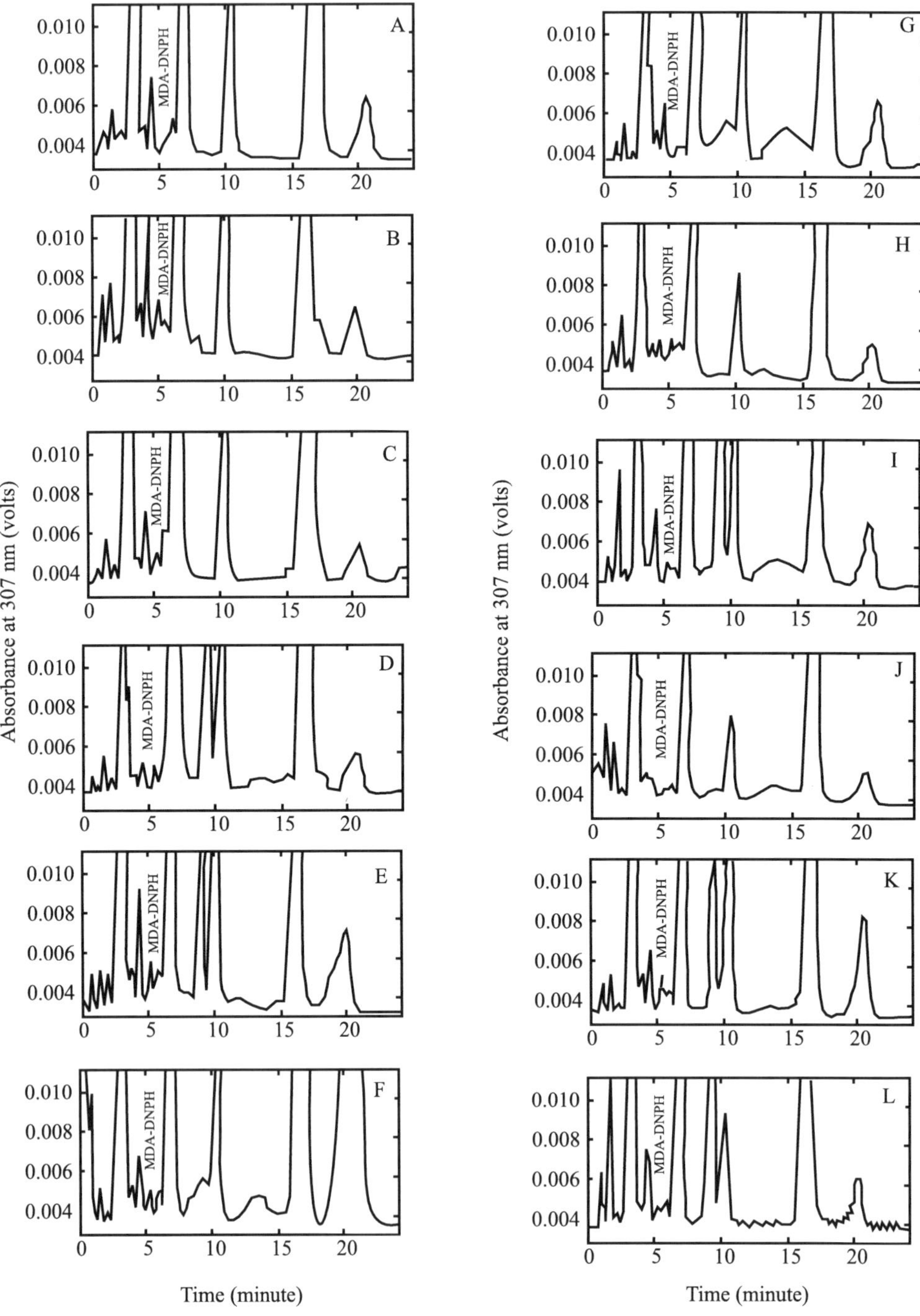

Fig. 5.38 Separation of FDA-DNPH, ADA-DNPH, Acetone-DNPH, and PDA-DNPH in rat heart perfusates under the same conditions described in Fig. 5.37, except that the absorbance was measured at 356 nm. (A) to (L), same as in Fig. 5.36 (Data reproduced with permission from *J. Chromatographer.*, 661, 181-191, 1994)

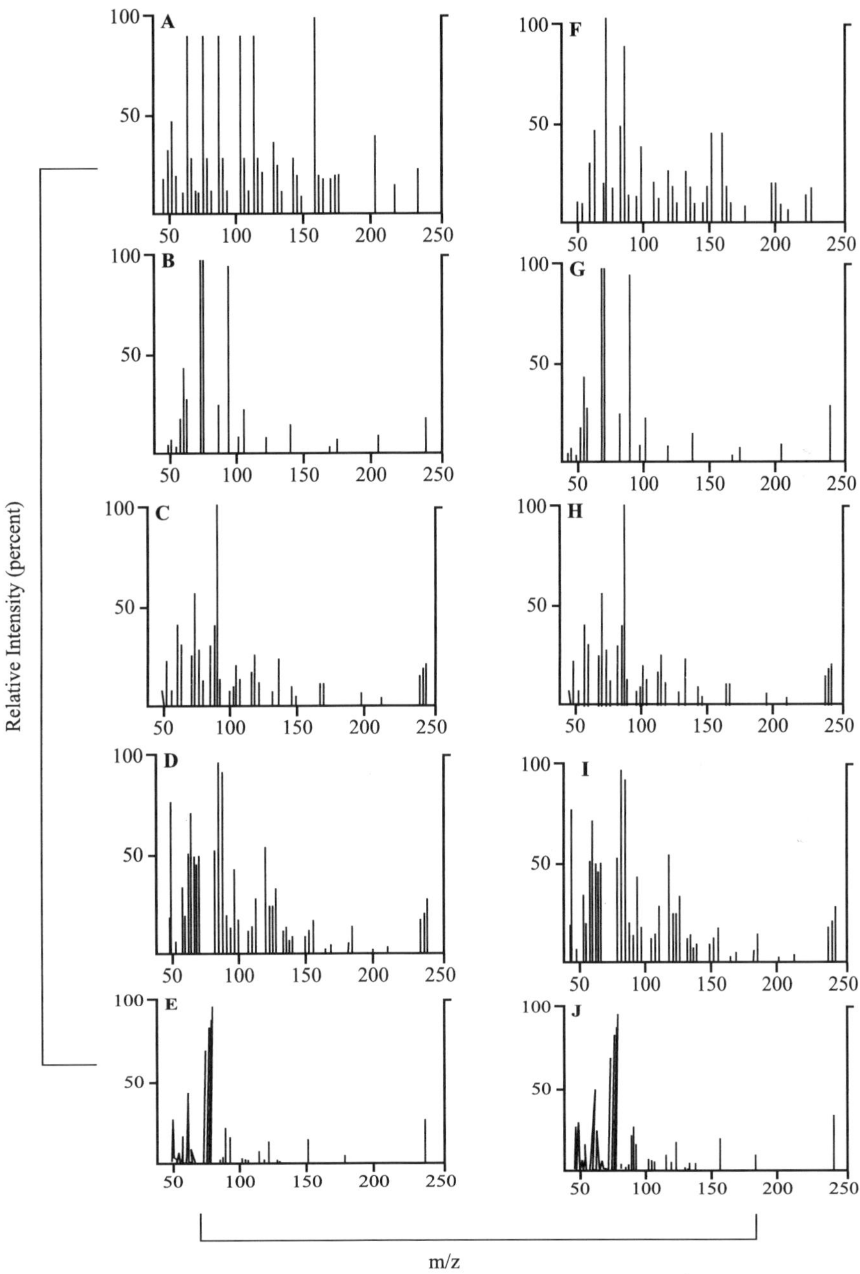

Fig. 5.39 Representative mass spectrum of DNPH derivatives of the standards for the five lipid metabolites and for the five lipid metabolites in rat heart perfusates. Mass spectra were obtained for: (A) MDA-DNPH standard; (B) FDA-DNPH standard; (C) ADA-DNPH standard; (D) Acetone-DNPH standard; (E) PDA-DNPH standard; (F) MDA-DNPH in rat heart perfusate; (G) FDA-DNPH in perfusate; (H) ADA-DNPH in perfusate (I) Acetone-DNPH in perfusate; and (J) PDA-DNPH in perfusate. (Data reproduced with permission from *J. Chromatographer.*, 661, 181-191, 1994.)

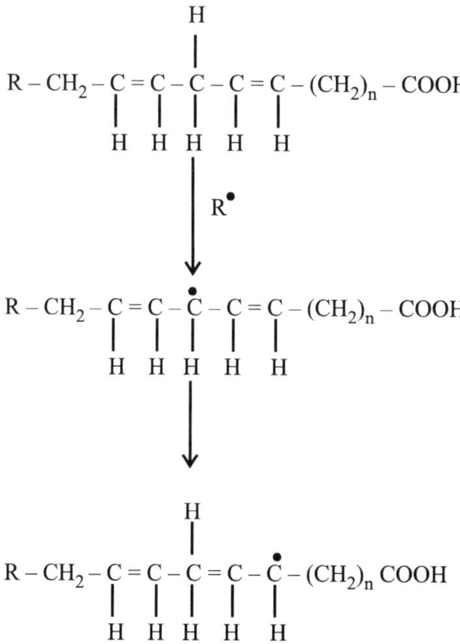

Fig. 5.40 Formation of conjugated dienes after hydrogen abstraction and rearrangement of C = C bonds

been developed to grow mammalian and plant cells on a small scale in the laboratory bioreactors. A mammalian cell culture begins with a mammalian tissue. The tissue is dissociated either mechanically or enzymatically, or by a combination of the two methods. This yields mixture of single cells and small clumps of cells. The mixture is inoculated into an appropnate liquid growth medium containing salts, glucose, certain amino acids, and blood serum. Although most mammalian cells need to be anchored to a solid support, cells that originate in blood or lymphatic tissue, along with most tumor cells and other transformed cells, can be adapted to grow in suspension. Such cells can be cultivated in spinner bottles. It has been reported that a Waldhof-type and bubble column oxygenation bioreactor with a draft tube in the middle of the vessel have also been used successfully.[95,99] Bioprocess engineering that involves mammalian cell culture has come to prominence recently with a growing number of bioproducts obtained from such bioprocesses.

In order to explain the mechanisms of cell loss in conventional agitated and sparged oxygenation bioreactors, many experimental studies have been carried out to investigate the influence of culture conditions on the susceptibility of cell damage. It has been proposed that bubbles of sparged air cause most of the losses as they disengage from the broth. Thus, conventional and novel oxygenation bioreactors for microbial, rnammalian, and plant cell culture systems possess several common and uncommon features.

5.16 MICROBIAL CELL CULTURE BIOREACTORS[101]

They can be defined as a system oxygenators of single or multiple vessels in which microbial reactions are carried out employing free or immobilized cells in batch, fed batch, or continuous operations. The system configurations are designed to take care of the reaction and transport processes adequately. Although these oxygenators relate to classical chemical reactors, from the point of view of reaction the basic difference lies in the living nature of the cells and their ability to initiate and conduct multiple reactions in most cases in series, consecutive, or sequential reactions. Various features and advances in microbial bioreactor oxygenators can be seen in the literature.

Classical microbial bioreactors have the following features:

- Closed, submerged upright cylindrical vessels
- Provision of air sparging
- Provision of mixing for mass, momentum, and heat transfer
- Aseptic operation

Problems with classical bioreactors include:

- Development of circulation zones in which intermixing between individual zones may become the limiting factor for adequate blending
- Clumping or overlay of mycelia
- Wall growth
- High power demand for adequate mass transfer rates
- Inhibition exercised by substrates, intermediates or their products

In view of these problems associated with classical bioreactors, new systems with several configurations were initiated in the early 1960s. External loop reactor and trickling filters are the two systems that require far less energy, mainly for hydraulic transport needs, than most other systems developed to date. Other loop systems like injector loop and internal loop systems, on the other hand, consume nearly two-thirds to three-fourths of the total energy input compared to the normal, widely used, multiblade STRs.

5.16.1 General Requirements and Features of Bioreactors

Bioreactors are required to perform a great number of functions to fulfill many requirements. The requirements are met partly or to a large extent in having incorporated configurational changes in the classical system of STR or PFRS. As a result several new reactor types have come into existence which are either being tried in prototypes or used in large commercial operations.

5.16.2 Stirred Tank Reactors

Principally, these are upright cylindrical vessels in which air is sparged through the agitated liquid medium. Various types of STRs are in use. Examples include single and multistage STRs and Waldhof reactors.

Generally in an STR specific power consumption is high. Comparatively, Waldhof reactors consume less specific power since the center of gravity of the liquid is lower. Gas hold-up is also high since a considerable volume of air is drawn and is finely dispersed through the turbulent agitator zone.

5.16.3 Surface Reactors

In physical configuration these are also cylindrical vessels rotating on the horizontal axis in which air is blown inside the vessel. Examples include the horizontal rotary reactor (HRR), disc reactors and film reactors. In extreme gas-liquid interactions this type of reactor has demonstrated its excellent suitability. It has been suggested that large inequalities in the distribution of DO in STRs, particularly in high viscous non-Newtonian broths, HRRs offer good solution. This reactor is significantly important on account of a number of outstanding performance.

5.16.4 Cyclone Reactors

In this system the cells are circulated around a closed loop to effect oxygen transfer, mixing, and homogeneous cultivation instead of agitation and stirring in a tank. Special advantages are: a high gas exchange, no use of antifoam, no wall growth, and operation suitable for cultivation of aerobic and anaerobic nonpathogenic microorganisms. This reactor can be used for batch and continuous growth of synchronous and asynchronous cultures.

5.16.5 Fixed-Film Reactors

These reactors have a performance behavior similar to that of trickling filters extensively used in waste water treatments. The ideal film thickness should correspond to the penetration depth of the limiting nutrient. Further increase in film thickness leads to no improvement in conversion efficiency.

5.16.6 Deep-Shaft Reactors

The principle of operation is similar to that of the pressure cycle reactor, except that all or most of the air is introduced into the downflow tube and no baffles are permitted to rise because of blockage risks. Depth is also considerably greater, normally in the range of 50-150 m. Air introduced in this way is at a lower pressure than if it were introduced at the bottom; this enables savings both in capital and operating costs. Liquid circulation is established by injection of compressed air through a sparger placed at relatively shallow depth in the upflow side. Air is then gradually switched to the downflow side. The gas voidage in the top part of the upflow tube continues to balance hydraulic friction losses and net voidage resistance in the lower part of the reactor. Bubble contact time, high pressure, and turbulence provide oxygen transfer as high as 3 kg of O_2/h-m^3. Energy requirement for this high degree of oxygen transfer is about 1 kWh.

5.16.7 Immobilized Cell Reactors

In these reactors, enzymes/cells are either attached by adsorption, chemical bonding (cross-linked or covalently bound), or entrapment on a suitable carrier, or are encapsulated and placed/packed in different types of vessel configurations to serve as a flow reactor. Reactors with physical adsorption of enzymes or cells encounter practical difficulties because the adsorbed enzyme or cell is weakly bound and is lost rather easily during operation. Gel-entrapped enzyme reactor systems are associated with severe problems of diffusional resistances more exercised by the substrate than the product. Covalently or cross-linked immobilized reactor systems require mild processing conditions. Large changes in pH and temperature are not permitted. A microencapsulated reactor system is subjected to the requirement of substrate diffusivity across the semipermeable membrane which contains the enzyme or cells. Despite these disadvantages, the greatest advantage offered by this system is high-productivity.

5.16.8 Membrane Reactors

Membrane reactors are one of the first novel immobilized enzyme reactors. More complex the reactor design is, the more changes of the coefficients and constants will be expected with scale-up or scale-down practices. This underlines the complicated similarity relationships of the standard STR configuration.

Although physical functions of bioreactors are determined by the geometry and mechanical inputs, the microbial activities are manifested by the established physiological and morphological picture. Total correlations between physical and mechanical functions against microbial functions are not completely available. The release of substances by the cells into the liquid bulk is generally associated with feedback mechanism controlling the changes in the input variable and thus resulting in an altered regulatory expression in the microbial mass. The release of surface active proteinous materials affects the rheological properties of the liquid medium and thus sets up a chain of changes in the environmental conditions such as air distribution, gas hold-up, diffusional mass transfer, bulk heat transfer, and so forth. These problems change the interrelationships of constants and coefficients of reactor functions. Problems associated with aggregated mycelia in many reactor systems are well known.

The oxygen transfer pathway in a typical bioconversion process is shown in Fig. 5.1. Transport of oxygen from air bubbles to the liquid and then to the cell through the liquid pathway poses some serious problems in some particularly immiscible systems. It is associated with the sparingly soluble oxygen and the rate-controlling step for oxygen is that from the bubble interface to the bulk liquid. The problem is aggravated by the rheological properties of the liquid. Power requirement in such a system is necessarily high. High and low power input in such systems create different mixing zones. Creation of mixing zones in turn may result in nonhomogeneity in the reaction rates.

5.16.9 Theoretical

The conversion in a bioreacter depends on the kinetics of the biological reaction, mostly determined by Monod-type rate expression, the distribution of the concentration of reactants, and their residence time in the reactor. This latter characteristic is related to the bulk flow regime. Bulk flow regimes have been analyzed on a thcorctical basis. Two idealized flow regimes describing performance characteristics include the perfectly mixed continuous bioreactor and the continuous plug flow reactor. As in chemical reactors cell nutrients fed into the perfectly mixed reactor are immediately mixed and uniformly distributed, so that the total reactor remains homogeneous. The bulk flow characteristics of this reactor are easily described by residence time distribution (t_R) of reactants (S) passing through it. It is apparent that in the perfectly mixed bioreactor, single reactant/nutrient do not have a defined residence time.

In plug flow bioreactors, no axial mixing occurs. Nutrients entering into the reactor have defined residence time and reactant concentrations are different in their special distribution within the system. The difference between perfectly mixed and plug flow reactor performance has been analyzed by some investigators for reactions following Monod's rate pattern at a given initial cell concentration in the feed. Substrate utilization and cell mass production are affected in a different manner in the two types of reactors. It has been stated that the perfectly mixed reactor in the region of short t_R gives rise to higher cell mass at lower substrate concentration than the plug flow reactor. With large t_R, however, the situation is reversed. The combination of perfectly mixed and plug flow reactors in a two-stage process provide the optimum performance, loop or recycle reactors provide a practical realization of this combination. Also, recycle reactors provide cases of maximum mixedness and plug flow. In the recycle system, recycle ratio (R) greater than 10 generally guarantees adequate mixing.

In practice the R is easily obtained and in fact, it can be much higher. Depending on the value of R, a minimum concentration profile is observed in the bioreactor. This concentration profile is successively folded over on itself. The time of a single passage through the reactor is $t_R/(1 + R)$ and this profile will also characterize the recycle reactor. The recycle-to-feed ratio is, therefore, an important criterion in the scale-up practice of a microbial reaction in a recycle reactor.

In mixing it is virtually impossible to maintain dynamic and geometric similarity on scale-up; one must decide whether circulation rate, power dissipation, or shear rate has more influence on the process result. Except for the biological characteristics of the bulk, there is hardly any difference in the scale-up approach between a chemical reactor and a biochemical reactor. To explain the principles and performance of circulation and agitation devices, the following points are important to remember.

Principle of circulation: The O_2 gradient has been shown in a confined circulation circuit in which the maximum O_2 availability takes place near the agitator and almost none takes place near the end of the system.

Emulsifying circulation stirrer : The system is shown as it exists. In fact, it represents two distinct but undivided zones: the contacting and emulsifying zone, and the other more stable zone at the top. Such circulation and mixing systems were in extensive use in the past in SCP processes based on *n*-alkane and gas oil.

Regime flow velocities: The velocity profile around a flat blade turbine stirrer with a tip speed of 130 cm/s in turbulent flow condition ($Re = 10^5$) is plotted against the distance of the indicator element from the central section of the paddle with its rotational speed fixed at 250 rpm.

Blending and contacting zones: In a highly viscous situation the ratio of impeller diameter (D_i) to tank diameter (D_t) plays a very significant role in determining the situation under which the reaction rates provide two distinct maxima, one in respect to mass flow and the other with regard to mixing (i.e., gas liquid contacting operation). In a given situation with D_i/D_t, of 0.25, mixing provides maximum reactor rate while at a D_i/D_t, of 0.75, mass flow or blending only brings about an almost equal rate of reactions.

A typical and widely used system in viscous fungal bioconversion systems with multiple blades properly spaced and submerged a classical system has been used in biochemical engineering over nearly the last four decades.

An approximate distribution of the extent of turbulence and mass flow takes place in a typical well designed bioreactor handling antibiotic and SCP production system. The classification ranges are related to impeller diameter and rpm for low, medium, and high ranges. This is what one would expect in most conversion systems of these two kinds (antibiotic and SCP). For mixing in multi-impeller bioreactors, impeller spacing has a significant ratio. For a three-impeller system the effect of impeller spacing on flow pattern and power adsorption could be seen when impellers are too close (0.3 D_i); the effect resembles that of a wide impeller. Flow to the middle is restricted, power input is reduced, and the tank liquid is inadequately agitated. A small increase (0.5 D_i) in impeller spacing does not increase power input but produces some independent flow to the other impellers, giving an overall reduction in the height of liquid agitated. When impeller spacing equals the impeller diameter, the height of liquid agitated is increased further, with again no substantial change in power input. At this condition impellers should be working nearly independently with the return flows touching. However, when the impellers are placed too widely apart, input reaches a maximum and is unchanged by further separation of impellers. The correct spacing of impellers is affected largely by the rheological characteristics of the reactor contents. For a given impeller spacing, of course, a transition from one flow pattern to another can occur as fluid characteristics change during bioconversion reactions.

Increase in K_La by increasing the number of impeller stages can also take place in water as well as in viscous mycelial suspensions. The importance and the problems of oxygen in biochemical reactions are well documented.[34] In almost all aerobic bioconversions, attainment of maximum oxygen absorption (K_La values) is one of the major requirements in obtaining maximum product yield in bioreactors. Agitation in turn is dependent on power and is critical in non-Newtonian broths. Conventional STRs are no longer considered to represent the optimal principle due to relatively high specific power demand.

The various configurations provided in the literatures indicate that surface and loop reactors provide the ability of drastic reduction of specific power input up to 1-2 kW/l. It is one of the major reasons of increased interests in the bioreactor design based on loop forms.

5.16.10 Aeration Economy in Conventional Bioreactors

The amount of oxygen that can be dissolved per unit of power expenditure to the aerated liquid is expressed in terms of *economy*. But *aeration economy* (AE) must be based on the oxygenation capacity (OC) of bioreactors. AE and OC are defined as follows:

$$AE = K_LaC^*/(P/v) = OC/P \tag{5.108}$$

The power requirement P is calculated from the following polytropic compression relation :

$$P = [7.32\ O\ N'\ \{(P_2 - P_1)^{0.23\ N'} - 1\}]/n \tag{5.109}$$

where O is the air flow at atmospheric pressure dropping from P_2 to a pressure P_1, N' is the number of compression stages and n is compressor efticiency. As an example, an aeration economy of 3.5 KgO_2/kWh could be obtained in SCP production from methanol in a 20-m^3 bioreactor using an air compressor having 70% efficiency. In such a case it has been observed that when dissolved oxygen in the reactor goes below 10% saturation level, the corresponding aeration economy being very low, an immediate buildup of methanol occurs causing a decrease in SCP productivity. Since AE depends on the power requirement, oxygen availability in a bioconversion reaction becomes a function of agitator power. Use of the ratio of impeller diameter to tank diameter as a parameter for novobiocin production provides a typical example.

5.17 MAMMALIAN CELL CULTURE BIOREACTORS

For mammalian cell cultures various types of bioreactors are currently available.[100] Many designs have ranges from modified microbial bioreactor vessels to compact process-intensified configuration systems with required features. Usually, two classes of mammalian cell culture bioreactors are in use.[101] The first category is used for the cultivation of anchorage-dependent cells. The second class is used for the cultivation of suspended mammalian cells. Perfusion type of bioreactors are usually used in the former systems. In the suspended mammalian cell cultivations, airlift bioreactors, stirred tank bioreactors, and so forth have been used. The airlift bioreactor has been scaled-up from the 101 level to the 20001 level. Improved oxygen transfer rates have been claimed at the larger scale. In this bioreactor, oxygenation is carried out by introducing air at the bottom of the vessel within the draught tube. A decrease in the density of the aerated contents in the draught tube results in a upward circulation behavior of the culture through the draught tube, and downward circulation in the outer zone of the reactor.

5.18 IMPORTANCE OF K_La IN CELL CULTURE PROCESS SCALE UP

Perform experiments on a small scale and obtain the profits on a large scale is the basic slogan for scale up. The approach to achieve this need is based on several criteria. Among the suggested criteria for scale up, volumetric oxygen transfer coefficient (K_La) has been given important emphasis in practice. Oxygenation is a critical and frequently a limiting process step so that oxygen transfer coefficients, K_L (m^3 of O_2 $m^{-3}s^{-1}$) constant volumetric oxygen transfer coefficient, K_La (s^{-1}) may be used as a process scale up parameter. The scale up relation between K_La, gassed power input per unit volume, P_g/D^3 (where P_g is gassed power and D is the vessel diameter) and superficial gas velocity (v_s) has been discussed in Chapter 8.

5.19 ACKNOWLEDGEMENT

The author likes to thank Dipak K.Das, Ph.D., Professor and Director, Cardiovascular Division, UCHC, Farmington, USA for providing facilities in using the library of the Health Centre and contributing fifteen text pages.

5.20 REFERENCES

1. Aiba,S., Humphrey, A. E., and Millis, N.F., *Equipment Design and Analysis in Biochemical Engineering*, 2nd ed., pp303, University of Tokyo Press, Tokyo, 1973, .
2. Daniels, W. F., and Browning, F. W., "An Apparatus for Aeration of Tissue Cells in Suspended Cultures with Controlled Gas Mixtures", *Biotechnol. Bioeng*, pp 4,79, 1962.

3. Matelova,V., "Investigations of Conditions for Production of Penicillin and Chlorotetracycline in Submerged Fermentation", *Biotechnol Bioeng*., pp 6, 329, 1964.
4. Ulrich, K., and Moore, G.E., "A Vibrating Mixer for Agitation of Suspension Cultures of Mammalian Cells", *Biotechnol. Bioeng.*, pp 7, 507, 1965.
5. Chain, E. B., Gualandi, G., and Morisis, G., "Aeration Studies IV: Aeration Conditions in 3000 Liter Submerged Fermentations with Various Microorganisms", *Biotechnol. Bioeng.,* pp 8,595, 1966.
6. Bailey, J. E., and Ollis, D. F., "Design and Analysis of Biological Reactors", *Biochemical Engineering Fundamentals,* 2nd ed., pp107, McGraw-Hill, New York, 1986.
7. Telling, R. C., Elsworth, R., "Submerged Culture of Hamster Kidney Cells in a Stainless Steel Vessel", *Bitechnol. Bioeng*, pp 7, 417, 1965.
8. Fowler, M.W.(ed.), "Natural Products and Industrial Application in Biotechnlogy of Higher Plants", *Plant Cell Culture,* pp 107, Dorset, U.K., 1983.
9. Prescott, S. C., and Dunn, C. G., *The Gluconic Acid Fermentation in Induatrial Microbiology*, 3rd edn., pp 578, McGraw-Hill, New York.
10. Ghose,T.K., and Mukhopadhyay, S.N., "Kinetic Studies of Gluconic Acid Fermentation in Horizontal Rotary Fermenter by Pseudomonas Ovalis", *J. Ferment. Technol.*, pp 54,738, 1976.
11. Moser, A., "Bioreactors with Thin-layer Characteristics", *Biotechnol*, pp 4,281, 1982.
12. Gorbach, G., Fette Slifen, *Austrichmitted*, pp 71, 98, 1969.
13. Techobanoglous, G., "Rotating Biological Contactors in Waste Water Engineering", *Treatment Disposal Reuse*, 2nd ed., pp 452, Metcalf & Eddy Inc., TMH Pub. Co., New Delhi, 1979,
14. Fried, D. W., and Thomson, J. B., "Oxygen Transfer Efficiency of Three Microporous Polypropylene Membrane Oxygenators", *Perfusion*, pp 6, 105, 1991.
15. Sittig,W., "The Present State of Fermentation Reactors", *J. Chem. Technol. Biotechnol*., pp 47, 1982.
16. Schugerl,K., "Some Basic Principles for the Layout of the Tower Bioreactors", *J. Chem. Tech. Biotechnol*., pp 32, 73, 1982.
17. Spier, R.E.,and Whiteside, J.P., "The Description of a Device which Facilitates the Oxygenation of Microcarrier Cultures", *Dev. Biol. Stand.*, pp 60, 283, 1985.
18. Sheritz, J., Reuveny, S., LaPorte, L. T., and Cho, H. G., "Stirred Tank Perfusion Reactors for Cell Propagation and Monoclonal Antibody : Production and Application", (Mizrani, A.,Alan R. Liss, eds.), New York, 1989.
19. Cox, S. C., Jr., Zwichenberger, J. B., and Kurusz, M., "Development and Current Status of a New Inracorporeal Membrane Oxygenator", *Perfusion*, pp 6, 291, 1991.
20. Pols, J. N., and Brands, W., "Clinical Evaluation of the Bentley Univox Membrane Oxygenator," *Perfusion,* pp 7, 59, 1992.
21. Heijnen, J. J., and Dijken, J. P., "In Search of a Thermodynamic Description of Biomass Yields for the Chemotrophic Growth of Microorganisms", *Biotechnol. Bioeng.,* pp 39, 833, 1992.
22. Minkevich, J. G., and Eroshin, V. K., "Productivity and Heat Generation of Fermentation Under Oxygen Limitation", *Folia Microbiol*., pp 18, 376, 1973.
23. Stouthamer, A. H., "In Search of a Correlation between Theoretical and Experimental Growth Yields", *Microbial Biochemistry*, Vol. 21, (Quayle, J. R., ed.), University Park Press, Baltimore, 1979.
24. Blakebrough, N., and Hamer, G., Resistance to oxygen transfer in fermentation broths, *Biotechnol. Bioeng*. pp 5, 59, 1963..
25. Finn, R.K., "Agitation and Aeration", *Biochemical and Biological Engineering Scienc*, Vol. 1, (Blakebrough. N, ed.), Academic Press, New York, 1967.
26. Hanhart, J., Kramers, H., and Westerterp, K. R., "The Residence Time Distribution of the Gas in Agitated Gas-liquid Contactor", *Chem. Eng.,* pp18, 503, 1963.
27. Whitman, W. G., "Diffusion of Binary Mass Transfer Coefficients in Two Phases at Low Mass Transfer Rates", *Chem. Met. Eng.,* pp 29, 146, 1923.

28. Bird, R. B., Stewart, W. E., and Lightfoot, E. N., *Interphase Transport in Multicomponent Systems in Transport Phenomena*, pp 636, John Wiley, New York, 1962 .
29. Aiba, S., Humphery, A. E., and Millis, N.F., *Aeration-agitation in Biochem. Eng.*, 1st ed., University of Tokyo Press, Tokyo, 1964,
30. Finn, R. K., "Agitation-aeration in the Laboratory and Industry", *Bacteriol. Rev.*, pp 18, 1954.
31. Mimura, A., Takeda, I., and Wakasa, R., "Some Characteristic Phenomena of Oxygen Transfer in Hydrocarbon Fermentation", *Advances in Microbnial Engineering,* Part I, pp 467, (Sikyta, B., Prokop, A., and Novak, M. eds.), Wiley-Interscience, New York, 1973.
32. Bailey, J. E., and Ollis, D. F., "Gas-liquid Mass Transfer in Cellulary Systems", *Biochemical Engtineering Fundamentals*, 2nd ed., pp 459 McGraw-Hill, New York, 1986.
33. Miller, D. N., "Scale-up of Agitated Vessels Gas-liquid Mass Transfer, *AIChE J.*, pp20, 442, 1974.
34. Mukhopadhyay, S. N., and T. K. Ghose, "Oxygen Participation in Fermentation, Part I: Oxygen-microorganism Interactions", *Process Biochem.*, pp 1,11, 1976.
35. Calderbank, P. H., "Physical Rate Process in Industrial Fermentation", Part I: "The Interfacial Area in Gas-liquid Contacting with Mechanical Agitation", *Trans. Instn. Chem. Eng.*, pp 36, 443, 1958.
36. Rols, J., Condoret, J. S., Fonate, C., and Goma, G., "Mechanism of Enhanced Oxygen Transfer in Fermentation Using Emulsified Oxygen-vectors", *Biotechnol. Bioeng.*, pp 35, 427, 1990.
37. Mttiason, B., and Adlercrautz, P., "Perfluorochemicals in Biotechnology", *Trends in Biotechnol.*, pp 5, 250, 1987.
38. Maclean, G. T., "Oxygen Transfer in Aerated Systems with Two Liquid Phases", *Process Biochem.*, pp 12, 22, 1977.
39. Higbie, R., "The Rate of Absorption of a Pure Gas into a Still Liquid During Short Period of Exposure". *Trans. A.I.Ch.E.*, pp 31, 365, 1935.
40. Danckwerts, P.V., "Significance of Liquid Film Coefficients in Gas Absorption", *Ind. Eng. Chem.*, pp 43, 1460, 1951.
41. Kishenevsky, M., Zhumal prikladnoy Khimii, 22, 1173, 1949; 24, 542, 1951; 27, 382, 1954; 27, 450, 1954.
42. Kafarov, V., Theory of Mass Transfer Accounting for Adsorption Phenomena", *Fundamentals of Mass Transfer Engineering*, pp249, MIR Pub., Moscow, 1975.
43. Hartman, R. J., *Colloid Chemistry*, 2nd ed., Houghton Mifflin Co., The Riverside Press, Cambridge, MA, 1947.
44. Philips K. L. "Reactor Systems for Process with Extreme Gas-liquid Transfer Requirements", *Fermentation Advances,* pp 465, (Perlman, D.,ed.,), Academic Press, New york, 1969.
45. Mukhopadhyay, S. N., and T. K.Ghose, Oxygen Transfer in Laboratory Horizontal Rotary Fermenter Under Varying Rotation Speed", J. *Ferment. Technol.*, pp 56, 558, 1978.
46. Mukhopadhyay, S. N., "Determination of Liquid Film Thickness and Volumetric Oxygen Transfer Coefficient in the Film in Horizontal Rotary Fermenter", Proc. 6th HMTC, Madras, IIT, F37-F41, 1981.
47. Okada,H., and H.O. Halvorson, "Uptake of a-thioethyl D-Glycopyranoside by *Saccharomyces cerevisae*. I. The Genetic Control of Facilitated Diffusion and Active Transport", *Biochem. Biophys, Acta*, pp 82,538, 1964.
48. Oginsky, E. L., and Umbreit, W. W., "Dehydrogenation and Respiration", *An Introduction to Bacterial Physiology,* 2nd ed., W.H. Freeman & Co., San Francisco, 1959.
49. Sawyer, C. N., and McCarty, P. L., *The Winkler Method in Chemistry for Environmental Engineering*, 3rd ed., pp 411, McGraw-Hill Kogakusha Ltd., Tokyo, 1978.
50. Johnson, M. J., Borkowski, J., and Engblom, C., "Steam Sterilizable Probes for Dissolved Oxygen Measurement", *Biotechnol. Bioeng.*, pp 6, 457, 1964.
51. Aiba, S., Ohashi, M., and Huang, S. Y., "Rapid Detention of Oxygen Permeability of Polymer Membranes", *Ind. Eng. Chem Fundam.*, pp 7, 497, 1968.

52. Krebs, W. M., and Haddad, I. A., "The Oxygen Electrode in Fermentation Systems", *Developmental Industrial Microbiology*, vol. 13, pp 113 (Murray, E. D.,ed.), American Institute of Biological Sciences, Washington, DC, 1972.
53. Brookman, J. S., and Owen, T. R., "A Description of Working Recommendation for Using a Modified Galvanic Cell Oxygen Electrode", *Biotechnol. Bioeng.*, pp10, 693, 1968.
54. Beechy, R. B., and Ribbons, D. W., "Oxygen Electrode Measurements", *Methods in Microbiology*, pp 25, (Norris, I. R., & Ribbons, D. W., eds.), Academic Press, London, 1972.
55. Kilburn, D. G., *Monitoring and Control of Bioreactors in Mammalian Cell Biotechnology*, pp159, (Butler. M. ed.), IRL Press at Oxford University Press, Oxford, New York, 1991.
56. Kilburn, D. G., and Webb, F. C., "The Cultivation of Animal Cells at Controlled Dissolved Oxygen Partial Pressure", *Biotechnol. Bioeng.*, pp 10, 801, 1968.
57. Karube, L, and Suzuki, S., "Applications of Biosensor in Fermentation Process, *Annual Reports on Fermentation Process,* Vol. VI, pp 203, (Tsao, G. T. ed.), Academic Press, New York, 1983.
58. Karube, L., Satoh, L., Araki, Y., and Suzuki, S., "Monosamine Oxidase Electrode in Freshness Testing of Nicat", *Enz. Microb. Technol.,* pp 2, 117, 1990.
59. Up dike, S. J., and Hicks, G. P., "The Enzyme Electrode", *Nature*, pp 214, 986, 1967.
60. Godman, R., Goldstein, L., and Katchalski, Eo., *Biochemical Aspects of Reactions on Solid Supports*, Academic Press, New York, 1971.
61. Pauling, L., *The Nature of the Chemical Bond,* 2nd ed., pp272, Comell University Press, Ithaca, NY, 1940.
62. Mukhopadhyay, S. N., "Studies on the Kinetics of Gluconic Acid Fermentation and Assessment of Volumetric Oxygen Transfer Coefficient by Oxygen Balance Technique", *Ph.D Thesis*, IIT Delhi, 1976.
63. Solomons, G. L., *Materials and Methods in Fermentation,* Academic Press, New York, 1969.
64. Cooper, C. M., Fernstrom G. A., and Miller, S.A., "Performance-of Agitated Gas Liquid Contactors", *Ind. Eng. Chem,* pp 36, 504, 1944.
65. Van't Riet, K., "Review of Measuring Methods and Results in Non-viscous Gas-liquid Mass Transfer in Stirred Vessels", *Ind. Eng. Chem. Proc. Des. Dev.*, pp 18,357, 1979.
66. Bertholomew, W. H., Karow, E.O., Sfat, M. R., and Wilhelm, R.H., "Oxygen Transfer and Agitation in Submerged Fermentation", *Ind. Eng. Chem.*, pp 42, 1801, 1950.
67. Bandyopadhyay, B., Humphrey, A. E., and Taguchi, "A Dynamic Measurement of Volumetric Oxygen Transfer Coefficient in Fermentation Systems", *Biotechnol. Bioeng.*, pp 9, 533, 1967.
68. Fujio, Y., Sambuichi, M., and Veda, S., "Numerical Methods of the Detennination of K_La and Respiration Rate in Biological System", *J. Ferment, Technol.*, pp 51, 154, 1973.
69. Tuffile, C. M., and Pinho, F., "Detennination of Oxygen Transfer Coefficient in Viscous Streptomycete Fermentations", *Biotechnol. Bioeng.*, pp 12, 849, 1970.
70. Mukhopadhyay, S. N., and Ghose, T. K., "A Simple Dynamic Method of K_La Determination in Laboratory Fermenter", *J. Ferment. Technol.,* pp 54, 406, 1976.
71. Heineken, F. G., "On the Use of Fast-response Dissolved Oxygen Probes for Oxygen Transfer Studies", *Biotechnol. Bioeng.,* pp 12, 145, 1970.
72. Linek, V., and Sobotka, M., "The Dynamic Method for Measuring of Aeration Capacity in Glucose-glucose Oxidase System", Collect. Czeck. Chem. Commun., pp 38, 2819, 1973.
73. Linek, V., Sobotka, M., and Prokop, A., "Measurement of Aeration Capacity of Fermenters by Rapidly Responding Oxygen Probes", *Biotechnol. Bioeng.* Symp. 4., (Sikyta, B., Prokop, A., and Novak, M., eds.), pp 429, 1972.
74. Kalyanraman, B., "Detection of Toxic Free Radicals in Biology and Medicine", *Reviews of Biochemical Toxicology,* Vol. IV, (Hodgson, E., Bend, J. R., and Philpot. R. M., eds.), Elsevier, North Holland, 1982.

75. Kalyanaraman, B., Mottley, P. C., and Mason, R. P; "A Direct Electron Spin Resonance and Spin-tapping Investigation of Peroxyl Free Radical Fonnation by Hematin/Hydroperoxide Systems", *J. Biol. Chem.*, pp 258, 3855, 1983.
76. Finkelstein, E., Rosen, G. M., and Rauckman, E. J., "Spin Trapping of Superoxide and Hydroxyl Radical: Practical Aspects", *Arch. Biochem. Biophys*., pp 200, 1980,
77. Rosen, G. M., and Rauckman, E. J., "Spin Trapping of Superoxide and Hydroxyl Radicals", *Methods in Enzymology,* Vol. 105, pp 198, Academic Press, New York, 1984.
78. Janzen, E. G., "Spin Trapping",(Packer, L.ed.) , *Methods in Enzymology,* Vol. 105, pp188, Academic Press, New York, 1984,
79. Tosaki, A., Haseloff, R. F., Hellegonarch, A., Scboenheit, K. Martin, V. V., Das, D. K., and Blasig, I. E., "Does the Antiarrhythmic Effect of DMPO Originate from its Oxygen Radical Trapping Property or the Structure of the Molecule Itself ?" *Basic Res. Cardio*l. pp 87, 536, 1992.
80. Arroyo, C. M., Kramer, J. H., Lelbof, R. H., Mergner, G. W., Dickens, B. F., and Weglicki, W. B., "Spin Trapping of Oxygen and Carbon Centered Free Radicals in Ischemic Canine Myocardium", *Free Rad. Biol. Med.*, pp 3, 313, 1987.
81. Das, D. K., Cordis, G. A., Rao, P. S., George, A., and Maity, S., "High Perfonnance Liquid Chromatographic Detection of Hydroxyl Radical in Heart: Its Possible Link with the Myocardial Reperfusion Injury," *J. Chromatogr*, pp 536, 273, 1991
82. Das, D. K., Engelnan, R. M., George, A, Lin, X., and Rao, P. S., Mitochondrial Generation of Hydroxyl Radical During Reperfusion of Ischemic Myocardium," *Biological Oxidation Systems*, Vol. II, pp 999 (Reddy, C. C., ed.,) Academic Press, 1990.
83. Grootveld, Me, and Halliwell, B., "Aromatic Hydroxylation as a Potential Measure of Hydroxyl Radical Formation in Vivo," *Biochem. J.*, pp 237, 499, 1986.
84. Tosaki, A., Bagchi, D., Pali, T., Cordis, G. A., and Das, D. K., "Comparisons of ESR and HPLC Methods for the Detection of OH. Radicals in Ischemic/Reperfused Hearts," *Biochem. Pharmacol.*, pp 45, 961,1993.
85. Bagchi, D., Bagchi, M., Douglas, D. M., and Das, D. K., "Generation of Singlet Oxygen and Hydroxyl Radical from Sodium Chlorite and Lactic Acid," *Free Rad. Res. Commun.*, pp 17, 109, 1992.
86. Ebert, M., Pulse Radiolysis, Academic Press, New York, 1965.
87. Prasad, M. R., and Das, D. K., "Effect of Oxygen-Derived Free Radicals and Oxidants on the *in vitro* Degradation of Membrane Phospholipids," *Free Rad. Res. Commun.*, pp 7, 381, 1989.
88. Maulik, N., Avrora, N., Denisova, N., Gaginoni, M. & Das, D. K., Free Radical Scavenging Activities of Gangliosides : A Sialic Acid Containing Glycosphin Golipid," *Active Oxygens. L. and Antioxidants*. pp 765. (Yagl, K., Kondo, M., Niki, E., and Yoshikawa, T., eds.), Excerpta Medica. Amsterdam, 1992.
89. Maulik, N., Das, D. K., Gogineni, M., Cordis, G. A., Avrova, N., and Denisova, N., "Reduction of Myocardial Ischemic Reperfusion Injury by Sialylated Glycosphingolipids, Gangliosides," *J. Cardiovasc. Pharmacol.* pp 22, 74, 1993.
90. Gutteridge, J. M. C., *Aspects to Consider when Detecting and Measuring Lipid Peroxidation,* pp 173, Free Rad. Res. Commun., 1986.
91. Cordis, G. A., Maulik, N., Bagchi, D., Engelman, R.M., and Das, D.K., "Estimation of the Lipid Peroxidation in the Ischemic and Reperfused Heart by Monitoring Lipid Metabolic Products Using High Performanc Liquid Chromatography," *J. Chromatogr*, pp 632, 97, 1993.
92. Cordis, G.A., Maulik, N., Bagchi, D., and Das, D.K., "HPLC Method for the Simultaneous Detection of Malonaldehyde, Acetaldehyde, Formaldehyde, and Acetone to Monitor the Oxiative Stress in Heart," *J. Chromatogr.,* pp 661, 181, 1984.
93. Douglas, D.M., Bandyopadhyay, D, Russel, J. C. Hoory, S., Antar, M., and Das, D.K., "Role of Oxygen Free Radicals in Wound Healing," *Surg, Res. Commun*, pp 9, 145, 1990.

94. Van Wezel, A.L., "Cultivation of Anchorage-Dependents Cells and their Applications," *J. Chem. Tchnol. Biotechnol.*, pp 32, 318, 1982.
95. Spier, R.E., "Animal Cell Technology: An Overview," *J. Chem. Tech. Biotechnol*, pp 23, 304, 1982.
96. Dodge, C.T., and Hu,S., "Growth of Hybridoma Cells Under Different Agitation Conditions," *Biotechnol, Lett.,* pp 8, 683, 1986.
97. Tramper, J., Wiiliams, J. B., Joustra, D., and Vlak, J.M., "Shear Sensitivity of Insect Cells in Suspension," *Enz. Microb. Technol.*, pp 8, 33, 1986.
98. Katinger, H. W. D., Scheirer, W., and Kromen, E., "Bubble Column Reactor for Mass Propagation of Animal Cells in Suspension Culture," *Ger. Chen. Eng.*, pp 2, 31, 1979.
99. Handa, A., Emery, A. N., and Spier, R. E., "On the Evaluation Gas-Liquid Interfacial Effect on Hybridoma Viability in Bubble Column Bioreactors," *Dev. Biol. Stand.*, pp 66, 241, 1987.
100. Thomas, C. R., and Zhang, Z., "Measuring Animal Cell Material Properties." *Biotechnolo.*, pp 24, 1, 1991.
101. Ghose T. K., and Mukhopadhyay, S. N., "Bioreactor-Recent Advances. Presented at the Symposium on Heterogenous Reactor Science and Practice," *32nd Annual Meeting, IIchE,* IIT Bombay, pp 25, *Dec.* 1979.

References for further reading

102. S. N. Mukhopadhyay and D. K. Das, *Oxygen Responses, Reactivitiy and Measurements in Biosystems*, Chapter 6, CRC Press, Boca Raton, Florida, 1994.
103. B. Halliwell and J. M. C. Gutteridge, *Free Radicals in Biology and Medicine*, 2nd edn., Chapter 1, Clarendon Press, Oxford, 1989.
104. S. N. Mukhopadhyay, *Process Biotechnology Fundamentals,* Chapter 11, 1st edn., Viva Books Pvt. Ltd., New Delhi, 2001.
105. J. O. Konz, J. King and C. L. *Cooney, Effects of Oxygen on Recombinant Protein Expression Biotechnol*, Prog. pp 14, 393-409, 1998.
106. B. Krems and V. C. Cullotta; "Oxidative Stress in Yeast," *Molecular Biology of the Toxic Response,* Chapter 27, (A. Puga and K.B. Wallace eds), Taylor & Francis, New York, 1998.
107. W. J. Kelly and A. E. Humptrey, "Computational Fluid Dynamics Model for Predicting Flow of Viscous Fluids in Large Fermenter with Hydrofoil Flow impellers and Internal Cooling Coils." *Biotechnol, Prog.* pp 14, 248-258, 1998.
108. Mixing Equipment (Impeller Type) In AIChE Equipment Testing Procedure, 3rd edn. 2001, *AICHE*, USA.
109. H. F. Bunand and R.O. Python, *Physical Rev.*, 76(3), pp 839-885, 1996.
110. S. I. Bibirov, R. Biran, K. E. Ruddund and J. S. Parkinson, J. Bact. 179 (2), 4075-1079, 1997.
111. K. Yadav *et al.* In abstracts *Microbiotech* 2000, pp. 65, AMI 41st Annual Conference, BISR, Jaipur.
112. K. L., S. Hein, W. Zou and G. Klug. The Glutathione Glutaredoxin System in Rhodobacter capsulatus: Part of a Complex Regulatory Network Controlling Defense against oxidative stress, J. Bact 186 (20) 6800-6808, 2004.
113. D. W. Green and R. H. Perry, Perry's Chemical Engineers' Handbook, McGraw Hill, New York, 2008, Chap. 7-18, 20-(71-79), 22-(48-50).
114. J. A. Muller, W. C. Boyle and H. J. Popel, AERATION : Principles and Practice, Voll 11, CRC Press, Boca Raton, Florida, USA, 2002.

Chapter

6

NEW BIOPROCESSING : ASPECTS AND STRATEGIES

6.1 ARCHAEBACTERIAL BIOPROCESSING : PROBLEMS AND DEVELOPMENTS

6.1.1 Introduction

"Methanogens no longer are second class citizens of the microbial world", is the classic statement by a renowned expert of *Archaebacteria*; R.S. Wolfe.[1] This statement was subsequently supported by convening two important international meetings e.g. "Genetics of Obligate Anaerobic Microorganisms", Chicago, Illinois, April 22, 1980 and "Genetic Approaches in the Study of Methanogenic Bacteria", Stockholm, Sweden, April 12-14, 1981.

The concept proposed by Woese[2-4] and his co-investigators led reclassification of all organisms into three primary kingdoms. The archaebacteria consists of methanogenic bacteria, the extremely halophilic bacteria, thermoplasma sp. and extreme thermophilic archaebacteria. Among the archaebacterial microorganisms methanogenic bioprocessing has gained highest interest. Methane production by methanogenic archaebacteria has been investigated by Wolfe and other investigators for many years. Enormous amount of scientific information in relation to bioprocessing of methane formers have been reported. As they are very slow growing organisms genetic approaches have also been used in more recent studies. Methane producing archaebacteria have surmounted enormous technical problems for describing their taxonomy, fine structure, physiology, growth requirements, developing recombinant DNA molecule and bioprocessing strategy decisions.[5-8]

6.1.2 Archaebacterial Bioprocessing

1. Biomethanogenesis

The bioprocessing in archaebacterial bioconversion process which occurs when refuse resources like domestic, municipal, agricultural and industrial organic waste materials in slurry are decomposed by mixed microbial growth comprising of acid forming bacteria and methane forming archaebacteria functioning in absence of dissolved oxygen and finally generating methane as major gaseous product thereby reducing environmental pollution strength of the waste to a significant level, has been defined, in general, as "anaerobic digestion" (AD). The hardware used for AD is called digester and the gaseous product obtained is called biogas.

Bioprocessing of biomaterials for conversion into methane by anaerobic archaebacteria is a process better understood each day. In bioprocessing the size and design of the digester should be such that it can handle soluble or insoluble materials available to produce the desired quantity of gas. Single or double chamber digesters are generally used. Methane production from organic waste resources depends largely on the degree of sophistication of the plant. While methane production efficiency is markedly increased in such plants the cost per therm rises substantially due to additional monitoring and control devices necessary. Methane gas production being not very rapid there is a point at which an optimum economic design must exist to take care of the three phasic complex bioconversion reactions. A schematic diagram of AD reactions sequence has been given in the literature [9] and reproduced in Fig. 6.1. It has been modelled on the basis of solid, liquid and gas phase of interacting substrates and products of anaerobic digestion of waste solids. Bioprocess engineering and technology approach to establish this point using $1 m^3$ volume plant has been given.[10]

The technology of archaebacterial methanation has taken this advantage primarily in three ways as below.[11]

First, the strategy of biomethanation has been conducted in continuous, completely mixed conditions without active biomass recycle. It has posed a bottleneck probably by permitting limited number of methanogenic bacteria to be present in the digester mixed liquor. As mentioned before since specific methane generation occured at a slow rate it has advanced design of second generation methane digesters. This design was to trap the methanogenic archaebacteria within the digester for accumulation of coenzyme P_{420} in methane digestion mixed liquor. P_{420} acts as shuttle for electrons from hydrogen and replaces ferredoxin in methanogens.

Second, for using insoluble organic substrate in biomethanation the preliminary solubilization of the substrate is often rate limiting. In such a situation the inverse of conversion varies linearly with the inverse of mean residence time. This allows calculation of ultimate conversion.

It is helpful in identifying problem of rate limitation and archaebacterial competency. Double chamber digestion strategy aids in overcoming the second bottleneck.

Third, improvements of monitoring of parameters like dry organic matter or COD by graphical correlation between heats of combustion, mean oxidation stages and specific COD with biomethanation efficiency. These advantages were in attempt to correlate the newer knowledge of methanogenesis with improved design of archaebacterial biomethanation technologies.[12]

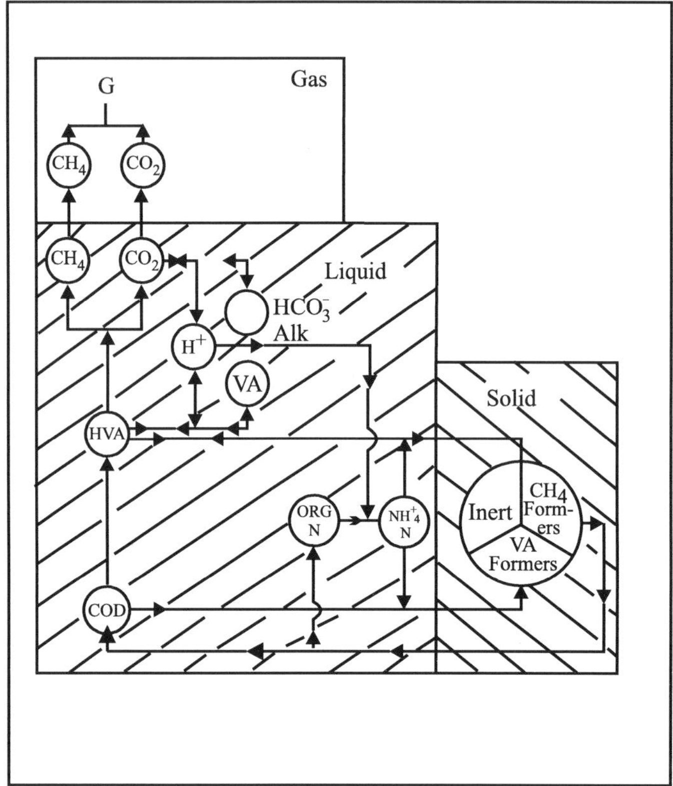

Fig. 6.1 Anoxic reactions with *Archaebacterial* participation

2. Biomethanation rate model

From the view point of biochemical reaction kinetics by mixed acidogens and archaebacterial flora of complex substrates involves sequential steps of hydrolysis, acidification and biomethanation. In biomethanation the conversion of acids to methane is the rate limiting step,[13-17] so the step of conversion of acetic acid (major acid) to methane is quite significant. The CO_2 produced can also participate in the reaction.[12] From the stoichiometric balance it could be seen that conversion of acetic acid should produce 50% CH_4 and 50% CO_2. So presumably, the CO_2 reduction route for methane formation is also involved. Accordingly the most probable mechanism of biomethanation which was noticed to give the best fit with experimental results was proposed to be[12]

$$A + X \rightleftharpoons AX \tag{6.1}$$

$$AX \rightleftharpoons B_1 + C_1 + C_2X \tag{6.2}$$

$$C_2X \rightleftharpoons B_2X \tag{6.3}$$

$$B_2X \rightleftharpoons B_2 + X \tag{6.4}$$

in which A is acetic acid, X is archaebacterial cell mass, AX is acetic acid-cell complex, B_1 is CH_4 produced directly from A, B_2 is CH_4 produced by CO_2 reduction. B_2X intracellular methane-cell complex produced from CO_2, C_1 is free CO_2, C_2 is the amount of CO_2 reduced to CH_4, C_2X intracellular bound CO_2. Analysis of this mechanism of biomethanation showed that in the conversion of A to methane the formation of CH_3-S-COM (AX) from A inside the cell is the rate limiting step. Then AX forms free CH_4 (B_1), free CO_2 (C_1) and a complex of CO_2 and COM inside the cell (C_2X). Next C_2X gets reduced intracellularly to methyl-COM complex (B_2X) which in turn produced free CH_4 (B_2) and cells (X) in the last step. It was clear that CO_2 which was reduced to CH_4 was not extracellular free CO_2 but was intracellular CO_2. Pictorial depiction of this mechanism is shown in Fig. 6.2. Further to this pictorial mechanisms the pathway of CO_2 reduction to CH_4 as it has been summarised[12, 18] is shown in Fig.6.3.

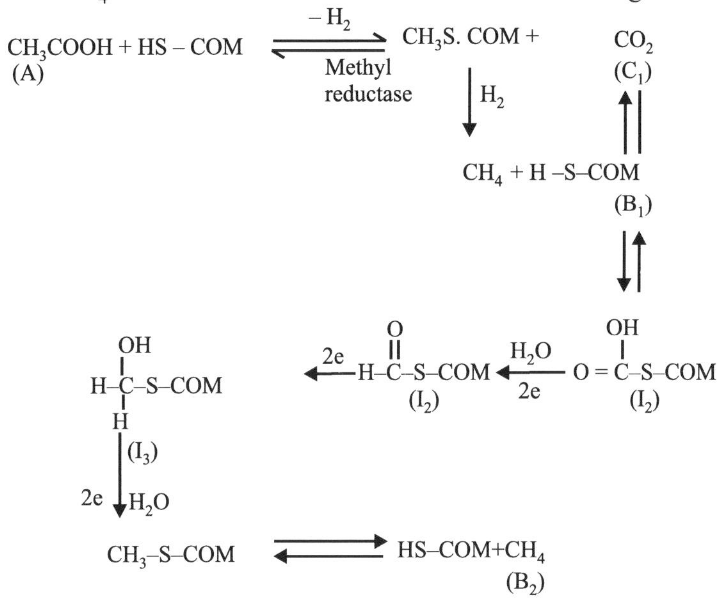

$CH_3COOH + HS - COM$ (A) $\underset{\text{Methyl reductase}}{\overset{-H_2}{\rightleftharpoons}}$ $CH_3S.COM$ + CO_2 (C_1)

$CH_3S.COM \xrightarrow{H_2} CH_4 + H-S-COM$ (B_1)

$O = C(OH)-S-COM$ (I_1) $\xrightarrow[2e]{H_2O}$ $H-C(=O)-S-COM$ (I_2) $\xrightarrow{2e}$ $H-C(OH)(H)-S-COM$ (I_3) $\xrightarrow[2e]{H_2O}$ $CH_3-S-COM$

$CH_3-S-COM \rightleftharpoons HS-COM+CH_4$ (B_2)

Fig.6.2 Pathway for methane formation reaction mechanism

The best fit rate model of this mechanism has been shown[12] to be

$$r = \frac{K_1 C_x \left(C_A - K_3 K_4/K_1K_2 C_{B_2} C_{C_1}\right)}{\left[1 + (K_3K_4/2) C_{n_1} C_{B_2} C_{C_1} + K_4 (1 + K_3) C_{B_2}\right]} \tag{6.5}$$

Here, K_1 to K_4 are rate constants. The rate constants which could fit well with experimental data for C_{B_1} from 0.5 to 0.9. C_{B_1} values of 0.71 C_B and 0.85 C_B gave very good matches.

Significance of B_1 and B_2 in the Rate Model : In the actual measurement of methane its total amount (i.e $B = B_1 + B_2$) is measured. In the total amount the part B_1 is the amount of methane produced via the route

$$A \rightarrow CH_3—S—COM \rightarrow CH_4 \tag{6.6}$$

and B_2 is the amount of methane produced from

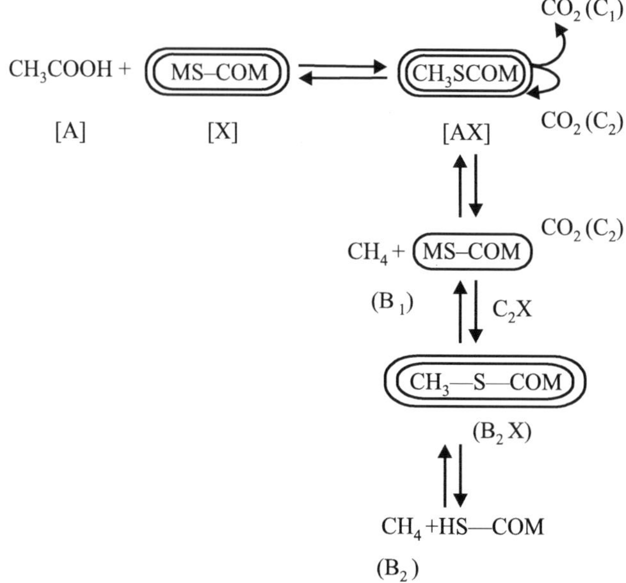

Fig. 6.3 Pictorial depiction of CO_2 reduction to CH_4

$$CO_2 \rightarrow (I_1 \rightarrow I_2 \rightarrow I_3) \rightarrow CH_3\text{—S—COM} \rightarrow CH_4 \qquad (6.7)$$

It indicated when B_1 moles of CH_4 are produced from direct decarboxylation of acetic acid (A), an equal amount of CO_2 should be produced. If the entire amount of CO_2 is reduced to CH_4 then an equimolal amount of CH_4 will be obtained, thereby $B_1 = 0.5$. If no CO_2 is reduced to CH_4 $B_1 = B$, B_1 should range from 0.5B to 1.0B.

3. Archaebacterial biomethanation parameters

The determination of basic biotechnological parameters of biomethanation from complex organic substrates should be based on the elemental analysis of the substrate. It yields the substrate formula referred to 1 carbon atom, values of degree of reducibility (v_a) and mass fraction of carbon in organic substrate (P_s). These values then aid in determining the $(Y_{CH4/S})_{theo}$, COD_{theo} and CH_4 per cent. Experimental determination of volatile substance (v_s), Y_{exp} and COD is also carried out. If the substrate composition is now known, the value of T_s for a moment can be determined from the experimental COD and v_s from the context of CH_4 in the gas. Measurement of these quantities in the course of biomethanation/digestion makes it possible to characterize semiquantitatively the course of individual phases of the process. From the values of Y_{exp} and Y_{theo} it is possible to determine the actual biological efficiency, η. Also, from the values of v_s determined from the % CH_4 in the gas and T_s assessed by means of COD one can obtain the Q_{theo} yields by combustion of CH_4 after digestion.

The mass and energy balance permitted the evaluation of the efficiency of bioconverion devices in the context of bioprocessing strategy of complex organic waste substrates.[13-15]

6.1.3 Chemicals from Archaebacterial Bioprocessing

Using methanogenic archaebacteria *Methanosarcina barkeri* efforts have been put to produce useful chemicals.[14,15] The potential of this archaebacteria as biocatalyst has been noticed for three major possibilities. First, the ability of the methanogen to reduce exogenous NAD(P) to NADPH with H_2, CO_2 or formate should render it an economic coupler of redox reactions requiring reduced cofactors. Second, formate production from pyrolysis gas (H_2, CO_2, CO) represent an alternative means of chemical conversion by archaebacterial methanogenic cells. Third, corrinoid production from methanol by this organism is specially promising for production of extracellular corrinoids. These have potentials for future developments.

6.1.4 Genetics and Molecular Cell Biology Concerns

In order to reduce technical problems in archaebacterial methanogenesis the molecular biotechnology of methanogens have started in late seventies.[10] Some of the technical difficulties in developing rDNA molecules of methanogens have been given.[6] Even though the possibility of using recombinant DNA techniques for improved bioprocessing of methanogens with increased growth rates, or higher methane yields or to transfer the ability to produce methane to other species currently appear remote, it cannot be ignored. Ribosomal characters of archaebacteria is useful for understanding the aspects of their metabolism. Archaebacterial ribosomes display characteristics of 70s and 80s types. Ribosomes being ribonucleoprotein particles consist of two subunits, one of which is twice as large as the other. The basic architectural features of each of the two subunits are formed by a single high molecular weight rRNA molecule. This rRNA is associated with a large number of ribosomal proteins (r-proteins). These rRNA species have been given with generic terms, small subunits (SSU) and large subunits (LSU)-rRNA. Complete SSU- rRNA and LSU-rRNA of few archaebacteria are given in the Table 6.1 with the lengths of the mature rRNA molecule.

Table 6.1 Nucleotide sequence length of a few *archaebacteria*

Archaebacterial	*Nucleotide Sequence Length*	
Organism	SSU–rRNA	LSU–rRNA
Methanococcus vannielli	1466	2958
Thermoprotens tenax	1604	3038
Halobacterium halobium	1473	2905
Methanobacterium hungatti	1664	—
Methanobacter autotrophicum	1496	3019

The availability of mutants of archaebacteria is the initial step in developing a genetic exchange system. A subsequent major problem relates to successfully transfer, and to recognize the transfer of DNA from the donor strain to the recipient. In relation to bioprocessing many of the technical problems as mentioned earlier associated with the direct genetic analysis of methanogenic archaebacteria may be circumvented by analyzing DNA derived from methanogens in a suitable host. By ligation of DNA derived from *Methanosarcina barkeri* to two different cloning vectors (Fig. 6.4) it has been possible to construct r-DNA molecules of this archaebacteria.

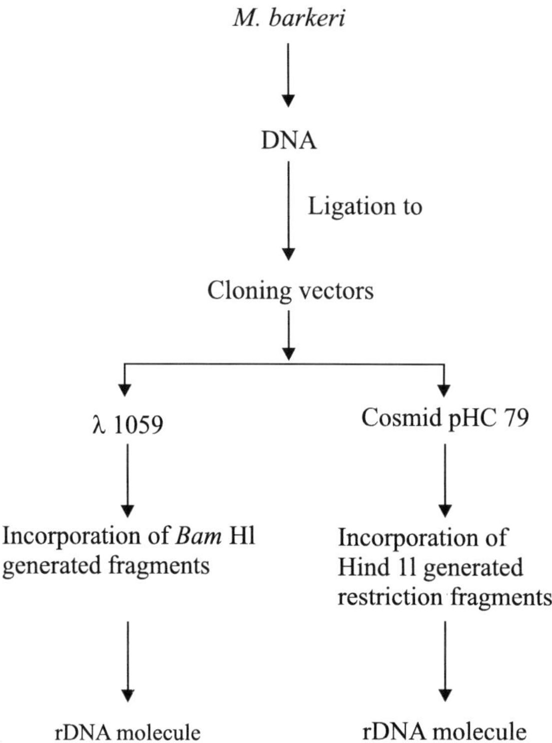

Fig. 6.4 Methanogen derived rDNA using r-DNA technology

This has enabled to proceed from molecular aspects, including transcription and DNA structure, to general metabolism, and, finally cellular lipids and envelops. However, two points are very important in designing potential transformation/cell fusion protocols. First, difficulty of non-availability of enzymes known equivalent to lysozyme which could be used to digest or weaken the cell envelop of methanogenic archaebacteria. Second, *M. vannietii* may be an absolute choice as the experimental system. This is because this species unlike other methanogenic archaebacteria is easy to lyse for obtaining high molecular weight DNA or for rapid screening for the presence of plasmids and should form protoplasts on careful handling. So designing of an *in vitro* protein synthesizing system derived from *M. barkeri* is an important development. However, in some archaebacteria the presence of modification and restriction endo-nucleases has been observed in recent years.

6.1.5 Stoichiometric and Performance Principles[16,17]

In biomethanation by anoxic bioconversion of many wastes and their admixtures have been used as substrates. For this, single-stage, two stage and multi-stage bioreactor system approaches have been used. In principle, there are two major types of organisms requiring different pH and temperatures for optimum growth in biogas production. The mesophilic organisms produce mostly fatty acids from the substrate and grow best at pH 5.0–5.8 and temperature 35°C. On the other hand for thermophilic organisms that convert acids into methane, optimum pH is 6.8 and temperature, 45-50°C. It has been reported that methane production drops by 50% for every 11°C change in temperature. Theoretically, in the slurry of biogas production plants, one gets an equal amounts of methane and carbon dioxide. In practice, however, a part of the carbon dioxide evolved remains fixed on organics or mineral bases or remains dissolved in the liquid. The carbon in carbon dioxide as dissolved $CO_2/HCO_3^-/CO_3^-$ has been shown to participate in and cause enhancement in biomethanation. The mass and energy balance analysis of the biogas production process is an important requirement for understanding its biological efficiency. For this, the primary requirement is to have an appropriate stoichiometry of biomethanation of the substrate. Considering C, H, O and N as the major elemental components in the substrate, the anoxic bioconversion stoichiometry may be written as follows :

$$C_nH_aO_bN_c + (n - a/4 - b/2 + 3c/4)\ H_2O$$

$$(n/2 - a/8 + b/4 + 3c/8)\ CO_2 + (n/2 + a/8 - b/4 - 3b/8)\ CH_4 + \text{Cell} \tag{6.8}$$

For this bioredox conversion of substrate, the electron balance with respect to *n* carbon atoms is given by

$$r_d = 4n + 1a - 2b - 3c \tag{6.9}$$

So for one carbon atom it is

$$r_d = 4 + a/n - 2b/n - 3c/n \tag{6.10}$$

where r_d refers to the degree of reducibility of the substrate. As the ultimate metabolic fate of the complex substrate is expected to go through anoxic glucose degradation, the simplified mass balance may be considered as

$$C_6H_{12}O_6 \text{ or } (CH_2O)_6 \rightarrow 3CH_4 + 3CO_2 \tag{6.11}$$

The r_d value of the substrate referring to 1 C atom of the products.

r_d remains between the two limits of 0 and 8. However, in anoxic bioconversion, yield coefficient is an important parameter. It depends on the mass fraction of carbon in organic substrate and products and the degree of reducibility. From the computed values of mass fractions and r_d the value of theoretical yield coefficient can be obtained. The experimental data likewise will provide experimental value of yield coefficient $Y_{(CH_4/S)_e}$. Now the value of biological efficiency, η of the anoxic bioconversion can be obtained as

$$\eta = \frac{Y_{(CH_4/S)_t}}{Y_{(CH_4/S)_e}} \tag{6.12}$$

The bioconversion engineering parameters (BEP) would serve in the evaluation of environmental engineering parameters (EEP) of the process.

Correlation between BEP and EEP in biomethanation

It is well known that anoxic bioconversion process can provide superior performance in terms of waste stabilization, i.e., significant reduction in COD/BOD value of the waste for environmental control through generation of biogas.

Taking a simple case of COD/BOD contributing stoichiometry of the waste as

$$C_nH_aO_b + (n + a/4 - b/2)\, O_2 \rightarrow nCO_2 + 1/2\, H_2O \tag{6.13}$$

the value of

$$COD_t = 0.67\, r_{ds}\, x_s \tag{6.14}$$

From this relationship the approximate value of BOD can be obtained. The heat energy available from the combustion of biogas (Q) produced by anaerobic bioconversion of organic substrate can be computed from

$$Q = \rho r_{ds}\, x_s \eta \tag{6.15}$$

where ρ is a factor involving the mean heat of combustion of a free electron.

6.1.6 Approach of Genetic Engineering

One of the major problems in a biogas system is the slow growth rate of methanogens, which, in turn, reduces methane yield. To overcome this problem, recombinant DNA technology approach of genetic engineering has been adopted in recent years to obtain methane formers with higher specific growth rates for getting improved efficiency. However; there exist several technical problems in using rDNA technology for methanogenic organisms. By overcoming some of these problems, it has been possible to develop rDNA molecule from *Methanosarcina* sp. Development of an *in vitro* protein-synthesising system derived from the above anoxic methanogen is an excellent achievement in the progress of biogas technology. Plasmids and phages of methnogenetic bacteria are currently unknown. Many active investigators and experts in the area, however, are very optimistic about their identification in the near future. Establishment of rDNA technology for enhancing biogas production in a short time by genetically redesigning methanogens having high growth rate is, therefore essential.

For advancement of biomethanation technology, the performance parameters of the anoxic bioreactor need to be integrated considering bioconversion and environemental and genetic engineering principles. Correlation of these parameters leading to application in optimization of the system is needed. Also, the numerous governmental and industrial interest in both rDNA research and the search for renewable energy sources are expected to ensure that rDNA technology will be focussed on and used to evaluate the potential of methanogenic species.

6.1.7 Thermophilic Methanogens

Thermophilic methane bacteria have been of great interest for many years. It is to enable development of improved or new biotechnology. Among the thermophilic methane forming bacteria *Methanobacterium thermoautotrophicum* has been reported to be an obligate anaerobe.[19] In more recent years a thermophilic *Methanobacterium* sp. has been isolated from cow dung which uses acetate as substrate.[19] Properties of a few thermophilic methanogenic bacteria are given in Table 6.2.

6.2 BIOPROCESSING BY CELL SYNCHRONIZATION

6.2.1 Introduction

Cells remaining in same physiological phase giving balanced growth is called synchronous culture.[20] Then, synchrony, no matter how achieved, will last for many generations in unlimited

Table 6.2 Properties of a few thermophilic methanogenic species

Thermophilic Methanogenic Species	*Response to Oxygen*	*Maximum Growth Temp. (°C)*	*Primary Habitat*	*Nutritional Class*	*Reference*
Methanobacterium thermoautotrophicum	Obligate anaerobe	70 – 74	Hot springs	Chemoauto-troph	18
Methanobacterium wolfei	"	55 – 65	Deep sea hydrothermal	"	11
Methanothermus fervidus	"	83	Vents	"	11
Mixed culture	Anaerobe	55 – 60	Slaughter house waste	Syntrophs	12
Methanobacterium sp.	"	65 – 68	Rumen of cow	Organotroph	19

growth medium under conditions met by atleast certain procaryotes. Efforts to produce the desired synchronization of cell division have been made in both microbial as well as in mammalian cell cultures. In both systems cells synchronization is carried out for various purposes. Also, in both systems synchronous cultures can be divided into two broad procedures. They are: physical method and chemical method. These are achieved by induction synchrony and selection synchrony. Induction synchrony makes use of inducing cells by some treatment to divide synchronously. But selection synchrony uses a fraction of cells of a growing culture at a particular phase of the growth cycle. This fraction of cells is then grown separately as a continuous culture. Each of the methods can have several techniqucs. Cells which could be synchronized are *E. coli, C. utilis, S. cerevisiae* and CHO (mammalian).

6.2.2 Microbial Cell Synchronization

1. Concepts

The induction synchrony used in microbial system can be carried out by three techniques e.g., inhibitor block, starvation and growth and multiple changes of temperature or light. Likewise the selection synchrony may also be achieved by three techniques. These are gradient separation, membrane elution and filtration. Besides these growth limitation by cell surface has also been used.

The dependency of specific growth rate (μ) on substrate concentration (s) followed Monod's law. Growth is first order at low and zero order at high concentration. One may consider μ_m to be independent of surface to volume (A/V = S) because at high substrate concentration the transport capability is high and unlimiting. However, the first order constant is dependent on S_0. This is because the rate of uptake of a cell suspended in a medium of low substrate concentration is proportional to the cell surface area. For augmentation of this concept K_s in Monod's Law is replaced by K'/S_0. The validity of this substitution is demonstrated by considering cells growing at very low substrate concentration or under starvation where cell surface area determines the growth rate.

Thus, the method of synchronizing which has been used widely with microorganisms is to starve a culture. It allows the culture to run into a stationary phase and then to add fresh medium, the culture usually grows synchronously for one or more divisions. This starvations synchrony has been best utilized in developing synchronous budding yeasts. The purpose of such synchronization has been for regulation of cell proliferation, biochemical and/or biological events in such phases.

2. *Theoretical aspects*

(i) Surface to Volume Ratio for Rods with Hemispherical Poles : In order to fix ideas and to indicate computational method, it is necessary to consider simplest case for an organism whose shape is a right cylinder with hemispherical poles. The volume is given by

$$V = \frac{4}{3}\pi R^3 + \pi R^2 (L - 2R)$$

or

$$V = \pi R^2 \left[L - \left(\frac{2}{3}R\right)\right] \tag{6.16}$$

and the area

$$A = 4\pi R^2 + 2\pi R (L - 2R)$$

$$A = 2\pi RL \tag{6.17}$$

where R = radius, L = end to end distance. The length of a cell of a particular volume can be found from a rearrangement of equation 6.16.

$$L = \frac{V}{\pi R^2} + \frac{2}{3} R \tag{6.18}$$

Then substituting L in equation 6.16, 6.17 and 6.17 the surface area to volume ratio becomes

$$S_0 = \frac{A}{V} = \frac{2\pi R\left[\frac{V}{\pi R^2} + \frac{2}{3}R\right]}{\pi R^2\left[L - \frac{2R}{3}\right]}$$

which is rearranged to give

$$S_0 = \frac{2}{R} + \frac{4}{3}\frac{\pi R^2}{V} \tag{6.19}$$

Using surface area to volume ratio through cell cycle as a parameter it may be possible to maintain synchrony of such cell growth.

(ii) Growth Limited by Cell Surface : The dependency of specific growth rate (μ) on substrate concentration may be expressed by Monod's model

$$\mu = \frac{\mu_m s}{k_s + s} \tag{6.20}$$

In analogy to Fick's diffusion law

$$\frac{dq}{dt} = D.A. \frac{dc}{dx} \tag{6.21}$$

one can unite

$$\frac{dV}{dt} = YPAs \tag{6.22}$$

In equation 6.21, q is the quantity transported, D is the diffusion constant, A is the surface area, and $\frac{dc}{dx}$ is the concentration gradient. In equation 6.22, Y is the yield coefficient (corresponding to the cellular volume produced by a unit amount of the limiting nutrient), P is the permeability constant (which is the diffusion constant divided by the thickness of the membrane, i.e. $\frac{D}{dx}$) and s is the external substrate concentration (since the internal concentration is presumed to be maintained at zero). For uptake always limited by an active transport system, P would not have the meaning of a permeability constant, but would have the significance of

$$\frac{n V_{max}}{k_m + V}$$

for the n permease assemblies on a unit surface area (V_{max} and K_m are the kinetic constants of the permease assembly). Dividing both sides of equation 6.22 by V and substituting S_0, with A/V, equation 6.22 becomes

$$\frac{dV}{Vdt} = YP\, s_0 \,.\, s \tag{6.23}$$

If the dilution cycle results in a high concentration for part of the cycle then for that part, this relationship would be

$$\frac{dV}{Vdt} = \mu_{max} \tag{6.24}$$

Equation (6.24) can be written in the form

$$m = \frac{dV}{Vdt} = m_{max} \frac{x}{(s'/s_0)} \tag{6.25}$$

where μ_{max}/k' has been substituted for YP. These two equations are the high and low substrate limits where diffusion through the medium is never limiting. The Monod relation of bacterial growth is a relationship analogous to the Michaelis-Menton enzyme law covering both extremes. In the present purpose it would be given by

$$\frac{dV}{V \cdot dt} = \frac{\mu_m s}{[(k'/s_0) + s]} \tag{6.26}$$

The Blackman "Law of the Minimum" formulation of growth is probably more generally pertinent instead of the hyperbola. Equations (6.24) and (6.25) apply as well in the intermediary concentration and growth as synchrony is determined by

$$\frac{dV}{V \cdot dt} = \frac{s}{(k'/s_0)}, \; s \le s_c \tag{6.27}$$

and

$$\frac{dV}{V \cdot dt} = \mu_{max} \; s > s_c \tag{6.28}$$

where s_c is the critical concentration such that uptake of the critical substrate just becomes nonlimiting i.e.

$$s_c = \frac{\mu_{max} k'}{s_0} \tag{6.29}$$

indicating transfer from starvation medium to growth medium.

(iii) Importance of Cell Synchronization : In starvation stress synchrony, the cells (*S. cerevisiae*) subjected to starvation induction degrade its existing proteins at considerable rate. This leads to the generation of an amino acid pool that is utilized to synthesize new proteins whose induction is unique to the maintenance of synchrony in starvation state. This method of synchronizing has been used widely with microorganism culture. The principle is to run the culture into the stationary phase and then add fresh synthetic medium. The starvation synchrony as used for budding yeasts has been depicted in Fig. 6.5. It shows in developing synchronized yeast growth the first cycle is very long, because of the long lag phase of about 75 minutes, which precedes the start of building. Using membrane elution technique its characteristics in comparision to other relevant types of culture can be realized[21-30] from the summarised form given in Fig. 6.6. Interesting implications of phased or synchronous culture may concern growth rate, cell composition, variability in the cell cycle of growing and non-growing cells.

In developing starvation synchrony in bacterial cultures like *E. coli* it has been observed that at the onset of starvation it undergoes a temporarily ordered program of starvation gene expression involving 40-80 genes which some four hours later yields cells possessing an enhanced general resistance. Two classes of genes are induced upon carbon starvation stress, the *cst* genes

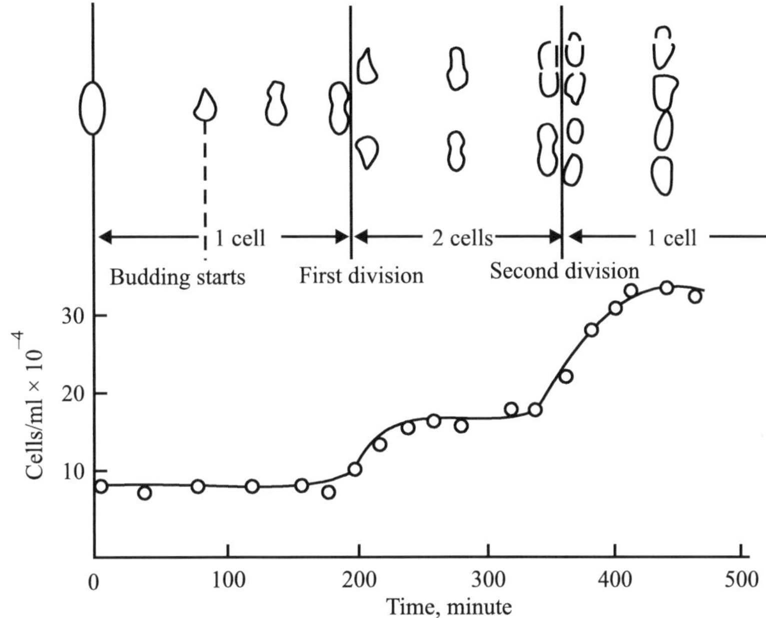

Fig. 6.5 Growth of a synchronised yeast culture (*Saccharomyces cerevisiae*) on inoculation into synthetic medium.

requiring cyclic AMP and *pex* genes not requiring this nucleotide for induction. On careful analysis of carbon starved synchronous culture of *E. coli* by 2D gel autoradiographs, it was revealed that upto 50 proteins are induced upon carbon starvation.

As depicted in Fig. 6.6 in membrane elution technique, a random growing culture (*E. coli*) is collected on a membrane filter. The filter is then inverted allowing fresh medium to run through and thus excess cells are washed off. The new born cells which are released from the filter surface are suitable for growing as a synchronous culture. The distribution of cell ages in a random culture appears as given in Fig. 6.7(a) and the relative concentration level of cells in the elute after loading and eluting shows the profile as in Fig. 6.7(b). If one follows the rate of synthesis of macromolcules and the elution pattern of radioactivity per cell from the membrane culture, which was radio pulse-labelled with a radioactive precursor of the macromolecules, the profile that appears to be as in Fig. 6.8 a and b. A fairly clear picture of the synthetic pattern of DNA in different media can be observed in this synchronization mode. Phased culture in comparison to other stratcgies is performed at steady repeated condition state as shown in Fig. 6.9. From this figure it can be observed that in batch and continuous cultures the individual cells are at different points of development in their replication cycles. However, in phased culture cells grow approximately in unison during the cell cycle. This enables cell size amplification.

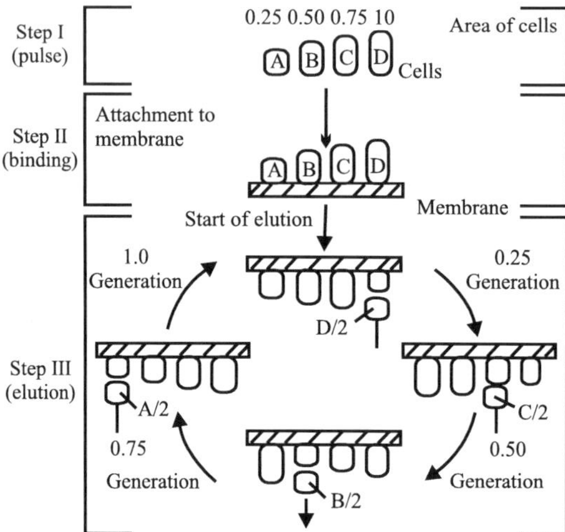

Fig. 6.6 Pulse-labelling before membrane elution with *Escherichia coli*. Outline of the procedure for determining the rate of incorporation of a labelled molecule into cells of different ages in an exponential unsynchronised culture

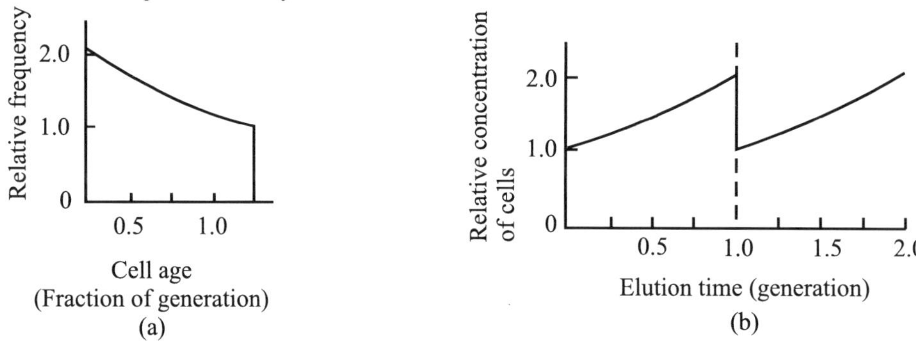

Fig. 6.7 Pulse-labelling before membrane elution with *Escherichia coli,* (a) idealised age distribution in an exponential phase culture containing no dispersion of generation times of individual cells. (b) Theoretical concentration of cells in the eluate from a membrane-bound culture with an age distribution as shown in Fig 6.7 (a)

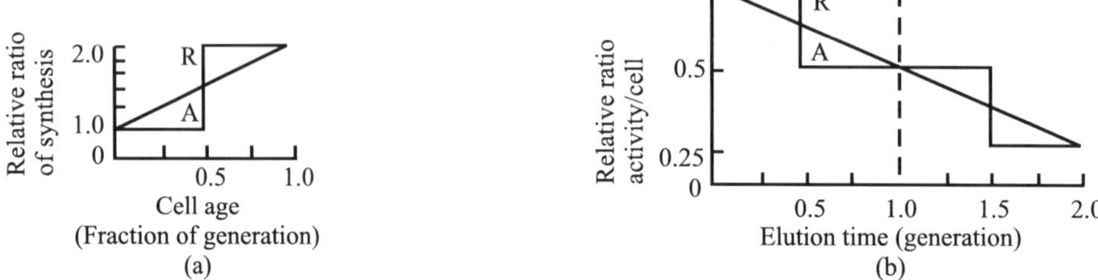

Fig. 6.8 Pulse labelling before membrane elution with *Escherichia coli.* (a) Rate of synthesis of two hypothetical macromolecules through the cell cycle. (b) Theoretical radioactivity per cell in the eluate from a membrane-bound culture if it has been pulse-labelled with the radioactive precursors of the macromolecules in (a)

6.2.3. Mammalian Cell Synchronization[21-31]

1. Purposes and methods

Like in microbial cells the methods of synchronizing mammalian cells in culture serve various purposes. The important purposes of mammalian cell synchronization relate to the regulation of the following:

1. Cell proliferation, biochemical and/or biological events in each phase.
2. Cell metabolism and other cell cycle-dependent events (protein, MAb synthesis)
3. Cell attachment

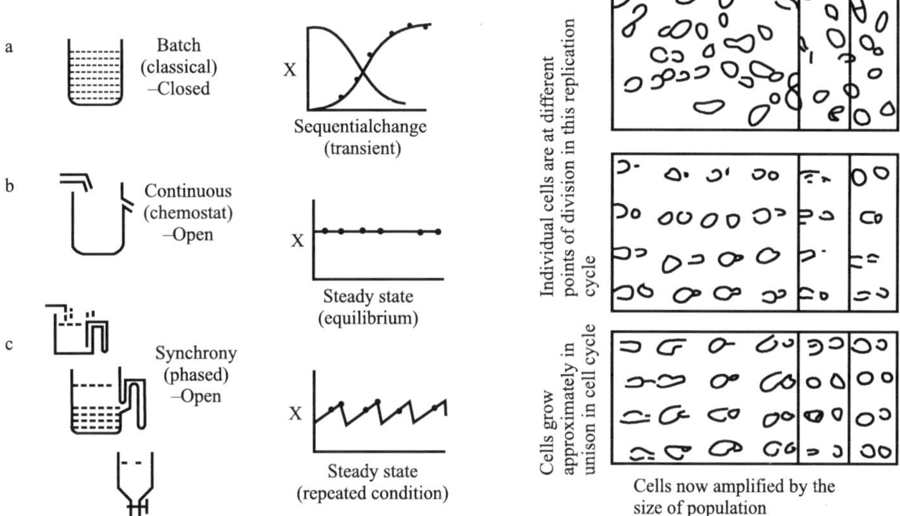

Fig. 6.9 Cell amplification[20]

In this system also method of synchronization can be divided into two broad classes.

I. Physical methods
  – mitotic attachment
  – ficoll gradient centrifugation
2. Chemical methods
  – double thymidine block (DTB)
  – isoleucine deprivation (ID)
  – serum deprivation (SD) and hydroxy urea (HU)

By double thymidine block synchronous DNA synthesis in mammalian cells (CHO) could be achieved. However, the degree of synchrony has been observed to be cell line dependent (Fig. 6.10 a and b)

In isoleucine deprivation cells (CHO) are incubated in F10 medium without isoleucine and glutamine plus 15% serum for 48 hrs, then isoleucine and glutamine are added to the normal concentration. The degree of synchrony is fair (Fig. 6.11).

In SD and HU method cells are incubated with low serum (1% or 0.5%) medium for 48 hrs, then serum-deficient medium is replaced by medium containing 10% serum, six hrs later HU is added to a final concentration of 1.5 mM and incubated for another 14 hrs. After that cells are resuspended in fresh medium. The degree of synchrony has been stated to be excellent for obtaining cells synchronized at G_1/S boundary (Fig. 6.12).

2. Comparison of the methods

Examination of figures 6.10 through 6.12 may reveal an inter-comparison of the methods as given in table 6.3.

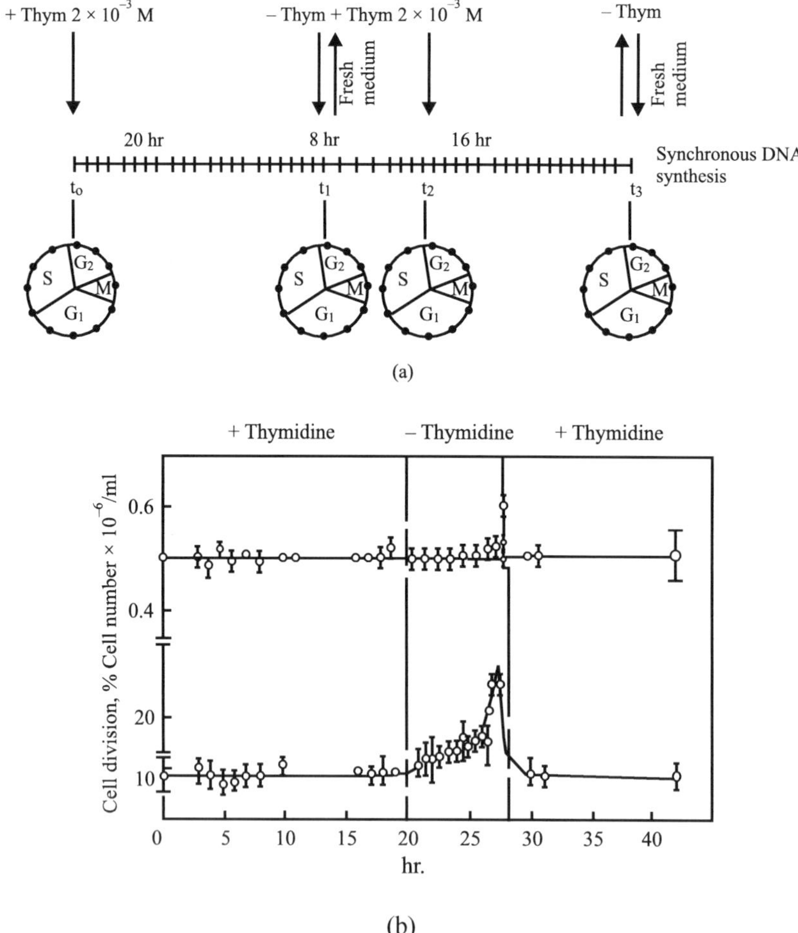

Fig. 6.10 Double thymidine block

The cells synchronized by above methods are characterized in terms of the following:

1. DNA synthesis (incorporating [^{3}H] thymidine into DNA.
2. Cell density and
3. Cell division (percent of double cells in population).

Table 6.3

Method	*Comparative*	
	Advantage	*Disadvantage*
DTB	Gives good synchrony in certain cell lines e.g. CHO	Cell line dependent
ID	Synchronizing large quantities of cells in suspension	Not applicable to all cell lines
SD/HU	Degree of synchrony is excellent for obtaining cells synchronized at G_1/S boundry	Needs longer time

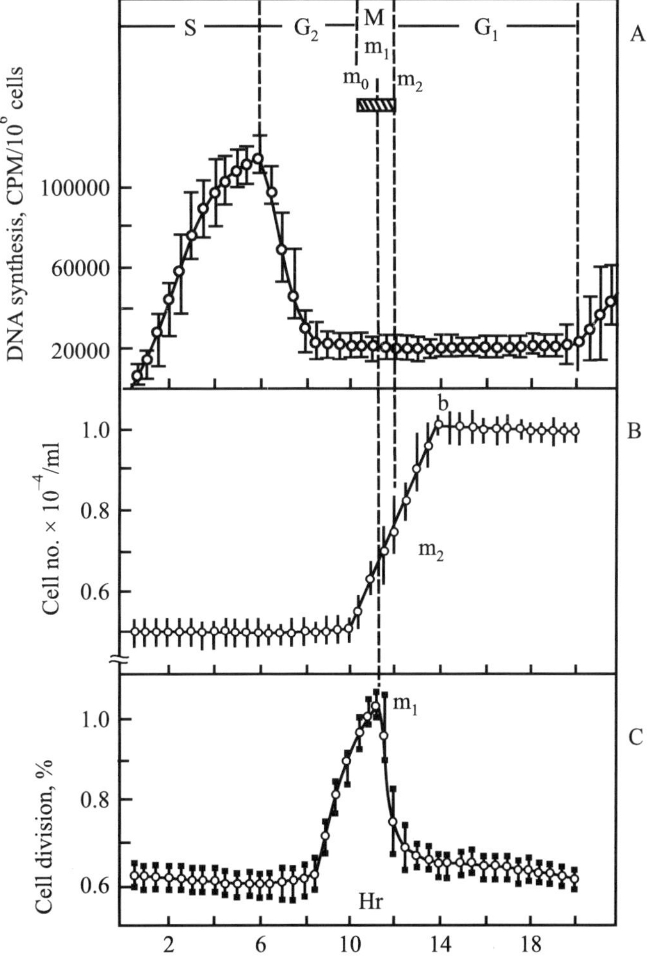

Fig. 6.11 Isoleucine deprivation to develop synchrony

6.3. RECENT ADVANCES OF YEAST BIOPROCESSING

6.3.1 Introduction

Yeasts are known to contribute significantly in the development of biotechnological processes. Both mesophilic and thermophilic yeasts are making extraordinary advances in the knowledge of fundamental and applied bioprocessing systems at cellular, molecular and production levels. Mesophilic yeasts like *Saccharomyces cerevisiae* containing covalently closed circular 2μ

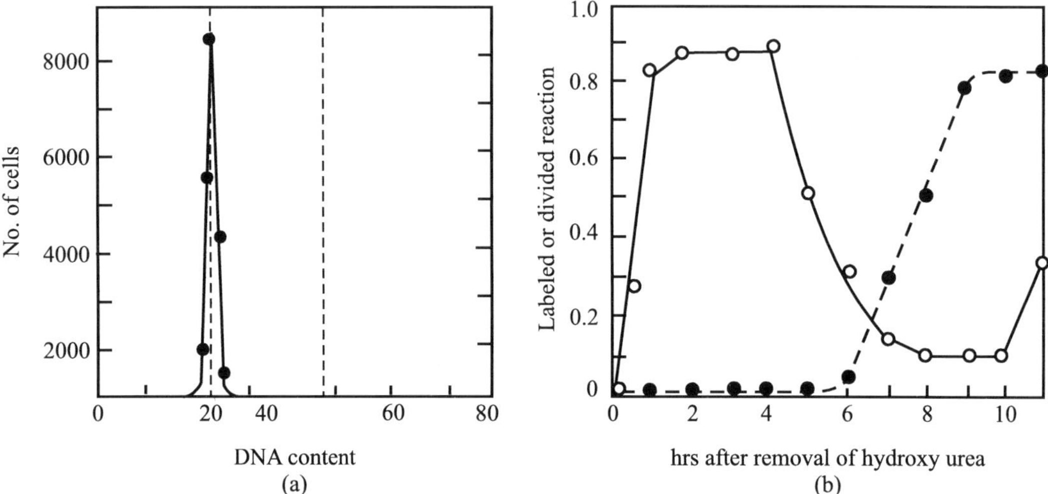

Fig. 6.12 Chemical methods of synchronization in mammalian cells (a) serum deprivation (SD), (b) hydroxy urea (HU) deprivation

plasmid has been attempted to be used as a source of cloning vehicle for upgradation of brewer's yeasts in terms of utilization of various carbohydrates like dextrin, maltose, lactose and flocculation characters. For this recombinational amplification of 2μ plasmid copy number increase has been attempted. This has added a new direction to yeasts technology. Therefore it has been necessary to examine the 2μ plasmid characters of the yeast in understanding this new direction. Also, several thermophilic yeasts which are found in digestive tract of wild and domestic animals as well as in nature are contributing significantly in the development of yeast biotechnology. Maximal growth temperatures of 40-50°C of thermophilic yeasts are not as high as those for thermophilic bacteria and fungi. *Candida brassicae, C. acidothermophilum, Pichia etchelsii, Kluyveromyces hennenbergii* etc. are few examples of thermophilic yeasts. In biotechnology these yeasts are playing significant role in overcoming many problems of product formation and giving newer *in vivo* proteolytic products using suitable bioprocessing strategy, and contributing towards downstream separation. Use of molecular biology techniques on these yeasts may add new dimensions towards new frontiers of industrial yeast biotechnology including the benefit in downstream separation.

6.3.2 More Recent Bioprocess Advances

Yeasts are heterogeneous group of fungi. In common they possess predominantly unicellular morphology in at least one phase of their vegetative life cycles. Nuclear DNA base composition has proven to be a valuable exclusionary criterion for characterizing yeasts. Likewise plasmid has a great role to play in recombinational amplification under certain circumstances in several yeast strains of *Saccharomyces* species.[32] Yeasts in nature and in bioprocessing circumstances may frequently encounter temperature shifts.[33] Temperature shift causes several changes in cellular metabolism. One of the manifestations being transmit decrease in the production of ribosomal proteins. Upon temperature shift strains of yeasts carrying *rna* mutations are known. It resulted different thermophilic strains of yeasts which are not true thermophilic but may belong to thermoduric. Both mesophilic and thermophilic yeasts show important characters of varying nature in terms of process biotechnology. Many yeasts of commercial importance have been shown to exhibit the flocculation property. This property has been used as an aid to downstream separation of bioproducts. Characteristic process biotechnology parameters of some thermophilic yeast has been used in newer bioprocessing for ethanol—a base chemical for product synthesis. In recent years using *in vitro-in vivo* events of cloning technology DNA recombination the flocculation characteristics of the yeast has been used to aid in quicker downstream separation of yeast cells.[34]

6.3.3 Secretion of Foreign Proteins

A great deal of advances in yeast genetics, molecular biology, physiological studies and cellular design engineering e.g. recombinational DNA technology have taken place in recent years. It has increased the interest in this microorganism as an alternate host to *E.coli* for the production of foregin proteins of commercial importance.

The development of transformation methods and identification of many strong constitutive or inducible promoters in yeast has allowed the construction of a number of convenient expression vectors. For example the PGK promoter from *Saccharomyces cerevisiae* can direct the synthesis of phosphoglycerate kinase to levels equivalent to 15-30% of total cell protein. Moreover, when the PGK promoter region is cloned into a high copy number, 2 μ plasmid, the synthesis of PGK reaches 50-80% of total cell protein. Vectors based upon this system have been used to direct the expression of several heterologons proteins. Also, *S. cerevisiae* secretes several enzymes to the medium offering possibilities of harnessing this feature to secrete foreign proteins. Yeasts are, therefore, capable to render additional advantages like safety in food and health care products.

6.3.4 Yeast Signaling System in Bioprocessing

The processing and secretion mechanism in yeast for the α mating factor involves synthesis of a large prepro 4α or prepro 3α subunit precursor. This is glycosylated in the endoplasmic reticulum (ER), translocated to the golgi apparatus and processed by a protease encoded by the KEX2 gene. Dipeptidy1 aminopeptidase encoded by STE 13 cleaves the Glu-Ala peptide from N-terminus of the polypeptide before the mature α-factor is secreted to the medium. In yeast for secretion of proteins export mechanism may use different signal sequence. However, self secretion may also be possible. Export using the α-factor singal and export using the SUC 2 signal sequence could be observed in *S. cerevisiae.* Few important foreign proteins expressed and produced through redesigning of *S. cerevisiae* and using different signalling methods are given in Table 6.4.

It is evident that yeast has many features as a host for the synthesis of foreign proteins of health care and commercial value. The organism is easy to cultivate on a large scale bioprocessing and the use of, for example, the α-factor preprosequence, spliced to the product of interest, offers a potentially efficient secretion/export mechanism. It has been indicated that it is possible to produce 10 mg per liter of a desired protein. By the advent of biomolecular redesigning it appears likely that this can be raised significantly by further molecular design engineering principles to increase the initial level of expression and by the use of mutants with hypersecretion activity.

Table 6.4 Examples of a few foreign proteins expressed and produced in *S. cerevisiae* using different signaling methods in bioprocessing

Sl. No.	*Protein*	*Estimated Proportion of Total Cell Protein, %*	*Signaling Method Used*
1.	Growth hormone releasing factor interleukin-2	5.0	a-factor prepro-sequence
2.	Calf prochymosin	0.5	SUC 2 signal sequence
3.	Invertase	—	α-factor preprosequence
4.	Human α-interferon	1.0	"
5.	Aspergillus glucoamylase	—	self secretion.

6.3.5 Advances in Yeast Brewing by Cloning Technology

In more recent years transformation of yeasts has been carried out. DNA is extracted and purified in an unmodified form from donor yeast cells. The native DNA has been modified with spheroplasts of the recipient yeast culture in presence of certain reagent and ion regenerating colonies. The regenerated colonies have been finally screened for obtaining successful transformants. Such a maltose/maltotriose system could be transformed. There are strains of *Saccharomyces* that ferment only maltose and not maltotriose. Such strains lack the ability for uptake of the trisaccharide. However, by overcoming this permeability barrier to trisaccharide, the β-glucosidase system within such maltotriose negative strains can readily hydrolyze maltotriose to glucose units. A maltose positive/maltotriose negative haploid yeast strain could be developed by sequential treatments. Maltotriose positive transformant could also be developed. However, this was similar to untransformed parent on wort-gelatin medium. These observations together with later findings indicated that successful transformations have been obtained for maltotriose uptake using native DNA as donor material into maltose positive/maltotriose negative yeast strains.[34,35]

6.3.6 Flocculation Property

1. Aid to process biotechnology

Cell recycle system has been reported to be a better processing strategy for alcohol production by yeast. In a cell recycle system the mash containing the cells are passed through a cell settler.

In the settler cells are allowed to settle by flocculation through hindered settling phenomena and liquid is sent to a mash collector prior to distillation. For efficient operation of a settler the yeast cells must flocculate and settle with a high setting velocity. It allows the dense viable cells to be recycled to the main fermenter to increase alcohol production. However, alcohol producting yeast strains are usually nonflocculating. Non flocculating strains take longer time to settle in the settler and required higher retention time of the cells in the reactor. For increasing settling velocity of yeast in the settler two approaches have been used. The first approach attempts to increase settling velocity in a settler by inducing flocculation of the cells by suitable processing condition. In the second approach, however, genetic change in yeast strain is carried out by flocculating gene cloning technology as stated in earlier section.

2. Characteristic analysis

In settler the flocculation of yeast is characterized through the estimations of floc diameter and floc density.[36] The floc diameter (d_f, cm) may be estimated from the relation

$$d_f = \frac{d_p}{A_1 A_2} \tag{6.30}$$

in which d_p is the projected floc diameter on the screen perpendicular to the direction of settling (cm). A_1 is the rate of enlargement on the film through the closeup photography of the settler. A_2 is the enlargement through the projection on the screen.

The floc density can be calculated from its size and settling velocity by using a suitable settling velocity equation if the water temperature is known. The general equation for the terminal free settling velocity (W) of a descrete particle in water is given by

$$W = \left[\frac{4}{3} \cdot \frac{g}{C_D} \left(\frac{\rho_s - \rho_w}{\rho_w}\right) d\right]^{1/2} \tag{6.31}$$

where g is the gravitational acceleration 98 cm sec^{-2}, C_D is drag coefficient, ρ_s and ρ_w are density of the particle and water respectively, g. cm^{-3}, d is the particle diameter (cm). As C_D is a function of Reynolds number (Wd_s/v) and sphericity (ψ), therefore it was shown that when all the flocs have Reynolds number (N_{Re}) less than 10^6 in their settling the general form of C_D is given by

$$C_D = \frac{k}{N_{Re}} \tag{6.32}$$

in which k is a constant depending on the sphericity. From available data on sphericity of ordinary floc its average value is known to be 0.8. Accordingly C_D for the floc particles has been given by (from plot of C_D vs N_{Re}).[36]

$$C_D = \frac{36}{0.8} \times \frac{1}{N_{Re}} = \frac{45}{N_{Re}} \tag{6.33}$$

So, the equation describing the settling velocity of floc takes the form

$$W = \left[\frac{4g}{3} \frac{N_{Re}}{45} \left(\frac{\rho_f - \rho_w}{\rho_w} \right) d_f \right]^{1/2} \tag{6.34}$$

or

$$W \approx \frac{g}{34\mu} (\rho_f - \rho_w) d^2_f \tag{6.35}$$

In these relations ρ_f is the density of the floc (g cm^{-3}). Considering buoyant force of liquid on the flocs, the effective buoyant density of floc

$$\rho_e = \rho_f - \rho_w \tag{6.36}$$

Since the change in value of ρ_f is between 1.01 to 1.02 g cm^{-3} the increasing rate of floc density is only 1% (1.02-1.01) × 100/100 = 1). Therefore it is difficult to make clear difference of floc density itself by experiment. On the other hand increasing rate of effective density ρ_e is 100% $\left(\frac{0.02 - 0.01}{0.01} \times 100 \right)$. It is, therefore, easy to evaluate the characteristic values of the effective density of floc from the floc density function

$$\rho_e = \rho_f - \rho_w = \frac{a}{(d_f/L)\, K_p} \tag{6.37}$$

where d_f/L is a dimensionless floc diameter (cm/cm), *a* and K_p are constants, the former has unit g cm^{-3} and later is unitless. The rate of flocculation can be increased by adding efective flocculant.[37, 38]

6.3.7 Advances in Nutrition in Relation to Bioprocessing

In ethanol production using *Saccharomyces cerevisiae* (ATCC 4126) it has been shown that an oxygen tension of 0.07 mm Hg was optimal. Below this oxygen tension the yeast becomes oxygen starved and ethanol productivity decreased. At high oxygen tensions the yeast metabolism began to shift from anaerobic to acrobic and less ethanol was produced with a corresponding increased cell mass production. In continuous ethanol fermentations sometimes low fermentation rate is shown to be due to the lack of oxygen. It appears that even though ethanol fermentation is anaerobic process trace amount of oxygen is required for biosynthesis. It is reported that as a substitute of this trace oxygen unsaturated lipid, ergosterol can be used to the fermentation broth.[39-42]

Likewise wort fermentation in beer production is largely anaerobic but this is not the case when the yeast is pitched into this wort and at that time some oxygen must be made available to the yeast. There is a need for oxygen because brewing yeasts in the absence of molecular oxygen are unable to synthesize sterols and unsaturated fatty acids. Sterols and unsaturated fatty acids are essential in membrane for efficiency and beer flavour. Underaeration leads to suboptimal synthesis of essential membrane lipids. In turn it is reflected in limited yeast growth, a low fermentation rate and concomitant beer flavour problems. Over aeration results in overexpending nutrients for the production of unnecesary yeast biomass, thus lowering fermentation efficiency because of the excess biomass and lower ethanol production.

6.3.8 Yeast Redesigning Advances

1. Noncommitted mutation

Yeast mutational redesigning is a common occurence throughtout the growth and fermentation cycle. The mutation is usually recessive in nature. This is because of the loss of function of a gene. Since industrial strains are usually at least diploid, the dominant gene will function adequately in the strain and it will be physiologically normal. Only if the mutation takes place in both alleles will the character be expressed. If the mutation weakens the yeast, the mutated strain will not be able to compete and will soon be out grown by the other yeasts.

Normally three characteristic groups are routinely encountered resulting from spontaneous mutational redesigning of yeast which can be harmful to a fermentation. These include (a) the tendency to the yeast strain to mutate from flocculescence to nonflocculescence, (b) the loss of ability to ferment maltotriose and components that are normally present in the worth in suboptimal quantities. They are abundant in malt. As normal manufacturing procedures prevent their passing into the wort, oxygen must be supplied to allow their synthesis by yeast when ergosterol and an unsaturated fatty acid like oleic acid are added to wort, the requirement for oxygen disappears. When a brewer's yeast is grown anaerobically it accumulates sterols and unsaturated lipids within the cells. These lipids can be diluted to a degree by subsequent growth without negative effects. So cells prepared aerobically can grow to some extent anaerobically also. However, if yeast is harvested at the end of fermentation and used to inoculate a second batch of wort then oxygen is required. This is because the new inoculum contains no reserves of the necessary lipids. Oxygen content of the wort at pitching is important to lipid metabolism in yeast fermentation. Another factor is the presence of respiratory deficient (R_D) mutants. The last group usually consists of cytoplasmic mutants.

The most commonly and frequently identified spontaneous mutant found in brewing yeast strains is the R_D or petite mutation. The R_D mutant arises spontaneously when a segment of the wild type mitochondrial genome, exercised by an illegitimate site, specific recombination is amplified. It is due to formation of a defective mitochondrial genome. The mitochondria are then unable to synthesize certain proteins. This mutation shows non-Mendelian seggregation when crosses of the wild type with the mutant are carried out and may be termed non-committed mutation.

2. Frequency level and characters

The R_D noncommitted mutational redesigning occurs at frequencies between 0.5% and 5% of the yeast population. In some strains, however, figures as high as 50% have been reported.[43] The mutant is characterised by deficiencies in mitochondria function resulting in a diminished ability to function aerobically. These redesigned yeast, are unable to metabolize nonfermentable carbon sources such as lactate, glycerol or ethanol. Many phenotypic changes occur because of the redesigning, including alterations in sugar uptake.

6.4 MULTIINTERACTING MICROBIAL BIOPROCESSING: THEORY, BENEFITS AND PROBLEMS

6.4.1 Introduction

Many types of multiinteraction biosystems are found in nature or during bioprocessing. Many of them may be homogenic while others are heterogenic character. These systems may be stress dependent or operational mode dependent. Some examples of multiinteracting biosystems include monoculture pellet forming systems like citric acid fermentation by *Asp. niger*, cellulase fermentation by *T. reesei* and in many multiculture systems like biological waste treatment, industrial mixed culture bioprocessing, soil microbial interactions etc.

6.4.2 Multiinteractions in Monoculture Biosystem

In microbial cell processing many cells have tendency to form flocks or pellets by multiple interactions due to turbulence.[44-46] They may also form pellets by multiple interactions in quiescent liquid by excreting tubulin proteins having chemotactic properties or by molecular motion.

Many yeasts and other cells form flocs during cultivation, processing for product formation and biocolloid formation.

1. Theory

The above observations led to conceive that microbial monoculture multiple interactions to form aggregates may occur by [47-49] (1) perikinetic attachment (peripheral); (2) orthodynamic collision (orthogonal) and (3) binary adhesion dynamics (adhesional). These multiple interactions between monoculture cells may result loose/ fluffy or dense/hard core pellets/flocs depending on microbial nature and operating conditions of temp., pH, turbulence, shear, etc.

(*i*) *Perikinetic Attachment* : In this interaction the particle/cell motion is affected by Brownian diffusion as a result of KT energy. The concentration of pellets at time t may be given by

$$N_t = N_0 \, (1 + t/t_{1/2})^{-1} \qquad (6.38)$$

where N_0 = initial conc./no. of colloid/pellet particles (Number/Vol) and

$$t_{1/2} = \frac{3\mu}{4\eta \, KTN_0} \qquad (6.39)$$

in which μ is the kinematic viscosity, η is the efficiency of attachment on collision, K is the Boltzmann constant and T is the operational temp. in absolute scale.

(ii) Orthodynamic Collision : It affects cells motion by physical agitation or turbulence of fluid mixing. The concentration of pellets at time *t* is given by

$$N_t = N_0 \exp\left(-\frac{4}{\pi}\eta\,\Omega\,\overline{G}\,t\right) \qquad (6.40)$$

Here, $\Omega = \frac{\pi d_c^3}{6}$ = Volume fraction of pellets/flocs

d_0 = Original diameter of the pellet of the monodispersed spherical particles

$\overline{G}$ = Mean velocity gradient

Comparative inference

From a comparision of the rate of pellets separation from the medium between perikinetic and orthodynamic collisions in pellet formation one can have

$$\frac{\left(\frac{dN_t}{dt}\right)_0}{\left(\frac{dN_t}{dt}\right)_p} = \frac{4\overline{G}\,\mu\, r_1^3}{kT} \tag{6.41}$$

which for equal rates indicates equal dominance.

(iii) Binary Adhesional Multiple Interactions : In cellulase production by *T. reesei* depending on processing conditions pellet formation has been observed.[47,48] The pellet diameter at any time was computed from that measured at any time from its growth analysis.

When a given conidia concentration (in inoculum) for pellet formation is used the increase in number of pellets in the agitated broth depended on the multiple number of adhesive collisions to form pellets. The increase in pellet number may be given by

$$\frac{dN}{dt} = \eta' N^2 \tag{6.42}$$

in which N = no. of pellets, η' = a constant under a given geometry of the vessel and bioprocessing conditions.

A. Significance of η'

Physically η' signifies homogenization efficiency because adhesive collision is dependent on the degree of homogenity of the broth. In turn it is a function of energy expenditure per unit mass of the charge in the batch.

If equation 6.42 is integrated between limits

$$N = N_0, \text{ at } t = t_1$$
$$N = N_t, \text{ at } t = t_2$$

one obtains

$$N_t = N_0\,[1 - N_0\,\eta'\,(t_2 - t_1)]^{-1} \tag{6.43}$$

The values of N_t and N_0 may be computed as[47]

$$\left.\begin{aligned} N_t &= \left(\frac{M_t}{\frac{4}{3}\pi r_1^3 \rho_t}\right) \\ N_0 &= \left(\frac{M_0}{\frac{4}{3}\pi r_0^3 \rho_t}\right) \end{aligned}\right\} \tag{6.44}$$

B. Value of η'

The value of η' in relation to energy expenditure is given by

$$\eta' = \frac{U}{E} \log \left[\frac{2}{x}\right]^3 \tag{6.45}$$

where x is the degree of homogenity; values of E and U are defined as

$$E = \frac{P \cdot \theta}{V \cdot P} \tag{6.46}$$

$$U = \frac{V}{\theta D_t^2} \tag{6.47}$$

E represents mean energy consumption per unit mass of the broth, U has dimension of velocity, θ is the mixing time and V is the broth volume. These concepts enabled to determine the pellet radius at any time from its initial value and has been reported in the literature.[47]

(iv) Observed Substrate Uptake Rate Behavior in a Single Species Multiinteractions : In bioprocessing for cellulase production by *T. reesei* QM9414 showing pellet formation it has been noticed that in the pellet formation by multiinteraction the proportional relationship in pellet forming period could be expressed by[47]

$$\frac{dC_s}{dt} = -kC_s \tag{6.48}$$

where C_s is the residual substrate concentration, k is the substrate uptake rate constant and negative sign indicates the decrease of substrate concentration. This relationship was further checked by determining value of rate constant at four different temperatures 23, 26, 29 and 34°C and checking the validity of Arrhenius equation to provide activation energy required for optimum substrate uptake. The determined value of activation energy 21,350 cals/mole was in the reasonable range in comparison with the other microbial bioprocessing reported in the literature.[45,46] Temperature effect on unit cellulose uptake time (t_u) showed a nearly constant ratio with pellet formation lag time (t_l) suggesting that lag can be a useful parameter on the effect of environment in microbial multiinteraction and specific substrate uptake rate.[47,48]

6.4.3 Prey-Predator (Host-Parasite) Biosystem

In multiinteractions of prey-predator biosystem the level of one population depends in an intimate way on the level of another population. A parasite is born from its cell/egg deposited on the host.[49] The host is killed in the process. It may completely jeopardize the product formation by the host.

1. Growth rate of prey-predator

At any time t, let

X_1 = Number of prey
X_2 = Number of predator

The number of eggs deposited by invading virus $\propto X_I X_2$ (assumed) parasites depends on the probability of the virus/parasite and hosts coming together.

Prey kill rate by virus/parasites $= -\alpha X_1X_2$

Prey birth rate $= K_b$

Natural death rate of prey $= K_d$

(exclusive of parasite)

So net rate of growth $= K_b X_1 - K_d X_1 = \beta X_1$

where $\beta = K_b - K_d$

As long as $K_b > K_d$, $\beta = +ve$

Considering all birth and death rates of prey & predator we may write

$$\frac{dX_1}{dt} = (\beta - aX_2)X_1 \tag{6.49}$$

Here, α = a +ve constant, –ve sign accounts for death rate. Similarly,
Natural death rate of predator $= K_d$
Growth rate of predator is

$$\frac{dX_2}{dt} = - K'_d X_2 + f\alpha X_1 X_2\ , \quad K'_d > 0,\ 0 < f \leq 1 \tag{6.50}$$

Equations (6.49) and (6.50) are basic equations for Prey-Predator system and are called Lotka-Voltera equations.
Considering following initial conditions

$$X_1 = X_0$$

$$X_2 = X_0$$

at $t = 0$

For stationary growth

$$X_1(\beta - \alpha X_2) = 0 \tag{6.51}$$

$$X_2(- K_d + \alpha f X_1) = 0 \tag{6.52}$$

The trivial solutions

$$X_1 = 0$$

$$X_2 = 0$$

The non-trivial solutions

$$X_1 = X_{1e} \equiv \frac{K_{d'}}{f\alpha} \tag{6.53}$$

$$X_2 = X_{2e} \equiv \frac{\beta}{\alpha} \tag{6.54}$$

Expanding (6.49 and 6.50) in Taylor series about (X_{1e}, X_{2e}) and retaining linear terms

$$f(X_{1e}, X_{2e}) = f(X_{1e},, X_{2e}) + (X_1 - X_{1e}) \left[\frac{d}{dX_1} f(X_1 X_2) \right]_{\substack{X_1 = X_0 \\ X_2 = X_0'}}$$

$$+ (X_1 - X_{2e}) \left[\frac{d}{dX_2} f(X_1 X_2) \right]_{\substack{X_1 = X_0 \\ X_2 = X_e'}} \tag{6.55}$$

From equations 6.51 and 6.52 we get

$$X_1 (\beta - \alpha X_2) = - \alpha X_{1e} (X_2 - X_{2e}) + \ldots \tag{6.56}$$

$$X_2 (- K_d + \alpha X_1) = f \alpha X_{2e} (X_1 - X_{1e}) + \ldots \tag{6.57}$$

So, from equation 6.49 and 6.50 and 6.56 and 6.57

$$\left(\frac{dX_1}{dt} \right) = - \alpha X_{1e} (X_2 - X_{2e}) \tag{6.58}$$

$$\left(\frac{dX_2}{dt} \right) = f\alpha X_{2e} (X_1 - X_{1e}) \tag{6.59}$$

For simplification of equations (6.58) and (6.59) change (X_1, X_2) to (ξ, η) using the following displacement

$$\xi = (X_1 - X_{1e}) \tag{6.60}$$

$$\eta = (X_2 - X_{2e}) \tag{6.61}$$

Now,

$$\frac{d\xi}{dt} = - \alpha X_{1e} \eta \tag{6.62}$$

$$\frac{d\eta}{dt} = f\alpha x_{2e} \xi \tag{6.63}$$

So,

$$dt = \frac{d\xi}{f a X_{2e} \eta} \tag{6.64}$$

and

$$dt = \frac{d\eta}{f a X_{2e} \xi} \tag{6.65}$$

$\therefore$

$$- \frac{\xi d\xi}{X_{1e}} = \frac{\eta d\eta}{f X_{2e}} \tag{6.66}$$

Integrating

$$\frac{\xi^2}{X_{1e}} + \frac{\eta^2}{f X_{2e}} = c = \text{constant} \tag{6.67}$$

Putting equations (6.60 & 6.61) in (6.67) we get

$$c = \frac{(X_1 - X_{1e})^2}{X_{1e}} + \frac{(X_2 - X_{2e})^2}{f\,X_{2e}} \tag{6.68}$$

2. Temporal course of events

The above equation indicates that it is an equation of an ellipse whose centre is at the origin in ξη plane (Fig. 6.13). The arrow head indicates temporal course of events. The prey-predator undergoes cyclic changes in growth, alternatively waxing and waning.

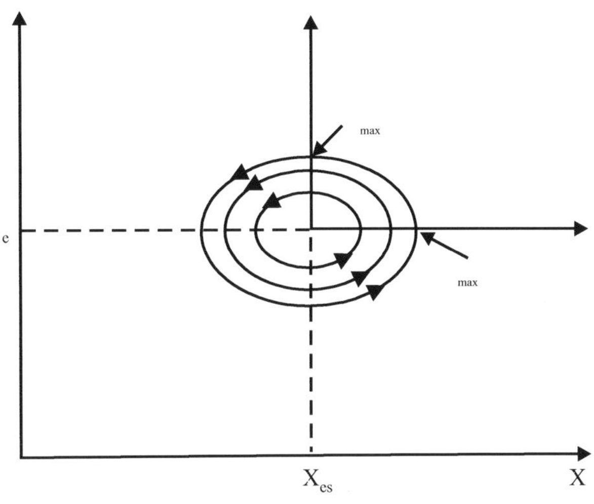

Fig. 6.13

3. Qualitative interpretation

The increase in the prey population favours an increase in predator population. The later increases at the expense of the host. They too must begin to disappear because of lack of food supply (for the predator larvae). This favors the recovery of the prey population and the cycle begin all over again. Knowing the inter-dependence of ξ and η and considering

$$dt = -\frac{d\xi}{aX_{1e}\eta}$$

and

$$dt = \frac{d\eta}{f\,aX_{2e}}$$

we can determine the explicit dependence of these variables on the time.

Value of ξ

For $t = t_0$, When $\eta = 0,\ \xi = \xi_m$

So,

$$\xi = \xi_m = \sqrt{X_1 C} \tag{6.69}$$

Thus from equations (6.64), (6.67) and (6.69)

$$\alpha X_{1e} \int_{t_0}^{t} dt = -\sqrt{\frac{X_{1e}}{f X_{2e}}} \int_{\xi_m}^{\xi} \frac{d\xi}{\xi_m^2 - \xi^2} \tag{6.70}$$

Integrating

$$\alpha \sqrt{f X_{1e} X_{2e}}\ (t - t_0) = \cos^{-1} \frac{\xi}{\xi_m} \Big|_{\xi}^{\xi_m} = \cos^{-1} \frac{\xi}{\xi_m} \tag{6.71}$$

Solving,

$$\xi = \xi_m \cos\left[a \sqrt{X_{1e} X_{2e}}\ (t - t_0)\right] \tag{6.72}$$

Value of η

As above we may have

$$\eta = \eta_m \sin\left[a \sqrt{f X_{1e} X_{2e}}\ (t - t_0)\right] \tag{6.73}$$

where

$$\eta_m = \sqrt{f X_{1e} c} \tag{6.74}$$

η_m and ξ_m are amplitudes of oscillations.

T = period of oscillation = time for the displacemet to return to a given value.

From equations (6.72 & 6.73)

$$T = \frac{2\pi}{a \sqrt{f X_{1e} X_{2e}}} \quad \text{or } T = \frac{2\pi}{\sqrt{\beta K_d'}}$$

It shows that the period is independent of initial conditions.

Since $\quad \cos\left(t - \frac{\pi}{2}\right) = \sin \pi\, t$

So, from (6.73)

$$\eta = \eta_m \cos\left[a \sqrt{f X_{1e} X_{2e}} (t - t_0) - \frac{\pi}{2}\right] \tag{6.75}$$

This equation when compared with equation (6.72) indicates that

(1) Peak of predator lag behind the peak of prey by $\frac{\pi}{2}$ or 1/4th the period of oscillation.

(2) $\frac{\pi}{2}$ = Phase angle = constant

(3) (X_{1e}, X_{2e}) = The point of neutral stability in the trajectory of the point (X_1, X_2).

6.4.4 Benefits of Multiinteraction

Depending on microbial system characteristics multiinteractions may render several benefits. These include :

(1) Reduction in bulk viscosity—examples are cellulase production in pellet forming system, citric acid production by pellet forming molds.

It causes easy separation of microbial biomass from culture fluid during downstream separation.

(2) Mutualistic interaction in biotransformation to produce products like (a) biofertilizer (b) yoghurt/*dahi* etc.

6.4.5 Problems of Multiinteractions

Multiinteracting species in microbial bioprocessing may pose problems depending on the system condition. Some examples are given below :

Problems in productivity

1. The acetone-butanol production by microbial fermentation is very prone to contamination by phages. In fermentative production of acetone-butanol by *Actinomycetes* species the actinophage is a common contaminant if the fermentation is not controlled strictly. In this system the virus/parasite causes ultimate killing of the *Actinomycetes* and spoil the fermentative production of solvents. Here *Actinomycetes* is the prey and actinophage is the predator.
2. In cellulase production by pellet forming *T. reesei* cells, depending on the pellet characteristics may create oxygen penetration problem which in turn may reduce enzyme productivity of the cells.

6.5 STRATEGIES OF CYCLING AND PROFILING OF VARIABLES IN BIOPROCESSING

6.5.1 Introduction

The environment of microbial cell processing plays significant role in determining the rates and yields of specific product formation. The regulatory influence of pH, temperature and pH cycling and temperature profiling indicated improvements in bioprocessing for certain product formation systems. Two well known examples of such microbial cell processing systems include cellulase enzyme production by *Trichoderma reesei* strain and propionic acid upstream bioprocessing by *Propionibacterium acidiopropionici.* In bioconversion of cellulose to ethanol by *Clostridium thermocellum* using pH and vacuum cycling indicated the merit of the strategy in bioprocessing.

6.5.2 pH Cycling

1. Mode in cellulase production by T. reesei

The importance of pH in cellulase production by organisms is known.[50-64] It was reported that cultivating *T. reesei* QM9414 in Mandel's medium containing 1% beech wood cellulose and 0.05% yeast extract for cellulases production showed a fall of pH to 3.0 (initial pH 5.7) in 18 hours. The increase of cellulase production by pH cycling during cultivation of *T. reesei* has been shown.[51,52] The cycling continued for three days and from fourth day pH started rising and was controlled at pH 5.7 to avoid inactivation of enzyme at higher pH due to heavy sporulation. The culture with above strategy showed high oxygen demand (2.1 mM02/g of cells/hr) compared to cells grown without pH cycling (1-1.2 mMO_2/g. cells/hr). Natural pH of fermentation medium after sterilization was 5.2 and in the first ten to fifteen hours pH increased to 6.2. At this stage 1 N hydrochloric acid was aseptically added to bring it back to 5.2 and maintained till pH start droping down.[52] It started from twenty to twenty five hours of age and reached 3.0 somewhere between forty to fortyfive hours of age of cell cultivation. As soon as pH reached 3.0 a peristaltic pump (Watson-Marlow) was actuated to add 2N NaOH at very slow flow rate 0.2 (ml/min) with the help of a circuit diagram for automatic pH cycling (Fig. 6.14). The addition of NaOH was stopped as soon as pH reached 5.2 and again natural fall to pH 3.0 was awaited. Normally the next cycling needed 18 to 30 hours depending upon physiological conditions of the fungal biocells in the fermenter. In cycling control of pH in gold 465 series

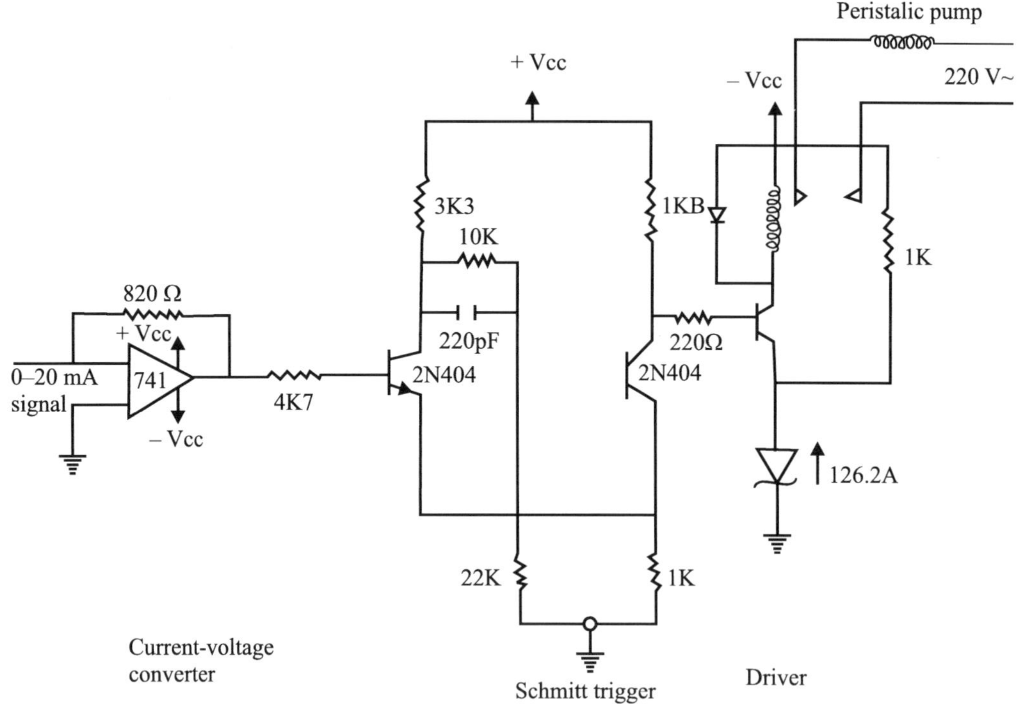

Fig. 6.14 Cicruit diagram for automatic pH cycling

sterilizable pH electrode with pressure assembly was used. The electrode was pressurised to 1.5 kg/cm^2 pressure during sterilization and 0.2 kg/cm^2 above residual pressure during the cycle. For fixing the frequency of addition of 2N NaOH in pH cycling, amplifying and controlling Mostech AG regler M7882 was used. The pH cycling output of the amplifier (0-20 mA) was received in a 741 IC to convert to volt signal and trigger a relay between two control pH point 5.2 and 3.0 to add 2N NaOH. Measured results of cell concentration, cellulase yield, and productivity during cell cultivation and given in Table 6.5 indicated that pH cycling favoured cell growth and increased cellulase yield and productivity. Under pH cycling data obtained with 30 and 40 gl^{-1} cellulose level (Fig. 6.15 and Table.6.6) were also in concurrence of the same.

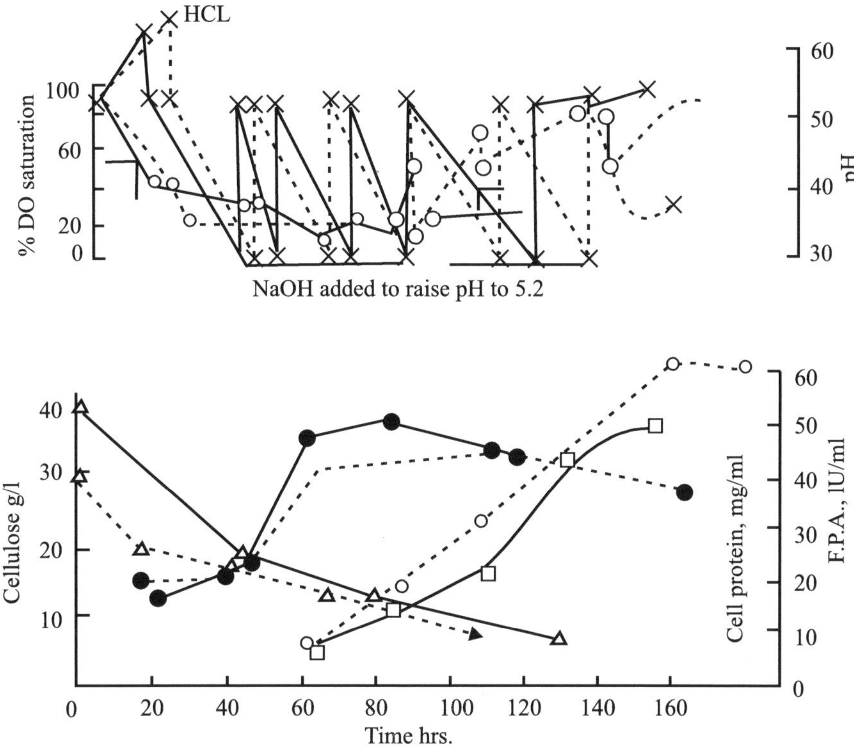

Fig. 6.15 Behaviour of *T. reesei* cultivation under pH cycling : (. . .) 30 g/liter; (—) 40 g/liter cellulose. (Δ— Δ) Residual cellulose (g/liter); (• – •) cell protein (mg/ml); (□ — □) filter paper activity. (IU/ml); (× — ×) pH cycle; (○ – ○) % DO.[52]

Table 6.5 *T. reesei* cultivation results obtained with and without pH cycling [52]

Run	*pH Condition During Cultivation*	*Total Culture Time (hr.)*	*Cell Conc. (g/liter)*	*Maximum Oxygen Demand Rate (mM O_2/g cell/hr.)*	*Cellulase*		
						Productivity	
					Yield (IU/ml)	*(IU/liter/hr.)*	*(IU/g cell/hr.)*
1.	No pH cycling (controlled at pH 3.0 after 40 hr.)	180	8.0	0.40	4.5	25.0	3.0
2.	pH cycled between 3.0 and 5.2 and 40–160 hr.	160	9.5	0.48	6.2	38.75	4.0

2. *Analysis in relation to cell growth*[58]

The analysis of results indicated that pH cycling in *T. reesei* cultivation favours enhanced cellulase production with less cell growth as compared to that controlled pH cultivation. The growth of *T. reesei* in the pH cycling environment could be expressed by a single species logistic equation containing a periodically oscillating parameter, ϕ (t), representing the reciprocal of the specific cell yield of *T. reesei.* From logistic law the growth rate X of *T. reesei* could be written as

$$\overline{X} = (b_1 X/b_2)(b_2 - X) \tag{6.76}$$

in which b_1 is the specific growth rate, b_2 is carrying capacity of cell mass formation. In principle b_1 and b_2 are functions of time. The physical significance of b_1 is as an expression of specific growth rate (μ), while b_2 represents the maximum level of cell mass formation. Assuming b_1 represents maximum specific growth rate (μm) and is constant but b_2 is a time dependent factor, depending on the substrate uptake rate, which oscillates periodically about a mean value due pH cycling in batch cultivation. So equation 6.76 can be expressed as

$$\overline{X} = \left[\frac{b_1 X}{b_2(t)}\right][b_2(t) - X] \tag{6.77}$$

Table 6.6 Growth of *T. reesei* and its cellulase production at different cellulose[52] concentrations under pH cycling condition (160 hr Cycle)

Cellulose Conc.	*Cell Conc.*	*Cellulose Uptake Rate*		*Cellulase*			
				Yield		*Productivity*	
(g/litre)	*(g/litre)*	*(g/litre/hr)*	*(g/g cell/hr)*	*(IU/ml)*	*(IU/g cellulose)*	*(IU/litre/hr)*	*(IU/g cell/hr)*
7.5	4.0	0.062	0.015	1.6	213	10.00	2.0
15.0	6.5	0.134	0.020	3.9	213	20.00	3.0
30.0	9.5	0.287	0.030	6.0	206	38.75	4.0
40.0	12.0	0.200	0.016	4.4	110	27.50	2.3
45.0	14.0	0.115	0.008	3.5	78	21.80	1.6

where

$$b_2(t) = b_2[1 + p\,\phi(t)] \tag{6.78}$$

Here p is a parameter representing the ratio of maximum value of the substrate uptake rate constant (K_T) to the specific growth rate (i.e., $p = K_T/\mu$), and ϕ (t) is a periodic function of t with period $\theta > 0$. Thus,

$$\phi\,(t) = \left(\frac{ds}{dt}\right)\Big/\left(\frac{1}{X}.\frac{dX}{dt}\right) = X\ \frac{ds}{dX} = \frac{1}{\left(\frac{1}{X}.\frac{dX}{DS}\right)} = \frac{1}{\text{sp. cell yield}} \tag{6.79}$$

So, ϕ (t) = reciprocal of specific cell yield. In *T. reesei* cell growth the magnitude of p is restricted by conditions b_2 (t) > 0 for all t values and |p| is small. Both the conditions are assumed satisfied in growth of *T. reesei* under pH cycling. It provides an assymptotically stable solution of the growth rate equation (6.76) to be

$$X = b_2 \tag{6.80}$$

Under above restricted conditions a solution of equation (6.77) may be obtained by standard mathematical procedure[58], which is θ periodic. This solution differs from the above solution (6.80) by an amount that tends to zero with p and may be expressed as a convergent series, as below

$$X\,(t, p) = b_2 + \sum_{n=1}^{\infty} p^n\ X_n\,(t) \tag{6.81}$$

provided p is small. Substituting Equations (6.78) and (6.81) into Equation (6.77) and equating coefficients of like powers of *p* provides a sequence of equations. The first equation of the sequence is

$$\overline{X}_1 + b_1 X_1 = b_1\ p\phi \tag{6.82}$$

It has a periodic solution X_1 (t). Considering

$$\phi\,(t) = \cos\,\omega\,t$$

$$\text{and } \omega = \frac{2\pi}{\theta} \tag{6.83}$$

one finds,

$$X_1\,(t) = \frac{b_1\,b_2}{b_1^2 + \omega^2}\ [b_1 \cos\,\omega t + \omega \sin\,\omega] \tag{6.84}$$

The mean value of *T. reesei* cell concentration can now be written by Equation below.

$$X\,(t) = b_2 \left\{1 - \left(\frac{p}{b_2}\right)^2 [b_2\,\phi - X_1]^2\right\} \tag{6.85}$$

which has second order smallness in p. The physical meaning of X_1 in this equation is that it indicates cell concentration in the terminal span in the range of pH cycling. Considering oscillatory parameter of *T. reesei* cell growth is given by equation (6.83), the equation (6.85) becomes

$$X\,(t) = b_2 \left[1 - \frac{p^2\,\omega^2}{2\,(b_1^2 + \omega^2)}\right] \tag{6.86}$$

Thus,

$$d = b_2 - X(t) = \frac{p^2 \omega^2}{2(b_1^2 + \omega^2)} \quad (6.87)$$

showing thereby that logistic law indicates that in a fluctuating-pH environment, the maximum cell concentration falls below the level attained in a constant pH environment. The amount of decrease (d) in cell concentration is proportional to the square of the amplitude of the oscillating parameter $\phi(t)$. Experimental results of the behaviour of *T. reesei* cell growth and its oscillatory parameter $\phi(t)$ at controlled pH 5.2 and with two different pH cycling spans (5.2-3 and 5.2-4) confirmed above theoretical analysis. Not only that but also the amplitude of the periodic variation of $\phi(t)$ decreases as the pH cycling span becomes narrower. Observations with the pH cycling span of 5.2 to 4.6 was also similar. The amplitude of periodic variation of $\phi(t)$ as measured were 0.075, 0.05 and 0.025 with the pH cycling spans of 5.2-3, 5.2-4 and 5.2-4.6 respectively. A plot of square of the amplitude of periodic variation of $\phi(t)$ for different pH cycling spans (ω^2) against the corresponding decrease is the mean value of the cell concentration (d) showed a proportional relation confirming thereby the validity of equation 6.87. The direct proportionality of d with ω^2 (Fig.6.18 and Table 6.7) indicated that a wider span (5.2-3) of pH cycling will increase cellulase production more than a narrow span. Table 6.7 also shows that an increase of pH cycling limits in *T. reesei* cell cultivation increases the amplitude of $\phi(t)$ and cellulase activity (FPA) but decreases cell growth. Thus, from this analysis it was clear that the maximum cell mass of *T. reesei* will not necessarily produce the maximum cellulase yield, rather, the proper cycling strategy of pH environmental condition during cell growth yield maximum cellulase enzyme at a considerable cell mass concentration.

Table 6.7 Growth, cellulase yield and amplitude of ϕ (t) in relation to pH-cycling limits

Run	*pH-Cycling Limit*	*Amplitude of ϕ (t)*	*X ($g.l^{-1}$)*	*FPA* ($IU . ml^{-1}$)*
1.	5.2 – 4.6	0.025	4.8	1.6
2.	5.2 – 4.0	0.050	4.5	1.9
3.	5.2 – 3.0	0.075	3.8	2.2

*Filter papaer activity
At controlled pH 5.2, X = 5.0 and FPA = 1.4 $IU.ml^{-1}$

3. Bioethanolation

The strategy of pH cycling was also helpful in single step bioethanolation of cellulose by *Clostridium thermocellum*. This was because *Cl. thermocellum* contained a system of enzymes and each of these enzymes was of different nature having their own pH optima. So pH cycling operation could increase ethanol productivity by periodically favouring the components of enzymes in the system. The pH of the medium was cycled between 5.2 (initial) to 7.0 by successive

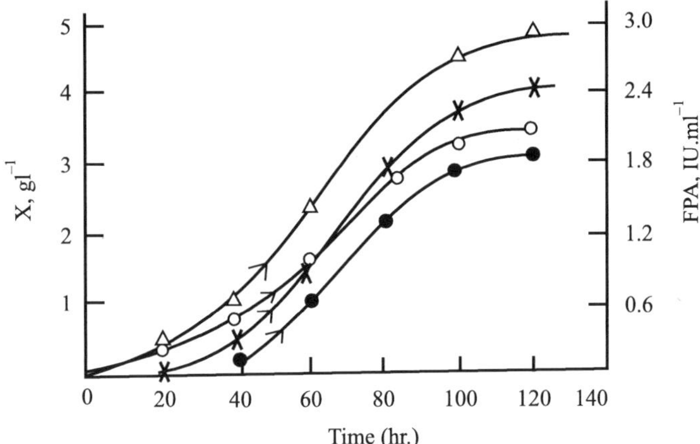

Fig. 6.16 Growth and cellulase yield of *T. reesei* under controlled pH 5.2 and pH-cycling. Δ, O: at controlled pH of 5.2, × , □ : at cycled pH from 5.2 to 3.0

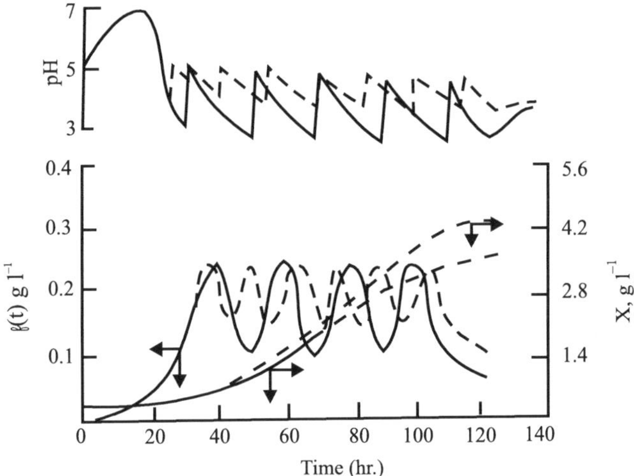

Fig. 6.17 Behaviour of oscillatory parameter ϕ (t) and cell growth with different pH-cycling span— pH 5.2 to 3.0, ... pH 5.2 to 4.0

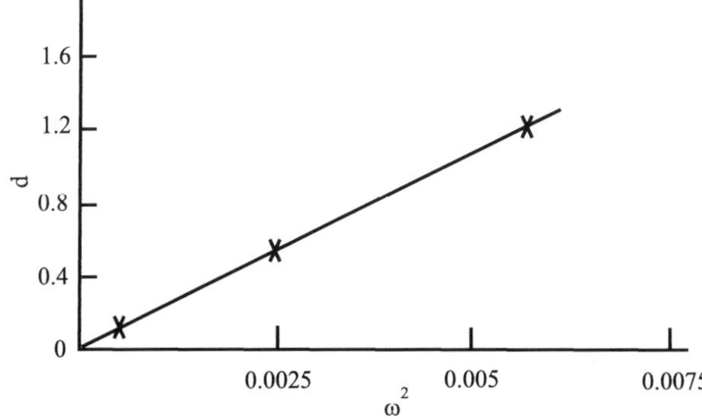

Fig.6.18 Decrease in cell concentration of *T. reesei* as a function of the square of the amplitude of ϕ (*t*)

addition of 3N NaOH solution.[54,55,65] In its reaction sequence this thermophile converts cellulose first into glucose and next through its glucose fermenting enzyme actions glucose is metabolized into multiproducts. Among the multiproducts ethanol yield is reported to be growth associated and the major one. Dynamics of this bioconversion in terms of cell growth, substrate conversion and product formation rates showed biokinetic informations of parameters which could reveal product inhibition characteristics. It led to the development of the concept of vacuum cycling process strategy to minimize product inhibition.

4. For enhancement of propionic acid fermentation

In propionic acid fermentation by *Propionibacterium acidipropionici* pH was found to influence the lag time, specific growth rate, yield of cells and product formation per gram substrate consumed.

pH could be influencing specific product formation due to the following reasons (Fig 6.19).

(1) pH optima of the enzymes involved in propionic acid pathway to be around 5.

(2) Influence of pH on redox potential which in turn affects the NAD^+/NADH ratio. This then determines whether acetic or propionic acid pathway will be followed.

(3) pH influences the CO_2 tension in the head space which controls the ratio of propionic to acetic acid (Johns, 1951).

(4) pH optima of the enzymes involved in *P. acidipropionici* pathway for acetic acid production to be around 7.

Ratio of propionic to acetic acid was also greatly influenced by pH. While lower pH gave better ratios of propionic to acetic acid (5 : 1), the propionic acid productivity was low (0.11 gl^{-1} h^{-1}) while at pH value above 6 (upto 7.5) lower ratios of propionic acid to acetic acid was

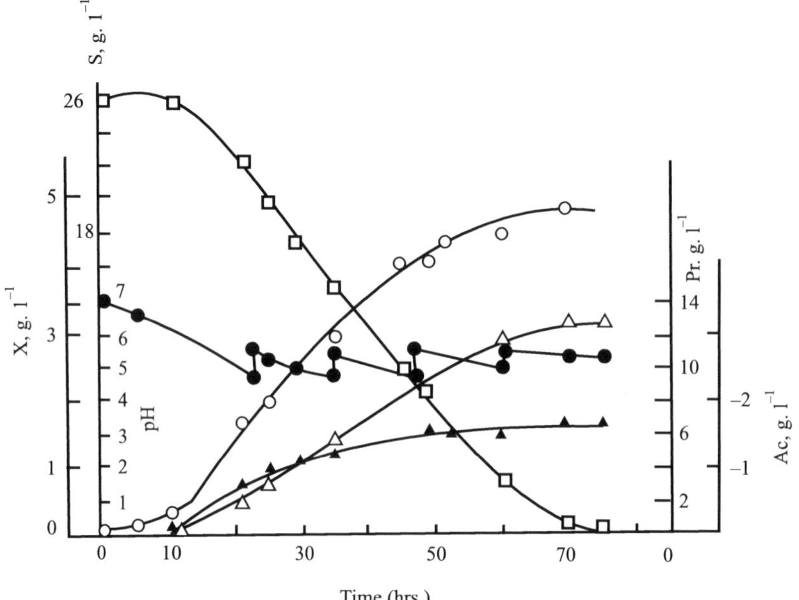

Fig. 6.19 Time profile of parameters under pH cycling conditions in glucose degradation by *P. acidipropionici*

obtained (2.5 : 1) but productivity of propionic acid was higher (0.2 g^{-1} h^{-1}). Therefore, a pH cycling strategy was adapted[55] which gave higher ratios of propionic acid to acetic acid (5.4) with appreceable productivity of propionic acid (0.22 gl^{-1} h^{-1}).

6.5.3 Temperature Profiling Mode[52]

1. Cellulase production

Four batch cultivation runs at 27, 29, 31, and 33°C were carried out in medium (pH 5.2) containing 30 g/litre cellulose. Cell protein and cellulase activity for each run were measured at different periods. In Fig. 6.20 the plot of cell protein and cllulase activity is shown as a function of cultivation age at different temperatures. For temperature optimization the data in Fig.6.16 were analyzed by logistic law equations 6.88 and 6.89 in the time range indicated.

$$dX_1/dt = b_1X_1\,(1 - X_1/b_2) \qquad (6.88)$$

$$0 \leq t \leq 30 \text{ hr}$$

and

$$dE/dt = b_3\,X_1 - b_5\,.\,1/X\,.\,dX_1/dt \qquad (6.89)$$

$$30 \leq t \leq t_f \text{ hr}$$

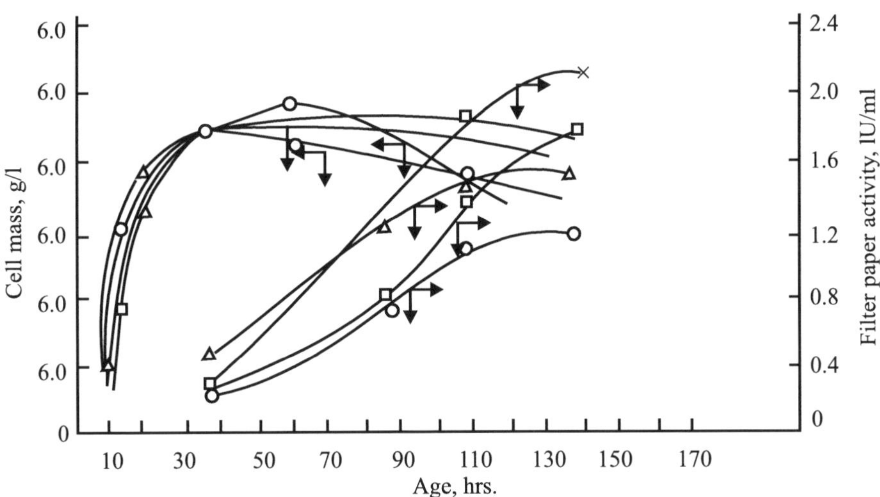

Fig. 6.20 Effect of temperature on cell mass and cellulase production without pH cycling, (Δ) 31°C; (O) 33°C; (□) 27°C; (×) 29°C[3]

Equations (6.88) and (6.89) represent cell growth and enzyme production, respectively. In these equations X_1 represents the cell concentration, b_1, b_2, b_3, b_4, and b_5 are parameters of the models, and E is the enzyme elaboration and only cell mass increases with cultivation age. The parameter b_1 is closely related to specific growth rate ($1/X_1\,.dX_1/dt$) in early stages of cultivation, i.e., when X_1 is low and b_2 represents maximum cell mass produced. In the region ($0 \leq t \leq 30$ hr) optimization of b_1 with respect to temperature will provide maximum growth rate and will give optimum,

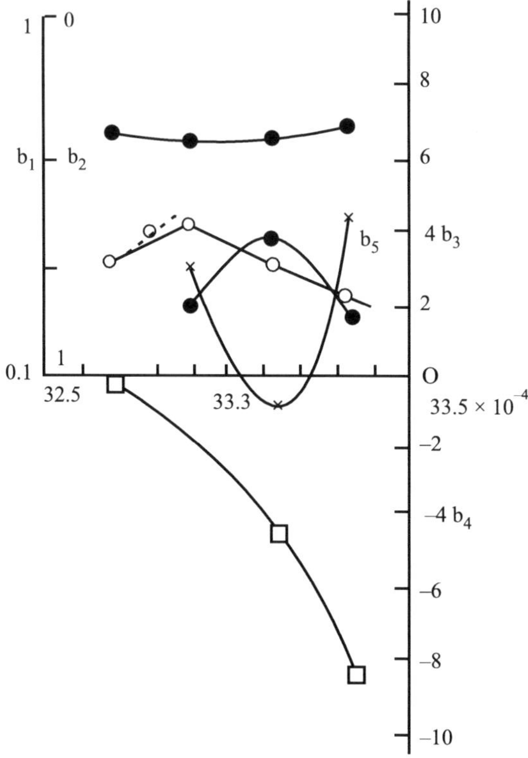

Fig. 6.21 Behaviour of parameters b_1, b_2, b_3, b_4 and b_5 as functions of 1/T. (O) b_1; (⊗) b_2; (•) b_3; (□) b_4; (×) b_5

temperature in this region. Equation 6.89 describes the behaviour of cellulase production in the region $30 \le t \le t_f$ hr. The factor b_3 describes the fact that the cellulase production in this period is associated with cell mass formation, b_4 takes into account the influence of enzyme level present in the reactor on its further synthesis, and b_5 incorporates the effect of μ on cellulase synthesis. The term containing b_5 is added to account for the fact that cellulase production was enhanced considerably when X_1 became equal to b_2 and μ becomes zero or slightly negative. The factors b_1, b_2, b_3, b_4, and b_5 are all functions of temperature. At each temperature the values of b_1 and b_2 were determined by plotting $1/X_1 \cdot dX_1/dt$ vs. X_1. The slope of this plot gives $(-b_1/b_2)$ and intercept b_1. Using eqation 6.89 between 30 hr and end of cultivation b_3, b_4, and b_5 were computed from simultaneous equations. The plot of b_1, b_2, b_3, b_4, and b_5 as a function of temperature is shown in Fig. 6.21. Negative values of b_4 indicate that the presence of cellulase concentration favors production of cellulase. It is because of the fact that cellulase hydrolyzes cellulose to small quantities of soluble substrate (below repression level) which enhances further synthesis of cellulase. Changes of b_5 from positive to negative and then to positive are indicative that cellulase elaboration is favored at zero or slightly negative growth rates. The data of Fig. 6.20 were analyzed following techniques used by Constantinides and Rai[66] to optimize temperature condition at different ages of cultivation. The optimum temperature profile obtained for cellulase production is given in Table 6.8.

Table 6.8 Optimum temperature conditions at different ages in cellulase production by *T. reesei*

Cultivation age (hr)	*Optimum Temp. Condition (°C)*	*Maximum Cellulase Activity Reached (IU/ml)*
0-30	31.3	0.04
30-120	28.7-29	5.00
120-160	28	6.43

2. In penicillin production optimization

Pontryagin's continuous maximum principle was used by Constantinides[66] and predict the optimum temperature profile for penicillin production by *Penicillium chrysogenum*. It could show that approximately 16% improvement in penicillin yield was possible if the optimum temperature profile were followed during penicillin fermentations[66] as shown in Fig 6.22. Using the directional integration method in combination with the Fabonacci[66,67] search in the penicillin model the above optimum temperature profile could be obtained. From their analysis Constantinides and Rai could show that the temperature remained at 27.2°C for the first 56 hours of fermentation, then dropped linearly to 18.7°C and remained constant between 84 to 184 hours. Next 24 hours it returned to initial temperature of profiling 27.2°C. With the help of vector of adjoint variables their profiling behavior in penicillin production could be explained satisfactorily.

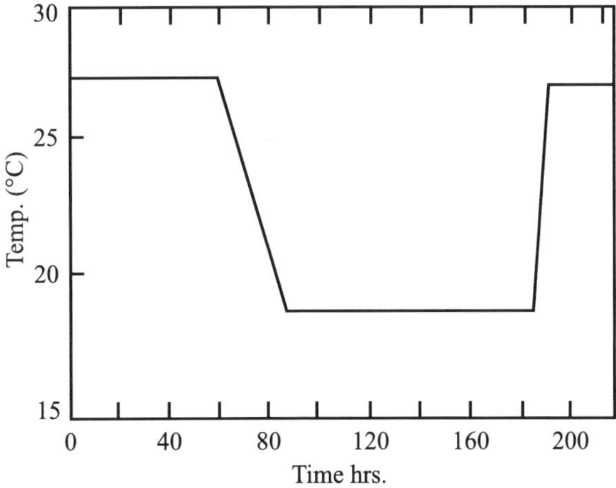

Fig. 6.22 Optimum temperature profile for the pencillin fermentation[66]

6.5.4 Simultaneous pH Cycling and Temperature Profiling

1. In cellulase enhancement

Cellulase production in 30 gl^{-1} cellulase medium was carried out under pH cycling condition as described earlier (Fig. 6.15) upto 80 hr of cultivation. Beyond 80 hr for pH cycling, 2N NH_4OH

was used instead of NaOH. During cultivation the temperature was also profiled as in Table 6.9. Cell protein, cellulase activity, and oxygen uptake pattern of the culture under simultaneous pH cycling and temperature profiling are shown in Fig. 6.23. At an oxygen supply rate of 22mM O_2/liter/hr (K_La = 124 hr^{-1}). the maximum oxygen demand rate of the culture 5.8 mM O_2liter/hr (0.58 mM O_2/g cell/hr) was attained during 55-70 hr of cultivation. These results when compared to that of earlier run (Tables 6.5 and 6.6) as shown in Table 6.10 it is seen that simultaneous pH cycling and temperature profiling strategy produced 13% higher cellulase productivity and 16% higher cellulase yield. Maximum oxygen demand rate was also higher. It appears that by simultaneous and frequent alterations in pH and temperature conditions during cultivations the cellulase-forming system tries to move from one quasi-equilibrium state to another by a path that causes an overshoot in cellulase yield and cellular metabolism of *T. reesei* for approaching a new equilibrium value. The possibility of such phenomena in other enzyme- forming system is known.[60]

2. Results compared to available reports

As high as 90 IU/liter/hr cellulase productivity is reported by Ryu *et al.*[61] from hyperproducing repression-free mutant MCG 77 in the second stage of the two-stage continuous cultivation. To obtain this productivity, the fermentable capacity for cell cultivation stage was 6.8 liter and for cellulase production it was 10 liter. On equal fermentable capacity basis, however, this productivity becomes 53.0 IU/liter/hr and 16% higher than the 44 IU/liter/productivity obtained in this investigation. The productivity of 44 IU/liter/hr is 1.5 times higher than reported from *T. reesei* QM 9414 in continuous cultivation.[2] A comparison of high cellulase productivities reported so

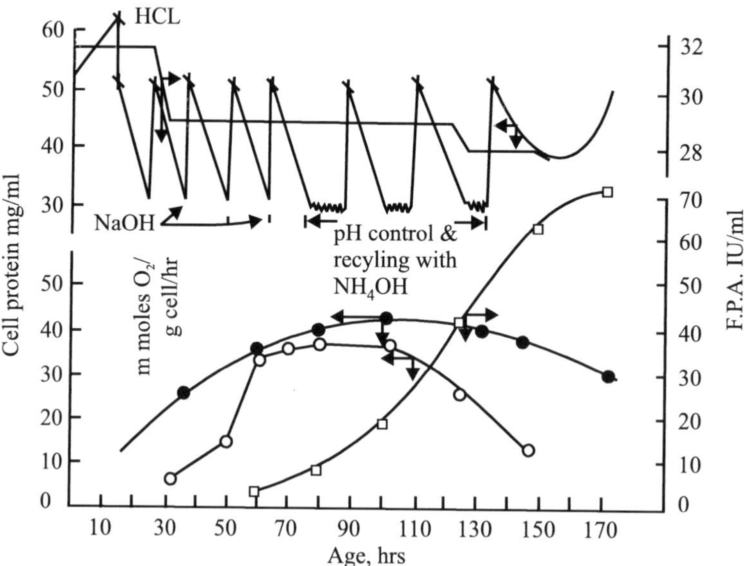

Fig. 6.23 Behaviour of cellulase production and oxygen demand of the culture under simultaneous pH cycling and temperature profiling. (•) Cell /; protein; (□) activity; (⊗) oxygen demand

Table 6.9 Comparison of run with and wtthout temperature profiling

Parameter	*Obtained Value Under* — *pH Cycling Only (No Temp. Profiling)*	*Simultaneous pH Cycling and Temp. Profiling*
Cellulase yield (IU/ml)	6.2	7.5
Average cellulase productivity (IU/liter/hr)	38.75	44.0
Productivity in cellulase production phase (30-160 hr) (IU/liter/hr)	55.40	61.82
Productivity (IU/g cell/hr)	4.0	4.5
Maximum oxygen demand rate (mMO_2/liter/hr)	0.48	0.58

far is presented in Table 6.10. It shows that appreciable cellulase productivity could be obtained from *T. reesei* QM 9414 by the present cultivation strategy.

The strategy of pH cycling and temperature profiling in cellulase production from *T. reesei* has a marked influence on the increase in cellulase synthesis. This technique may increase in cellulase synthesis. This technique may increase cellulase productivity of hyperproducing mutant strain.

3. Effect on RQ behaviour of T. reesei [59]

The strategies of improving both strain of *T reesei* and technology of processing are vital in relation to cellular physiological behavior and yield of its product. As simultaneous pH cycling

Table 6.10 Higher cellulase productivities of different investigators

Culture	*Cultivation mode*	*Cellulose Level (%)/Dilution Rate (hr^{-1})*	*Maximum Productivity Liter (IU/Liter/Hr.)*	*Ref.*
Trichoderma MCG-77 (hyper producing)	Two-stage continuous	0.028	53	61 (90 in second stage only)
Trichoderma	Batch (with pH cycling and temp. profiling)	3	44	52
T. reesei QM 9414	Batch	5	30	62
T. reesei QM 9414	Continuous (cell recycle)	0.025	30	63
Trichoderma MCG 77	—	—	100	64

and temperature profiling strategy of cellulase production did show appreciable improvement in enzyme yield and productivity its influence on RQ behavior of the cell was also followed. In order to follow RQ behavior during cell cultivation on 3% cellulose medium (C/N 8.5) in automated bioreactor (301, Bioeng AG. Switzerland) exit gas off line estimations of O_2 and CO_2 were made by Maihak's Oxygen Analyser and I.R. Analyser. Estimated parameters are shown[59] in Fig. 6.24. As seen in this figure the highest respiration quotient (RQ) 0.84 was exerted at 64 hours of age. The fermentation has just entered into cellulase production phase and cell growth was passing from exponantial phase towards zero specific growth rate phase at this age. At this RQ condition the dissolved oxygen (DO) had dropped below 20% saturation level. The flow rate of air had to be increased to 6l/min from 5l/min to maintain DO at 20% level. There was a steady decrease of RQ from 0.84 to 0.575 by the cultivation age of 110 hours. RQ remained at 0.575 till 140 hours and slowly decreased to 0.40 by 180 hours i.e. end of the fermentation cycle. This behavior showed that the biggest productivity of the enzyme was attained when RQ was constant and maintained at 0.575. The productivity decreased on RQ falling below 0.50. This behavior of RQ in cellulase production is an indication that in fermentation RQ can be used as single parameter for control of complete fermentation process biotechnology.

6.5.5 Simultaneous pH and Vacuum Cycling in Carbohydrate Bioconversion

In ethanol production by *Clostridium thermocellum* it was observed that 50 gl^{-1} substrate (MCCP, Cellulose Product India, Ltd, Ahmedabad, India) was a critical substrate concentration above which severe reduction in ethanol production rate takes place due to substrate inhibition. Therefore, in vacuum bioconversion of cellulose to ethanol by *Cl. thermocellum* initial substrate level should be within critical limit otherwise productivity decreases to a great extent. Consequently attempts were made to increase the final concentration of the product by vacuum cycling with cellulose fed batch (19 gl^{-1} to 33 gl^{-1}) bioconversion (60°C, pH 7). In the fed batch, substrate concentration was maintained nearly at 50 gl^{-1} level to eliminate the substrate inhibition. The bioconversion lasted for 115 hours but cell lysis began after 90 to 100 hours perhaps due to accumulation of some metabolic inhibitors. The final concentration of ethanol and reducing sugars were 25.57 gl^{-1} and 19.27 gl^{-1} respectively. A total of 129 gl^{-1} of cellulose was fed in 115 hours out of which 14.5 gl^{-1} remained unconverted hence representing a 88.76% degradation. It showed that the product yield could be enhanced by vacuum cycling. Further investigations showed that in non-vacuum cultivations increase of substrate level upto 10 g/*l* increased yield of ethanol above which ethanol yield decreased. However, when the same cultivations were repeated using vacuum cycling (VC) amplitude 220-240 mmHg and frequencies 20-15 hrs the tolerence limit of substrate level in the cultivation system could be increased to 50 g/*l*. More than 5 fold increase of substrate level exercised inhibition on ethanol yield in vacuum cycling process (VCP) as well. In NVB system yield of ethanol was only 0.17 g and 0.19g per gram of raw and partially refined bagasse (PRB). By using VCP 0.22 g ethanol per gram PRB was obtained. It was indicative, therefore, that substrate level inhibition was exercised in bioethanolation. As it is a well known product inhibition system it was necessary to carry out the cultivation experiments by adding initially different concentrations of ethanol in the cellulose medium (2-20 g/*l*) for checking simultaneous substrate and product inhibition nature. For this μ and γ values were

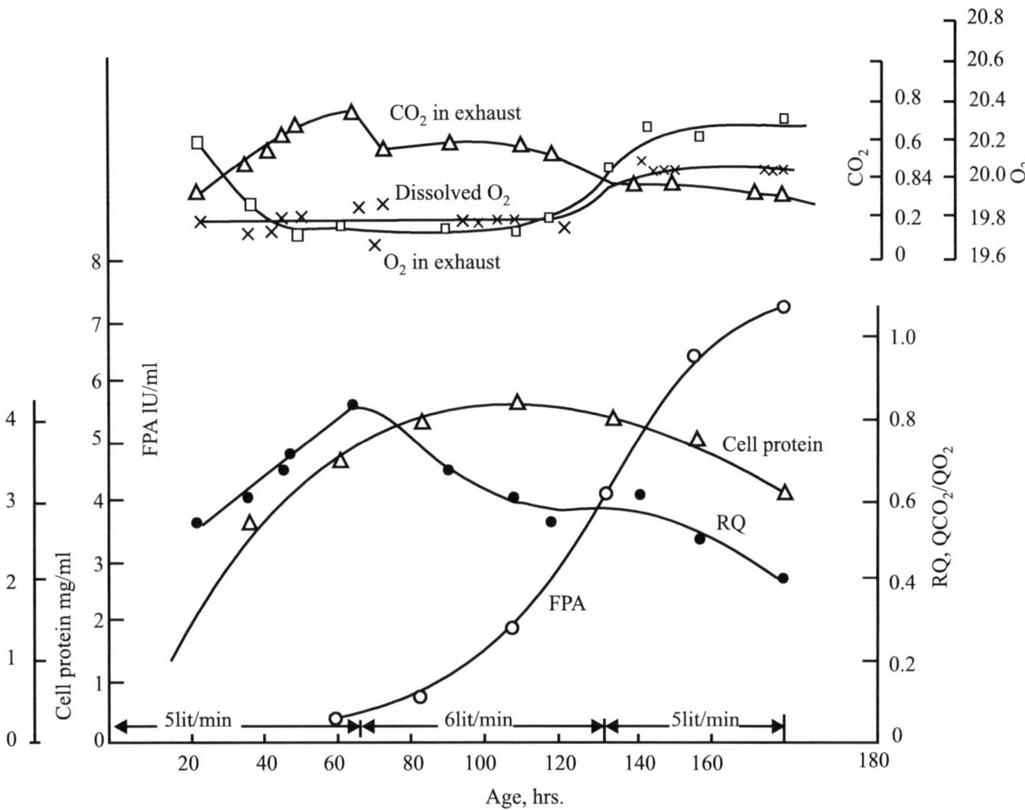

Fig. 6.24 Batch run with *T. reesei* Q 9414 pellets in STR under pH 4 temp. profiling

followed as functions of intracellular ethanol concentrations. It was seen that above 8.7 g/l initial ethanol level in the medium μ_m and γ_m decreased to a great extent. Possibility of change in the cell membrane fluidity being available in the literature one could measure the increase in cell membrane pore size in relation to increase in initial ethanol level in the medium based on the following diffusion linked osmotic permeation equation,[65,68]

$$\frac{P_0}{P_d} = 1 + \frac{r^2 RT}{8\eta \overline{V} D^0} \tag{6.90}$$

where

$$P_0 = \frac{kT}{h}\left(\frac{\lambda^2}{t}\right) e^{-\Delta H/RT} e^{-\Delta S/RT} \tag{6.91}$$

$$P_d = \frac{v_1 \Delta C_1}{A\,(C_2 - C_1)\,\Delta t} \tag{6.92}$$

In these relations the values of different constants and parameters used are given below.

$k = 1.30 \times 10^{-16}$ erg/°k $\quad h = 6.63 \times 10^{-27}$ erg. sec
$\lambda = 6$ Å $\quad R = 1.98$ cal/g mole/°k
$T = 333$°k (60°C) $\quad t = 100$Å
$\Delta H = 6.2$ cal/mole $\quad \Delta S = -12.2$ cal/mole/°k

V_1 is the volume of cell, C_1 and C_2 are ethanol concentrations inside and outside the cell respectively. The values of $\Delta C_1/\Delta t$ were obtained from the slope of the plot of increase in intracellular ethanol concentration as a function of time witi initial ethanol concentration as a parameter. It was shown that pore radius obtamed from equation 6.90 at 20 g/*l* initial ethanol level was 1.7 times higher than the radius at 2.0 g/*l* level of initial ethanol in the medium. It was therefore indicative that above 8.7 g/*l* ethanol level in the medium growth was inhibited by ethanol due to diffusion linked osmotic disbalance in the cells. Since *Cl. thermocellum* contained a system of enzymes and each of these enzymes was of different nature having their own pH optima so simultaneous vacuum and pH cycling operation was carried out for further increase in ethanol productivity. The pH of the medium was cycled between 5.2 (initial) to 7.0 by successive addition of 3N NaOH solution as shown in Fig. 6.25. The redox potential (E_h) value changed from 0 to 300 mv and cycled between -200 to -300 mv with the addition of alkali for pH cycling. In this strategy with monoculture system maximum productivity of ethanol obtained was 0.241 g/*l*/h. In coculture cultivation of *Cl. thermocellum* with *Cl. thermosaccarolyticum* at 60°C however, further improvement in productivity to 0.55 g/*l*/h could be seen. It showed that fed batch mode and coculture processing by simultaneous vacuum and pH cycling is a better approach as compared to product inhibited batch culture using only vacuum cycling with *Cl. thermocellum* alone. However, energy balance of the total process need to be worked out for indepth analysis of the access of the process in industry.

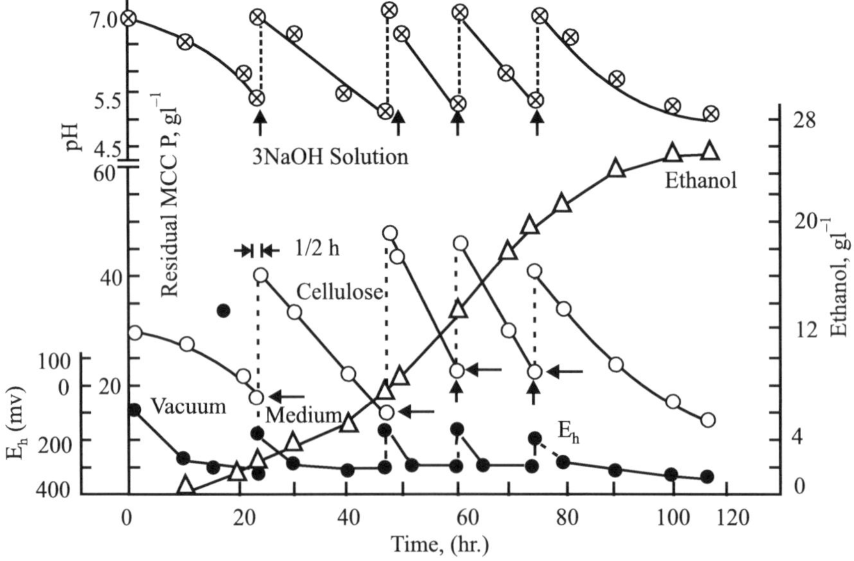

Fig. 6.25 Fed batch bioconversion of cellulose by *Cl.thermocellum* under simultaneous pH and vacuum cycling[68]

Nomenclatures

P_0-osmotic permeability coefficient, P_d-diffusion permeability coefficient, r-pore radius, R-ideal gas law constant, T-operating temperature, η-viscosity, V-partial molal volume, D_0 Stokes-Einstein selfdiffusion coefficient, K-Boltzmann constant, h-Plank's constant, X-molecular jump, t-cell wall thickness, H-enthalpy of activation, S-entropy of activation.

6.5.6 Pressure Cycling Strategy in Membrane Bioreactor Operation

A new operating procedure for the multimembrane bioreactor eliminating diffusion limitation frequently associated with the operation of a bioreactor has been reported in more recent years.[69] This new mode of operation has been claimed to increase the bioreactor productivity by almost an order of magnitude and also eliminated the need of periodical nutrient additions. A schematic diagram of this multimembrane bioreactor and the membrane unit is shown below Fig. 6.26 (A&B)

In order to circumvent feedback inhibition and to integrate production and recovery this strategy offering minimization of diffusional limitation has been stated to have advantage.

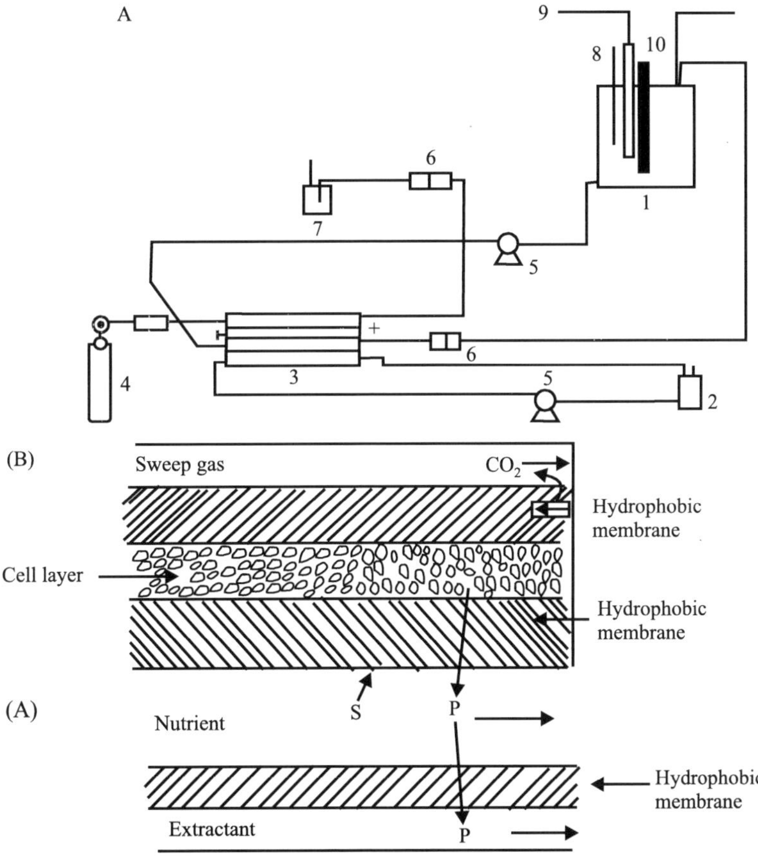

Fig. 6.26 Schematic diagram of the multimembrane bioreactor set up (A) and multimembrane unit (B) (1) Nutrient recycle vessel, (2) TBP, Recycle vessel, (3) Multimembrane bioreactor, (4) Gas cylinder (5) Pump, (6) Solenoid valve, (7) Trap, (8) Thermometer, (9) pH probe, (10) heater

6.5.7 Anaerobic Pure Culture Bioprocessing

Anaerobic growth and product formation on glucose in a pure culture of *Clostridium thermocellum* has been investigated. Cell mass formation on glucose medium of this organism in logistic form is given by

$$\frac{dx}{dt} = f(x) = \mu X\left[1 - \frac{X}{X_{max}}\right] \tag{6.93}$$

from which one gets

$$\text{In}\left[\frac{\bar{X}}{1-\bar{X}}\right] - \text{In}\left[\frac{\bar{X}_o}{1-\bar{X}_o}\right] = \mu t \tag{6.94}$$

where $\bar{X} = \dfrac{X(t)}{X_{max}}$

Using Luedcking-Piret (L-P) model equation one has for product formation rate

$$\frac{dp}{dt} = n\, X(t) + m\left[\frac{dX(t)}{dt}\right] \tag{6.95}$$

For multiproduct formation above equation (6.95) requires simply a separate equation of the above form for each product, i. Thus,

$$\frac{dpi}{dt} = n_i X(t) + m_i\left[\frac{dX(t)}{dt}\right] \tag{6.96}$$

Expected sinks for substrate(s) being, biomass, product and cell maintenance one may write the substrate balance rate equation for multiproduct bioconversion as below

$$\frac{ds}{dt} = -\frac{1}{Y_x}\cdot\frac{dx}{dt} - \sum_{i=1}^{N}\left|\frac{1}{Y_{Pi}}\cdot\frac{dpi}{dt} - KeX\right| \tag{6.97}$$

(biomass) (products) (maintenance)

Combining equations (6.96) and (6.97) the modified form of L–P model equation becomes

$$\frac{ds}{dt} = -\frac{1}{Y_x}\cdot\frac{dx}{dt} - \sum_{i=1}^{N}\left(\frac{1}{Y_{Pi}}\left[niX + mi\frac{dX}{dt}\right]\right) - KeX \tag{6.97a}$$

or

$$\frac{ds}{dt} = -\left[\frac{1}{Y_x} + \sum_{i=1}^{N}\left(\frac{mi}{Y_{pi}}\right)\right]\frac{dX}{dt} - \left[Ke + \sum_{i=1}^{N}\left(\frac{ni}{Y_{pi}}\right)\right]X \tag{6.97b}$$

or $$\frac{ds}{dt} = \alpha\left(\frac{dx}{dt}\right) - \beta X \tag{6.97c}$$

The form of parameters α and β indicates that products which are growth associated, nongrowth associated or both are all properly included in equation (6.97c). In other words, the timing in the fermentation of the use of metabolic path leading to each product pi is reflected in the values of ni and mi, these in turn make appropriate contributions of substrate utilization. The product formation is given by integration of equation (6.96) as below.

$$P(t) = P_o + n\int_o^t X(t')at' + m[X(t) - X_o]$$

$$= P_o + n\frac{X_{max}}{\mu}\ln\left(1 - \frac{X(1.0 - e^{\mu t})}{X_{max}}\right)$$

$$+ mX_o\left(\frac{e^{\mu t}}{\left(1 - \frac{X_o}{X_{nax}}\right)\left(1 - e^{\mu t}\right)} - 1.0\right) \tag{6.98}$$

Similarly,

$$S(t) = S_o + (-\beta)\int_o^t X(t')dt' + (-\alpha)[X(t) - X_o] \tag{6.97}$$

$$= S_o - \beta\frac{X_{max}}{\mu}\ln\left(1 - \frac{X_o\left(1 - e^{\mu t}\right)}{X_{max}}\right)$$

$$-\alpha X_o\left(\frac{e^{\mu t}}{\left(1 - \frac{X_o}{X_{max}}\right)\left(1 - e^{\mu t}\right)} - 1.0\right)$$

Validity of these models, in *Cl. thermocellum* grown on glucose and other sugars producing ethanol, acetic acid, lactic acid, formic acid and biomass were tested.

6.6 REFERENCES

1. Wolfe, R.S., "Methanogens: A Surprising Microbial Group." *Antonie Van Leewenhoek,* pp 45, 353-64, 1979.
2. Batch, W.E., G.E. Fox, L.J. Magrum, C.R. Woese and R.S. Wolfe, "Methanogens: Reevaluation of a Unique Biological Group," *Microbiol. Rev.,* pp 43, 260-96, 1979.
3. Woese, C.R. "The Primary Lines of Descent and the Universal Ancestor," (Bendall, D.S. ed.), *Evolution from Molecules to Men.,* pp 209-33, Cambridge Univ. Press, Cambridge, 1983.
4. Fox, G.E., E. Stackebrandt, R.B. Hespell, J. Gibson, J. Manloff, T.A. Dyer, R.S. Wolfe, W.S. Batch, R.S. Tanner, L.J. Magrum, L.B. Zablen, R. Blakmore, R. Gupta, L. Bonen, B.J. Lewis, D.A. Stabl, K.R. Luehrsen, K.N. Chen, and C.R. Woese. "The Phylogeny of Eukaryotes," *Science,* pp 209, 457-63, 980.
5. Kenealy, W. and J.G. Zeikus. "Influence of Corrinoid Antagonists on Methanogen Metabolism," *J. Bact.* pp 146, 133-40, 1981.
6. Mukhopadhyay, S.N. "Bioprocessing Properties and Application of *Bam* H1," *Bioprocess Engineering-The First Generation,* pp 227, (Ghose T.K. ed.), Ellis Horwood Pub., West Sussex, Chichester, 1989.
7. Zeikus, J.G. and V.G. Bowen, "Fine Strcuture of Methanospirillum Hangati," *J. Bact.* pp 121, 373-80, 1975.
8. Ghosh, S. and D.L. Klass. "Two Phase Anaerobic Digestion Process," *Biochemistry,* 1978.
9. Ghose, T.K. and S.N. Mukhopadhyay, "Some Basic Engineering Considerations to Maximize Bioenergy Production," *Ind. Chem. Engr.* pp 28 (4), 12-16, 1976.
10. Hawkes, *D. Process Biochem,* 12 (2), 32, 1976.
11. Melchior, J., R. Binot. I.A. Perez, H. Naveau, and E. Nyns. "Biomethanation: Its Future Development and the Influence of the Physiology of Methanogenesis," *J. Chem. Tech. Biotechnol.* pp 32, 189-97, 1982.
12. Bhadra, A., S.N. Mukhopadhyay and T.K. Ghose, "A Kinetic Model for Methanogenesis of Acetic Acid in a Multireactor System." *Biotechnol. Bioengg.* pp 26, 257-64, 1984.
13. Wolfe, R.S. and I.J. Higgins. "Microbial Biocbemistry of Methane-A Study in Contrast." *Int. Rev. Biochem.* pp 21, 267-50, 1979.
14. Nagai, S. and N. Nishio, "Applications of Methanosarcina Barkeri Cells for the Production of Useful Chemicals," *Bioprocess Engineering: The First Generation,* (Ghose, T.K. ed.), pp. 291-302 Ellis Horwood, Ltd, Chichester, 1989.
15. Majumdar, T.K. "Application of Methanogens to the Production of Useful Chemicals and Fuel Gas," *Ph.D. Thesis,* Faculty of Eng. Hiroshima Univ. 1987.
16. Mukhopadhyay, S.N. and T.K. Ghose. "Integration of Bioconversion, Environmental and Genetic Engineering Concepts in Bioenergy System." *Proc. BESI Second Convention,* pp 260-263, (O.P. Vimal ed.), 1985.
17. Sobotka, M., J. Votruba, I. Havlin and I.G. Minkevich. "The Mass-Energy Balance of Anaerobic Methane Production," *Folia Microbiol,* pp 25, 195-204, 1983.
18. J.G. Zeikus; "Thermophilic Bacteria: Ecology, Physiology and Technology," *Enz. Microb. Technol.* pp 1, 243- 52, 1979.
19. N. Saha and S.N. Mukhopadhyay, "Studies on Thermophilic Bioconversion of Waste Material Into Methane," *Proc. ICFB-97, Advances in Biotechnology,* pp 503-508, (A. pandey ed), Edu. Pub.& Distrib., New Delhi, 1998.
20. Dowson, P.S.S. "Continuous Phased Culture–Some New Perspectives for Growth with *Candida utilis,*" *Proc. Biocon. & Biochem. Engg.* Vol. 2, pp 275- 93, (Ghose, T.K., ed.), BERC, IIT Delhi, 1980.

21. Glacken, E. Adema, and A.J. Sinskey. "Mathematical Descriptions of Hybridoma Culture Kinetics: 1. Initial Metabolic Rates." *Biotechnol, & Bioeng.*, pp 32, 491-506, 1988.
22. Harbour, C., J .P. Barford and K.S. Low. "Process Development for Hybridoma Cells," *In Adv. in Biochem, Engg/Biotechnol.* pp. 1-40, (A. Fiechter ed.) Vol. 37, Springer Verlag, Berlin, 1988.
23. Miller, W.M., C.R. Wilke and H.W. Blanch. "Transient Responses . . . In Continuous Culture: I. Glucose Pulse and Step Changes," *Biotechnol. & Bioeng.*, pp 32, 947-965, 1988
24. Miller, W.M. *et al.* "The Transient Responses of Hybridorna Cells to Nutrient Additions in Continuous Culture: II Glutamine Pulse and Step Changes," *Biotechnol. & Bioeng.* pp 33, 487-99, 1989.
25. Dowson, P.S.S. "The Average Cell— A Handicap in Bioscience and Biotechnology," *TIBTECH* pp 6, 87-90, 1988.
26. Dalili, M. and D.F.Ollis. "Transient Kinetics of Hybridoma Growth and Monoclonal Antibody Production in Serum-Limited Cultures." *Biotechnol. Bioeng.*, pp 33, 984-90, 1989.
27. Glaeken, M. W., E.A. Dema and A.J. Sinskey; "Mathematical Description of Hybridoma Culture kineties: The Relationship Between Thiol Chemistry and the Degradation of Serum Activity," *Biotechnol. and Bioeng.*, pp 33, 440-50, 1989.
28. Miller, W.M., H. W., Blanch and C.R. Wilke; "A Kinetic Analysis of Hybridoma Growth and Metabolism in Batch and Continuous Suspension Culture: Effect of Nutrient Concentration Dilution Rate and pH," *Biotechnol. and Bioengg.*, pp 32, 947-65, 1988.
29. Miller, W.M., C.R. Wilke and H. W. Blanch; "Transient Response of Hybridoma Cells to Nutrient Additions in Continuous Culture: I. Glucose Pulse and Step-Changes," *Biotechnol. and Bioengg.* pp 33, 477-86, 1989.
30. Glacken, M.W. R.J. Fleischaker and A.J. Sinskey; "Reduction of Waste Product Excretion Via Nutrient Control: Possible Strategies for Maximizing Product and Cell Yields on Serum in Cultures of Mammation Cells," *Biotechnol. and Bioengg.* pp 28, 1376-89, 1986.
31. Humphrcy, A.E. "Personal Communication," 1989.
32. Rebinoss, C.F. "The View Through Microscopes," *Adv. in Biotechnology* Vol. 1, pp 623-634, (Mooyoung, Gen. Ed.) Pergamon Press. Toronto, 1950.
33. Payne, W.J. *Annual Rev. of Microbiol* (ed. C.T. Clifson), pp 17, 1970.
34. Miki, B.L.A., N.H. Poon, A.P. James and V.L. Seligy, "Flocculation in Saccharomyces Cerevision: Mechanism of Cell-Cell Interactions," *Current Developments in Yeast Research*, (G.G. Stewart and I. Russal eds), *Adv. in Biotechnol*, Pergamon Press, Toronto, 1981.
35. Stewart, G.G. and I. Rund Can. *J. Microbiol*, pp 23, 441, 1377.
36. Tumbo, N. and Y. Wantabe. "Physical Characteristics of Flocs I," *The Floc Density Function and Al floo Water Res.* pp 13, 409, 1979.
37. Shuler, M.L. and F. Kargi, *Biochemical Engineering: Basic Concepts,* pp 320-323, Prentice Hall, Englewood cliffs, New Jersey, 1992.
38. Broachs, J.R. and J.R. Pringh, *The Molecular and Cellular Biology of the Yeast Socchoromyces,* Vol. 1 CSHL Press, 1991.
39. Cowland, T.W. and D.J. Maule, *J. Inst. Bioeng.,* pp 72, 480, 1966.
40. Andreas, A.A. and T.J.B. Stier, *Cell comput. Phys.,* pp 41, 23, 1953
41. Cysewske, O.R. and C.R. Wilke, *Biotechnol. Bioeng.,* pp 16, 1297, 1974.
42. Cysewske, O.R. and C.R. Wilke, *Biotechnol and Bioeng.,* pp 19, 1125, 1977.
43. I. Russell. *Yeasts in Hand Book of Brewing.,* pp 169-202, W.A. Hardwiched. Mercel Dekker Ine, New York,
44. Pirt, S.J. *Principles of Microbe and Cell Cultivation*, pp 230, Blackwell Sci. Pub., Oxford, 1970.
45. Aiba, S., A.E. Humphrey and N.F. Millis, *Biochemical Engineering*, 2nd Edn., Univ. of Tokyo Press, Tokyo, 1972.

46. Bailey, J.E. and D.F. Ollis, *Biochemical Engineering Fundamentals*, 2nd edn. McOraw Hill Book Company, N.Y., 1986.
47. Mukhopadhyay, S.N. and T.K. Ghose, *Proc. Biocom. Sympo.*, pp 97-107, IIT Delhi, 1977.
48. Mukhopadhyay, S.N. and T.K. Ghose, *Proceed. AP Biochem,* pp 162-165, (F. Furusaki, I. Endo and R. Matsunoeds), Springer-Verlag, Tokyo, 1992.
49. Rubinow, S.I. *Introduction to Mathematical Biology*, pp. 23-28, John Wiley & Sons, New York, 1975.
50. Mukhopadhyay, S.N, A. Fiechter and T.K. Ghose, "Abstracts of Poster Papers," *First Euro. Congress on Biotechnol.*, pp. 9-10, Switzerland, 1978.
51. Mukhopadhyay, S.N., T.K. Ghose, and A. Fiechter. *Biotechnol. Lett.* pp 1, 217, 1979.
52. Mukhopadhyay, S.N. and R.K. Malik, *Biotechnol. & Bioengineering* pp 22, 2237, 1980.
53. Kundu, S., "Microbial Conversion of Cellulose to Ethanol," *Ph.D. Thesis,* IIT Delhi, 1983.
54. Seshadri, N. "Regulation of an Anacrobic Mixed Acid Fermentation to Accumulate Propionic Acid," *Ph.D. Thesis,* IIT, Delhi. 1989.
55. Seshadri, N. and S.N. Mukhopadhyay, "Influence of Environmental Parameters on Propionic acid Upstream Bioprocessing by Propionibacterium Acidi-Propionici," *J. Biotechnol.,* pp 29, 321, 1993.
56. Mukhopadhyay, S.N., S. Kundu and T.K. Ghose, *Proc. Biotech.* 85, Asia, Singapore, London, pp 445-49, 1985.
57. Mukhopadhyay, S.N. and T.K. Ghose. *Proc. Bioconv. Sympo.*, IIT Delhi, pp 97-102, 1977.
58. Mukhopadhyay, S.N. "Growth of *Trichoderma Reesei* in a pH Cycling Environment: Application of a Single Species Logistic Law," *J. Ferment. Technol,* pp 59 (4), 309-13, 1981.
59. Malik, R.K. and S.N. Mukhopadhyay, Unpublished Data,
60. Duysens, L.N. and J. Amery. *Biochem. Biophys. Acta,* pp 24, 19, 1957.
61. Ryu, D., R. Andreoti, M. Mandels, B. Gallo, & E.T. Reese. *Biotechnol. Bioeng.*, pp 21, 1887-1903, 1979
62. Nystrom, J.M. and H.P. Diluca. *Proc. Bioconv. Sympo.*, pp 293, T.K. Ghose (ed), IIT Delhi, 1977.
63. Ghose, T.K. and V. Sahai *Biotechnol. and Bloeng.*, pp 21 283, 1979.
64. Spano, L., A. Allen, T. Tassinari, M. Mandels and D. Ryu. Proc. *Fuels from Biomass Sympo.*, pp 671, Vol II, Troy, N. Y. 1978.
65. Kundu, S. and S.N. Mukhopadhyay, Unpublished Data.
66. Constantinides, A. and V.R. Rai, "Application of the Continuous Maximum Principle to Fermentation Process," *Biotechnol and Bioeng. Symp.* pp 104, 663-680, 1974.
67. Wilde, D.J., "*Optimum Seeking Methods,*" Prentice-Hall, Englewood Cliffs, N.J. 1964.
68. Kundu, S. S.N. Mukhopadhyay and T.K. Ghose, "Studies on Direct Bioconversion of Cellulose to Ethanol," *Clostridium thermocellum Under Vacuum Cycling* Proc. National Sympo., pp 58-68, Biotechnology (ed. S.C. Lain), Dept. of Chem. Eng. & Technol., P.U. Chandigarh, 1982.
69. Efthymiou, G.S. and M.L. Shular, "Elimination of Diffusional Limitations in a Membrane Entrapped cell Reactor by Pressure Cycling," *Biotechnology Progress,* pp 3 (4), 259-64, 1987.

Chapter

7

BIOREACTORS AND BIOSENSORS

7.1 INTRODUCTION

The importance of bioreactors in bioprocess engineering and process biotechnology is well known. A large number of contributions addressed process engineering aspects of bioreactror systems with particular bioreactor type and performance parameter of reactor systems were emphasized. Importance of mass transfer effects, overall reaction kinetics, biocatalytic loading capacity and reactor fluid flow patterns have been given in various literatures. Also, bioprocess optimization and bioreactor operation strategies have been presented.[1-4, 9, 10] For many reasons, the manufacturers of bioproducts need a bioreactor which can meet a number of different running conditions, such as viscosity, aeration rate, intensity of mixing and reaction volume. Many of these running conditions often pose problem or become limiting in conventional stirred tank bioreactors. Also, it is often necessary to carry out different types of bioproduct formation in the same plant having flexible layout. In such bioprocessing plant a certain ease of modifications is necessary for bioreactor designers. Looking at the modern trends in biotechnological concepts and products many types of novel/non-conventional modern bioreactors and designs have been developed to suit the system processing.

7.2 BIOREACTORS IN BIOPROCESSING OF BIOCELLS

7.2.1 Microbial Cell System

1. Newer concepts in microbial processing

There has been substantial progress over the past two decades in the fermentation bioreactors. This is mainly for increased capacities of microbiological industries and for production of newer high value pharmaceutical and other important products. Also many microbial processes are run at limited and low substrate concentration to avoid substrate and/or end product inhibitions. This not only leads to lower reaction rates and thus slow cell growth but also to more difficult downstream processing resulting in increased energy consumption. Thus integration of microbial unit and fermentation bioreactor design with downstream processing has become important.[1-4] Newer advances have occured in these areas.

Modern bioreactors for microbial processing have many components and aspects. Usually there are two general options in all microbial processing in bioreactors. One is to use strategy for technologically redesigned super microbioreactor strain or rDNA (recombinant DNA) fermenter. In such strategy physical containment requirements for fermentations using redesigned microorganism containing recombinant DNA molecules is important. As per NIH guidelines the bioreactor size greater than 10 *l* is generally considered as large scale; smaller scale than this is taken as pilot plant scale. For the purposes of large scale research or production two or three physical containment levels have been established. One such containment bioreactor has been called P1-LS. Therefore, biological containment[5] in bioreactor operation of such organisms needs to be kept in view.

2. Progress in bioreactor operational engineering

(*i*) *Conventional* : Keeping in mind the bioreactor design cardinal rules[6] and provisions of whole set of parameters influencing the processes of microbiological product formation, several improvements and concepts in conventional bioreactor designs have been incorporated depending primarily on a limiting stage of a process.[3,4,6,7] Performance of conventional bioreactors for microbial processing have also been examined for bioprocessing of cell lines of organisms like mammalians[8] and plants.[9,10] It has been revealed that many differences between mammalian and plant cell cultures with microbial cultures have direct implications for the design and scale up of suspension cell reaction systems.[10] However, in conventional bioreactor designs for microbial processing major progress has been towards its instrumentation, automation and computerization. Computer instrumented bioreactor operation and control has become a normal practice in recent years. For this various types of biomonitors and biosensors have been developed through years. A computer instrumented bioreactor set up including conventional bioreactor has many components, e.g. the vessel, the agitation system, process monitoring and control system (including computer system) and miscellaneous parts.

In a highly computer instrumented bioreactor purely formalistic quantitative description of the process are more easily made. At the same time, it is quite evident that in order to ensure optimum control which would react flexibly to different perturbations, it would be preferable to use mathematical model having an adequate physical model as their basis.

For microbial bioreactors besides improving mechanical and operational designs[11] now computers are available which are able to process and act on data and render/reach conclusions which are beyond human comprehension.[12] Computers are greatly used in feed-back control of fermentations and in analysing and controlling fermentation by indirect means. Not only one can achieve better control, better reproducibility and greater reliability but one can also achieve in the future on-line dynamic optimization of microbial process biotechnology.

It has been hoped that use of computer instrumented bioreactors in microbial processing will have greatest influence in process biotechnology with regard to automation particularly in processes supporting *in vivo* gene machines. Automated analysis of the DNA sequence of gene fragments and automated synthesis of gene fragments from nucleic acids has now become a routine matter. As computers are becoming a more and more creative element in microbial processing research and process development their importance is becoming more and more prominent.

(*ii*) *Non-conventional* : Model configurational reactor modification by changing the type of reactor have been used in smaller scale mainly to alleviate accumulation of products of the reaction due to flow distribution. Both the methods of adding the substrate and product removal and the flow around the bioreactor could be altered. Vacuum cycling bioreactor operation and three phase extractor bioreactor are typical cases. Significant improvements in productivity are obtained compared to microbial product formation without vacuum cycling or extraction. Simultaneous fermentation-saccharification (SFS) of cellulose[13] and extractive microbial processing[14] for lactic acid are two examples of the same.[15]

7.2.2 Mammalian Cell System

1. General

Mammalian cells are of three types. The first type are anchorage dependent cells, e.g. cells that require a surface or support for growth such as vero cells, human fibroblast cells WJ 38, FS4, etc. The second type are suspension cells, i.e. they are non-anchorage dependent like Hela cells, a tumerogenic cell line and the hybridomas. The second type of cells, being able to multiply in suspension culture, may be cultivated in bioreactors similar to those used in microbial fermentation.[16,17] For production of anchorage dependent cells, however requires novel bioreactor designs. Based on the nature of mammalian cells a plethora of novel bioreactors are now available for their cultivations. The bioreactor designs vary from modified bacterial cell culture vessels of 1-10,000 l (e.g. stirred tank bioreactor and airlift bioreactor) to compact need-dependent bioreactor system like hollow fibre, perfused flat membrane bioreactors, etc.[16,18] In developing mammalian cell bioreactor, vero cell is playing a great role. Vero cell has been selected for many reasons in developing a bioreactor given in Table 7.1.

Table 7.1. Vero cell line–why ?

- Vero is a diploid and characteristically anchorage dependent fibroblast.
- Vero cell after its passage from the origin could form established cell line.
- Attachment of vero cell to microcarrier surface is multistep adhesion process.
- Its attachment on specific surface is affinity base.
- It has high affinity and spreading on cytodex microcarrier thereby high cell-substrate interactions.
- In producing viral vaccine using diploid cell or established cell line with high affinity, cell-microcarrier system is preferred.
- It grows continously in culture.
- It supports the propagation of numerous viruses like poliovirus, vaccinia virus which have been approved for human use.
- It is a good system for developing mammalian cell bioreactor.

The vero cell, after its passage from origin to establish cell line, manifests several characteristics of physical, chemical and biological nature which help in its attachment/anchorage on inert solid supports (like cytodex microcarriers).[18-21] Vero cell line has been accredited for heteroploid vaccine production using microcarrier support in bioreactors. These vaccines, like polio are suitable in clinical use. Polio vaccine and beta subunit of human corionic gonadotropin (βhCG) from vero cells attached and grown on microcarrier can be cultured in bioreactors for transfectional fermentation biotechnological (TFB) product formation.[19] Vero cell adhesion to a microcarrier is a selective process where the cells show performance to certain specific surfaces over others. Vero cell lines are found to spread much faster on uncharged cytodex 3 (collagen coated) microcarrier than charged (positively) cytodex land 2 microcarriers. The kinetics of attachment of vero cells to cytodex 3 was not a function of the concentration of free cells. However, cytodex 1 was found to be the best choice for vero cells as the attachment rate constant and final cell growth were higher than in the other two cases. [18-20] Cytodex supported vero cell culture bioreactor operation using transfectional molecular blending redesigning principle can produce desired bioproduct. Production of βhCG is a classical example of the same. Metabolic labeling and pulse experiments indicated that synthesis is of 'zero order' kinetics. Vero cell culture bioreactor characteristics have not been analysed critically so far. The third type of mammalian cells are established cell lines or transformed cells. They are heteroploid having unlimited life span and often anchorage independent. So for culture purposes cells are distinguished as being capable of growing free in suspension or requiring a solid growth support surface. They are further differentiated as being of fibroblast or epithelial origin. This differentiation correlates strongly with differences in cell behaviour under cultivation conditions.

2. Screening of cells

In order to locate the best cells to produce a desired product, different cell types were screened for their ability to produce the bioproduct. It has been observed that isolates of the same cell type produce differently. This necessitates extensive screening process of cells. So like in microbial cell screening productive mammalian cell screening is equally important.

3. Bioprocessing: Concerned advantages and disadvantages of mammalian cells vis-a-vis microbial cell systems

Both microbial and mammalian cells show many advantages in bioprocessing. For example, microbial cells can adjust expression system for inserted gene. Mammalian cells also have unique properties as an expression system for inserted genes. In microbes expression of viral protein genes may overcome several transgenic problems although not easily. But in mammalian cells expression of viral envelop protein genes avoid the problems of aggregation and insolubilization in many cases. Microbial cells are able to synthesize and secrete proteins encoded by inserted foreign genes. Mammalian cells are able to properly process, fold, glycosylate, transport, assemble and secrete proteins encoded by inserted foreign genes. Although both biocells have many advantage, they are associated with several disadvantages as well in terms of bioprocessing. Microbial bioprocessing, being less time consuming for process development studies, validation is not so accurate. Mammalian cell bioprocessing is time consuming but being more stringent the screening of the donors of the starting material provides a degree of confidence further supported by validation of the production process. However, although validation is more reliable but very expensive.

4. Media formulation

The composition of the majority of mammalian cells media in use were formulated many years ago. The formulations were based entirely on biological fluids like plasma and embryonic extracts. Chemically difined and undefined media were used. The former media were based on analysis of plasma and is complex formulation. Most chemically defined media contain over sixty ingredients. Chemically undefined media are more complex. The use of undefined media suffers from the disadvantages of batch to batch variation and prone to contamination. Examples of a few chemically designed media for cell culture are: DMEM (Dulbecco's Modified Eagles's Medium), BME (Basal Medium of Eagle), EMEM (Eagle's Minimal Essential Medium) and many others. Like in many microbial bioprocessing use of separate media for growth and production has been seen to be advantageous in many mammalian cell processing. Growth media, in general, are complex in construction, rich in nutrients and usually supplemented with 5-15% sera. Usually production media are less complex, less rich and have less sera. Newer media have begun to be designed in more recent years. They are termed serum free medium or reduced serum medium. Mostly these are mixture of the basic salt portion of older, conventional media supplemented with newly discovered growth and attachment factors. These new media are designed to provide a single defined medium for growth and production phases. These are less expensive media. In order to solve several problems in culture operation the present trend is to formulate serum free media.

Cell counting:

Before animal/mammalian cells can be subcultured or used in an experiment, they must be counted. This is usually done with a *haemocytometer* with 'improved Neubauer' markings: this is a specialized microscope slide and coverslip. It gives cell conc. per ml = cell count* × 2(if typan blue used) × 10^4
Confluent culture/primary culture of suspension cells.

The count in one square or an average of a count if more than one square is used. For example, a total of 210 cells were counted in three squares, this gives a cell density of $\frac{210}{3} \times 10^4 = 7 \times 10^5$ per ml.

[Ref. S. J. Morgan and D. C. Darling: Animal cell culture, Chapter 5, Bios Sci Publishers Ltd., Oxford, 1993 (pp 37-50)].

5. Cell behaviour in cultures

In suspension culture the growth of many mammalian cells may exhibit typical pattern as that of microbial cells. In this growth process, in general, serum free media have performed very well. In some cases cells need three to four passages for adaptation when moving to the new medium.

This has a similarity to the lag phase exhibited in microbial growth. This adaptation is needed to allow expression of new enzymes. A typical example of this behaviour has been noticed in vero cells. The vero cell line was initiated from the kidney of a normal adult african green monkey in the early sixties. The cells are anchorage dependent fibroblasts and grow continuously in culture. Vero cells are often selected to produce human vaccine. The cells support the propagation of numerous viruses. Vero cells can grow and produce virus very well. In a serum free medium as they do in their preferred conventional medium supplemented with 10% foetal bovine serum. Similar results have been reported with BHK 21 (Bovine Hamster Kidney) cells.

6. Growth rate

After cell inoculation in culture medium growth follows the typical pattern as observed for microbial cell growth. Like in microbial growth the exponential law

$$x = x_0 2^n \tag{7.1}$$

follows in which *x* is the final cell number at time t. Here x_0 is the initial cell number and n is the number of generations of exponential growth. It shows the value of n to be:

$$n = \frac{\log x - \log x_0}{\log 2} = \frac{1}{0.3010} \log \frac{x}{x_0} \tag{7.2}$$

For mammalian cells the estimation of cell weight is not a convenient method of cell mass determination. Cell number determination by a microscope or a coulter counter is often used. Now one can calculate the average generation time during the exponential growth by using the relation

$$t_g = \frac{\text{Time elaspsed}}{\text{Number of generations}} = \frac{t}{n} \tag{7.3}$$

or

$$t_g = \frac{0.3010\, t}{\log x - \log x_0} \tag{7.4}$$

The relation of cell concentration increase (dx/dt) and cell concentration (x) or biomass is defined as specific growth rate (μ). So,

$$\mu = \frac{1}{x} \cdot \frac{dx}{dt} \tag{7.5}$$

or

$$\ln x = \ln x_0 + \mu t \tag{7.6}$$

The value of μ can be obtained from the slope of the plot of ln x vs time. Like in microbial growth process mammalian cell growth continues in a batch culture till typical cell density is sustainable by available medium design. At this point the depletion of nutrients or the accumulation of metabolic product concentration or inhibitor metabolite may cause cessation of cell growth.

7. Substrate uptake and product yield

The substrate(s) uptake rate or consumption is related to cell concentration and product yield by the following equation:

$$\frac{ds}{dt} = \frac{\mu x}{Y_{max}} + mx \frac{P}{\left[Y_{p/s}\right]_{max}} \tag{7.7}$$

in which m is the maintenance coefficient (g substrate/g cell-hr), $Y_{p/s}$ is apparent yield of product per unit substrate uptake, Y_{max} is apparent cell growth yield, P is the product concentration.

8. Passage number in cell growth

It denotes the number of subcultures performed after the original isolation of the cells from a primary source. It relates to the generation number (n) of the cell as follows:

$$n = \text{Passage number} \times \frac{\text{Split ratio}}{2} \tag{7.8}$$

The split ratio is the number of new cultures established at each stage of subculture. The simplest case occurs where a confluent culture is subcultured into two cultures, i.e. split ratio of 2.

Although some reports provide applicability of Monod growth model for mammalian cell growth, however, this has not been confirmed by testing with different cell lines.

9. Anchorage dependent cell character

Mammalian cells of anchorage dependent type need a substratum for cell growth and monolayer formation of cells covering the available solid surface. For this type of cells the interaction between the cell membrane and the solid surface is critical. In order to culture such type of cells the ratio between surface area available for growth and the total culture volume serves as a very important parameter. For this reason anchorage dependent cells have been traditionally grown on a large scale on the inner surface of rotating bottles. The phenomenon of adhesion between two solid surfaces of carrier and the negatively charged cell cations, basically proteins, form a layer between the substratum and the cells. In the two solid phase adhesive interaction a combination of elctrostatic attraction and van der Waal's forces have been stated to be present. In roller glass bottles negative charges on its inner surface may be provided by alkali treatment. In subculture of anchored cells their detachment from the substratum prior to reinoculation in a fresh culture is mandatory. Thus, using proteolytic enzyme like pronase or dispase anchored cell culture could render many advantages e.g. (a) high surface to volume ratio, (b) support of high cell density and (c) homogeneous cell population in the system allows easy monitoring and control of environment and several others. Kinetic cytodex microcarrier has been reported to give primarily first order attachment with respect to concentration of free cells.

10. Culture systems

Like in microbial cell culture, three types of culture systems can be used in mammalian cells. These are batch, fed batch and perfusion systems. In batch mode nutrients are not replenished and the only addition to the medium is oxygen. The parameters that can be controlled are pH, temperature and oxygenation. In fed batch culture system only vital components are fed as per need and thus maintain a constant nutrient concentration. Although cellular waste products are not removed, their accumulation may be limited by adjusting nutrient flow rate. In perfusion culture system both nutrient and waste product concentration can be controlled by varying dilution rate. In this system the environment can be highly controlled.

11. Persisting limitations

Contamination in mammalian cell cultivation poses a problem which can occur at all stages of operation in a bioreactor. Also, criteria of defining predictable or engineered enhancement in production capacity from one scale to a higher scale is not still well established. So scale up in mammalian cell culture has been given high importance in solving various barriers existing. Among these barriers a few important ones are (a) shear and oxygen transfer limitations, (b) accumulation of toxic wastes, (c) lack of regulatory hardwares and softwares for process control and (d) high cost of serum. Approaches to overcome some of these limitations to some extent have been shown. The approach of development of serum free medium may contribute towards reducing oxygen transfer limitation by minimizing diffussional resistance. The limitation of low surface to volume ratios of the systems for anchorage dependent cells has been overcome to some extent introducing novel methods.

Reactors have been designed for growing large quantities of health care and medically important bioproducts such as hormones, interferons and monoclonal antibodies. For this purpose a plethora of bioreactors are now available. Their designs range from modified microbial bioreactors (STR; ALB, 1-10,000 l) to rotary, compact process intensified designs like hollow fibre and flat membrane bioreactors. However, any successful asceptic cell cultivation at any scale requires a combination of highly skilled cell culturists and optimally designed bioreactors. The selection of bioreactor for a particular mammalian cell depends on several factors namely, the cell nature and type, the nature of the product, operational scale, space and service facilities available and process economy.

7.2.3 Plant Cell System

Extensive efforts in development of plant cell culture in a bioreactor is evident from literature. This is because defferentiated cells of higher plants have an awesome ability to synthesize diverse types of bioproducts, many of which form the basis of existing agricultural, forestry and pharmaceutical industries. More recent developments in tissue culture techniques in bioreactors have made it possible to use less differentiated plant cells to produce some of the more valuable phytochemicals and agrochemicals under controlled conditions. This has offered the prospects of higher productivity and greater flexibility in production of secondary metabolities. In cultivation of plant cells major concerns involve the following.

1. Making plant tissue suitable to plant cell culture.
2. Culture medium design.
3. Cell propagation.
4. Plant cell culture type.

5. Bioreactors for plant cell cultivation.
6. Plant cell culture products.
7. Plant cell culture rheology.
8. Recombinant plant cells.

1. Plant tissue to cell culture

In this transfer, the following steps are involved

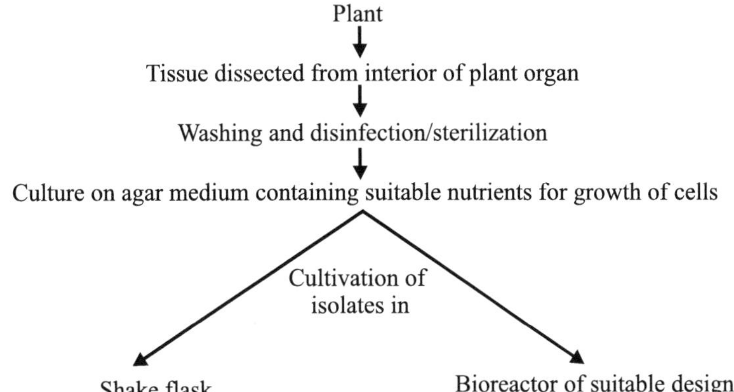

2. Culture medium design

It consists of sucrose or glucose (as carbon source), a mixture of mineral salts and growth regulators like phytohormones, vitamins, amino acids, sugar alcohols, etc. In the prepared liquid medium oxygen is supplied by diffusion from top surface of the culture or by a gas sparging device. White medium is a typical medium for plant cell culture.

3. Cell propagation mode

Plant cells using the nutrients in the medium utilize the propagation mode which is said to be chemoautotrophic rather than photoautotrophic.

4. Plant cell culture type

The strategy of plant cell culture may be as below.

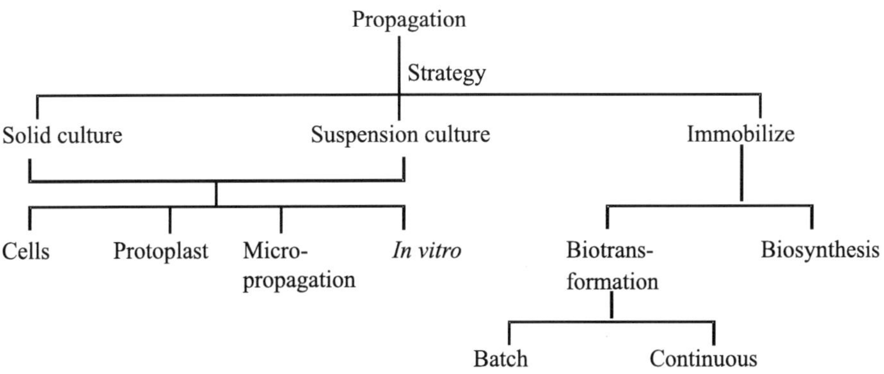

5. Bioreactors

In plant cell cultivation the choice of bioreactors depends on whether the system is to be processed in (a) suspension culture or (b) solid and/or immobilized cell culture.

(*i*) *Suspension Culture* : It is a free cell suspension system and is comparable to microbial cell-liquid and gas contact processing system. Culture residence time in this system can be analysed in three modes of bioreactor operation, e.g. continuous stirred tank bioreactor (CSTBR), plug flow bioreactor (PFB) and batch. For such operation, CSTBR, Bubble column, Air lift (internal loop or external loop) and horizontal drum reactor (static or rotary) types have been used depending on the nature I of the cells to be cultivated with special care to cells hydrodynamic stress sensitivity.

(*ii*) *Immobilized Cell Culture* : In practice immobilized plant cells have been formed in either particles or sheets. The particles or beads of different dimensions are very versatile. They can be packed into columns or beds of different sizes. However, good flow distribution, important in maintenance of cell viability, can be difficult to achieve. In down flow system compaction can occur while in up flow bioreactors, particularly with gas sparging system buoyancy of bubbles could resist flow rates and may cause channelling. This in turn results in imperfect flow distribution causing low productivity. Fluidized or expanded bed reactors are expected to be more convenient for particulate packing system although the reduced biocatalyst density in these bioreactors is a disadvantage. Cells immobilized on sheets or membranes provide an alternative method of deploying biocatalysts and are more convenient to handle in the processing than are beads. Sheets, however, being rarely self supporting, need secondary structure within the reactor. Also, it must be custom made for each reactor design. A good advantage of them is that they can be packed so as to provide a lumen of controlled dimensions, giving more defined fluid flow through the reactor. Coaxially wound sheets as in hollow fibre membrane IWC (immobilize whole cell) reactor, baffled tanks, flat plate reactors or modified plate and frame presses have been used for immobilized biocatalysts and provided convenient reactor design using existing process plant.

7.2.4 Fundamentals of Fermentation Process Design

Introduction

A large number of materials are produced by fermentation processes. Fermentation process design should be such that the product may be obtained efficiently and economically. Any fermentation process design must consider three major aspects: (i) Value creation opportunity, (ii) Process design analysis and (iii) Objectives of the design project.

These objectives are discussed in brief below.

(i) Value Creation Opportunity: It concerns mostly establishment of microbial reaction process and its development recognizing economic opportunity.[21] Recognition of economic opportunity relates to the appropriateness of the following: (i) selection of microbial strains (ii) selection of appropriate fermenter design (iii) scope of product utilization.

A. Microbial strains

Exploitation of microbial activity is done considering the following important aspects:

(a) Selection of new stable strains for getting a share in the market by producing useful new products using modern fermentation plant.

(b) Selection of stable strain for known product of the established equipment.

B. Fermenter design

For production of a substance having established market, combination of an existing stable strain and a simplified fermenter together with new devices need to be used. In almost all fermentation processes the fermenter configuration plays the part of a mediator between energy input variables and physiological reactions of microbial cultures. As microbial behaviour vary widely, it is difficult to design a versatile fermenter for multipurpose use. This limitation led to the development of various conventional and non-conventional fermenter designs.

However, attempts in all designs have been made to meet the requirements as listed in Table. 7.2. High power demand and underutilization of impeller energy input are the two important weak points of conventional designs. In any new design principles of unconventional fermenter

Table 7.2 Desirable requirements of a fermenter

Kinetic/Physiological-Biological	*Operational*	*Economic*	*Scale up*
• Ideal flow regime (i) perfectly mixed CSTR (ii) Continuous PFR (Small RTD) • Easy vent out of gaseous products (to minimize hold up effects on the kinetics) • must carry chemical transformation reactions in biological fashion • Provide conditions for biological stability	Adequate macro and micro mixing High gas-liquid mass transfer with negligible foaming Uniform energy distributions in liquids Adequate hold-up of required phase No dead zone in mixing No cell damage or undesirable flocculation Adequate heat transfer provision	Simple design and easy to fabricate Simple and easy aseptic operation Flexible to various process condition Low specific power demand Stable at fluctuating process conditions	Simple mechanical design Well understood design ratios Selection of most suitable scaleup criterion

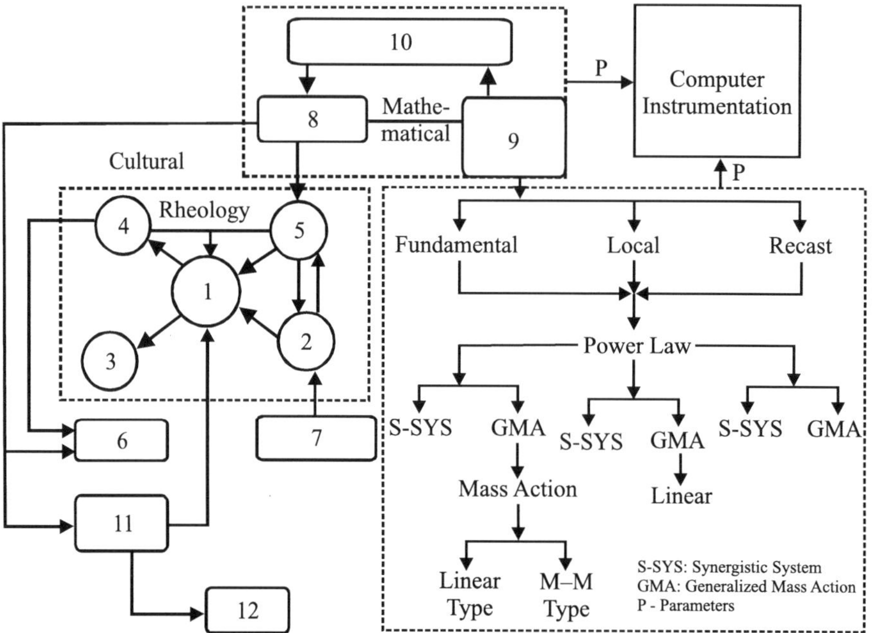

1. Microbial unit, 2. Chemical input, 3. Physiological reaction output, 4. Morphological reaction output, 5. Physical fermenter input, 6. Fermentation process output, 7. Nutrients/raw material energy, 8. Fermenter configuration, 9. Constants characterising physical input variables, 10. Model experiment, 11. Downstream processing, 12. Product

Fig. 7.1 Integration of microbial unit and fermenter design with downstream processing

have been to minimize these shortcomings of conventional fermenters. Also, care is needed in the interaction between fermenter design and microbial unit at used physiochemical environment as depicted in Fig. 7.1 to make the downstream processing of the product easier.

C. Scope of the product

It is associated with the mode of utilization of the product to get an adequate fitness of the product on human needs.

(ii) Process Design Analysis: In fermentation process analysis major requirements include the following:

(a) Design variables to which similarity concepts are applicable, most important among them requires:
   (i) fermentation time course and profiles of *state and control variables*.
   (ii) determination of most favourable control variables condition to obtain maximum product yield.

(b) Design variables to which innovation concept is applicable. It requires:
   (i) pilot plant studies for new process development thereby aid in innovation in scale up.

(ii) investigating possibilities of innovation by the process simplification and by adopting high technology easily and successfully.

(iii) product development such that marketing is decisive.

(c) Design variables in relation to optimization concept. These concern

(i) yield equilibrium specific rates of fermentation and growth profiles.

(ii) product concentration in finished broth, fermentation cycle or fermentation rate and product recovery process.

(d) Process economics: Evaluation of the fermentation process design has to be done on economic basis. As indicated[21] the concept based on financial cash flow and discounted cash flow are useful in economic evaluation of the process. Considering capital cash flow *C* earns the present value P in n years at a nominal interest rate i and compounding and discounting occurs m times per year

$$P = C\left(1 + \frac{i}{m}\right)^{-nm} \tag{7.9}$$

n may be plus or minus according to the past or future respectively. If compounding or discounting occurs continuously

$$P = \lim_{n \to \infty} C\left(1 + \frac{i}{m}\right)^{-nm} = C\,e^{-ni} \tag{7.10}$$

However, the useful economic index for the optimization of fermentation process is rate of return r based on discounted cash flow. The relation between r and c considering its uniform flow for p years is given by

$$\sum_j C\,j^{-n_j r}\,\frac{e^{P_j r} - 1}{P_j\,r} = 0 \tag{7.11}$$

Here, C = Cash outflow or inflow, n = Period between the time of cash flowing and the present time, P = Period through which cash flows uniformly and r = Rate of return by discounted cash flow method expressed as a decimal.

(iii) Objectives of Design Project: The fermentation process design project deals with:

(i) Aims of

– product development
– possibilities of producing new type of microbial group in a known fermenter design
– efficiency of new fermenter for known fermentation
– process improvement

(ii) Procedure of design project for

– organization of basic idea
– structure of design project
– other process design requirements

(iii) Projected design and development programme

A systematic analysis of the points discussed above are essential in developing fermentation processes in bioreactors.

7.3 ENZYME BIOREACTORS

Reactors making use of biocatalytic functions of enzyme in bioprocessing for bioconversions are termed as enzyme bioreactors. Both enzymes *in vitro* and whole cells (both viable and lysed) have been used in bioreactor operations. Free enzyme and immobilized enzyme have been used in bioreactor development for carrying out biochemical reactions. Immobilized bioreactors have been observed to offer many advantages over free enzymic bioreactors that have been successfully developed at industrial scale. In immobilized enzyme bioreactors the support used for immobilization may be porous or nonporous. The characteristics of both these support media have been described in a more recent book.[17] The advent of immobilized bioreactor has increased the role that sophisticated techniques of optimization can play in decreasing the bioreaction costs.[23] Immobilized enzyme bioreactors have opened avenues for the utilization of continuous reaction systems in bioconversions and/or biotransformations. In immobilized enzyme bioreactors the substrate usually in an aqueous medium, is passed over the enzyme immobilized by adsorption, or by covalent binding to solid supports or by other means. Based on the bioreactor operation mode, the reaction rates may vary to a great extent. For example, based on the following standard enzyme reaction model

$$E + S \underset{K_2}{\overset{K_1}{\rightleftharpoons}} ES \xrightarrow{K_3} E + P$$

reaction rates can be shown to be several times higher than in continuous stirred tank reactor (CSTR) in the following way. The general equation for a CSTR is given by

$$S_x + K_m \left(\frac{x}{1-x}\right) = K_3\, E_0\, \sigma \tag{7.12}$$

in which S_0 is initial substrate concentration, E_0 is initial total enzyme, x is fractional conversion $[= (S_0 - S_1)/S_0]$, S_1 is final substrate concentration, K_3 is reaction rate constant, K_m is Michaelis-Menten (M – M) constant and $\sigma = V_R/Q$ i.e. reaction rate per unit volumetric flow rate.

The equation for an immobilized enzyme reactor (or plug flow reactor) is given by

$$S_0 \times - K'_m \ln(1 - x) = K_3\, E_1\, \sigma\, \xi \tag{7.13}$$

In this relation ξ is the reactor porosity and E_1 is total enzyme. Assuming steady state condition to prevail in the reactor, the reaction velocity is

$$v = \frac{V_{max}\, S}{K_m + S} \tag{7.14}$$

When S >> K_m, v = V_{max} and the reaction is zero order. But when S << K_m equation 7.14 may be written as

$$K_m \left(\frac{x}{1-x}\right) = K_3 E_0 \ \sigma \tag{7.15}$$

and equation 7.13

$$K'_m \ln (1 - x) = K_3 E_1 \ \sigma \tag{7.16}$$

Dividing equation 7.15 by equation 7.16

$$\frac{E_{CSTR}}{E_{PFR}} = \frac{X}{\ln (1 - x)} \tag{7.17}$$

It shows that when conversion x is 90% the amount of enzyme required in CSTR (E_{CSTR}) is four times as that required in a PFR (E_{PFR}). Also, when conversion is 99% the amount of enzyme required in CSTR is 22 times as that required in a PFR enzyme bioreactor type and operational parameters of reactor systems are bound by several resistances. The following resistances are encountered in packed bed type reactors.

(a) External diffusion or film diffusion
(b) Internal diffusion or pore diffusion
(c) Bulk mixing

Film resistance is characterized by the bed height required where as pore diffusion is characterized by Thiele's modulus or effectiveness factor. However, for bulk mixing the dispersion number characterize the performance of the bioreactor.

The governing equations of performance of the above cases are given below.

For film diffusion controlled enzyme bioreactor

$$Z = \frac{\varepsilon (N_{Re})^{2/3} (N_{sc})^{2/3}}{1.09 \, a_v} \ln \frac{\gamma_1}{\gamma_2} \tag{7.18}$$

in which Z is the bed height, ε is void fraction, a_v is surface area per unit volume, γ_1 is inlet mole fraction of substrate, γ_2 is mole fraction of substrate in product. $N_{Re} = \frac{DG}{\mu}$ where D is particle diameter, G is mass velocity, μ is liquid viscosity and $N_{sc} = \frac{\mu}{\rho D_v}$, where D_v is the effective diffusivity and ρ is liquid density.

In pore diffusion controlled enzyme bioreactor

$$\text{Rate} = \eta \frac{KE_0 \, S_s}{K_m + S_s} \tag{7.19}$$

If pore diffusion is controlling in packed bed and the reaction is of first order, the bed height is given by the following relation

$$Z = \frac{1}{A} \cdot F \cdot \frac{\tau}{\varepsilon} \tag{7.20}$$

where F is flow rate (c. c./hr)

$$\tau = \text{reactor space time} = -\frac{\ln(1-x)}{K_f}\left[\frac{1}{\phi}\left(\frac{1}{\tan 3\phi} - \frac{1}{3\phi}\right)\right] \tag{7.21}$$

Here ϕ is Thiele's modulus, x is fraction conversion and K_f, is intrinsic dissociation constant. In a bulk mixing controlled enzyme bioreactor,

$$\text{Dispersion number} = \frac{D}{uL} = \left(\frac{1}{N_{pe}}\right)\left(\frac{dp}{\varepsilon L}\right)\left(\frac{\tau}{\tau_p}\right) \tag{7.22}$$

in which N_{pe} = Peclet number = $\frac{udp}{D\varepsilon}$, where L is bed height. Equations 7.18, 7.20 and 7.22 can be used for determining which resistance is predominant in the immobilized enzyme bioreactor performance.

7.4 BIOSENSORS IN BIOPROCESSING[24-32]

7.4.1 Biocell Systemic Estimation

1. Substrate

Increase in respiration activity of cells by assimilation of substrate (glucose) is monitorable by oxygen electrode. Based on this microbial electrode sensor for glucose has been constructed (Fig 7.2) using immobilized whole cells that utilize mainly glucose and oxygen.

Components of the electrode system: It consists of the following:

a. Immobilized whole cells of *Pseudomonas fluorescens.*
b. Oxygen eloctrode.
c. The bacteria-membrane in contact with O_2 electrode is tightly secured with rubber O-rings.

Working: In working of microbial glucose sensor the following steps are involved.

- The sensor assembly is inserted into a glucose sample solution.
- The solution is saturated with dissolved oxygen by stirring at fermentation temperature 30° ± 1°C prior to insertion of electrode.
- The bacteria in the membrane begin to utilize glucose and oxygen in sample solution and current of the sensor markedly decreased with time until a steady state is reached.
- The current is measured by a milliammeter and signal is displayed on the recorder as response curve. (Fig. 7.2 b and c).

- The steady current is attained within 10 mins at 30°C. It is dependent on the concentration of glucose (Fig 7.2 b).
- When the sensor is removed from the sample and placed in a solution free from glucose the current of the microbial sensor gradually increases and returns to the initial level within 15 minutes at 30° ± 1°C (Fig,.7.2 b).

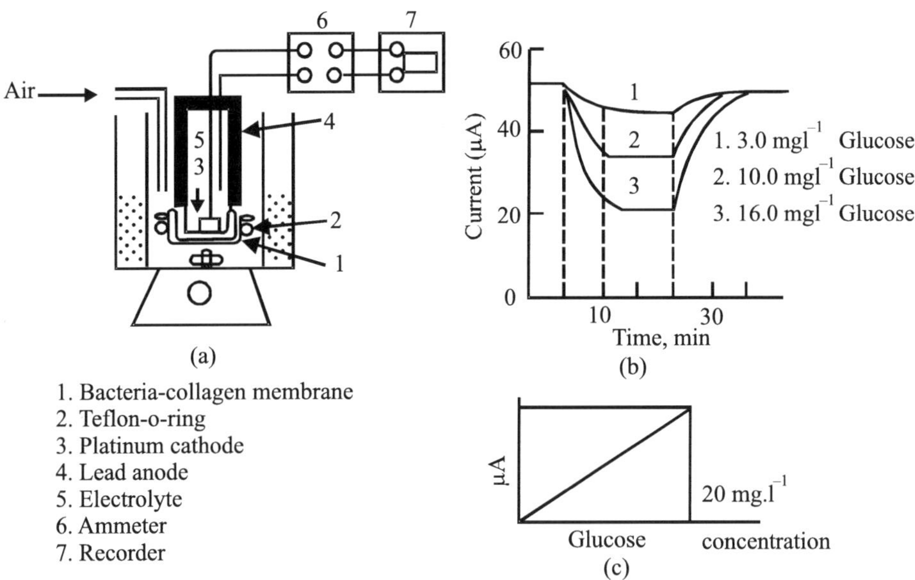

Fig 7.2 Biosensor for substrate (glucose) estimation

Advantages: Advantages of the biosensor are given below:

- It can be used for continuous determination of glucose in molasses broth.
- Reusable several times.
- No response to aminoacids.
- Satisfactory sensitivity

Disadvantage: It responded slightly to fructose, galactose, mannose and saccharose.

2. Cell population

(*i*) *Direct Method* : Principle: It was found that bacterial oxidation occured directly on the surface of the anode and a current was generated. This electrochemical system has been applied to determine microbial cell populations.

Electrode system: It is composed of two similar electrodes as shown in the Fig. 7.3 namely

(a) the determination electrode
(b) the reference electrode.

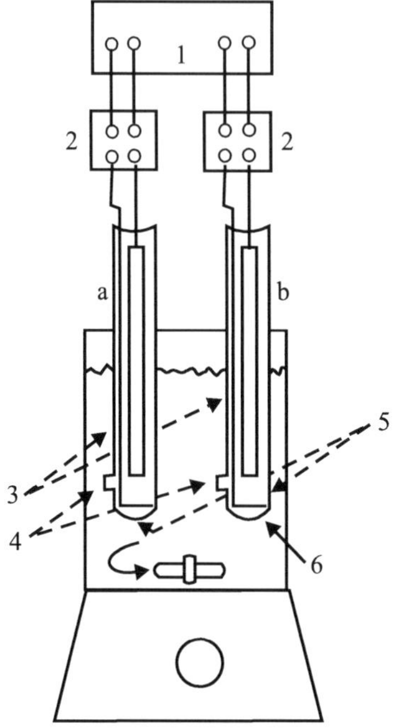

1. Recorder,
2. Ammeter,
3. Cathode (Ag_2O_2)
4. Anion exchange membrane,
5. Anode (Pt)
6. Cellulose dialysis membrane.

Fig. 7.3 Cell population sensor

Each electrode is composed of platinum anode (ρ_t) and the silver peroxide (Ag_2O_2) cathode. Phosphate buffer (0.1M, pH 7.0) is used as catholyte. An anion exchange membrane is used as a separator. The current is measured by a milliammeter and signal is displayed on a recorder. *Working:* Both the electrodes are inserted into a culture broth. The current of the determination electrode (I_1) resulted from microbial oxidation and of electro active substances is obtained. The current of the reference electrode (I_2) is due to oxidation of electroactive substances only because cells could not penetrate through cellulose dialysis membrane. Thus, the current difference between the two electrodes is as below.

$$\Delta I = I_1 - I_2 \tag{7.23}$$

This ΔI is proportional to the number of microbial cells in the broth (Fig. 7.4). So one can write

$$\Delta I = KN \tag{7.24}$$

where N is the number of cells and K is a constant. Fig 7.4 provides calibration curves for microbial cell population. However, the response time of the electrode system varies with temperature and pH as illustrated in Figs. 7.5 a-d for *Saccharomyces cerevisiae* which was centrifuged at 8000 × *g* for 10 minutes to be used in calibration.

(*ii*) *Indirect Method*: An indirect method of electrometric detection and counting of *E. coli* in the presence of a reducible coenzyme, lipoic acid (LA) has been reported.[25] In this method reduction of LA by bacteria coupled to oxygen consumption during uptake of glucose has been followed

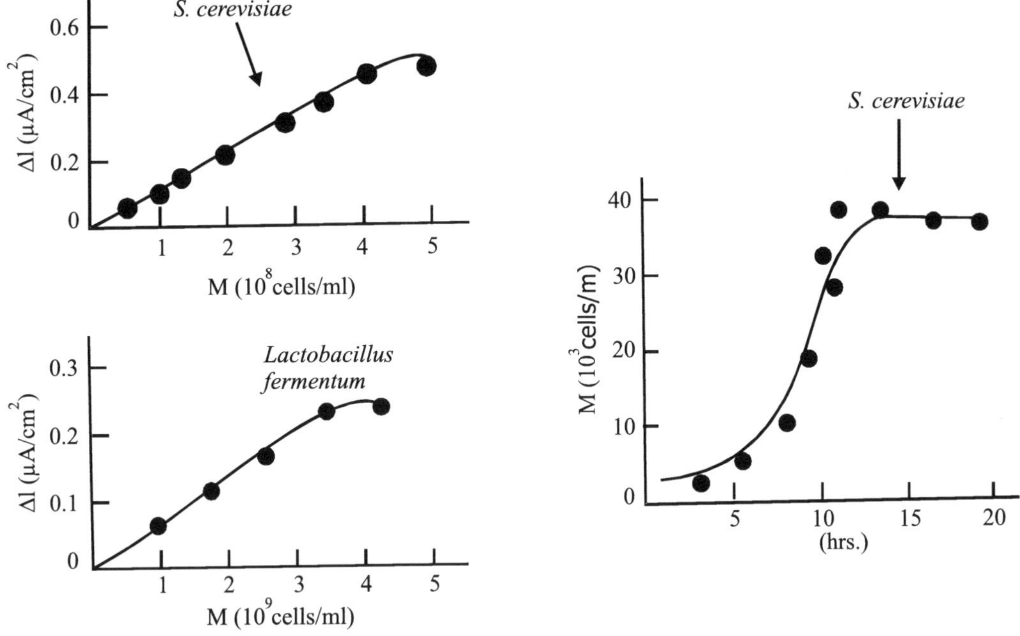

Fig. 7.4 Calibration curves for microbial cell population

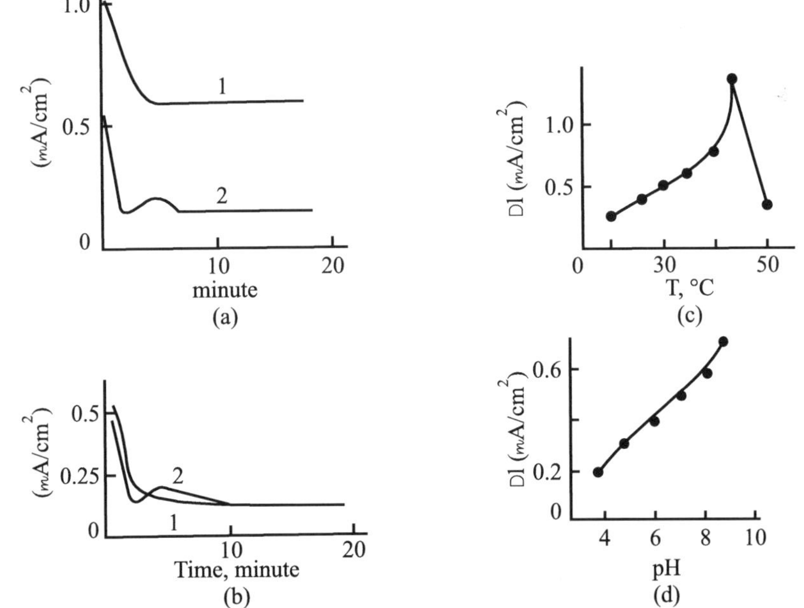

Fig. 7.5 (a) Time course of current determination electrode (line 1) & ref. electrode (line 2), (b) Time course of current from both the electrodes (pH 7.0, 30°C), (c) Effect of temperature on ΔI, (d) Effect of pH on ΔI

potentiometrically with a pair of gold and reference electrodes in a minimal culture medium. From the variation of potential as a function of time, a theorectical relation could be derived between inoculum size and the time preceding the appearance of the wave. Making reasonable assumptions the theoretical minimum lag time, t_l (TMLT) was developed from the law of cell growth and consequent dissolved oxygen (DO) consumption in the following form.

$$t_l = \frac{t_g}{\ln 2} \ln\left[1 + \frac{(Q_2)_0}{Q'_m\, x_0}\right] \tag{7.25}$$

In this relation Q'_m is maximum specific oxygen uptake rate, $(O_2)_0$ is the DO at time $t = 0$, x_0 is the cell concentration and t_g is generation time. This potentiometric method relies on the choice of an adequate culture medium (minimal glucose medium, with or without yeast extract) and a natural oxidation-reduction indicator (LA) which is reduced without degradation during bacterial growth.

3. Product

(*i*) *Alcohol Biosensor* : On line measurement of ethyl alcohol or methanol in 1. ethanol/methanol fermentation and 2. yeast cultivation is very much required to (i) minimize product inhibition and (ii) increase yield. In cultivation of microorganisms using methanol or ethanol as carbon source, its concentration must be maintained at the optimal level to overcome product inhibition.

Principle: As many microorganisms can use alcohols as carbon source, its concentration can be determined from the respiration activity of cells. The respiration activity is directly measured by oxygen electrode. It has thus been possible to construct microbial sensor for alcohols using immobilized microorganisms and oxygen electrode.

Biosensor system: It consists of the following components.

(i) immobilized yeast (e.g. AJ 3993) or bacteria (e.g. *Trichosporon brassicae*, CBS 6382), (ii) a gas permeable membrane (teflon) and (iii) an oxygen electrode.

Porous membrane retaining microbial cells is fixed on the surface of the teflon membrane of the electrode. So, the cells are trapped between the two membranes. Also, a gas permeable membrane is placed on the surface of the electrode and covered with a nylon net. These membranes were fastened with rubber o-rings. The steady state current obtained depended on the concentration of ethanol/methanol. The response time is within 10 mins at 30°C.

Modification: Since steady state method required long response time, a pulse method was used for the determination. The assay can be done within 6 mins. by this method. The total time required by steady state method was 30 mins while it took only 15 mins. by pulse method. The current difference was reproducible within ± 6% using 16.5 mgl^{-1} ethanol. The standard deviation a was 0.5 mgl^{-1} in 40 experiments.

For sensing bioproducts, oxygen probe biosensors having characteristics as given in Table 7.3 have been developed in more recent years.

Table 7.3 Oxygen probe biosensors in sensing bioproducts

Biosensor System		*Sensing*		*Response Time*	*Stability*
Type	*Device*	*Bioproduct / Range item*			
A. Immobilize whole cell (IWC)	Oxygen probe "				
Trichosporon brassica	"	Ethanol	$4 \times 10^{-5} - 4 \times 10^{-4}$	10 mins	21 days
Trichosporon brassica	"	Acetic acid	$5 \times 10^{-5} - 1 \times 10^{-3}$	8 mins.	30 days
Trichosporon enterium	"	BOD/Phenol	$10^{-4} - 1.8 \times 10^{-3}$	18 mins.	30 days
Bacillus subtilis	"	α-amylase	–	–	–
Pseudomonas fluorescens	"	Glucose	$10^{-5} - 10^{-4}$	10 mins.	30 days
Unidentified	"	NO_2(gas)	0.51 - 255 ppm	3 mins.	30 days
B. Immobilized Enzyme (IE, Amperometric)					
Ascorbate oxidase	"	Ascorbic acid	$2 \times 10^{-5} - 8 \times 10^{-4}$	1-2 mins.	7 months
Alcohol (ethanol) oxidase	"	Ethanol	$5 \times 10^{-6} - 2.5 \times 10^{-5}$	1-2 mins.	14 days
L-amino acid oxidase	Graphite H_2O_2	L-amino acid	$10^{-5} - 10^{-2}$	25 secs.	30 days
Glucose oxidase	Pt-H_2O_2	Glucose	$5 \times 10^{-5} – 4 \times 10^{-3}$	10 secs.	60 days

4. Bioprocess effluent BOD

(*i*) BOD *Sensor Electrode* : Scheme of BOD sensor microbial electrode consists of the following components (Fig. 7.6.a)

1. Bacteria-collagen membrane (50 μm thickness)
2. Teflon membrane (27μm)
3. Pt-cathode
4. Electrolyte (KOH)
5. Lead (Pb)-anode
6. O-ring

Its measuring circuit components consist of the following items (Fig. 7.6.b)

1. Microbial electrode, 2. Recorder, 3. Amplifier, 4. Air, 5. Magnetic stirrer, 6. O-ring.

Response curves of the sensor in 60 ml standard solution containing 0.1M Phosphate buffer (pH 7.0) and varying BOD sample between 2.5% to 10% at 30°C is shown in Fig.7.6. c. Current (μA)-Concentration (%) and BOD (ppm) relationship of this BOD sensor electrode is shown in Fig. 7.6.d. It indicates that when BOD < 22 ppm i.e. in the region of concentration <10% can be estimated by this electrode. A standard relation of current-BOD in waste water is shown in Fig. 7.6d. Good reusability pattern of BOD sensor electrode given in the figure shows reliability of its response.

Reusability: The current of the microbial BOD sensor is determined after it had been immersed in the standard solution. It is repeated three times per day. The repeated use shows response as given in Fig. 7.7.

(*ii*) *Biofuel Cell BOD Sensor*: As shown in Fig. 7.8 the sensor components are numbered. The sensor was calibrated using 200 ml 0.1 M phosphate buffer with different concentration of glucose (2.5 – 400 gm/ml) and gluconic acid. The electrode output in μA is obtained after 40 mins.

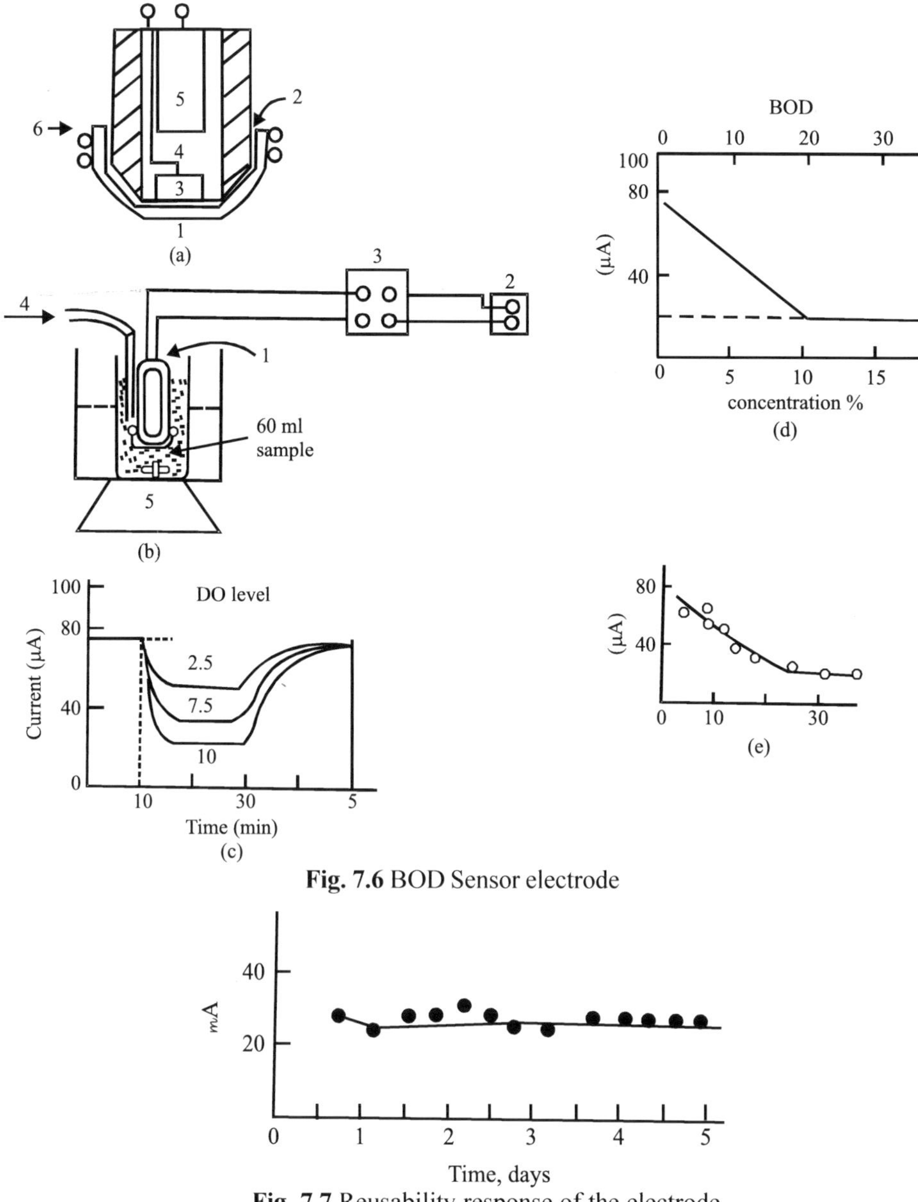

Fig. 7.6 BOD Sensor electrode

Fig. 7.7 Reusability response of the electrode

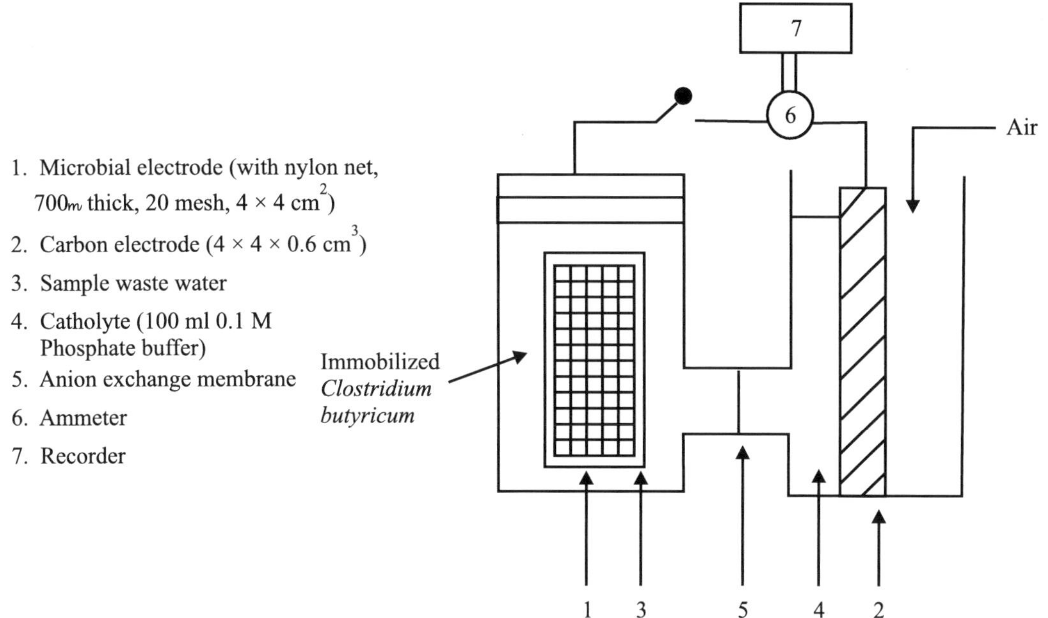

Fig. 7.8 Schematic of a biofuel cell BOD sensor

From the above section it is clear that biosensor technology is advancing very fast. The area of patterning self assembled monolayers (SAMS) using microcontact printing (μcp) is an example of new technology for novel biosensors.

5. Enzymic biosensors [6,9,10,26-29,]

The development of enzymic biosensors as integral component of process biotechnology is progressing rapidly. These biosensors are being used to measure either substrate or bioproduct concentrations in samples. Two examples of these biosensors are glucose oxidase and urease immobilized on the electrode membranes.[10] Another important enzymic biosensor, very useful in food industry is monosamine oxidase electrode sensor. It is used in freshness testing of meat. Various compounds such as amines, carboxylates, aldehydes, ammonia and carbon dioxide are produced in the meat putrefaction process. The conventional method of testing meat freshness is the measurement of volatile basic nitrogen in meats. However, this method is complicated involving many operations. This complicated method has been replaced by determination of monosamines using biosensor. Monosamine oxidase (monooxygen oxidoreductase EC 1.4.3.4 from *Aspergilus niger* and beef plasma) has been immobilized in a collagen membrane. The biosensor, consisting of a monosamine oxidase-collagen membrane (10 units) and an oxygen electrode, could be developed and used to determine monosamines in meat and meat products by determining oxidation of monosamines with dissolved oxygen in the presence of monosamine oxidase as per following reaction

$$R \cdot CH_2 \cdot NH_2 + O_2 + H_2O \xrightarrow{\text{Monosamine oxidase}} RCHO + H_2O_2 + NH_3$$

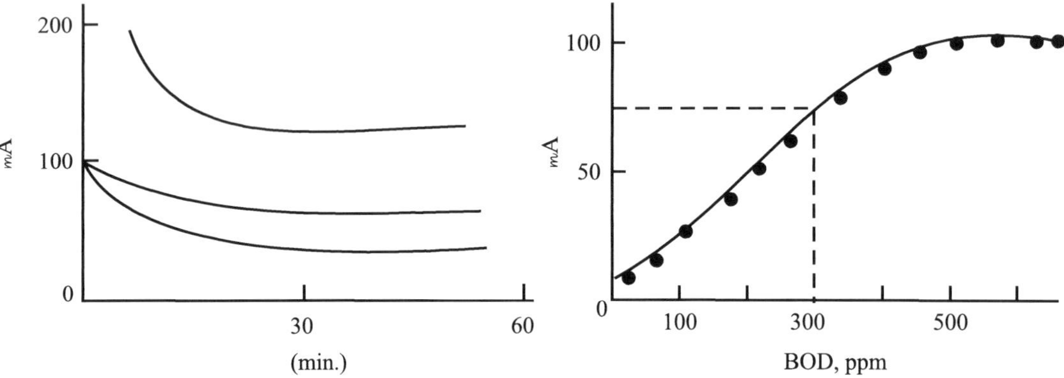

Fig. 7.9 Current-time relation of the biofuel cell BOD sensor

Fig. 7.10 BOD-current output relation

The principle of this bioassay is based on monitoring the decrease in dissolved oxygen resulting from the above enzymatic reaction in the presence of monosamines and the oxygen electrode determines dissolved oxygen.[24] A few of the oxygen probe immobilized enzyme (IE) biosensors have been listed in Table 7.3.

7.5 REFERENCES

1. Ghose, T.K. "Special Design Problems of Microbial Reactors," *Indian Chem. Engr.,* pp 14, 6, 1972
2. Ghose, T.K. and S.N. Mukhopadhyay, "Bioreactors—Recent Advances," *Sympo. Heterogeneous Reactions Science and Practice*, 32nd Annual Meeting 11ChE, IIT Bombay, Dec. 25, 1979
3. Mukhopadhyay, S.N. and D.K. Das, "Microbial Cell Culture Bioreactors," *Oxygen Responses, Reactivities and Measurements in Biosystems*, pp 167-172, CRC Press, Boca Raton, Florida, 1994.
4. Mukhopadhyay, S.N. "Fundamentals of Fermentation Process Design," *Proc. DAE Sympo on Newer Approaches to Biological Applications*, pp 201-206, MS Univ. Baroda, Dec. 19-21, 1984.
5. Kendrew, S.J. (ed), *Biological Containment*, pp 115, The Encyclopedia of Molecular Biology, Blackwell Sci., Oxford, 1994.
6. Aiba, S., A.E. Humphrey and N.F. Millis, *Biochem. Engg*. 2nd edn. Univ. of Tokyo Press, 1973.
7. Prince, M.J., J.F. Walter and H.W. Blanch, "Bubble Break up in Air Sparged Bioreactors," *Bioprocess Engineering: The First Generation*, pp 160-173, (T.K. Ghose ed), Ellis Horwood, West Sussex, England, 1989.
8. Reiter,M., A. Buchacher, G. Bliuml, N. Zach, W. Steinellner, C. Schmatz, T. Gaida, A. Assadian and H. Katinger, "Production of the HIV-I Neutralizing Human Monoclonal Antibody, 2F 5: Stirred Tank *vs* Fluidized Bed Culture," *Animal Cell Technology*, pp 333-335, (R.E. Spier, J.B. Griffiths and W. Berthold), ESACT Butterworth Heinemann, Oxford, London, 1994
9. Bailey, J.E. and D.F. Ollis; *Biochem. Engg. Fundamentals*, 2nd edn. McGraw Hill Book Co., New York, , 1986
10. Shuler, M.L. and F. Kargi, *Bioprocess Engineering: Basic Concept*, chapter 14, Elsever Sci. Pub. 1994.
11. Sittig, W., "The Present state of Fermentation Reactors," *J. Chem. Tech. Biorechnol.*, pp 32, 47-58, 1982
12. Humphrey, A.E., *Biotechnology : The Way Ahead*, Ibid pp 25-32

13. Kundu, S. "Microbial Conversion of Cellulose to Ethanol," *Ph.D. Thesis*, IIT Delhi, 1984.
14. Srivastava, A., "Extractive Lactic Acid Bioconversion Using Ion Exchange Resins," *Ph.D. Thesis*, IIT Delhi, 1994.
15. Mukhopadhyay, S.N. *Bioreactors for Microbial Processing*, Lecture Delivered for UNESCO Sponsored Workshop, DBEB, IIT Delhi, Dee. 5-10, 1994.
16. "Process Biotechnology Fundamentals", Chp. 16., Corrigan, A.H. "Bioreactors for Mammalian Cells," *Mammalian Cell Biotechnology: A Practical Approach*, pp 139-158, (M. Butler ed), IRL Press at Oxford Univ. Press, Oxford, 1991.
17. Chotteau, V. and O. Bastin., "A General Two Step Procedure for the Kinetic Modelling of Animal Cell Cultures", *Animal Cell Technology: Products for Today and Tomorrow*, pp 545, (R.E. spier et. al eds.), Butterworth-Heinemann Pub., 1994.
18. Mukhopadhyay, A., S.N. Mukhopadhyay and G.P. Talwar, "The Influence of Serum Protecins on Attachment of Vero Cells on Cytodex Microcarriers," *J. Chem. Tech. Biotechnol.*, pp 56, 369-74, 1993.
19. Mukhopadhyay, S.N. *et al; Indian Chem. Enggr.,* pp 38(4), 104-144, 1996.
20. Mukhopadhyay, A., S.N. Mukhopadhyay and G.P. Talwar, "Studies on the Synthesis of βhCG Hormone in Verocells by Recombinant Virus," *Biotechnol. Bioengg.* pp 48, 158-68, 1995.
21. Nolan, E.J. and A.E. Humphrey; "Economic Opportunities for Biological Conversion of Biomass to Liquid Fuels," *Bioconversion and Biochemical Engineering,* pp 1-29, Vol. II. (T.K. Ghose, ed), 1980.
22. Kleinstpruer, C., "Analysis of Biological Reactors," *Advanced Biochemical Engineering,* pp 38-78, (H.R. Bungay and G. Belfort eds), John Wiley and Sons., New York, 1987.
23. Reilly, P.J. "Optimization of Mono and Dual Enzyme Reactor systems in Biochemical Engineering," W.R. Vieth, K. Venkatasubramanian and A. Constantinides, *Annals,* N.Y. Sci. pp 326, 97-103, 1979.
24. Karube, I., I. Satoh, Y. Araki and S. Suzuki, "Monosamine Oxidase Electrode in Freshness Testing of Meat," *Enz. Microb. Technol.* pp 2, 117-20, 1980
25. Junter, O.A., J.F. Lemel and E. Selegny, "Electro-chemical Detection and Counting of *Escherichia coli* in the Presence of a Reducible Coenzyme, Lipoic acid," *Appl. Environ. Microbiol.* pp 39(2), 307-316, 1980
26. Karube, I. and K. Sode, "Microbial Sensors for Process and Environmental Control," *Bioinstrumentation and Biosensors*, pp 1-18 (D.L. Wise ed), Marcel Dekkar Inc. N.Y., 1991.
27. Jacob, J.W. and S.P.A. Fodor. *TIBTECH,* pp 12, 19-26, 1994.
28. Loung, J.H.T., A. Mulchandani and G.G. Guilbault, "Dev. and Appl. of Biosensors," *TIBTECH*, pp 6, 310-326,1988.
29. Karube, I. and M. Suzuki, "Microbial Biosensors," *Biosensors: A Practical Approach*, pp 155-70, (A.E.G. Cass ed.), IRL Press/Cambridge Univ. Press, 1990.
30. Mrksich, M. and O.M. Whitesides., *TIBTECH*, pp 13, 228-35, 1995
31. Van't Riet, K. and J. Tramper, *Basic Bioreactor Design*, Marcel Dekkar Inc., New York, 1991
32. Blanch, H.W. and D.S. Clark, *Biochemical Engineering*, Marcel Dekkar, New York, 1996.
33. M. Bartow and E. Spark, Bioreactor Design for Mammalian Cell Culture, Chem. Engg. Jan. 2004., p 49-54.
34. K. Baily, W.R.Victh and G.K. Chotani, Analysis of Bioreactors Containing Immobilized Recombinant Cells, Anals of NYAS vol 506, Biochemical Engineering V. M.L Shnler and W.A. Weigand Eds, New York, 1987 pp 196-207.
35. R. Freitag, Biosensors in Analytical Biotechnology, R.G. Landers, Acad Press, Austin, Texas.
36. S. Ghose, G.M. Forde and N.K.H. Slater, Affinity Adsorption of Plasmid DNA, Biotechnol. Prog 20, 841-850, 2004.

Chapter

8

BIOPROCESSING SCALE UP: CONCERNS AND CRITERIA

8.1 INTRODUCTION

The aim of scaling up a bioprocess in a bioreactor is to obtain microbial or biochemical reaction results efficiently on each scale, essentially in large scale bioreactors. Moreover, engineering steps have to be undertaken to guarantee the economy of industrial processes by high yields and productivities. "Make experiments on a small scale and obtain profits on a large scale on the basis of specific criteria" is the basic principle of scale up. So in effect it transfers the experimental results of bench scale into large scale to obtain profits. The approach to achieve this transfer is based on different parameters or criteria used in scaling up.[1–8]

8.2 SCALE UP CONCERNS OF MICROBIAL, MAMMALIAN AND PLANT CELL PROCESSES

Scale up concerns with transferring of optimum process results from laboratory or pilot plant equipment of kinematically or dynamically similar industrial size equipment. However, physical conditions in a large bioreactor can never exactly be same to those in a smaller bioreactor even though geometrical similarity in small and large systems remains same. Other concerns as pointed out relate to wall growth in bioreactor. During bioprocessing, if biocells adhere to surfaces of bioreactor, or its accessories, these cells may alter metabolic characteristics mainly due to limitations like mass transfer, substrate uptake etc. Thus data obtained in a small bioreactor may be unreliable in predicting culture behaviour in a large bioreactor. Advantage in scale up, of 10 *l* to 2000 *l* airlift bioreactor for bioprocessing of hybridoma cell has been reported to provide improved oxygen transfer rates in larger scale.[9] The increase in hydrostatic pressure resulting from increased biorector height did not have detrimental effects on the cells. In conventional stirred tank bioreactor (STBR) for microbial cell cultivation it is a common practice to increase the OTR (oxygen transfer rate) by increasing bubble surface area by break up with impeller rotation speed. For mammalian cell cultivation has increased bubble break up results in excessive foaming and losses of cells and proteins at the medium surface. Many mamalian cell culture sytesms have therefore been scaled up by maintaining constant K_La using bubble free aeration by perfusion technique. In scale up of plant cell culture systems it has been stated to be necessary to know in which way yield, oxygen transfer and uptake rate, actual pH and pO_2 are interlinked.[10,11] From various analysis it has been noticed that it is virtually impossible to reproduce identical conditions and environments on different scales. As such the problem resolves into one of identifying key parameters involved in a bioprocess and select the best on which it is designed to maintain this key parameter is then used as "Criterion of scale up." Also, the system is designed to maintain this key parameter at the same value at all scales of operation. In bioprocessing, therefore, the purpose of any process biotechnology scale up procedure is to reproduce a given bioproces on a large scale to achieve a predictable process result. Scale up, thus, has been defined as the predictable (engineered) increase in production capacity. Ideally what the scale up engineer would like to do is to simulate and predict the performance of a large scale bioreactor (e.g. 5000 l and above) using only data from a laboratory bench scale (5 l) vessel. In order to do this equations are required that correlate the performance of bioreactor with its size.

8.3 SCALE UP CRITERIA

8.3.1 Mircobial Cell Process

Theoretically the following criteria were assumed suitable basis for scale up of bioreactors.

A. Constant power input per unit volume (P/V = constant).

B. Constant K_La

C. Constant mixing quality

D. Constant momentum factor ($MF = ND.\ NWL\ (D - W)$) = constant)

E. Similar drop size distribution (d_s = constant)

F. Constant impeller tip speed ($\pi\, ND_i$ = constant)

G. Constant mixing rate number = $\left(\frac{N}{K}\right)\left(\frac{D_i}{D_t}\right)^{\alpha}$ constant

Short accounts of scaling up of bioreactors of fermenters on the basis of these criteria are discussed in the following sections.

1. Constant power input per unit volume

For scaling up based on this criteria it is necessary to consider whether it is gassed or non-gassed system. From the work of Rushton and his associates,[12] for geometrically similar, fully baffled vessels with turbulent conditions, it may be noted that if scale up should be based on maintaining a constant power input per unit volume considering no gassing in the system one may have the following.

(*i*) *Non-gassed System* : When there is no gassing in the system then based on constant *P/V* has the power number, N_p as

$$N_p = \frac{P \cdot g_c}{N^3 D_i^5 \rho} \tag{8.0}$$

or

$$N_p = \frac{P}{D_i^3}\left(\frac{g_c}{N^3 D_i^2 \rho}\right) = \frac{P}{D^3}\left(\frac{A}{N^3 D^2}\right) \tag{8.1}$$

$$[\because D_i \propto D]$$

where D_i is impeller diameter, D is vessel tank diameter, P/D^3 is power per unit volume i.e. P/V and A is a constant. So, when P/D^3 i.e. P/V = constant = K'

$$Np = K'' \frac{1}{N^3 D^2}, \text{ where } K'' = K' A = \text{constant} \tag{8.2}$$

For scale up,

$$N^3 D^2 = \text{constant} \tag{8.3}$$

or

$$N_1^3 D_1^2 = N_2^3 D_2^2 \tag{8.4}$$

or

$$N_1 = N_2 (D_2/D_1)^{2/3} \tag{8.5}$$

Thus to scale up a non-gassed fermentation system (anaerobic) on the basis of constant P/V the relation between impeller speed of bench scale fermeter to that of scale up fermenter is given by equation (8.5).

(*ii*) *Gassed System* : From the results of Cooper *et al*[13] and Ohyama and Endoh[14] it was observed by Michel and Miller[15] that the relation between power consumption in gassed and non-gassed system can be expressed as below.

$$\frac{P_g}{P} = \text{constant}\left(\frac{N^{1/2} D^{3/2}}{Q^{1/4}}\right) \tag{8.6}$$

where P_g is gassed power and Q is volumetric gas flowrate.

From equation (8.6)

$$\frac{P_g}{D^3} = \frac{P}{D^3} \text{ constant}\left(\frac{N^{1/2}\, D^{3/2}}{Q^{1/4}}\right)$$

or
$$\frac{P_g}{D^3} = N_P N^3 D^2 \text{ constant } \left(\frac{N^{1/2}\, D^{3/2}}{Q^{1/4}}\right)$$

or
$$\frac{P_g}{D^3} = \text{constant } \left(\frac{N^{7/2}\, D^{7/2}}{Q^{1/4}}\right) \tag{8.7}$$

So, for scale up

$$\frac{P_g}{D^3} = \frac{P_g}{V} = \text{constant}$$

Thus, from equation (8.7)

$$\frac{N^{\frac{7}{2}}\, D^{\frac{7}{2}}}{Q^{1/4}} = \text{constant}$$

or
$$\frac{N_1^{7/2}\, D_1^{7/2}}{Q_1^{1/4}} = \frac{N_2^{7/2}\, D_2^{7/2}}{Q_2^{1/4}} \tag{8.8}$$

from which

$$N_1 = N_2\, (D_2/D_1)\, (Q_1/Q_2)^{1/14} \tag{8.9}$$

Equation (8.9) is showing the relation of impeller speeds between two scale bioreactors.

2. Constant $K_L a$

The relations between $K_L a$ with gassed power input per unit volume, (P_g/D^3) and superficial gas velocity, (υ_s) have been given as below.

$$K_L\, a = \text{constant } (P_g/D^3)^{0.95} \tag{8.10}$$

and
$$K_L\, a = \text{constant } (\upsilon_s)^{0.67} \tag{8.11}$$

combining equations (8.10) and (8.11)

$$K_L a = \text{constant } \left(\frac{P_g}{D^3}\right)^{0.95} (\upsilon_s)^{0.67} \tag{8.12}$$

but $$\upsilon_s = K_L a \left(\frac{Q}{D^2}\right) \tag{8.13}$$

Therefore, from equations (8.12) and (8.13)

$$K_L\, a = c\left(\frac{P}{D^3}\right)^{0.95} (K_L a)^{0.67} \left(\frac{Q}{D^2}\right)^{0.67} \tag{8.14}$$

where c is constant

From equation (8.14) one may write

$$K_L\, a = c\left(\frac{P_g}{D^3}\right)\left(\frac{Q}{D^2}\right)^{3/2} (K_L\, a)^{2/3} \; [\because 0.95 \approx 1, 0.67 \approx 2/3] \quad (6.15)$$

So, for scale up, $K_L a$ = constant, equation (8.15) gives

$$\left(\frac{P_g}{D^3}\right)\left(\frac{Q}{D^2}\right)^{3/2} = \text{constant} \tag{8.16}$$

But for gassed system

$$\frac{P_g}{D^3} = \text{constant}\ \frac{N^{7/2}\, D^{7/2}}{Q^{1/4}} \quad \text{(from equation 8.7)} \tag{8.17}$$

or $$N_1^{\ 7/2}\, D_1^{\ 13/6}\, Q_1^{\ 5/12} = N_2^{\ 7/2}\, D_2^{\ 13/6}\, Q_2^{\ 5/12} \tag{8.18}$$

This gives

$$N_1 = N_2\, (D_2/D_1)^{13/21}\, (Q_2/Q_1)^{5/42} \tag{8.19}$$

Equation (8.19) provides the relation between impeller speeds of two scale fermenters based on K_L a = constant as a scale up criteria.

3. Constant mixing quality

Constant mixing quality in otherwords indicates constant Reynolds number, N_{Re}. From the power curve relation when

$$N_{Re} = \text{constant}$$

then the power factor ϕ = constant

So, $$\phi = \frac{t \cdot (ND_i^2)^{2/3} \cdot g^{1/6} \cdot D_i^{1/2}}{H_l^{1/2}\, D^{3/2}} = \text{constant} \tag{8.20}$$

in which H_L is liquid height = 1.2 D, D_i is impeller diameter = 1/3 D, t is mixing time and g is gravitational factor. Putting these values in equation (8.20) one has

$$\frac{t \cdot (ND_i^2)^{2/3} \cdot g^{1/6} \cdot \left(\frac{1}{3}D\right)^{1/2}}{(1.2D)^{1/2}\ D^{3/2}} = \text{constant} \tag{8.21}$$

Simplifying equation (8.21)

$$t\ .\ N^{3/2}\ D^{-1/6} = \text{constant} \tag{8.22}$$

Also, from equation (8.3)

$$N^3D^2 = \text{constant}$$

Taking 18th power of equation (8.22)

$$t^{18}\ N^{12}\ D^{-3} = \text{constant} \tag{8.23}$$

and taking 4th power of equation (8.3)

$$N^{12}\ D^8 = \text{constant} \tag{8.24}$$

Dividing equation (8.23) by equation (8.24)

$$t^{18}\ D^{-11} = \text{constant} \tag{8.25}$$

or

$$t_1^{18}\ D_1^{-11} = t_2\ D_2^{-11} \tag{8.26}$$

from which

$$t_2 = t_1 \left(\frac{D_2}{D_1}\right)^{11/18} \tag{8.27}$$

Equation (8.27) provides the relationship between mixing time in two scales fermenters when constant mixing quality is the basis of scale up.

4. Constant momentum factor (MF)

Blakebrough and Sambamurthy[6] found that $K_L\,a$ in a broth of three phase systems can be computed by the following equation.

$$K_L\ a = 152 \left[\frac{t^{0.203}\ (P_g/V)^{1.79}}{MF^{1.05}\ N^{0.459}}\right] \tag{8.28}$$

where MF is momentum factor (= ND. NWL (D – W)), t is mixing time, N is impeller speed and P_g/V is power input per unit volume.

In MF, ND represents mean velocity of the liquid leaving the impeller, cm. sec^{-1}, and NWL (D – W) is the volumetric flow rate from the impeller, cm^3 sec^{-1} which in turn is the measure of mass flow rate. Thus the product of ND and NWL (D – W) represent momentum factor.

From equation (8.28)

$$MF^{1.05} = 152\left[\frac{t^{0.203}(P_g/V)^{1.79}}{K_La \cdot N^{0.459}}\right] \quad (8.29)$$

Approximating,

$$MF = c'\left[\frac{t^{1/5}(P_g/V)^{1.8}}{K_La \cdot N^{1/2}}\right] \quad (8.30)$$

where c' is a constant.

For scale up MF = constant. So, from equation (8.30)

$$\frac{t^{1/5}(P_g/V)^{1.8}}{K_La \cdot N^{1/2}} = \text{constant} \quad (8.31)$$

However, $K_La \propto (P_g/V) = K'(P_g/v)$

Now, equation (8.31) can be written as

$$\frac{t^{1/5}(P_g/V)^{1.8}}{K'(P_g/V)\,N^{1/2}} = \frac{t^{1/5}(P_g/V)^{1.8}}{N^{1/2}} = \text{constant} \quad (8.32)$$

From which

$$N_1 = N_2\left(\frac{t_1}{t_2}\right)^{2/3}\left[\frac{(P_g/V)_1}{(P_g/V)_2}\right]^{1./6} \quad (8.33)$$

5. Similar drop size distribution

Bajpai *et. al.*[7] proposed an oil drop size distribution in hydrocarbon fermentation as

$$d_s \propto We^a\,\psi(C_x)\,f(\phi') \quad (8.34)$$

where d_s is the saueter mean drop size, We $(= D^3 N^2 \rho/\gamma)$ is the Weber number, $\psi(C_x)$ represent a function of cell concentration (C_x) and $f(\phi')$ gives the measure of dispersed phase change. It was found that

$$f(\phi') = 1 + b\phi' \quad (8.35)$$

where ϕ' is the dispersed phase fraction (volume of dispersed phase/total volume), which is a linear relation with ϕ as a constant. Also,

$$\psi(C_x) = e^{-C.C_x^n} \quad (8.36)$$

where C is a constant. It was shown that for low cell concentration in the system $\psi(C_x)$ has significant contribution but for high cell concentration range $\psi(C_x)$ becomes insignificant.

It was also apparent that in an oil drop dispersion system d_s could serve as an important criteria for scale up. The value of '*a*' in equation 8.34 depends on the type of agitator used in the system. For turbine impeller $a = -0.6$ whereas for draft tube fermenter its value ranges between -0.15 to -0.35.

6. Constant impeller tip speed[1]

It was rather surprising to recognize that most of the data on impeller tip speeds collected were in the range 5–7 m sec^{-1} indicating the predominant importance of this parameter in scale up. Specially in antibiotic production plants constancy in tip speed (πND_i) was encountered in several cases. For scale up

$$\pi N D_i = \text{constant} \tag{8.37}$$

or

$$\pi N_1 D_{i_1} = \pi N_2 D_{i_2} = \text{constant}$$

∴

$$N_1 = N_2 \left(\frac{D_{i_2}}{D_{i_1}}\right) \tag{8.38}$$

In equation (8.37) N represents impeller tip speed and D_{i_1} impeller diameter.

7. Constant mixing rate number[8]

In scale up of bioreactors mixing time is often used as a criteria. Mixing time (t_{mix}), defined as the period of time required for the homogeneous distribution of a small volume of pulsating material in the bulk of the liquid, was used for scale up to adjust proper mixing conditions in large vessels. However, limitation of using t_{mix} as scale up criteria is that it increases markedly with the size of the vessel and it is difficult to maintain t_{mix} constant in both vessels at reasonable power expenditure. In mixing a fermentation broth two vital questions to be answered are : (1) what size of motor is needed for a given impeller rotation speed? and (2) how long the broth must be mixed to achieve a required degree of homogenity?

From the present knowledge the first question can be answered using $N_p - N_{Re}$ relations of Rushton[16] and Bates *et al.*[17] The answer of the second question has been provided[8] by introducing a new dimensionless term mixing rate number $[(N/K)(D/D_t)^\alpha]$, N_{MR} in the $N_P - N_{Re}$ profile to characterize the rate of approach to uniformity in mixing vessels. This profiles as shown in Fig. 8.1 a and b indicate that for large impeller Reynolds number ($N_{Re} > 10^4$) the following correlations will be applicable depending on the type of mixer used.

For turbine impeller mixer

$$N_{MR} = \left(\frac{N}{K}\right)\left(\frac{D_i}{D_t}\right)^{2.3} = 0.1 \frac{P_{g_c}}{\rho N^3 D_i^5} = 0.5 \tag{8.39}$$

or

$$N_{MR} = 0.1\, N_P = 0.5$$

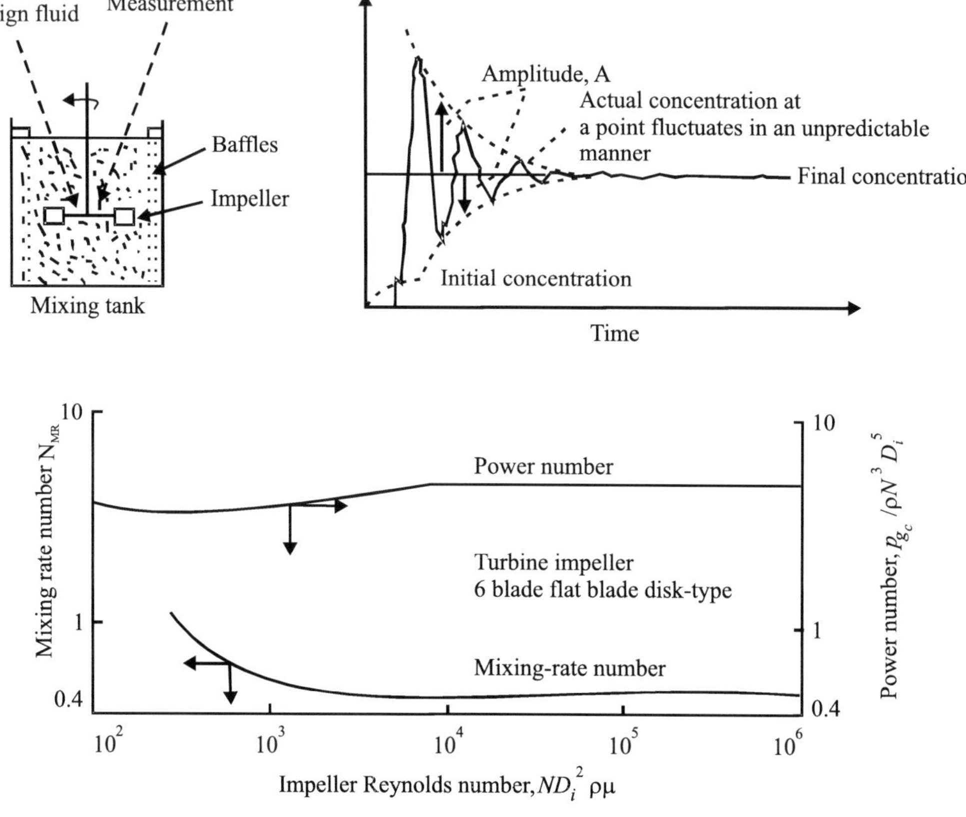

Fig. 8.1 (a) Typical behaviour when blending a quantity of foreign fluid into the bulk liquid contained in a mixing tank, (b) Dimensional correlations for turbine mixers speed scale up and design procedures for agitated systems

For propeller mixer

$$N_{MR} = \left(\frac{N}{K}\right)\left(\frac{D_i}{D_t}\right)^{2.0} = 1.5\left(\frac{P_{g_c}}{\rho N^3 D_i^5}\right) = 0.9 \tag{8.40}$$

or

$$N_{MR} = 1.5 \ N_P = 0.9$$

These correlations of mixing apply only to fully bafffled vessels with vertical impellers at the centre.

In most Newtonian fermentations $N_{RE} > 10^4$ in laboratory scale. For scale up such systems using N_{MR} as criteria in STF having turbine impeller one can write

$$\left(\frac{N}{K}\right)\left(\frac{D_i}{D_t}\right)^{2.3} = \text{constant} \tag{8.41}$$

where K is tracer amplitude decay rate constant in mixing vessel. From equation (8.41)

$$\left(\frac{N}{K}\right)_1 \left(\frac{D_i}{D_t}\right)_1^{2.3} = \left(\frac{N}{K}\right)_2 \left(\frac{D_i}{D_t}\right)_2^{2.3} = 0.1 \left(\frac{P_{g_c}}{\rho N^3 D_i^5}\right) \tag{8.42}$$

From this equation

$$\frac{N_1}{N_2} = \left(\frac{K_1}{K_2}\right)\left(\frac{D_{i_2}}{D_{i_1}} \cdot \frac{D_{i_1}}{D_{i_2}}\right)^{2.3}$$

Since for similar operation $K_1 = K_2$

So,
$$N_1 = N_2 \left(\frac{D_{i_2}}{D_{i_1}} \cdot \frac{D_{t_1}}{D_{t_2}}\right)^{2.3} \tag{8.43}$$

8.3.2 Scale Up of Filamentous Cell Fermentation[13]

Aerobic fermentative bioprocessign using filamentous microorganisms cover a wide range of industrially important bioproduct formation systems. Various *Streptomyces* sp. antibiotic fermentations fall in this group. Such bioprocessing exhibit viscous and non Newtonian behavior following Power law fluid characters. These processes are typical and present considerable problems in mixing and mass transfer for scale up purpose. Thus, agitator power number (N_P) and impeller diameter (D_i) are important case factors towards implications of Power law fluid on scale up along with liquid volume (V_L) and (H_L/D_t) ratio.

Case 1. Agitator power ($P_{t'}$) number influence

a. Provided with same geometry, υ_s, (P_t/V_t), V_L and D_i manipulation of volumetric mass transfer equations show

$$\frac{K_L a_1}{K_L a_2} = \left(\frac{N_{P_1}}{N_{P_2}}\right)^{\frac{n-1}{3}} \tag{8.44}$$

It shows that if $n < 1$ and $N_{P_1} < N_{P_2}$ then

$$K_L a_1 > K_L a_2$$

hence $K_L a$ increases with decreasing N_P.

b. Provided with same geometry, υ_s, (P_t / V_L), V_L and N_P gives

$$\frac{K_L a_1}{K_L a_2} = \left(\frac{D_{i_1}}{D_{i_2}}\right)^{\frac{5(n-1)}{3}} \tag{8.45}$$

It shows that if $n < 1$, $D_{i_1} < D_{i_2}$ then

$$K_L a_1 > K_L a_2$$

meaning thereby, $K_L a$ increases with decreasing D_i. However, use of this influence should be tested by the need of uniform mixing.

c. Provided with same geometry, VVM (volume per unit volume per minute), (P_t/V_L), (D_i/D_t) and N_P leads to

$$\frac{K_L a_1}{K_L a_2} = \left(\frac{V_{L_1}}{V_{L_2}}\right)^{\left[0.1+\frac{2(n-1)}{9}\right]} \tag{8.46}$$

Index = 0, when n = 0.55 thus

(i) if n = 0.55, K_L a is constant at all scales.
(ii) if n < 0.55, K_L a decreases with increasing scale.
(iii) if n > 0.55, K_L a increases with increasing scale.

Case 2. Influence of (H_L/D_t) ratio.

Special case with change of (H_L/D_t) from 1 to 3 and provided with same (D_i/D_t), with VVM, (P_t/V_L), V_L and N_P leads to interesting observations. it is found that the predicted decrease in K_L a is effectively cancelled out by the change in superficial gas velocity which is $3^{2/3}$ times higher in the $H_L = 3\ D_t$ vessels. This may put a question mark on the use of V_s for the gassing term in the K_L a model. This leaves only the viscosity term to account for which one has

$$\frac{K_L a_3 D_t}{K_L a\, D_t} = 3^{\frac{5(1-n)}{9}} \tag{8.47}$$

Thus, if n < 1, K_L a increases with increasing aspect ratio.

8.3.3 Mammalian Cell Processing Scale Up[19–27]

In scaling up bioreactors of mammalian cell bioprocess most of the correlations are based on laboratory models alone and still awaits confirmation of their utility in industrial production concern. For mammalian cell bioprocessing current industrial scales typically involve bulk liquid volume of 25*l* per day per bioreactor for continuous or semicontinuous systems. In batch processing this bioreactor volume ranges between 500-5000 *l* capacities, operating over 1-3 weeks. There are no established scale up criteria for scaling up mammalian cell culture process. Cell culture engineers therefore, still largely depend on concepts and scale up procedures developed for chemical or microbial/biochemical processes to begin with. However, an engineering body of experience and data will increasingly enable more specific design engineering and scale up procedures for mammalian cell culture bioprocesses in which kinetics is likely to be influenced by many factors and associated with many problems and limitations. In scaling up procedures specific to animal cell culture, effect of scale on oxygen mass transfer through microporous membranes like silicone tubes for supplying bubble free oxygenation has been investigated. In order to aerate cell cultures, the membrane is immersed in the medium and the gas mixture (e.g. air, CO_2 and O_2) is passed through the tube under pressure. Depending on the difference in pressure between the gas and the medium, gas flows through the membrane tube. Bubble free aeration is achieved if the internal gas pressure does not exceed the pressure at which bubbles will form. Correlation for bubble free oxygenation through membrane tubes has been developed.[24,25] For this, novel bioreactors have been designed for cell culture engineering in large quantities of the fragile complex mammalian cells that synthesize commercially and medically important proteins such as interferon and monoclonal antibodies.[26,27] The correlation for bubble free oxygen using silicone microporous tube for oxygen mass transfer in this novel bioreactor has been given by the following correlations.

$$\mathrm{Sh} = \frac{\mathrm{Kd}}{\mathrm{D_0}} \tag{8.48}$$

or

$$\mathrm{Sh} = \mathrm{e}\ \mathrm{N_{Re}}\mathrm{f}\left[\frac{\mathrm{d^g}}{\mathrm{D_t}}\right] \tag{8.49}$$

In these correlations, Sh is Sherwood number, K is film mass transfer coefficient (m s^{-1}), d is tube diameters, D_0 is molecular diffusivity of oxygen ($m^2\ s^{-1}$), e, f, g are specific constants, D_t is bioreactor diameter (m) and N_{Re} is impeller Reynolds number.

The provision of an adequate oxygen supply to large volumes of mammalian cells is the most crucial barrier to scale up, especially in suspension systems. Oxygen is only sparingly solube in cell culture medium (0.2 m mole O_2l^{-1}). Oxygen demand of a culture (10^6 cells per ml) ranges between 0.053 m mole $O_2\ l^{-1}\ h^{-1}$ and 0.59 m mole $O_2\ l^{-1}\ h^{-1}$ depending on the type of cell. Scale up of mammalian cell cultures are, therefore, bound by several barriers as shown in Table 8.1.

Table 8.1 Species barriers in scale up of mammalian cell cultures

Barrier Type	*Barrier Species*
A. Still to be overcome	Oxygen transfer limitation. Accumulation of toxic product. Lack of regulatory hardware and software for process control. High cost of serum.
B. Already overcome to some extent	Low surface to volume ratios of systems for anchorage dependent cells. Shear sensitivity of mammalian cells.

As d, D_0, N_{Re} and D_t are given and e, f and g are determined experimentally, then equation 8.48 enables calculation of the oxygen mass transfer coefficient from impeller speed. With the assumption that gas velocity and composition within the silicone tube are constant, one may calculate the power required for this form of aeration at the large scale using the correlation given below.

$$N_{Re} = \frac{P_i \cdot V \cdot D_i \cdot \pi^3}{\mu \, N_P} \tag{8.50}$$

In this correlation P_i is the power input per unit mass of liquid (W.kg^{-1}), V is the reactor volume (m_3), D_i is impeller diameter (m), μ is the kinematic liquid viscosity ($m^2 \, s^{-1}$) and N_P is the power number. Thus, scale up might be carried out on the basis of impeller speed to yield a constant oxygen mass transfer rate, but the power input per unit mass will vary with scale. It will need to check the power against an upper limit which will be determined by the shear sensitivity of the mammalian cells.

Lavery and Ninow[26] in their study of the conventional power input versus mass transfer relation in sparged mammalian cell culture indicated the necessity of consideration of both the effect of head space aeration and the effect of added antifoam. This could account for the deviations from the expected values of K_L a in their result.

A number of serious problems associated with the design and scale up of high density perfusion cultures of mammalian cell bioprocessing have been pointed out.[25] For overcoming the associated problems in cultivation of animal cells and their scale up the following usage has been suggested.

1. Microbubble technology and soluble surfactants for meeting cellular oxygen uptake rate (OUR).
2. Turbine or low shear impellers for achieving well mix cultures, such that it provides independent requirements of mixing and bubble aeration.
3. Minimization of ammonia accumulation by low glutamine supplemented media design.
4. Appropriately sized microfiltration hollow fibre cartridges which are steam sterilizable and easily cleaned after repeated uses.

8.3.4 Plant Cell Processing Scale Up

A typical plant cell culture manufacturing process is shown in Fig. 8.2. The great upsurge of interest in process biotechnology in the 1970's carried plant cell culture with it. This is primarily because of centuries plants have been an important source of drugs and chemicals.[2,5,28] The extensive effort in development of plant cell culture is evident from the literatures on the subject.[27-30] As plant cell cultures have many differences in comparison to microbes the design and scale up of suspension cultures bioreactors for plant cells also differ to a great extent. This becomes more pronounced as plant cell cultures can achieve high cell densities and viscosities. In such systems need for good mixing must have a compromise to shear sensitivity of plant cells. Thus, in plant cell culture scale up system information is very important. Useful system informations for scale up of plant cell culture as proposed by Goldstein[29] is presented in Table 8.2. In addition to these quantitation of entities as effected through bioprocess engineering studies at laboratory scale needs information on operational variables as listed in Table 8.3.

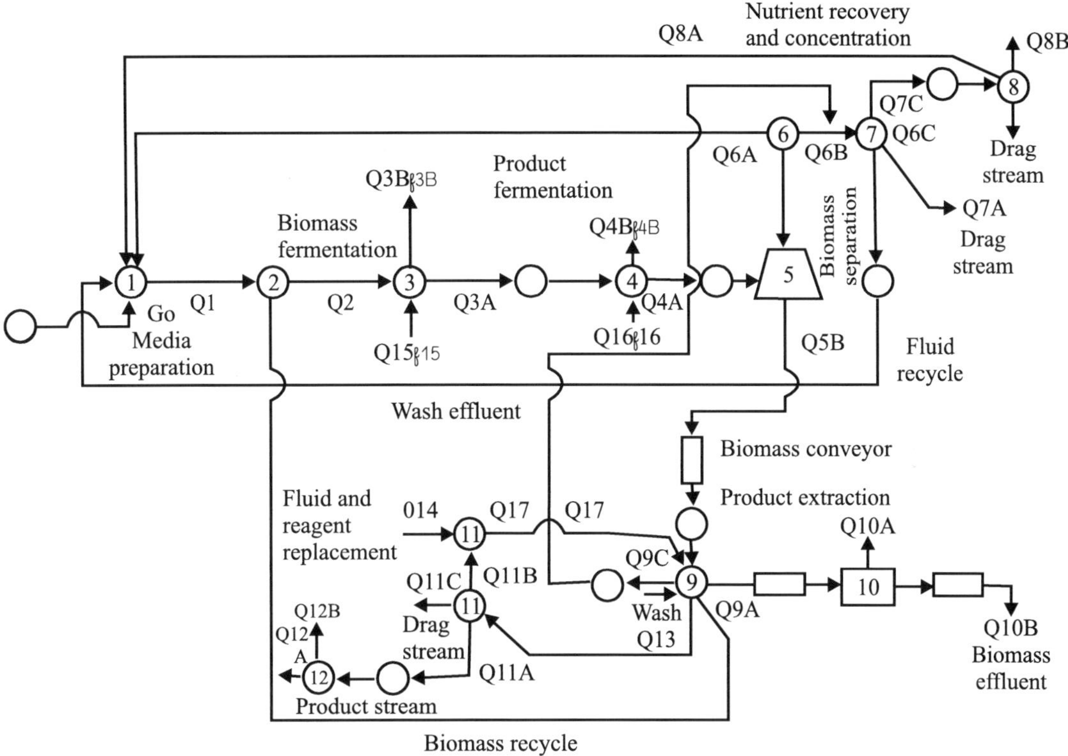

Fig. 8.2 A representation of plant cell culture/product manufacturing process[29]

Table 8.2 System information for scale up[29]

- Organism growth rate
- Product formation rate
- Means of detection
- Programming needs for nutrients and conditions
  - Repression nutrient or product limitation of an entity
    - Constant
    - Variable
- Control in processing
  - pH
  - Temperature
  - Nutrients
  - Treatments
  - Product
  - By-products
  - Asepsis
- Media cost Projection and final product value

The first consideration in generating these informations is the selecion of a suitable bioreactor type. Continuous stirred tank bioreactor (CSTBR), air lift bioreactor (ALB), immobilized plant cell bioreactor etc. have been used in plant cell cultivations either in batch, plug flow or in continuous modes. In these three modes culture residence time is analysed based on the relations given in Table 8.4. Assuming autocatalytic growth these relations emerge from classical catalysis.

Table 8.3 Information from laboratory-scale bioengineering

- Projected stoichiometry
- Project heat genertion from stoichiometry
- Oxygen requirements
  - Rheology
  - Dissolved oxygen
  - Respiration
  - Off-gass
- Fermentation
- Sterilization needs & conditions
- Recovery
  - Biomass as product
  - Intracellular metabolite
  - Extracellular metabolite
  - Process definition
  - Product stability

Table 8.4 Residence times for suspension cell culture[29]

Process Parameters for Fermenters

Residence Time

Biomass Formatin

Idealized Autocatalytic Growth

$$\frac{V}{Q} = \frac{1 - \frac{C_{BI}}{C_{BO}}}{\mu_B} \qquad \text{CSTR}$$

$$\frac{V}{Q} = \frac{\text{l N}\, \frac{C_{BI}}{C_{BO}}}{\mu_B} \qquad \text{Plug Flow}$$

$$\tau = (1 + \psi)\, \frac{\text{l N}\, \frac{C_{BI}}{C_{BO}}}{\mu_B} \qquad \text{Batch}$$

Product Formation

In Proportion to Biomass Present (Zero Order)

$$\frac{V}{Q} = \frac{C_P}{\gamma_P\, C_{BO}\, \mu_P} \qquad \text{CSTR Plug Flow}$$

$$\tau = \frac{C_P}{\gamma_P\, C_{BO}\, \mu_P} \qquad \text{Batch}$$

The process parameters for scale up of plant cell cultures as listed in Table 8.5 demand low shear bioreactor for plant cell aggregates. As reported in literature plant cell cultures often form aggregates in suspension cultures in bioreactor. It can make the provision of oxygen difficult: the high aeration or mechanical agitation necessary can both cause shear damage to the cells.

Table 8.5 Process parameters for scale up of plant cell culture[29]

- Rate of product effluent from process
- Yield of product/unit of biomass
- Maximal biomass concentration in the fermenter
- Fraction of biomass that can be reused
- Consumption of nutrients to form biomass
- Consumption of nutrients to form product
- Inlet concentration of nutrients to the fermentations
- Liquid removal ratio at the biomass separator
- Extractant needs per quantity of biomass
- Washing needs of biomass
- Disposition of fluids for recycle or waste after product extraction
- Fluid removal needs for biomass and product
- Specification of drag streams, constituents, and fluid

For overcoming the above difficulty and to facilitate scale up of plant cell culture bioreactor a design of low shear bioreactor has been reported.[32] This design is stated to create separate cell growth and aeration zones. The bioreactor design is analogous to fluidized bed columns except that the cells are immobilized naturally (by aggregation).

8.4 SELECTION OF SCALE UP CRITERIA[3,4]

In microbial bioprocessing scale up although many criteria have been provided as discussed earlier but among them only four criteria as given in Table 8.6 are widely selected in practice. Of these most emphasis has been given to specific power input, oxygen transfer and impeller tip speed. However, there still exists a gap between the theory and practice of scale up. For example, in theory constant power input per unit volume is assumed to be very useful in earlier practice of penicillin fermentation but in reality P_g/V is normally not a constant. In the light of failures of scale up of prototype into large systems more recent studies based on biological test systems suggest the need for serious engineering investigations on more precise biological data for use as scale up criteria. General data from industrial plants need to be correlated with hydrodynamic specifications. When these data are available scale up of bioreactors would be more realistic.

8.4.1 Microbial Process Scale up Example

Production of kilogram quantities of daunorubicin an antibiotic for cancer chemo therapy has been produced by a *Streptomycete* fermentation scale up procedure as shown in Fig. 8.3 flow chart. In the scale up of this process biotechnology in addition to fermenter operating parameter values shown in this figure, operating parameters values for the scale up/production fermenter are 1/2 *vvm* sparge rate, 10 psig back pressure, and 125 rpm (impeller tip speed of 750 ft/min). Under these parameteric conditions in the scale up fermenter, the sulfite oxidation rate in water is 2.0 m moles O_2 l^{-1} min^{-1}. A time course of a typical daunorubicin scale up fermenter (10,000 l) run is shown in Fig.8.4. The results indicated that harvest titers in the scale up fermenter have increased from run to run. This was due to the fermentation improvement program including scale up strategy.

In non-Newtonian microbial fermentation process scale up considerations for fermentation mixer scale up play a key role.[34] In general, in the first stage in scale up procedure, only the gross responses of the microorganisms to the external environment are established.[5] Also, to minimize effort and material costs experiments are carried out in bench scale fermenters. However, the scale up relationships developed should be independent of scale, i.e. size of the fermenter/ bioreactor. Thus, the equipment used for the experiments should be selected or designed to ensure artifacts, for example, due to poor mixing are not inadvertently introduced into the results. Based on the results of experiments and an economic assessment, which takes into account the likely heat and mass transfer constraints of the large scale bioreactor, a scale up target for the process performance and the range of environmental conditions necessary to achieve the target is determined. The scale up

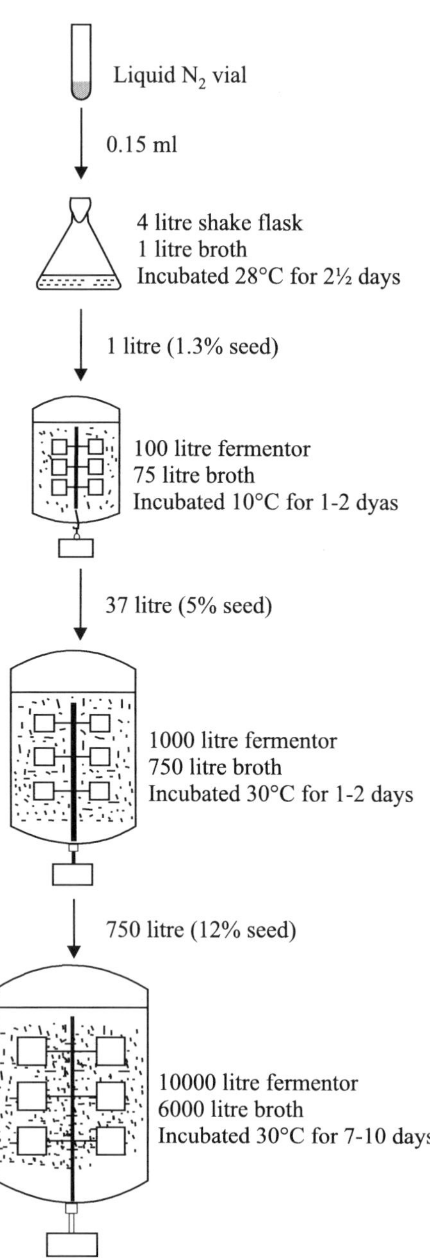

Fig. 8.3 Flowchart of basic fermentation process scale up[33]

process performance is usually specified in terms of one or more of the following: product concentration, productivity, yield of purity. However, classical scale up of process biotechnology is always associated with problems related to microkinetics, thermodynamics and transport phenomena.

Table 8.6 Selection of scale up criteria in bioprocessing industry

Criteria selected	% Scale up achieved
P_g/V (KW/m^3)	30
K_La (hr^{-1})	30
PO_2 (mM, ppm)	20
Tip speed (NDi)	20

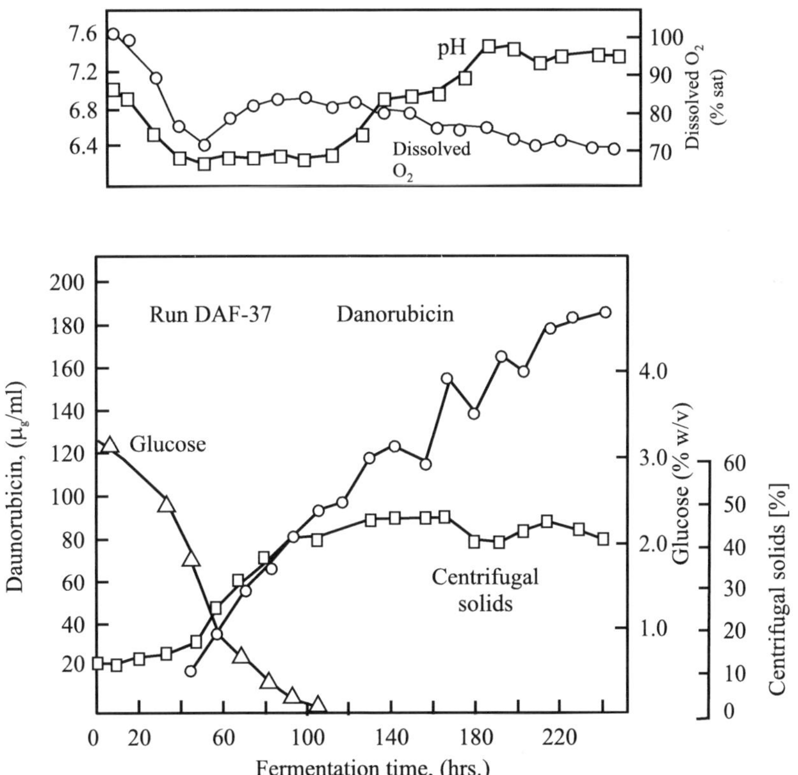

Fig 8.4 Time course of a typical daunorubicin production fermentation run in the 10.000 litre fermenter[33]

8.5 SCALE UP OF GENETICALLY ENGINEERED CELL CULTURE FERMENTATION[36]

One of the major breakthroughs of exploitation of genetically engineered cell culture fermentation is the development of a stable redesigned cell using recombinant plasmid vector for production of a metabolite in large scale fermenter. It involves keeping plasmid barriers most favourable in cell population when recombinant plasmid technique is used in fermentation industry. A typical series steps that has been followed in scale up of such host-vector fermentation process is as below.

(a) Transfer of cells asceptically from slant to conical flask in 20 ml of liquid medium.
(b) Transfer of inoculum from (a) in medium of larger conical flask (250-300 ml).
(c) Asceptic transfer of inoculum from (b) into the medium of a jar fermenter (101).
(d) The seed culture from (c) is transfered to a pilot scale fermenter (3000 l).
(e) Finally, from the seed culture vessel in (d) the transfer was made asceptically into the production scale fermenter (100,000 I) medium.

Considering inoculum size in each step is 3% v/v, the number of cell generations (*n*) needed from step to step may be computed to be 5 and supposing that cells to be harvested in each culture be around 1.0 ($\approx 0.03 \times 2^5$) the total number of n required for scale up would be

$$n = \frac{\ln 2}{\ln \dfrac{N}{N_0}}$$

In case of rDNA (recombinant DNA) fermenter scale up with physical containment requirement, however, the pilot plant is generally considered to be large scale (greater than 10 l). The host-vector system to be used mainly determines the level of physical containment required. As per NIH guidelines of 1978 for recombinant DNA research, genetically engineered cell fermentation scale up is restricted to 10 L or less in P-3 level containment conditions.[37]

Scale Down

By scale down it is meant in bioprocessing that a microbial production rate of a specific metabolite in a full scale plant is reproduced by some means to pilot plant vessels (i.e. transfer from production scale to pilot scale maintaining some criteria constant). Identities in both systems/scales with respect to time dependence of sugar consumption rate, pH, dissolved oxygen concentration etc. must be underlying the identity of product accumulation pattern.

Criteria: Referring to the criteria on scale up one may choose again either one of the following as constant

(i) power input per unit volume of liquid
(ii) shear rate of impeller
(iii) volumetric oxygen transfer coefficient
(iv) momentum transfer etc.

in scale down.

However, a proper selection can not be made a priori, because a direct correlation between microbial activity and environmental conditions, which are represented by the above scale up (and/or scale down) criteria still seems prohibitive.

8.6 REFERENCES

1. Aiba, S., A.E Humphrey and N.F. Millis, *Biochemical Engineering*, 2nd edn. Univ. Tokyo Press, Tokyo, 1973
2. Bailey, J.E. and D.F. Ollis, *Biochemical Engineering Fundamentals*, 2nd edn. McGraw Hill Book Co., New York, 1986.
3. Ghose,T.K. and S.N. Mukhopadhyay, *Bioreactors- Recent Advances*, Lecture delivered at the Sympo. Heterogeneous Reactions-Science and Practice, 32nd Annual Meeting, I.I.Ch.E., IIT Bombay,1979.
4. Mukhopadhyay, S.N. and D.K. Das, *Oxygen Responses, Reactivities and Measurements in Biosystems*, CRC Press, Boca Raton, Florida, 1994.
5. Shular, M.L. and F. Kargi, *Bioprocess Engineering: Basic Concepts*, Prentice Hall, Englewood Cliffs, N.J., 1992.
6. Blakebrough, N. and K. Sambamurthy, "Mass Transfer and Mixing Rates in Fermentation Vessels", *Biotechnol. and Bioengg* pp 8, 25-44, 1966.
7. Bajpai,R.K., A.Prokop and D. Ramakrishna, "Dispersions in Hydrocarbon Fermentation: A Retrospective Study", *Biotechnol. and Bioengg*. pp 17, 541-556, 1975.
8. Khang, S.J. and O. Levenspiel, "The Mixing Rate Number in Chem. Engg." pp 141-143, 1976.
9. Corrigan, A.H., "Bioreactors for Mammalian Cells", *Mammalian Cell Biotechnology—A Practical Approach*, pp 139-158, (M. Butler ed.), IRL Press/Oxford Univ. Press, Oxford, 1991.
10. Vogelmann, H. "Aspects on Scale up and Mass Cultivation of Plant Tissue Culture", *Advances in Biotechnol*, pp 117-122, (M. MooYoung, Gen.ed.), Pergamon Press, Toronto, 1981.
11. Winkler, M.A. "Application of the Principles of Fermentation Engineering to Biotechnology",*Principles of Biotechnology,* pp 94-143,(A Wisemann ed.), Surrey Univ. Press, N.Y, 198.
12. Rushton, J.H., E. W. Costich and H.J. Everett, "Power Characteristics of Mixing Impellers" *Chem. Eng. Prog*. pp 46,467, 1950.
13. Cooper, C.M., G.A. Fernstrom and S.A. Miller, "Performance of Agitated Gas-liquid Contactors", *Ind. Eng. Chem*. pp 36, 504, 1944.
14. Ohyama, Y. and K. Endoh; Power Characteristics of Gas-liquid Contacting Mixers", *Chem. Eng*. (Japan), pp 19, 12, 1955.
15. Michel, B.J. and S.A. Miller "Power Requirements of Gas-liquid Agitated Systems", *A.I.Ch.E. Jr*, pp 8,262, 1962.
16. Rushton, J.H. "How to Make Use of Recent Mixing Developments", *Chem. Engr. Prog*. pp 50, 587-89,1954.
17. Bates, R.L., P.L. Fondy and Corpstein., *Ind. Eng.Chem.: Process Design Develop*. Vol 2. pp 310, 1963.
18. Cooke, M. "Application of Model Suspensions in the Design of Fermenters", *Processing of Solid-liquid Suspensions*, (P.A. Shamloe ed.), Butterworth-Heinemann Ltd, 1993.
19. Arathoon, W.R. and J.R. Birch, "Large Scale Cell Culture in Biotechnology", *Science*, pp 23, 1390-95, 1986.

20. Glacken,M.W., R.J. Fleischaker and S. Sinskey, "Mammalian Cell Culture Engineering: Principles and Scale up", *TIBTECH*, pp l(4), 100-108, 1985.
21. Mukhopadhyay, A., S.N. Mukhopadhyay and G.P. Talwar, "Influence of Serum Proteins on the Kinetics of Attachment of Vero Cells to Cytodex Microcarriers", *J. Chem. Tech. Biotechnol.*, pp 56, 369-74, 1993.
22. Mukhopadhyay, A., S.N. Mukhopadhyay and G.P. Talwar; "Studies on the Synthesis of βhCG Hormone in Vero Cells by Recombinant Vaccine Virus", *Biotechnol. and Bioengg.*, pp 48(2), 158-68, 1995.
23. Mukhopadhyay, A. "Microcarrier Culture of Vero Cells for Bioprocessing of βhCG Expressed by Recombinant Vaccinia Virus", *Ph.D. Thesis*, IIT Delhi, 1996.
24. Annis, J.G., M.S. Croughan, D.I.C. Wang and J. Goldstein, *Biotechnol. and Bioengg. Sympo.*, pp 17, 699- 723, 1986.
25. Bliem, R. and H. Katinger, "Scale up Engineering in Animal Cell Technology", Part I, *TIBTECH*, pp 6, 190- 193, 1988
26. Lavery, M. and A. W. Nienow, *Biotechnol. & Bioengg.*, pp 30, 368-73, 1987
27. Corrigan, A.H., S.Nikolay and S.Zhang, "Rationalization of the Design of High Density Perfusion Cultures for Suspended Animal Cells", *Animal Cell Technology*, pp 309-312, (R.E.Spier, J.B.Griffiths and W. Berthold eds.) Butterworth-Heinemann Ltd., Oxford, 1994.
28. Anderson, L.A., J.D. Phillipson and M.F. Roberts "Aspects of Alkaloid Production by Plant Cell Cultures", *Secondary Metabolism in Plant Cell Cultures*, pp1-4,(P.Morris, A.H. Scragg, A. Staffordand M.W. Fowler eds.), Cambridge Univ. Press, Cambridge, London, 1986.
29. Goldstein, W.E. "Large Scale Processing of Plant Cell Culture", *Annals,* pp 394-408, N.Y.A.S., 1984.
30. Panda, A.K., S. Mishra, V.S. Bisaria and S.S. Bhojwani, "Plant Cell Reactors—A Perspective", *Enz. Microbiol. Technol*. pp11, 386-97, 1989.
31. Pace, G.W. *Scale up Of Fermentation Processes*, pp 249-63,On line Pub. Printer, U.K., 1985.
32. Higglin M., J.E. Prenosil and J.R. Borne; *Proc. 4rth Euro. Cong. on Biotechnol.* Vol.2, pp 400, Elsevier. Chem. Eng. Dept. (TLC), SFIT Zurich, 1982.
33. Hemilton, B., R. White, J. McGuire, P. Montgomery, B. Stroshane, C. Kalita and R. Pandey, "Improvement of the Daunorubicin Fermentation at 10,000 Liter Fermenter Scale", *Advances in Biotechnol*. M. Moo Young (Gen ed). Vol. I. Pergamon Press, Toronto, pp 63-68, 1981.
34. Oldshue, J .Y. "Some Scale up Considerations for Fermentation Mixers", *Advances in Biotechnol.* Vol.1, pp 517-522, (M. Moo Young. Gen.ed.), Pergamon Press, 1981.
35. Kossen, N.W.F. "Problems in the Design of Large-scale Bioreactors" , *Biotechnology and Bioprocess Engineering*, pp 365-380 (T.K. Ghose ed.), United India Press, Link House, New Delhi,1985.
36. Imanaka, T. and S. Aiba, *A Perspective on Application of Genetic Engineering: Stability of Recombinant Plasmid*, pp 369, N.Y. Acad. Sci., 1981.
37. W.L. Muth, "Scale up Biotechnology Safely", *CHEMTECH*, pp 352-61, June 1985.

Chapter 9

BIOPRODUCTS: MODERN ESTIMATION AND BIOASSAY

9.1 INTRODUCTION

In the progress of bioengineering and biotechnology, measurement/assay of bioproducts is very important. Most large scale oxic bioprocesses like fermentations are complex and difficult to optimize. As a typical example, the production of a typical secondary metabolite like antibiotic involves the growth of a mycelial culture on an assortment of nutrients. In many cases these nutrients include starch, soyabean meal, vegetable oil, yeast extracts, etc, which are not well defined in composition and are often insoluble. Cell-nutrient interactions give rise to product. Analysis of individual interactions within the resulting biologically and chemically complex and physically viscous broth containing bioproduct is a difficult task. The bioproducts may appear in solution phase as well as in gas form. Many on line and off line biosensing instruments have been developed and used for measurement and analysis of bioproducts.[1-5]

9.2 ON LINE MS INSTRUMENTAL ANALYSIS

In on line systems environment and products need to be measured and are particularly valuable because the information can be sent directly to a computer. During production important environmental data analysed routinely throughout bioprocessing include dissolved oxygen (DO), pH and exhaust/effluent gas besides bioproduct(s). Measurement of many bioproducts could be done as described in Chapter 7, by sensing through oxygen probe biosensors (Table 7.3) having varying stability. Through years infrared analyser has been used to measure CO_2 concentration in bioprocessing exhaust gas. Similarly a paramagnetic analyser has been used to measure the O_2 concentration in bioreactor effluent gas. However, both instruments suffer from the same disadvantages, e.g. difficulty of maintenance, severe calibration drift and slow response time (r.t). One of the versatile instruments, e.g. mass spectrometer (MS) has been made available since the middle of the 1970's and improvised gradually. It has been used in bioproduct data analysis in more recent years. This more modern instrument runs unattended and measure CO_2, O_2, N_2 and many other volatile bioproducts with a high degree of accuracy. An illustration of measurement by GCMS is provided in the literature.

In principle the gas molecules entering the mass spectrometer are ionized and accelerated through a magnetic field. The flow paths of gas molecules of different masses bend to different degrees and are collected on prepositioned Faraday collector cups. An amplified signal output, proportional to the number of molecules collected, is sent to the process gas analysis instrument. The number of gas components that can be analysed depend on the preselection and analyser design. For fermentation process biotechnology CO_2, O_2 and N_2 are the essential gases to be estimated. In MS the response time of gas passing being fraction of a second for 0 to 90 percent response the analysis in the analyser is not only fast and specific but also has provision for on line data analysis of many process parameters, e.g. CO_2 concentration (CDC), oxygen concentration (xc, % O2), RQ, CO_2 evolution rate (CER), oxygen uptake rate (OUR), volumetric oxygen transfer coefficient (K_La), total oxygen consumed, cell dry weight and specific growth rate. In this instrument at room temperature the 90% restore time is defined by the length (L) and radius (r) of the tubing connecting the MS and the analysis probe by the relation below

$$t_{90} = 7.4 \times 10^{-5} L^2 r^{-1} \tag{9.1}$$

Here, t is in seconds and L and r are in centimeters. For instance, when L = 10 m and r = 0.8 cm, t_{90} = 90s consequently 2 minutes is a reasonable switching time where permanent gases are concerned.

Besides on line analysis of permanent gases and vapours (like ethanol, methanol, aldelydes, formic acid, propanol, acetone, butanol, acetic acid, butyric acid etc.) many non volatile components can be analysed off line.[3] Therefore the MS is a versatile instrument for both aerobic and anaerobic fermentation processes. Although this instrument is associated with many advantages in terms of accuracy calibration drift, response time, reliability, computer interfacing and operation, the major disadvantage lies in the fact that the instrument is expensive to purchase and its maintenance is complicated as well as expensive.

9.3 LIGHT SCATTERING INSTRUMENTAL ANALYSIS

The instruments like turbidometer, differential light scattering (DLS) photometer and quasielastic light scattering (QLS) photometer have been used for the estimation of cell/virus process parameters for different types of microorganisms and viruses.[3,5,7]

A list of these light scattering techniques for measuring/obtaining different informations is given in Table 9.1.

Table. 9.1 Light scattering instrumental analysis mode and available information

Analysis Mode	*Type of Microbial System*	*Measuring Item(s)*	*Need Information*	*Analytical Information (s) Obtained*
Turbidometric	Any Motile	Total loss in intensity through scattering	Refractive Index (R.I.) Increase	Molecular weight (M. Wt.)
DLS	Virus	Angular dependence of scattered intensity		M.Wt., radius of gyration second virial coefficient.
	Spore	"	–	R.I. Profile of internal structure.
QLS	Virus	Time resolved intensity fluctuations (TRIF)	Sedimentation coefficient	Translational diffusion coefficient (TDC) Rotational diffusion coefficient (RDC)
	Spore	"	"	TDC
		Angular dependence of TRIF	"	Asymetric internal structure
	Motile cells	TRIF	–	Velocity distribution effects of environmental conditions

For more than four decades this analytical estimation has been useful for elucidating the conformation of biomolecular systems in solution. The estimation techniques involving the elastic or quasielastic scattering of visible radiation have been applied mainly to the study of the mass and gross conformation of biological macromolecules in solution. For example, a widely used light scattering (differential) equipment has been the 'Zimm plot' method.[8] This method has been used to determine the molecular weight, radius of gyration, and second virial coefficient of a wide range of biopolymeric molecules.

In simplest light scattering estimation of turbidity of a suspension of cells, the total loss of intensity is measured through scattering of the incident beam, using a conventional spectrophotometer. In fact this is a 'Zero Scattering angle' measurement. So, turbidity provides a conventional way of measuring the relative molecular mass, M_r of biomolecular assemblies (with $M_r \geq 10^6$) including viruses, yeasts, bacteria etc. Based on Rayleigh-Gaus-Debye (RGD) approximation and Camerini-Otero-Debye (COD) concept the value of M_r has been correlated with turbidity (τ) of the cell suspension. The value of M_r measured at a finite concentration needs to be extrapolated to infinite dilution and expressed by the following relation in which C is the

$$M_r^{-1} = HQ \lim_{c \to 0} \left(\frac{C}{\tau} \right) \quad (9.2)$$

cell concentration (gl^{-1}), $\tau = 2.303$ (O.D.), H is a factor dependent on R.I. (n), wave length (λ) in vacuo (λ_0) and integrating Avogadro number (N_A). The factor Q is defined as particle dissipation factor depending primarily on the size and shape of the cellular particles. This method has been applied to a range of bacteriophages (T_2, T_4, T_5 and λ) to determine their molecular weights and also has been compared with values determined by other methods, which showed accuracy better than ± 10%.

The simple useful turbidimetry has been applied to both the vegetative cells and spores of bacteria with the aim of (i) estimating the concentrations of microorganisms and (ii) estimating their masses. Therefore, this technique monitors changes in cell number and mass. The DLS method has also been a valuable technique for determining M_r of viruses and bacteria using laser light source. The advantages of lasers over traditional light sources are very high intensity, high collimation and narrow spread of wavelength, which give much improved angular resolution in intensity envelopes. The basic equation for angular dependence of light scattering by cells is given by

$$\frac{KC}{R_\theta} = \frac{1}{P(\theta)} \left\{ \frac{1}{M_r} + BC \right\} \quad (9.3)$$

Here R_θ is called the 'Raleigh Ratio' which is determined by

$$R_\theta = \frac{I_\theta \, r^2}{I_0 \, (1 + \cos^2 \theta)} \quad (9.4)$$

in which r is the hydrodynamic radius of the cell particles (microms), I_0 is the scattering intensity at scattered angle θ. In equation (9.3) K is related as below,

$$K = \frac{2\pi^2 \, n_0^2 \, (\delta n/\delta c)^2}{N_A \, \lambda_0^4} \quad (9.5)$$

where n_0 is the R.I. in vacuo, $\frac{\delta n}{\delta c}$ is the refractive index increment, P(θ) is the ratio of the actual scattered intensity without interference. The value of P(θ) depends on the shape of the scattering cell particle or for flexible particles on the average shape. Based on RGD scatters, such as viruses, its value is seen to be related to the root mean square (rms) radius about the centre of mass of the virus, R_g. Thus the value of P(θ) is

$$P(\theta) = 1 - \frac{16\pi^2}{3\lambda^2} R_g^{\,2} \sin^2(\theta/2) + O(\theta)^2 \quad (9.6)$$

Use of this relation is consistent, no error is introduced and has been done in form of a biaxial extrapolation, 'Zimm plot' which shows a log relation of (C/R_θ) in the ordinate and $\left[\sin^2 \theta/2 + 1 \times 10^2\, C\right]$ in the abscissa. The 'Zimm plot' carried out for vaccinia virus generated parametric values for this biosystem as given in Table 9.2. DLS technique has been used for application to bacteria like *Serratia marcescens* also.

9.4 CHROMATOGRAPHIC INSTRUMENTAL ANALYSIS [9-11]

In chromatographic instrumental analysis chromatographic separations involve the retardation and separation of solutes from each other while flowing through a porous media by some carrier fluid. Depending on the dominant interactions chromatographic separation can be of several

Table 9.2 'Zimm plot' parameters

Biosystem	M_r *(Relative Molecular Mass)*	*X(g)*	R_g*(nm)*	*Hydrodynamic Diameter*	*Ref.*
Vaccinia virus	$2.7 \pm 2 \times 10^9$	$4.5 \pm 0.3 \times 10^{-15}$	144 ± 2	373 ± 4	8
Serratia marcescens	1.0×10^{11}	1.7×10^{-13}	340	880	11

processes. For example, the separation by ion exchange chromatography relies on the electrostatic interaction between a charged molecule (e.g. protein) and a stationary ion exchange resin carrying a charge of opposite sign. In this resolutional analysis for molecular separation, selecting a column begins with understanding that it is composed of two parts. The first is the resoluting packing material and second the container (stainless steel or plastic wall). The goal of all separations in this instrumental analysis is resolution of peaks as related by the resolution equation.

$$R = \left(\frac{\sqrt{N}}{4}\right)\left(\frac{\alpha - 1}{\alpha}\right)\left(\frac{K_2'}{K_2' + 1}\right) \tag{9.7}$$

where α is the selectivity, N is efficiency, giving the number of theoretical plates and K'_2 is the capacity factor of the later eluting compound. Here

$$\alpha = \frac{K_2'}{K_1'} = \frac{V_2 - V_0}{V_1 - V_0} = \text{Selectivity}$$

$$K'_2 = \frac{V_2 - V_0}{V_0} = \text{Capacity factor}$$

and

$$N = 16\left(\frac{V_2}{W_2}\right)^2 = \text{Efficiency}$$

In the above relations V_0 is the volume of the system, V_1 and V_2 are the retention volumes at the apex of each peak, W_i is the peak width (i = 1, 2, ...etc), K' is the measure of retention, α describes the relative retention of the components by the stationary phase and N relates band broadening and retention volume. In HPLC α and K' are the major controlling influences on resolution. Most HPLC packings today are made from silica, a durable and economical adsorbent.

The advantages of using high performance liquid chromatography (HPLC) in experiments like cloning include increased speed of separation, increased resolving power and increased cloning efficiencies. In experiments where all vectors, linkers and DNA fragments to be inserted into the vectors were purified by HPLC stearic exclusion chromatography. Cloning could yield the number of transformants per microgram of vector DNA which was nearly 100 fold as measured by HPLC. Separation of tRNA molecules and restriction fragments by HPLC is now in common use. This separation based on size does not, of course, separate the individual tRNA species. Reverse phase chromatography on octadecyl silica column, equilibrated with ammonium acetate buffers, has achieved separation of individual tRNA species to a limited extent. Usually tRNAs are eluted and separated by an acetonitrite gradient.

More recent developments in HPLC estimation technology used for bioproducts relates to protein engineering cloning experiments. In this amino acid sequence of a known protein is especially redesigned in a predetermined manner at one or more amino acid residues. The purified cloned DNA specifying a protein is altered in a defined manner biochemically and this redesigned DNA will then direct the synthesis of the desired modified protein when expressed in the usual microbial culture.

9.5 FLOW INJECTION INSTRUMENTAL ANALYSIS (FIIA) [12-15]

The characteristic of FIIA is based primarily on a combination of the following aspects:

(a) Reproducible injection of the sample to be analysed into a nonsegmented continuously flowing carrier stream.

(b) Control of the dispersion of the injected sample on its way from the point of injection to the detector.

Disperson is the diffusion and dilution of the sample in the chosen system. Also, the dispersion degree allows the calculation of the necessary reagent concentrations and the optimization of the system regarding sensitivity and sample throughout. The techniques of FIIA systems are predominantly used as automated continuous flow analyzers, operating with well established methods for providing rapid and reliable results. One of the examples of FIIA system is "The Aquatech System." It is a modular and fully integrated microprocessor controlled FIIA system. In operation it includes fully automatic operation and data reporting. It consists of a specific controller and analyser with a built in detector unit (spectrophotometer, 400-600 nm) and a specific sampler. This system could be operated with manual or automatic sample introduction. The chemical manifold in this instrument is an integral part of the 'Method cassette'. Each dedicated 'Method cassette' contains the chemical manifold, optimized preinstalled pump, tubes and reagent bottles. This feature and construction allows for a very quick change of analysis.

In most of the analytical laboratories FIIA systems are mainly used as automated continuous flow analysers, operating with well established methods and providing rapid and reproducible results. In such analysis a reaction column can be integrated into a normal FIIA system at the , required point. There are a number of literature reports where immobilized enzymes have been used in reaction column. A typical example is provided in the following (Fig. 9.1) flow scheme for FIIA determination of starch in grain and feed using reaction columns with immobilized enzymes. The original sample for FIIA analysis was treated with termamyl (amylase) at 95°C. Various components are shown in Fig. 9.1.

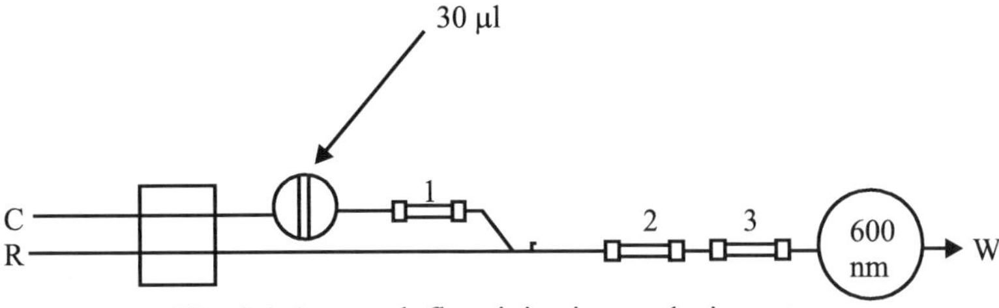

Fig. 9.1 Aquatech flow injection analysis system

A list summerizing few areas for which FIIA application data are available is given in Table 9.3.

Table 9.3 Few claimed application areas of FIIA

Assay Species	*Area of Application*		
	Water	*Agriculture*	*Food/Fermentation*
Alkalinity	Drinking/Waste	–	–
Copper	Waste, Sea	Plant	Fruits
Bitterness	–	–	Beer
Calcium	Drinking	Feed, Soil, Plant	Milk
Manganese	Drinking	Plant	Coffee, Rice
Nitrate	Drinking/Waste/Surface	Fertilizer	Milk
Urea	Drinking	Feed, Fertilizer	–

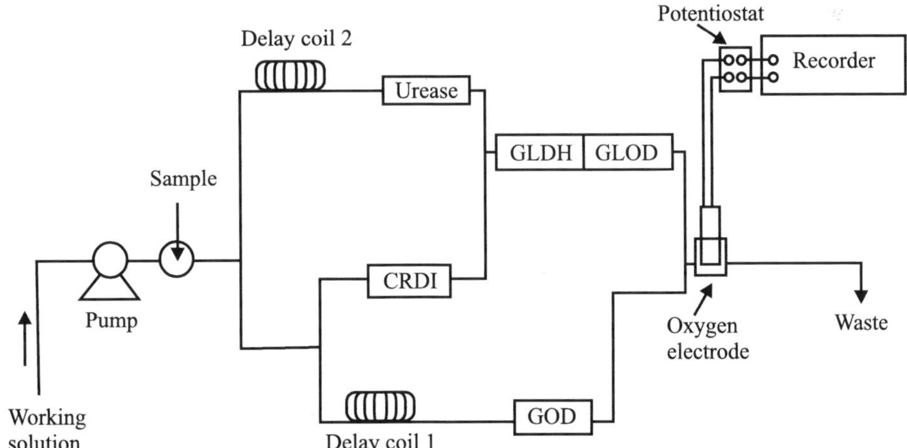

Fig. 7.2 Schematic diagram of the FIIA system for the simultaneous determination of urea, creatinine and glucose. Size of enzyme reactors and delay coils (i.d. × length, mm); GOD 2.4 × 46; CRDI 3.4 × 20; urease 3.4 × 23; GLDH 3.4 × 30; GLOD 3.4 × 20; delay coil 1, 0.8 × 1200; delay coil 2, 0.8 × 1500. Enzyme reactors and oxygen electrode were kept at 25°C with a water bath. Samples (50μl) were injected with a microsyringe through the injection port. Total flow rate was 2.0 ml/min. Working solution: 67 mM phosphate buffer (pH 8.0) containing 0.1 mM EDTA, 0.3 mM NADH and 5 mM 2-oxoglutarate

More recently, an amperometric flow injection biosensor has been developed consisting of three channel FIIA system. This FIIA system involved a peristaltic pump, an injection port, enzyme reactor, a galvanic oxygen probe with a flow cell, a potentiostat and a 3-pen recorder. This FIIA system was developed in Japan which has a schematic diagram as shown in Fig. 9.2. This system was used for simultaneous estimation of urea, creatinine and glucose with a single sample injection and one recorder. In this FIIA system the flow stream was split into three channels with a four direction connection after the sample injection. The channels involved urease and creatine deiminase (CRDI) for rejoining before L-glutamate dehydrogenase GLDH/ GLOD (L-glutamate oxidase). The mixed flow was further joined with GOD (Glucose oxidase) channel before electrode. For obtaining separate peaks corresponding to each channel, two delay coils of different lengths were set as in Fig. 9.2. Developments in FIIA Systems are occurring very fast.

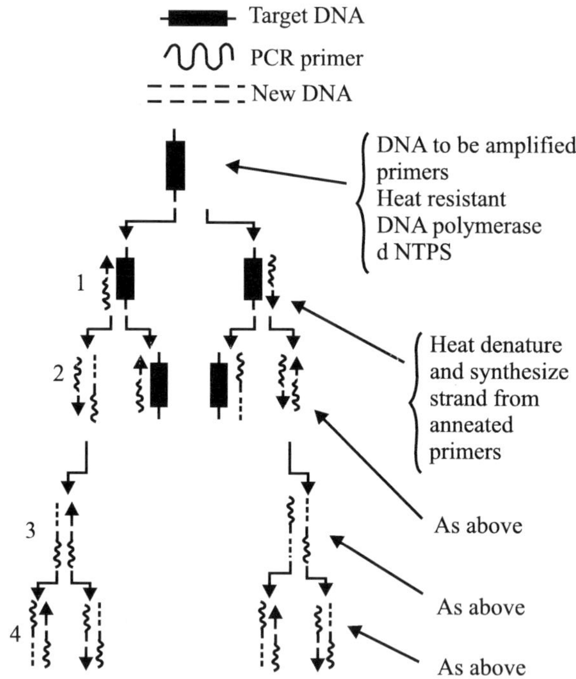

Fig. 9.3 Polymerase chain reaction (PCR): The basic technique

9.6 PCR INSTRUMENTAL ANALYSIS[16,17]

In 1984 a team of scientists in Cetus Corporation developed the method of polymerase chain reaction (PCR). This method can produce large amounts of a specific DNA fragment from a complex DNA in a simple enzymatic reaction. The method is unique in selectivity, sensitivity and speed. It was devised quite a few years ago. It involves an oligonucleotide-mediated enzymic amplification of a sample sequence in genomic DNA, resulting in an exponential increase of target DNA copies. In PCR instrumental analysis a DNA polymerase (usually the temperature stable *Taq* DNA polymerase) and dNTP are used to replicate a segment in a double stranded DNA, the procedure is carried out in presence of a large excess of two different synthetic oligonueleotides (extension primers), which anneal to the two sites flanking the segment of interest to initiate the replication. This method is based on the cyclic repetition of a set of basic three steps. The first step of the reaction is annealing of the oligonucleotide primers to denatured (95°C single stranded) genomic DNA followed by extension with Klenow DNA polymerase and deoxynucleotide triphosphates. In the second step temperature is lowered (37 to 72°C, depending on experimental condition and purpose) to allow annealing of the primers to the separated strands of the DNA. In the third step DNA polymerase-mediated extension of the primer-template complex is allowed to proceed 1 to 4 min. at 72°C. This three step cycle is repeated in succession for 25 to 30 cycles.

PCR analysis has been used for RNA blot analysis (Northern, Western and Southern blottings), m-RNA phenotyping, and nuclease protection analysis for the study of short lived, low copy number m-RNA transcripts. Essential power of PCR method: (1) It is possible to amplify any small segment of DNA (e.g. < 5kb) if the 18-28 bp sequences at either end of the DNA sequence to be amplified are known. (2) Ready changes can be made in the flanking ends of the amplified genes to introduce suitable restriction endonuclease sites without the need for the extra steps involved in the site directed mutagenesis techniques. A schematic of the method is shown in Fig. 9.3.

9.7 FEW BIOASSAY PROCEDURES[18-25]

9.7.1 Antibiotic Bioassay Method[18]

1. Agar diffusion

In this method of bioassay of antibiotics first a standard dose response profile between known stock solution of antibiotic and dilutions is prepared. For example in penicillin bioassay a stock solution of Na-penicillin G (1 mg/ml) is prepared in 0.1 M phosphate buffer (pH 7.0). The stock solution is diluted with phosphate buffer to 5 different concentrations within the range of 1.0-5.0 µg/ml.

For bioassay an inoculum is prepared. A slant culture (24 hr.) of *Bacillus subtilis* is transferred to 50 ml of nutrient broth bioassay medium in a 250 ml Erlenmeyer flask (sterile). It is incubated at 37°C for 24 hrs. The cells are thoroughly shaken for preparing a homogeneous suspension. The bioassay medium consisted of beef extract 0.3 g, peptone 0.5 g, glucose 1.0 gm, agar 3% and water 100 ml (distilled). In each test tube 15 ml of this medium is transferred, plugged with cotton and then sterilized at 15 psi pressure in autoclave for 15 minutes and cooled to room temperature.

In each test tube containing sterilized molten agar medium at normal temperature 0.5 ml of inoculum is transferred asceptically. The tubes are shaken and then poured into each petridish (4"dia). When the medium gets set, 5 cups are cut with the help of a sterilized cork borer (12 mm media). Experiment in triplicate is performed. In different cup of the same petri dish 0.5 ml of penicillin standard of different concentrations is poured. Five different concentrations are used on the same petriplate. The petriplate are kept in a refrigerator for 1 hr and then put in incubator at 37°C for 18-24 hrs.

After incubation the zone of inhibition of bacterial growth is measured with a mm scale. A standard dose-response plot is prepared with zone of inhibition of the microorganism as the ordinate and different concentrations of penicillin as the abscissa. The same procedure is followed for an unknown concentration of penicillin sample. Knowing its zone of inhibition, its concentration is determined from the standard plot.

2. Serial dilution

In this bioassay all steps are as above excepting that method of assay is as follows. Different volumes of nutrient medium (9.1, 9.2, 9.3, 9.4, 9.5, 9.6, 9.7, 9.8, 9.9 and 10 ml) are taken separately in 10 test tubes and are sterilized. Zero to 1.0 ml of antibiotic stock solution (0.2 mg/ml) is added to each test tube so as to make a final volume of 10 ml. One drop of inoculum is then introduced to tubes with the help of a pipette and then thoroughly mixed. The tubes are then incubated at 37°C for 18-24 hrs. Observation is made for the lowest concentration of the antibiotic that would inhibit bacterial growth. Results are tabulated under the heads as given below.

Tube No.	*Vol. of Antibiotic Solution (ml)*	*Volume of Medium (ml)*	*Concentration of Antibiotic (µg/ml)*	*Growth + ve or – ve*

9.7.2 Bioassay of Vitamins

1. Vitamin B_{12}

For bioassay of vitamin B_{12} a mutant strain of *E. coli* is cultured at 37°C on agar slant medium having following composition: Acid casein hydrolyzate–6.0 g, K_2HPO_4–0.2 g, $MgSO_4\ 7H_2O$ – 0.2 g, $FeSO_4\ 7H_2O$ – 5.0 mg, L-Asparagine – 0.15 g, Vitamin B_{12} – 0.4 mg and Distilled water–1 liter. The constituent minus vit. B_{12} are dissolved by gently heating with a few drops of HCl to dissolved the asparagine. The pH is adjusted to 7.2 ± 0.1 and heated slightly. Next 2.5% agar is added and the solution steamed to dissolve it. 400 microgram of vitamin is then added and after thorough mixing the medium is dispensed in the test tubes (sterile) in amounts of 5 ml, plugged and sterilized at 15 psig for 15 mins.

A 24 hrs subculture of the organism from the agar stant is grown in a 250 ml flask containing 50 ml sterile medium (peptone 2.0g, NaCl 0.5g, distilled water 200 ml, pH 7.2) broth and shaken on a rotary shaker for 24 hrs at 37°C.

For actual bioassay 100 ml of bacterial suspension is mixed with 15 ml of molten assay medium (45°C) having composition as given in the Table 9.4. It is placed in a petridish. After the medium sets filter paper discs (10-12 mm dia) saturated with the vitamin B_{12} solution of different concentrations (range 0.2-1.6 microgram/ml) are placed on the surface of seeded agar plate. 4 to 5 discs are used per plate. The petriplates are kept for 1 hr at 0°C and then inculcated at 37°C for 24 hrs. Next after incubation zone diameter of growth are measured and a standard plot of zone diameter vs conc. of vitamin B_{12} is prepared.

Table 9.4 Composition of bioassay medium of vitamin B_{12}

K_2HPO_4	—	7.0 g
KH_2PO_4	—	3.0 g
Na-citrate	—	0.5 g
$MgSO_4$, $7H_2O$	—	0.1 g
Dextrose	—	10.0 g
Glycine	—	0.1 g
Asparagine	—	4.0 g
Arginine	—	0.1 g
Histidine	—	0.1 g
Glutamic acid	—	0.1 g
Proline	—	0.1 g
Tryptophane	—	0.1 g
Agar	—	2.5 %
Na-thioglycollate	—	0.1 g
Distilled water	—	11.0 *l*
pH	—	6.8
Sterilized at	—	10 psi for 10 mins.

2. Bioassay of biotin

Assay range > 0 to 0.2 μg/ml.

Assay organism: Lactobacillus arabinosus

(*i*) *Preparation of the Inoculum* : Transfer a loopful of the assay organism to inoculum broth (Yeast extract 20.0 g; Proteosepeptone 5.0 g; Dextrose 10.0 g; KH_2PO_4 2.0 g; Water 1000 ml, autoclave at 121°C for 15 min). Incubate at 25-37°C for 16-24 hrs. Centrifuge under asceptic conditions, resuspend in 10 ml of sterile isotonic saline. Dilute 1 in 100 ml physiological saline. One drop of the diluted suspension is added per tube.

(*ii*) *Preparation of the Standard Curve* : It is essential that standard is run every time as assay is made (conditions of autoclaving and incubating affect the turbidity readings).

(*iii*) *Biotin Standard* : Prepare a main stock of 100. μg/ml (dissolve 0.1 g of biotin in 1000 ml. H_2O). Dilute 1 ml of the main stock to 100 ml to get the first working standard (1 μ/ml). Dilute 1 ml of the first working standard to 500 ml to get the second working standard (2 mμ/ml). To get the final working standard dilute 20 ml to 100 ml (0.4 mμ g biotin/ml). Dissolve carefully if necessary boil for a few minutes. Add 5.0 ml per tube; add the appropriate amount of the biotin standard, and sufficient water to make volume to 10.0 ml.

Assay Medium :

Vitamin free-casaminoacids	12.0	L-cystine	0.2
Dextrose	40.0	Tryptophane	0.2
Sod. Acetate	20.0	Adenine sulfate	0.02
K_2HPO_4	1.0	Guanine HCl	0.02
KH_2PO_4	1.0	Uracil	0.02
$MgSO_4$	0.4	Thiamine	0.002
NaCl	0.02	Riboflavine	0.002
$FeSO_4$	0.02	Niacine	0.002
$MnSO_4$	0.02	Pyridoxine HCl	0.004
		p-aminobenzoic acid	0.0002
		Calcium pantothenate	0.002
		Distilled water	1000 ml

The Standard Curve :

Tube No.	*ml of Final Working Standard (0.4 μm/ml)*	*Distilled H O*	*Biotin/ mμ/ml.*	*Per Tube mμ*
1, 2	0.0	5.0	0.0	0.0
3, 4	0.0	5.0	0.0	0.0
5, 6	0.5	4.5	0.02	0.2
7, 8	1.0	4.0	0.04	0.4
9, 10	1.5	3.5	0.06	0.6
11, 12	2.0	3.0	0.08	0.8
13, 14	2.5	2.5	0.1	1.0
15, 16	3.0	2.0	0.12	1.2
17, 18	4.0	1.0	0.16	1.6
19, 20	5.0	0.0	0.20	2.0

Plug and autoclave the tubes at 121°C (15 psig for 15 min) avoid over sterilising.

Use tubes 1 and 2 as uninoculated controls to adjust for blank. Inoculate each tube with 1 drop of inoculum. Incubate at 30°C for 16-20 hrs. After incubation refrigerate for 2 hrs to arrest growth. Read turbidity at 540 mμ.

To assay an unknown, it is better to check with 3 to 4 concentrations. Prepare suitable dilutions of the sample to get an approximate biotin concentration of 0.2 mμ/ml.

Tube No.	*ml of Sample Solution*	*Distilled H_2O*
21, 22	0.0	5.0
23, 24	1.0	4.0
25, 26	2.0	3.0
27, 28	3.0	2.0
29, 30	5.0	0.0

As usual the total volume per tube is 10 ml. Inoculate with one drop of inoculum and proceed as above. Calculate the exact amount of biotin with the help of the standard curve.

9.7.3 Bioassay of Aminoacid

1. Lysine bioassay [19,20]

Assay organism: Leuconostoc mesenteroides p 60
Assay range: > 0.0 to 30.0 μ/ml.

Preparation of the Inoculum : Methods are similar as in the case of biotin, except for the assay organism.
The Standard Curve :
Standard lysine: Dissolve 0.30 g of L-lysine in 500 ml of H_2O (stock solution of 600 μ/ml). Dilute 10 ml to 100 ml (60 μ/ml).

Assay Medium (mg):

Dextrose	50.0	dl-Alanine	0.4	Proline	0.2
Sod. Acetate	40.0	Arginine HCl	0.484	Serine	0.1
Amm. Chloride	6.0	Asparagine	0.8	Threonine	0.4
KH_2PO_4	1.2	Aspartic acid	0.2	Serine	0.08
K_2HPO_4	1.2	α-Cystine	0.1	Tyrosine	0.2
$MgSO_4$	0.4	Glutamic acid	0.6	Valine	0.5
$FeSO_4$	0.02	Glycine	0.2	Adenine SO_4	0.02
$MnSO_4$	0.04	Histidine HCl	0.124	Guanine HCl	0.02
NaCl	0.02	dl-Phenylanine	0.2	Uracil	0.02
		Thiamine HCl	0.001	Xanthine	0.02
		Pyrodoxine HCl	0.002	Methionine	0.02
		Pyridoxiamine HCl	0.0006	Isoleucine	0.05
		Pyridoxal HCl	0.0006	Leucine	0.05
		Ca-pantothenate	0.001	Water	1000 ml.
		Riboflavine	0.001		
		Nicotinic acid	0.002		
		p-Aminobenzoic acid	0.0002		
		Biotin	0.002		
		Folic acid	0.02		

Tube in 5.0 ml amounts.

(*i*) *Preparation of the Standard Curve* : Prepare tubes containing 0.0 to 30.0 μ/ml of lysinetube with suitable controls.

Tube No.	*Volume of Standard*	*Vol.* H_2O	*Conc. of Lysine μg/ml*
1, 2	0.0	5.0	0.0
3, 4	0.0	5.0	0.0
5, 6	0.5	4.5	3.0
7, 8	1.0	4.0	6.0
9, 10	1.5	3.5	9.0
11, 12	2.0	3.0	12.0
13, 14	2.5	2.5	15.0
15, 16	3.0	2.0	18.0
17, 18	4.0	1.0	24.0
19, 20	5.0	0.0	30.0

Keep tubes 1 and 2 as uninoculated controls.

(*ii*) *Preparation of the Unknown* : Dilute the unknown to come within the assay range. If approximate assay is known, prepare at least 3 different concentrations about the middle of the assay range. Add suitable concentrations and make up the volume to 10.0 ml in each tube. Sterilize by autoclaving at 121°C fcr 10 min.

(*iii*) *Assaying the Unknown* : Inoculate each tube with a drop of the made up culture suspension. Incubate at 35-37°C for 16-24 hrs. After incubation arrest growth by chilling the tubes and read turbidity at 600 nm.

Maintenance of Stock Culture : The assay organisms can be obtained from National College of Industrial Microorganisms, (N.C.L.) Pune. They can be conveniently maintained in the following medium :

Yeast extract	20.00
Protease Peptone	5.0
Dextrose	10.0
KH_2PO_4	2.0
Sorbitol Monooleate	0.1
Agar	10.0

Sterilize at (15 psig) 121°C, for 15 minutes and prepare deep tubes (do not slant). Lactic cultures are best maintained by stab inoculation. Keep at least 3 tubes for each culture. One for maintaining the stock, the other two for preparing inocula. Transfer at least once a month. After each transfer incubate at 35-37°C for 2 days and then store in a refrigerator.

2. Non-microbiological methods

Besides the bioassay procedure there are a number of methods available for quantitative determination of lysine. Among them Chinard's method [21] has been used widely. However, this method being associated with certain limitations some chemically improved methods [22] of lysine estimation have been introduced [23] in more recent years.

9.7.4 Bioassays of More Recent Bioproducts[24]

For evaluating the effects of biologically active compounds like interferons and interleukins rapid bioassays are vital. For mammalian cell culture bioproduct scientists have developed a rapid, accurate colorimetric method of evaluating the cellular response in bioassays that quantifies the concentration of secondary cellular metabolite lactic acid. The amount of lactic acid can reflect not only cell biomass growth but also subtle changes in the cell's metabolism that might occur when it is exposed to lymphokines or other biological response modifiers.

The coupled colour reaction involving lactic acid, contained in a biological sample, and the cofactor NAD^+ are enzymatically converted to pyruvic acid and NADH respectively by LDH. NADH, in the presence of the electron carrier PMSP readily reduces INT, a clear tetrazolium dye, to a coloured formazan as per following scheme. In this bioassay the colour change and intensity are proportional to the concentration of lactic acid produced by the assay cells and could be easily quantified in a 96-well microliter plate reader.

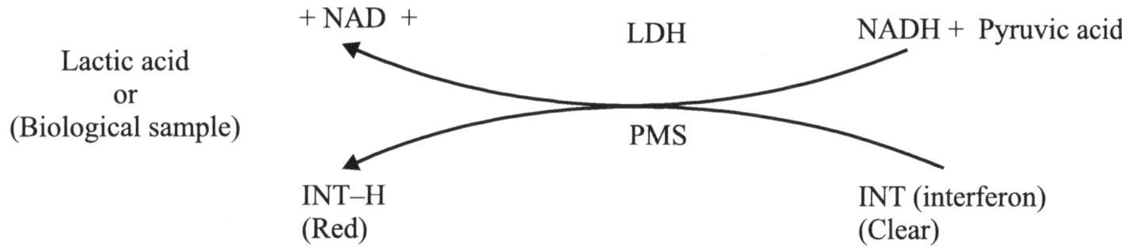

9.7.5 Bioassay by Blotting and Hybridization Techniques

They are frequently used for visualization of a specific DNA or RNA fragments among the many thousands of "contaminating" molecules.[25] It requires the convergence of a number of bioassay techniques, which are collectively termed blot transfer bioassay as illustrated in the following figure (Fig. 9. 4). In the bioassay the Southern (DNA), Northern (RNA) and Western (Protein) blot transfer procedures are useful in the assay of how many copies of gene are in a given tissue or whether there are any gross alterations in a gene (deletions, insertions or rearrangements).

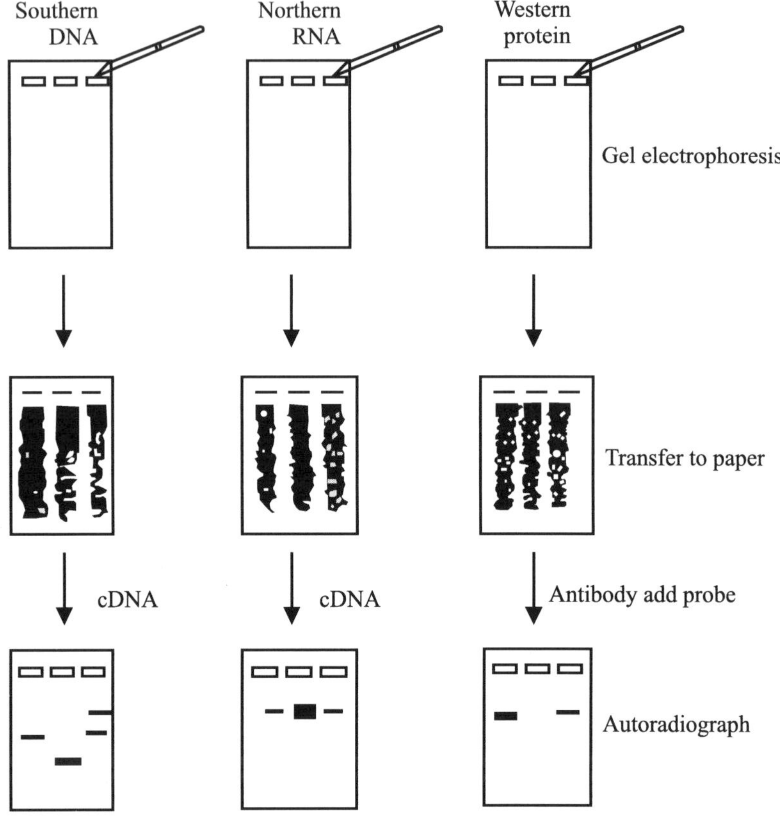

Fig. 9.4 Steps in blot transfer bioassay

9.8 REFERENCES

1. Lloyd, D., S. Bohatka and J. Szilagyi, *Biosensors I*, pp 179-212, 1985.
2. Ruess, M., H. Piehl and F. Wagner, *Euro. J. Appl. Microbiol. Biotechnol.*, pp1, 323-25, 1975.
3. Lloyd, D. and R.I. Scott., *J. Microbiol Methods*, pp 1, 313-28, 1983.
4. Buckland, B., T. Brix, H. Fastert, K. abewongo, G. Hunt and D. Jain, *Biotechnology*, pp 3, 984-88, 1985.
5. Harding, S.E. *Biotechnology and Applied Biochemistry*, pp 8, 489-509, 1986.
6. Mukhopadhyay, S.N. and D.K. Das, *Oxygen Responses: Reactivities and Measurements in Biosystems*, p-147, CRC Press, Boca Raton, Florida 1994 .
7. Chen, S.H. and P.C. Wang, *Biomedical Applications of Laser Light Scattering*, (D.B. Sattelle, W.I. Lee and B.R. Ware eds.) Elsevier, Amsterdam, 1982.
8. Fiel, R.J., E.H. Mark and B.R. Munson, *Arch. Biochem. Biophys*, pp141, 547-51, 1970.
9. Livingston, A.G. and H.A. Chase, *J. Chromatog*, pp 481, 159, 1989.
10. Janson, J.C. “Process Scale Chromatography of Proteins”, Lecture Notes of Course *Downstream Processing in Biotechnology*, Coordinator G.P. Agarwal, Sponsored by DBT, GOI, BERC, IIT Delhi, Dec 3-8, 1991
11. *Water Source Book for Chromatography: Columns and Supplies*, Waters Div. of Millipore, Millipore, Corporation, USA, 1986.

12. Tao, *Y. J. Flow Inj. Anal*, pp 2, 115, 1985.
13. Alsson, B.P. *An Introduction to the Use of Flow Injection Analysis*, Tecator, Sweden, 1988.
14. Rui, C.S., H.I. Ogawa, Y. Kato and K. Sonomoto, "Multi-Functional Flow Injection Biosensor for the Simultaneous Assay of Urea, Creatinine and Glucose", *Proc. Int. Sympo. on Advanced Computing for Life Science,* pp 12-15, 1992 (ISKIT'92).
15. Loibner, A.P., N. Zach; O. Doblhoff-Dier; M. Reiter; K. Bayer and H. Kaitinger, "On Line Glucose Control of Animal Cell Cultures in Fluidized Beds", *Animal Cell Technology*: *Products Today, Prospects for Tomorrow*, pp 372-375, (R.E. Spier, J.B. Griffiths and W. Berthold, eds.) Butterworth-Heinemann Pub., Oxford, 1994.
16. Innes, M.A., D.H. Gelford, J.J. Sinsky and T.J. White (eds.), *PCR Protocols : A Guide to Methods and Applications*, Acad. Press, N. Y., 1990.
17. Hsu, J.T.S. Dasand, S.N. Mohapatra, *Biotechnol. and Bioeng*. pp 55(2), 359-66, 1997.
18. Grove and Randall, *Assay Methods of Antibiotics*.
19. Broquist, H.P. "Lysine Biosynthesis (yeast)", *Methods Enzymol*, pp 17B, 112, 1971.
20. Dunn, M.S., M.N. Camein, S. Shankman, W. Fraukh and L.B. Rockland *J.Biochem*, pp 156, 715, 1944
21. Chinard, F.P., *J. Biol. Chem*., pp 199, 91, 1952.
22. Obei, I.U., *Agri. Biol. Chem*., pp 46 (1), 15, 1982.
23. Ganguli, S., J.K. Deb and S.N. Mukhopadhyay, "An Approach Towards Improvement in Lysine Estimation Method", *Indian Chem. Engr*.; Sec. A., pp 41(2), 101-104, 1999.
24. Familletti, P.C., A. Judith and A. W. Swanson, "A Novel Approach to Bioassays", *Biotechnology* Vol. 6, pp 1169-72, 1988.
25. Watson, J.D., T. Tooze and D.T. Kurtz; *Recombinant DNA*: *A Short Course*, Freeman, 1983.

Chapter

10

BIOPRODUCTS RECOVERY: CONVENTIONAL AND NEWER METHODS

10.1 INTRODUCTION

The increasing demand for enzymes and biocellular products as highly specific and active biocatalysts for a variety of processing and analytical applications depends on the ready availability of reasonably pure and low cost enzymes and biocells. This inevitably entails the development of large scale processes and equipment. Progress in this direction depends not only on the refinement of individual separation technique but also on engineering advances in the application of these procedures to large scale continuous flow or batch processing.

The approach used in this technical evaluation of the situation was as follows:

(i) Identification of existing methods of purification.

(ii) Establishment of criteria for scale up of the techniques with a view to identifying the potential of these techniques.

(iii) Analysis of the engineering problems involved in scale up.

(iv) Identification of the methods most suitable for large scale operation and comparison with existing processes if possible.

It is appreciated that these would be more meaningful if a technoeconomic study were available. Unfortunately due to limited resources and other restraints meaningful economic data is scanty.

10.2 CONVENTIONAL RECOVERY METHODS

A preliminary assessment of the techniques developed up to 1968 was obtained from a summary of detailed isolation procedures published in the *Journal of Biological Chemistry* in 1968. This survey was carried out by Dunnill *et al.*[1] and is given in Table 10.1. In the left hand column are the main isolation steps that were used, followed by a percentage of published reports in which those isolation steps occurred more than once. On the right hand side are the most common methods or materials for each isolation step and the percentage of occasions when they were applied at a given step. From the survey the most common set of five steps following extraction is nucleic acid removal, protein precipitation, ion-exchange, gel filtration and adsorption. The average yield is between 58 and 90%. The average overall yield is 18% and the average overall purification of cells need five steps.

Table 10.1 Survey of isolation procedures[1]
(Reported in the *Journal of Biological Chemistry,* 1968)

*Isolation Process**	%	*Common Methods / Materials*	%
Extraction	95	Ultrasonics	57
Nucleic acid removal	80	Protamine	70
Precipitation	90	Ammonium sulphate	100
Desalting	21	Dialysis	69
Gel filtration	58	Sephadex, Biogel	62
Ion-exchange	86	DEAE-cellulose	92
Adsorption	28	"Calcium phosphates"	86
Electrophoresis	11	Disc electrophoresis	73
*Average number of stages	=5		

To date many more techniques have been developed on a laboratory scale and could be considered for large scale application. It must be emphasised that the technology indicated in this chapter is based on published data and as a result is some-what limited as most information relating to large scale equipment and processes is still being treated as proprietary information by suppliers. Table 10.2 summarises the main classes of separation techniques available today.[2–4]

The degree of separation attained by these different methods depends upon the contribution made by the forces F_1 and F_2 to their net difference ΔF. Thus, in chromatography for instance, the F_1 forces are mainly hydrodynamic and are very similar for all molecules. The high selectivity of the process depends to a large extent on the types of forces involved in separation. Table 10.2 shows the different conventional separation processes available for the separation of components of a mixture along with the types of forces (F_1 & F_2) involved in each of the processes.

10.2.1 General Factors Related to Large Scale Purification Procedures

The main criteria for the scale up of any process are technical viability and economic feasibility. The main unit operation for the purification of enzymes are basically the same for both the

Table 10.2 Conventional separation methods and their features

	Methods	*Impelling Force, F_1*	*Retarding Force, F_2*	*Predominant Force*	*Separation Depends on*
1.	Chromatography				
(a)	Adsorption	Hydrodynamic	Surface energy Van der Waals force steric specificity	F_2	Polar and steric factors
(b)	Ion exchange	Hydrodynamic	Electrostatic polarizability molecular sieve effect	F_2	Ionic nature molecular dimension
(c)	Partition	Hydrodyanamic	Osmotic dipole interaction , association and dissociation effects	F_2	Polar factors
(d)	Molecular sieves	Hydrodynamic	Osmotic	F_2	Molecular
2.	Counter-current distribution	Mechanical	Osmotic association and dissociation effects	F_2	Polar factors
3.	Electric field				
(a)	In true solution	Electrostatic	Molecular friction force polarizability electrokinetic	F_1	Ionic nature
(b)	In porous supporting media	Electrostatic	Molecular friction force, polarizability electrokinetic surface energy	F_1	Ionic nature
(c)	Gel supporting media	Electrostatic	Molecular sieve effects	F_1 and F_2	Ionic nature molecular dimension
(d)	Isoelectric focussing	Electrostatic	None	F_1	Ionic nature
(e)	Electro-phoresis convection	Electrostatic Electrokinetic, Gravity	Molecular friction effects	F_1	Ionic nature
(f)	Electro-dialysis	Electrostatic electrokinetic	Molecular sieve effects and electro-kinetic	F_1 and F_2	Ionic nature and molecular dimension
4.	Diffusion				
(a)	Dialysis	Osmotic	Molecular sieve effects	F_2	Molecular dimensions
(b)	Ultrafiltration	Hydrostatic	Molecular sieve effects and surface energy	F_2	Molecular dimensions

Methods	Impelling Force, F_1	Retarding Force, F_2	Predominant Force	Separation Depends on
(c) Thermal diffusion in solution	Thermal gradient gravity	Molecular friction effects	F_2	Molecular dimensions
5. Crystallization	Crystal lattice energy	Diffusional	F_1	Molecular dimensions
6. Sedimentation				
(a) Kinetic	Gravity, Centrifugal	Molecular friction effects	F_1	Molecular dimensions
(b) Isopyknic	Centrifugal	None	F_1	Molecular dimensions

laboratory and large scale operations. However, certain problems which are inherent in large scale operations are often not noticeable in the smaller scale. Some of these problems are foaming, temperature control, high shear stresses and extended process time. Aeration of solutions during transfer, mixing or centrifugation may generate considerable foam and unit operations such as pH adjustment or the addition of reagents may become difficult. Large centrifuges, for instance, generate a considerable amount of heat and temperature control is maintained by the circulation of a coolant in a jacketed tank and by the use of special equipment. Control of process time is a most frequent problem. Certain steps require a longer period to complete on a large scale than in the laboratory, and cause enzyme instability, which may not be apparent in the laboratory, becomes evident and a problem. Once a particular step is recognised as being time-sensitive, the preparation is either divided into several batches or a continuous process is employed at that point. Ideally, the ultimate minimization of process time could be achieved with the development and utilization of a completely continuous process. These problems and others which are characteristic of certain steps will be discussed in greater detail in this chapter. The options available for scale up are:

(i) Large scale batch equipment.

(ii) Large scale semi-continuous or batch-continuous operations.

(iii) Large scale continuous operations.

There can be no rigid set of rules as to the best system, as in many cases the level of development of the technology and the related economics often dictate the final decision. It would be appropriate at this stage to briefly examine the use of batch and continuous systems for enzyme purification.

It is much simpler to initiate a batch process than a continuous one. However, once in operation, the continuous process can operate automatically whereas the batch process requires constant attention, especially during time sensitive stages. The development of a truly continuous process requires the co-ordination of every stage so that desired conditions prevail. This inevitably involves the use of automatic controls. It must be borne in mind that most analytical procedures developed at the laboratory scale for enzymes involve the degradation of at least part of the sample. Adaptation of such procedures for on stream analysis and process control would be very difficult. The technical problems of instrumentation are outside the scope of this chapter and as a result are only briefly mentioned.

10.2.2 Selection of Purification Methods

The criteria for selecting purification methods are largely dependent on the final use intended for the enzyme and the purity required. The important considerations are:

(i) Proposed use of the enzyme, e.g. L-asparaginase must be void of pyrogens and toxins; detergent enzymes must satisfy FDA standards with a microbial count of less than 50,000.
(ii) Cost of production.
(iii) Enzyme stability: This is particularly important as it dictates the entire course of purification. It must be emphasized that the stability conditions found with crude extracts will only be valid during the early stages of purification as the apparent chemical properties of the enzyme may change during the course of isolation, owing to progressive removal of substances which complex or interact with it. Enzyme stability will be discussed in greater detail later in this chapter.
(iv) Relative location of the enzyme: Apart from intracellular or extracellular, the enzyme may be part of a complex or agglomerate.
(v) Nature of the organism: The final yield of a particular enzyme from a process may be greatly influenced by the choice of organism and the growth conditions. Several techniques such as strain selection; modification of genetic composition; induction; etc., are available for improving enzyme yields.

The following basic data should also be known about the enzyme:

1. Solubility
   a. In water or dilute solutions
   b. In polar solvents such as methanol, ethanol, acetone
   c. In weakly polar solvents such as chloroform and hydrocarbons
2. Stability
   a. pH range
   b. Temperature effect
   c. Effects of organic solvents
3. Stability in the solid state
   a. Temperature effect
   b. Effect of moisture content
4. Physical properties
   a. Dialysability through membranes of different pore sizes
   b. Adsorption on solids
   c. Migration in an electric field as a function of pH
   d. Sedimentation in a centrifuge

5. Chemical properties
   a. Stability towards proteolytic enzymes
   b. Stability after acetylation under mild conditions
   c. Stability to esterification under mild conditions

The stability data 2.a-2.c, are the most important preliminary investigations. Most of the enzymes of biochemical importance are stable over a limited pH range and prolonged separation processes may require to be carried out at reduced temperatures.

Generally, the successive stages should be based on the different properties of the enzyme. Thus, if purification has been achieved by making use of the anionic properties of the enzyme further purification is more likely to be successful by making use of some other property of the enzyme such as its cationic properties. Fig. 10.1 summarises the general purification steps which may be used. A technique which would reduce the final cost of the enzyme is to design the purification stages so as to purify several enzymes from one source. This is practical, however, only when use exists for many enzymes from the same source.[5] This system is not considered in this chapter.

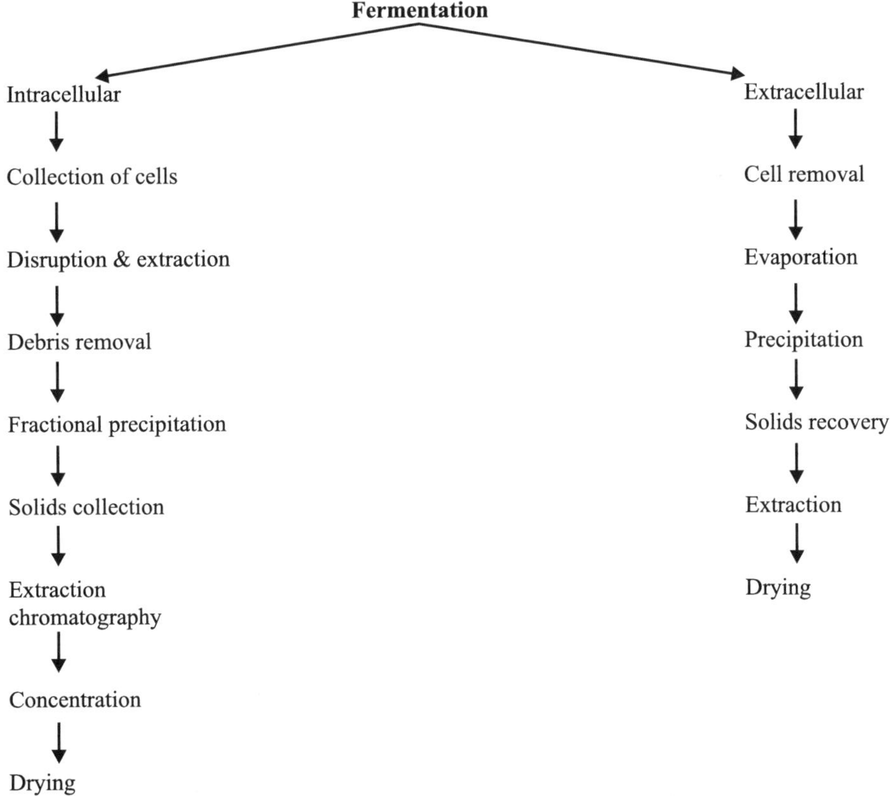

Fig. 10.1 Purification of enzymes

10.2.3 Scale up of Specific Purification Procedures

1. Cell disruption

(i) General : The techniques for cell breakage are summarised in Fig. 10.2.

Table 10.3 gives a synopsis of the relative effectiveness of some of the methods of cell disruption.

(ii) Theoretical Background : The non-mechanical models are limited in application to large scale protein release and will not be discussed here. The approach to data, has to use data, collected on laboratory devices for the adaptation of industrial machines already used extensively in the chemical process field. Sonication, too, is limited with regards to the high capital investment involved when related to separation efficiency. Such a system may only be feasible when a battery of units in parallel are considered. Equipment design must be accounted for adequate exposure and mixing of the fluid/cell mixture.

The machines available for mechanical disruption are:

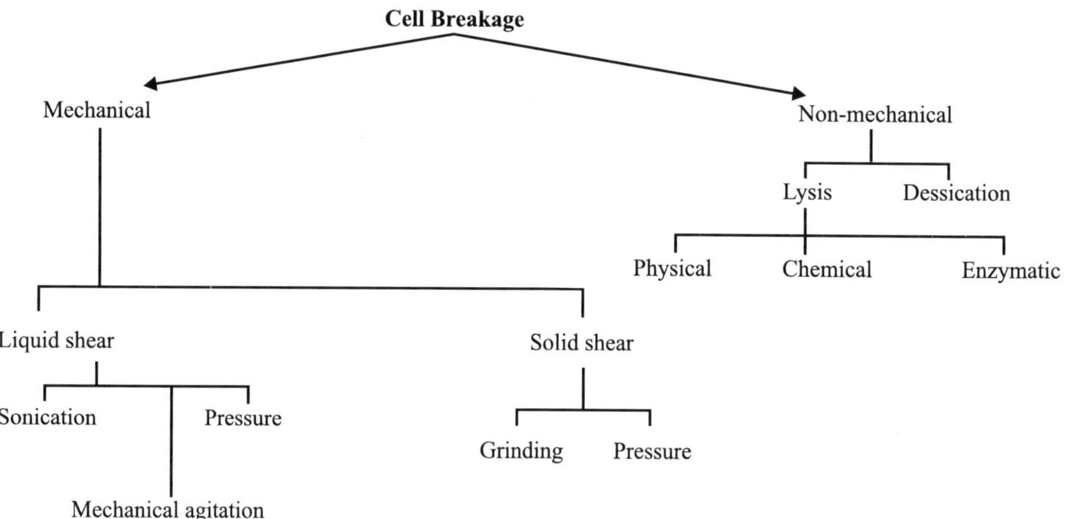

Fig. 10.2 Classification of disruption methods

(i) Colloid mill
(ii) Ultrasonic probe
(iii) Homogenizer
(iv) High speed ball mill
(v) Extreme pressure pump

Table 10.3 Scaled up production of soluble protein using APV Homogenizers

Machine	*Throughput l/hr.*	*Throughput Sol. Protein kg/hr**	*Pressure kg/cm^2*
APV – 15M	54	1.2	550
APV – K3	280	2.4	550
APV – MC45**	4500	100	550

* 60% w/v yeast 90% disrupted

** Projected from 15M & K3 data

Only (iii) to (v) will be considered as the rest are limited to pilot scale.

Dunnill *et al.*[6,7] carried out detailed studies on protein release on cell disruption using a Manton-Gaulin APV homogenizer (The APV Co., Ltd., Crawley, Surrey, U.K.). They obtained the following correlation:

$$\log\left[\frac{R_m}{R_m - R}\right] = KN \tag{10.1}$$

where R – Amount of soluble protein released after N cycles through the homogenizer

R_m – Maximum release of soluble protein

K – kP^x [fn(T)] – A temperature dependent 1st-order rate constant

P – Operating pressure

k, x – Constants for a given microorganism grown under particular conditions, *x* for yeast was 2.9.

They found no evidence of protein denaturation during multiple passes. Increase in cell disruption with pressure was supported by Brookman ,[8] who obtained 100% cell breakage at a pressure of 1750 kgf/cm^2. He produced evidence to indicate that the main mechanism responsible for the cell breakage was pressure. He also observed a linear increase of temperature with pressure (1.5°C/70 kgf/cm^2) at a flow rate of 59 *l*/hr, and a 60% w/v yeast suspension. Several factors influence the performance of homogenizers of different size.

The main factors concerning the use of these machines in large scale operations are:

(a) The correlation given as in equation 10.1 is applicable up to pressures of 1200 kgf/cm^2, and is useful in determining the required number of passes for a particular degree of disruption.

(b) The increase in temperature at increased flow rates and pressure must be well known. There must be adequate cooling between passes if protein denaturation due to heat is to be avoided.

(c) Commercial homogenizers working with high pressures are available with nominal capacities up to 9000 *l*/hr and there is a possibility that these could be adapted for use.

(d) Power efficiences (% disruption/kw), at different operating pressures must be carefully analysed before the decision is made to use machines of higher capacities and operating pressures.

(e) This system could be operated on a continuous basis as indicated in Fig. 10.3.

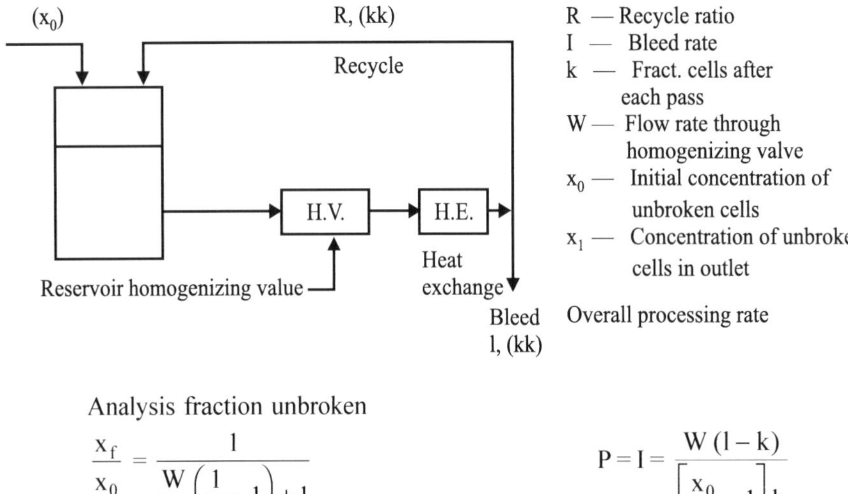

$$\frac{x_f}{x_0} = \frac{1}{\frac{W}{1}\left(\frac{1}{k} - 1\right) + 1} \qquad P = I = \frac{W(1-k)}{\left[\frac{x_0}{x_f} - 1\right]k}$$

Fig. 10.3 Manton-Gaulin homogenizer operated as a continuous system

Mogren *et al.*[9] obtained data for the use of a high speed ball mill for cell disruption. The machine used had a capacity of 180 *l*/hr (Model KD5 Dyno-Mill, W.A. Eachofen, Easel, Switzerland). 85% cell disruption and an electricity requirement of 0.3 kwH/kg of dry yeast were observed. Cooling was provided by an outer jacket to the grinding chamber. The main factors of interest here are:

(a) Cooling facilities would be inadequate as the equipment size is increased. Although different cooling media could be used, heat exchange surface area would be limiting. Provision must be made for the inclusion of an external heat exchanger in system so as to minimize the risk of denaturation.

(b) This system may produce high enough shear forces on a large scale to cause denaturation.

(c) Rotary mills tend to produce size segregation which could affect mixing, and even more–so at larger diameters. This would reduce the overall breakage efficiency.

(d) Power efficiencies must be compared with other classes of machines as well as other sizes of the same design. The efficiencies would be higher than for a homogenizer.

(e) Adhesion of the suspension to the walls of the containing vessel will be more significant on a large scale operation. The design may become too intricate if baffle/scrapers have to be used.

(f) Recovery of solid particles used to enhance grinding would require additional unit operations which could add significant costs to a large scale operation.

Brookman *et al.*[10] investigated the use of a high pressure pump (700-3100 kgf/cm^2) for pumping the cell suspension through a needle valve 90% cell breakage was obtained at flow rates of 2 *l*/hr (60% W/V yeast suspension). The main considerations here are:

(a) Increase in temperature will be due to the reduction in volume at high pressures in the needle valve. Cooling could be provided by jacketing the line from the pump up to end including the valve. Heat exchange surface area would be the limiting factor on large scale operation. A large pump coupled to a manifold leading to a battery of valves may be a possible solution.

(b) Capital investment may be higher for this system.

(c) Power efficiency will be lower.

(d) Maintenance costs due to the repair and replacement of valves will be significant.

2. Enzyme purification

(i) General Background : The main methods of enzyme precipitation are[11, 12, 15] :

(i) Isoelectric point—At the isoelectric point there are no electrostatic repulsion forces between neighbouring enzyme molecules that coalesce and precipitate. When the pH of the enzyme mixture is adjusted to the isoelectric pH of one of its components, much or all of that components will precipitate leaving behind in solution enzymes with pH values above or below that pH. The precipitated isoelectric protein remains in its native conformation and can be redissolved in a medium having an appropiate pH and salt concentration.

(ii) Salting out—At low concentration, certain salts increase the solubility of most enzymes. The ability of neutral salts to influence the solubility of enzymes is a function of their ionic strength, a measure of both the concentration and number of electric charges on the cations and anions contributed by the salt. As the ionic strength is increased the solubility of the enzyme begins to decrease. At a sufficiently high concentration the enzyme may be almost completely precipitated from the solution–an effect called salting out.

(iii) Solvent—The reduction of the effective dielectric constant of a solution of a polar solute in a polar solvent by the addition of a weakly polar solvent will frequently result in the precipitation of the solute. When applied to enzymes however, caution must be exercised, since a medium of low dielectric constant increases electrostatic interactions between ionic groups and reduces dispersion interactions between nonpolar groups. Denaturation may result.

(iv) Thermal differential denaturation—If the extraneous enzymes denature more rapidly than the desired enzyme, they precipitate, leaving the desired enzyme in solution.

(ii) Discussion : Precipitation is basically a simple first stage tool for the purification of enzymes from solution and allows further fractionation to be carried out with smaller volumes leading to

decreased processing time. Important to large scale operation are the physical characteristics of the final suspension. The following general problems must be considered:

(i) The rate of addition of the precipitating agent affects the particle size.

(ii) The rate of mixing (turbulence created) affects the particle size and also leads to heat generation in the system. A high degree of turbulence would ensure homogeneity of the mixture but may lead to protein denaturation.

(iii) Heat removal from the system must be efficient (especially so when organic solvents are used).

(iv) The high viscosity of crude protein extracts compounds poses the problems of adequate mixing and efficient heat removal.

(v) A method of agitation which may be suitable on the laboratory scale may not be on the large scale.

Methods (i)—(iii) could be carried out in similar equipment, although (iii) is applicable in special cases due to the problem of denaturation mentioned above. Only (ii) and (iv) will be discussed here.

On salting out Dixon and Webb[13], investigated the mechanism involved and put forward the following equation relating the solubility of a protein, s(gm/*l* of soln.) with the ionic strength:

$$\log s = \beta - K_s \frac{\Gamma}{2} \qquad (10.2)$$

where β and K_s are constants and $\frac{\Gamma}{2}$ the ionic strength in moles/*l* of solution. Hence, if an enzyme is present at a concentration s_1 and requires an ionic strength of salt I_1, for precipitation to occur, once the specific constant K_s is known, then the ionic strength I_2 required for precipitation of the enzyme at concentration s_2, could be calculated from the following relation:

$$\log \frac{S_1}{S_2} = K_s (I_2 - I_1) \qquad (10.3)$$

The work of Foster *et al*[(14)], at a later date indicated that equation (10.2) was useful for the purposes of estimation but they emphasized the need to study these systems in the regions where the equation was not valid and salting out occurs at lower ammonium sulphate concentrations as the enzyme concentration increases.

The following factors are particularly relevant to large scale operation:

(i) The temperature must be carefully controlled. Variation of temperature introduces a difficulty in the use of percent saturation as a measure of salt concentration since the solubility of the salt will vary. In addition, since the effects of a change of temperature are different with different enzymes the order of precipitation of a given series of enzymes as the salt concentration is increased, may be quite different at different temperatures. In large scale operation temperature control is not instantaneous and adequate cooling capacity must be provided.

(ii) Protein concentration is an important variable. Excess dilution must be avoided since dilute solutions require considerably more salt to achieve the same degree of precipitation.

(iii) Control of pH is difficult e.g. ammonium sulphate is slightly acidic, is not a buffer and there is always a slight loss of ammonia. Special pH control instruments would be required for a large system.

(iv) In the design of large systems using high concentrations of salts, allowance must be made for the fact that there are considerable volumetric changes when amounts of salt of the required order are dissolved in water.

(v) Repeated fractionation using the same conditions is of limited value and higher separating efficiences are obtained by repeating the fractionation under different conditions.

(vi) The rate of addition of salt may affect the equilibrium state.

(vii) Residence time required for the process would be important in equipment selection.

The following types of equipment are suggested for large scale operation:

(a) CSTR—The degree of mixing is the important consideration here. A mixing parameter is defined by the following equation:

$$\phi = \frac{t\,(ND_i)^{2/3}\,(g)^{0.16}\,(D_i)}{(H_L)^{0.5}\,(D_t)^{0.5}} \tag{10.4}$$

where t – Mixing time

N – Impeller speed

D_i – Impeller diameter

g – Gravity constant

H_L – Liquid depth in vessel

D_t – Vessel diameter

This mixing parameter ϕ could be correlated with the Reynolds number $\left(N_{Re} = \frac{ND_i^2\,\rho}{\mu}\right)$ to give a means of scale up. The main problem in this system would be foaming and equipment size above a certain plant capacity. Ideally, a battery of tanks should be used to allow time for precipitation.

(b) Column operation—The intrinsic problem here is the difficulty of obtaining equilibrium between liquid and solid phases sufficiently quickly to permit efficient cascade operation. The continuous extraction of a precipitated material with a gradient of increasing solvent properties is possible, e.g. a gradient of salt precipitant such as ammonium sulphate could be established in a molecular sieve column of suitable porosity so that the salt concentration increases downwards towards the outlet. This method as applied to large scale operation would be discussed later in the section of this chapter dealing with column chromatography.

(c) Cyclone mixers—A simple system which could probably be used in this type of application is a modified forced circulation crystalliser as indicated in Fig. 10.4. This system would, offer the following advantages.

(i) Adequate mixing

(ii) Adequate residence time

(iii) Continuous flow

(iv) Good temperature control.

(v) Low cost preliminary separation after precipitation.

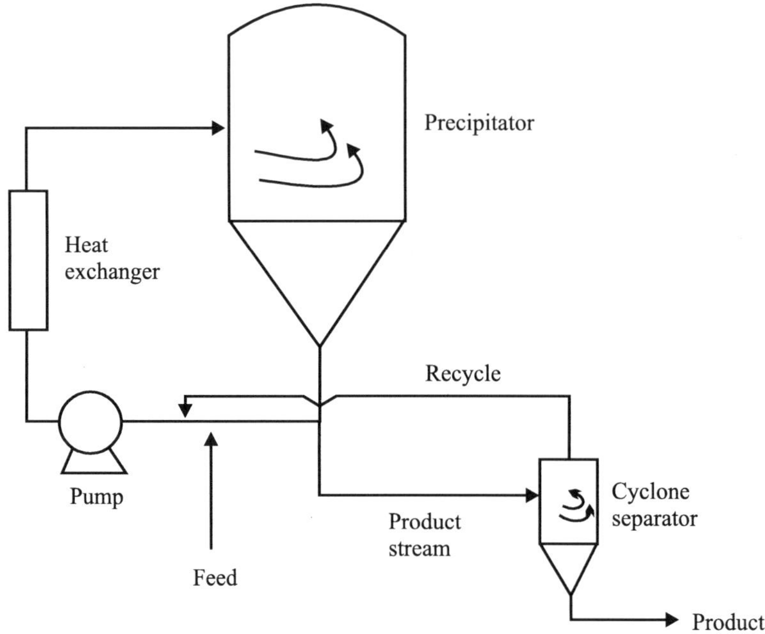

Fig. 10.4 Enzyme separation and precipitation using cyclone mixers

On thermal denaturation following equations were developed for scale up based on the assumptions that thermal denaturation is a first order reaction.[11]

If the protein concentration of a given species remaining undenatured at time θ is x, and if x_0 is the initial concentration, then

$$\ln (x/x_0) = k\theta \tag{10.5}$$

where k is the Arrhenius constant given by

$$k = A \exp(-H/RT) \tag{10.6}$$

Here H is the energy of activation for denaturation. The relation which could be used for scale up is therefore:

$$\frac{x}{x_0} \text{ (lab. scale)} = \frac{x}{x_0} \text{ (large scale)} \tag{10.7}$$

The activation energy for denaturation for a particular enzyme may be determined from the rate of loss of activity at two different temperatures:

at T_1 . . . $$k_1 = \frac{\ln(x/x_0)}{\theta}$$

at T_2 . . . $$k_2 = \frac{\ln(x/x_0)}{\theta}$$

Therefore, $$H = \frac{R\ln(k_1/k_2)}{\frac{1}{T_2} - \frac{1}{T_1}} \quad (10.8)$$

A mean value for H for several proteins is 82000 cal/mole. The equipment which could be used for this system is as follows:

(i) A battery of stirred jacketed vessels using steam, ethylene glycol, etc., as heating medium in the outer jacket: These vessels are standard equipment used in most food industries and selection could be based on standard heat exchange principles.
(ii) Shell and tube heat exchangers: These too are standard equipment.

The overall heat transfer coefficients for these systems could be determined by simple heat balance experiments (some data are given in reference 11). The main limitation to the use of shell and tube heat exchangers is the possible denaturation of the required enzyme due to shear forces at the turbulent Reynolds numbers required for efficient heat transfer. There would obviously be an optimum balance. In addition there may be a maintenance cost due to the plugging of the heat exchanger although this may be partially solved by passing the enzyme suspension on the shell side of the exchanger. The use of this system is, of course, limited to particular enzymes e.g. glucose isomerase.

10.2.4 Chromatography

1. General concepts

Chromatography is defined as the uniform percolation of a fluid through a column of more or less finely divided substance, which selectively retards, by whatever means, certain components of the fluid. The following types of systems are of interest for the large scale purification of enzymes:

(i) *Adsorption*—The solute is retained on an adsorbent surface as a result of dipole interactions, Van der Waals or London dispersion forces, and hydrogen bonding between solute and adsorbent. The principal environmental factor influencing the interaction between a solute and adsorbent is the solute-solvent interaction. Both forces are similar and energy changes are of the same magnitude. The extent of adsorption is influenced by a small change-in one of them.
(ii) *Partition*—The basic mechanism is the partition of the solutes between two immiscible liquid phases. Selection of solvent systems which will provide suitable distribution ratios (D) or partition coefficients (α) is essential for good separation ($\alpha = D\,(V_m / V_s)$ where V_m and V_s are the volume of mobile and stationary phases respectively).

(iii) *Ion-exchange*—This involves the stoichiometric exchange of ions across the solid-liquid interface. Exchange can involve either anion or cation. It is based on the principle that different enzymes have different ionic charges at different pH values and are attracted or repelled accordingly.

(iv) *Affinity*—This method is based on the attachement of one of the reactants to an inert, non-adsorbent and insoluble supporting matrix and the use of this matrix for the selective removal of the other reactant. After thorough washing to remove retained contaminants, the retained reactant could then be removed by elution under suitable conditions. This method is particularly appealing for industrial application since:

a. Purification in a single step may be as much as 4000.

b. Complete biological purity may be achieved.

c. Can be operated at very high loading.

d. It may be directly applicable to clarified cell extract.

The disadvantages are:

a. It must be developed afresh for each product or group of products.

b. The bound component causing specific retention is often costly.

c. The solid chromatographic phase must be highly porous and hydrophillic so that its mechanical strength tends to be poor.

d. Elution conditions tend to be harsh or expensive. Special eluent is required.

(v) *Molecular sieve*—This is based upon separation due to the different sizes of different enzyme molecules.

Of particular interest in large scale chromatography are the concepts of zonal separation and gradient solution. Zonal separation is ideally the resolution of the components of a mixture into discrete zones which are separated by regions of solute free solvent. The components become separated into discrete zones on account of diffusing affinities for the stationary phase. When gradient elution is used, the eluting power of the solvent is gradually and continuously increased by an automatically programmed change in some property such as solvent composition, ionic strength or pH. In this way, the solutes which are firmly retained by the stationary phase under the initial eluent conditions can be eluted as sharp separation zones. The following equations are useful for initial scale-up of the column:

$$V_e = V_0 + a\,V_s \tag{10.9}$$

$$D = \frac{1-R}{R} \tag{10.10}$$

where D – Distribution ratio, ratio of mass of solute in the stationary phase to the mass of solute in the mobile phase ($D = t_s/t_m$).

V_e – Elution volume ($V_e = Ft_e$)

V_0 – Column void volume: total mobile phase volume in the column.

a – Partition coefficient, ratio of solute concentrations in stationary and mobile phases.

V_s – Total stationary phase volume in the column.

R – Solute relative parameter, ratio of the linear rate of movement of a solute zone maximum to the linear rate of movement of the solvent (dimensionless).

t_e – Total time taken for a solute molecule to traverse the column.

t_s, t_m – Time spent by solute in stationary and mobile phases

F – Volumetric flow rate in column.

2. *Different chromatography methods*[15-22]

(i) Column Chromatography : The chromatographic methods identified in the previous section could all be applied to a large scale column and the important scale up parameters are the same. The major causes of increased zone dispersion are:

(i) Longitudinal diffusion of solute in both phases

(ii) Lack of attainment of equilibrium due to resistance to mass transfer

(iii) Dispersion phenomena arising from non-uniform liquid flow through a cross-section of column

The dispersion effects depend on the following:

(i) Flow rate

(ii) Stationary phase particle size

(iii) Column dimensions

The most important parameters which could be manipulated to optimise resolution are:

(i) Column geometry

(ii) Column packing

(iii) Particle size

(iv) Flow rate

(v) Solvent properties

(vi) Temperature

(vii) Inlet flow distribution

Scale up must, therefore, take into consideration the following:

(A) Column geometry

Considering the zone spreading characteristic equation in the following form

$$\sigma = \left[L \left(\frac{2D}{V} + 2R\,(1-R)\,V\,.\,t_d + d_p \right) \right] \tag{10.11}$$

where

σ – Zone spreading factor

L – Column length

D – Solute diffusivity in the mobile phase

R – Ratio of zone velocity to mobile phase velocity

V – Mobile phase or liquid velocity

t_d – Time between sorption and desorption

d_p – Particle diameter.

It is significant to note that is directly proportioned to $L^{1/2}$. It indicates that while the differential migration of different components in the mixture are proportional to L the overall resolution is only increasing by a factor of $L^{1/2}$. An approach to scale-up is to use constant L/D (length to diameter) ratio and Reynolds number (N_{Re} = DV r/m where V = superficial liquid velocity; m, r = viscosity and density of eluting fluid respectively), creating a situation of dynamic similarity between columns. Since porosity and packing are the same in each case, then the term DV is of particular significance. Charm *et al.*[16] used this approach for scaleup of molecular sieve chromatography but it should be applicable to columns using other methods, with slight modifications. They concluded that if these two dimensionless groups were kept constant, then the quality of the elution pattern will be the same in each column. They also found that for a molecular sieve system the following relationship is applicable:

$$\log ((L/D) / DV) = A (\Sigma \max / \text{minute}) + B \qquad (10.12)$$

where A and B are constants and Σ max/minute is a measure of the degree of separation achieved in the column (this is obtained by summing the maximum values of the second and third peaks of the elution pattern and dividing the total by the minimum value between them).

(B) Column packing

The column must be packed to avoid seggregation of the particles according to size, both longitudinally and laterally. This could lead to channelling in the bed.

(C) Particle size

Ideally there should be uniformity of particle size. Uneven reduction of particle sizes will occur due to attrition. Use of small particles leads to increased pressure drop and decreased flow rate. Size need to be optimized considering surface area and hydraulic problems.

(D) Flow rate

High flow rates are required in most situations but care must be exercised to always operate below the "flooding velocity".[17, 18] High flow rates lead to bed compaction and increased pressure drop. The two methods of introducing the feed into the column are by a positive pressure at the top of the column or by a section at the bottom of the column. The latter method is expensive and may result in the formation of gas bubbles in the section of the packed bed near the outlet. Although excess pressure applied to the solvent inlet stream may produce a similar effect on the upper section of the packing, this is less harmful as it alters the local column volume before the zones of the individual components have been separated. With the advent of mechanically stronger particles high pressure chromatography could be used in some cases.[18, 19] High pressure systems would require the use of reciprocating pumps and surge tanks or pressure transducers to reduce pulsations.

(E) Inlet distributor

Distribution becomes more problematic as the column diameter is increased. Charm *et. al.*[16] investigated the design of inlet distributors for large scale columns. Open cones of small diverging angles were found to be poor inlets. Multiple screens gave good velocity distribution but poor dispersion performance. Inlet cones packed from the larger end with 70-80% of their volume gave adequate distribution and exhibited excellent dispersion properties. A system which was not investigated (according to the literature) but which may be suitable is the use of an annulus with open cone nozzles so located that their range of spray overlap.

(F) Solvent properties
Low viscosity solvents reduce the pressure drop across the bed and enhance distribution.

(G) Temperature
Increase in temperature reduces the partition coefficient and causes a decrease in resolution with reduced enzyme stability.

(H) Mass transfer
The two basic mechanisms are longitudinal and lateral. These processes serve to establish local equilibrium within the column and affect the resolution. Hamilton *et al*[20] suggested the following equation for the height of the theoretical plate in ion-exchange chromatography (a modification of this equation should be applicable to other systems):

$$H = 4\lambda\, d_p + \frac{kD}{(D+1)^2} \cdot \frac{d_p^2\, F}{D_s} \tag{10.13}$$

where H – Height of the theoretical plate
λ – Constant
k – Mass transfer coefficient
D_s – Diffusion coefficient of the solute and the stationary phase
F – Linear flow rate
D – Distribution ratio
d_p – Exchange particle diameter

The role of lateral diffusion was investigated by Giddings,[21] who suggested various coupling mechanisms and emphasized the importance of analysing each system individually.

(I) Collection attractions
This would require a sophisticated control system if the column is operated continuously. The best approach would be the use of a battery of columns operating as a batch continuous system so that flow could be continuous downstream of the chromatographic section of the plant.

(ii) Continuous Gel Chromatography : A diagram of such a system is given in Fig. 10.5. In this system, the solute mixture is fed continuously while the individual solutes are recovered continuously from suitable ports.

An annular bed of the stationary phase is contained in the space between two concentric cylinders A and B, and packed in it to the level C. After passage through the "column" the eluent is removed at a series of equidistant drip points E, arranged at the bottom of the annulus.

This system was investigated by Fox *et al.*[22] who applied it successfully in the purification of skim milk proteins. This system is limited for large scale operation; however, it is believed that at high rotational speeds separation may be hindered by the resulting centrifugal forces.

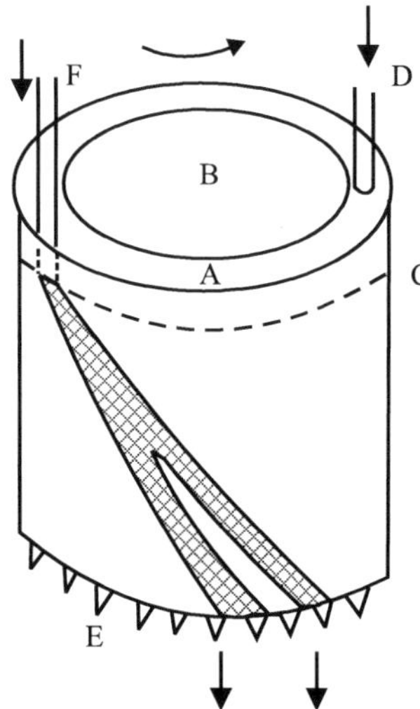

An annular bed of the stationary phase is contained in the space between two concentric cylinders A and B, and packed in it to the level C. After passage through the "column" the eluent is removed at a series of equi-distant drip point E, arranged at the bottom of the annuls.

Fig. 10.5 Continuous chromatography

3. Fluidized bed chromatography

The use of fluidized bed system was considered for counter current ion-exchange chromatography.[23] Although this was eliminated in preference to a packed bed, it is believed that there is potential in the use of fluidized beds for chromatographic separations. This is so, as such systems offer a high degree of mixing and expose greater surface area for mass transfer. The main limitation may be denaturation due to high shear forces.

10.2.5 Filtration

1. Membrane ultrafiltration (UF)

(i) General Background : This is the hydraulic pressure mediated separation of solutions into their individual components by passage through synthetic membranes. The process depicted in Fig. 10.6 utilizes specially constituted polymeric films as molecular screens which discriminate between solute and solvent molecules on the basis of size, shape or chemical structure. UF offers the following advantages for industrial application:

(i) The process is athermal and permits the removal of water up to 90% at ambient and other selected temperatures, avoiding thermal and oxidative degradation of the product. However in such cases solute diffusion coefficient is temperature dependent.

(ii) Since there is no phase change, it avoids collapse of gels, breaking of emulsions and mechanical damage associated with freezing.

(iii) No solvents or other precipitating agents are required for the concentrating process.

The types of membranes available will not be discussed in any great detail, as this subject is considered to be outside the scope of this chapter. The basic mass transfer mechanism involved

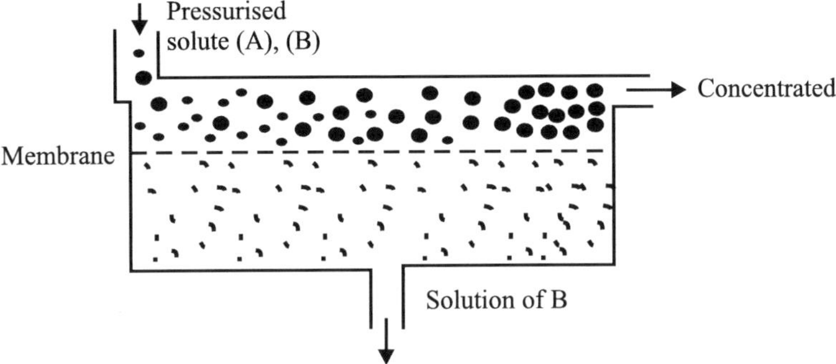

Dissolved molecular species above preselected cut off size are rejected by UF membrane while small material passes through.

Fig. 10.6 Ultrafiltration basic system

with tight membranes (those capable of retaining solutes whose molecular diameters are about 10 Å or less) is diffusive transport (Fickian). In these membranes both solute and solvent migrate by molecular diffusion within the polymer; driven by concentration gradients established in the membrane by the applied pressure difference. Loose membranes (those retaining particles larger than 10 Å) appear to function as molecular screens. Solvent moves through the membrane micropores in essentially viscous flow while solute molecules are carried convectively with solvent, but only in those pores whose dimensions are large enough to accommodate them.

(ii). Influencial Factors : The following factors are important for scale up:

(A) Concentration polarization

This is the major hindrance to the use of *UF* on a large scale. The criteria for local steady state mass transfer of solute require that the rate of convective transport of solute towards the membrane surface be equal to the rate of transport (by diffusive and convective mechanisms) of solute away from the surface. This condition can only be satisfied if the solute concentration in the layer of solute adjacent to the membrane surface is higher than in the bulk of the solution within the channel. This is the concentration polarization which is common to every mass transfer process occurring across a semi-permeable membrane. The consequence of polarization is the formation of a boundary layer of substantially more concentrated solution (relative to mid-channel concentration) adjacent to the membrane. As the fluid moves down the channel and becomes more and more solvent depleted, the bulk and boundary layer solute concentrations increase and the thickness of the solute enriched boundary layer increases. This process is depicted in Fig. 10.7 and 10.8.[23, 24] The following adverse effects of concentration polarization are important:

(i) If the membrane is not completely retentive for solute, the ultrafiltrate will contain a substantially higher concentration of solute that would be predicted from the bulk excellent dispersion properties for a system which has solute concentration in the upstream solution. Hence the membrane's apparent rejection efficiency will be substantially reduced relative to its rejection efficiency.

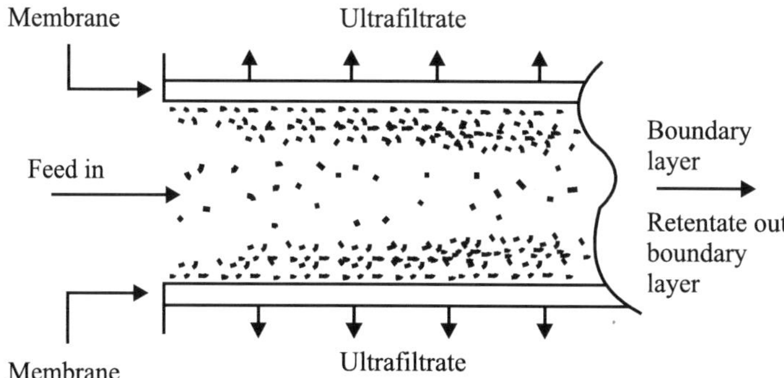

Fig. 10.7 Development of the polarised boundary layer

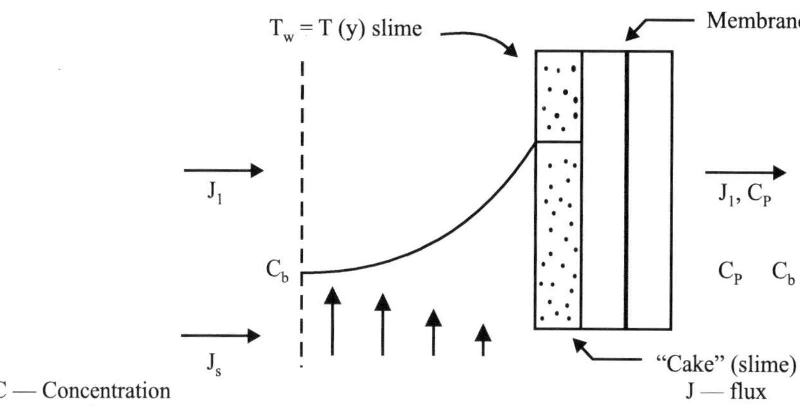

Fig. 10.8 Boundary layer formation in UF of macrosolutes

(ii) If the solution is sufficiently concentrated and the solute of relatively low molecular weight, the high solute osmotic pressure in the boundary layer will reduce the effective pressure for UF, thereby reducing the UF flux.

(iii) If the solution contains a high molecular weight solute, accumulation at the membrane surface produces a large hydraulic flow resistence.

This system has been analysed by several worker,[24-26] and the following equations could be applied for scale up of channel flow:

Turbulent flow (well stirred batch cell)

$$\frac{C_w}{C_b} = \exp \frac{J_1 r}{\left(\frac{v}{D_s}\right)^{0.3}\left(\frac{w r^2}{v}\right)^{0.75} 0.0443\, D_s} \tag{10.14}$$

Laminar flow

$$\frac{C_w}{C_b} = 1 + \frac{V_w^2 \cdot h^2}{3\, D_3^2} \tag{10.15}$$

where J_1 – Solvent flux
C_b – Upstream solute concentration
C_w – Solute concentration at the wall
r – Cell radius
w – Stirrer speed
v – Kinematic viscosity
D_s – Solute diffusivity
V_w – Wall permeation velocity
h – Half channel height

It should be noted that these equations do not consider molecular or eddy diffusion in the boundary layer.

(B) Salt concentration

In the preparation of enzymes, the aqueous suspension often contains a combination of salts. Membrane manufacturers often report the performance of their products in terms of filtration rates for distilled water. This method of reporting the performance index is almost meaningless for biological solutions.[27,28] The *UF* rate decreases with increasing molar concentration. The membrane does not usually retain the salts but due to their ionic nature some intramolecular association occurs and the UF rate is ultimately decreased. This problem would lead to serious discrepancies in equipment capacity on a large scale.

(C) Effect of pressure and temperature on the UF rate

The effect of pressure and temperature are important for several reasons. If the rate can be increased by a proportional increase in pressure, this would allow one to use a smaller *UF* unit to accomplish a given task. Thus the gain in the filtration rate could lead to a reduction in the equipment cost. Thermal instability of enzymes will dictate the upper operating temperature so that it is desirable to know the effects of temperature changes on the membrane behaviour. Generally, there is an increase in filtration rate with pressure. However, this is not a linear increase in rate and the linearity *decreases with increasing temperature* and pressure. This suggests that membranes may become deformed with increasing pressure and so carcful selection must be made.

(D) Effectiveness of shear in clearing membrane surface

The greatest shear rate does not necessarily produce the greatest filtration rate.[29] When shear strength of the resistance cake is the dominating factor limiting filtration, then high shear rate and the associating high shear stress at the membrane surface should be the effective means for reducing the resistance. High shear rates tend to inactivate the enzyme. Table 10.4 gives an idea of the effect of different systems on the enzyme at different shear rates.[30] However, as turbulence[31] and vibration are effective in improving the flow rate, an optimum balance between effective flow rate and inactivation must be obtained.

Table 10.4 Inactivation of catalase

Type of System	*% Inactivation*	*Shear Rate, sec.$^{-1}$*
Thin channel	7	10,000
Turbulent	26	22,000
Vibrating plates	46	81,000

(E) Simplified filtration model for scale-up

This model is applicable to *UF* and other types of filtration systems which will be mentioned later in this section in the context of cell debris removal.[32] The flow of filtration through a filtration medium is given by:

$$\frac{dV}{dt} = \frac{R_m}{A\Delta P} + \frac{K_1 V}{A\Delta P} \tag{10.16}$$

where V – Volume of filtrate
A – Area of membrane
P – Pressure drop across membrane
K_1 – Constant characteristic for a given material deposited
R_m – Resistance of membrane
t – Time

2. Equipment

UF could be used in anyone of the following systems on a large scale operation[33-36]:

(i) Batch
(ii) "Feed and bleed" operation
(iii) Multi-stage continuous

Multistage continuous operation, could be used for both purification and concentration or as a continuous counter current system as indicated in Fig. 10.9 and 10.10. This is most suitable for large scale operation. In recent years protein transmission capacity of *UF* membranes has been reported.[35]

3. Other filtration techniques

The following methods are available for the filtration of cell debris and precipitated protein:

(i) Rotary vacuum[31]
(ii) Filter press (Leaf and Plate and Frame)[31]

These systems could use filter aids such as charcoal to assist in the filtration process. A technique which is applicable to the removal of solids at this stage of the purification process is cross flow filtration.[36] This basically involves the retention of undissolved (particulate) material by the filtration barrier with tangential suspension flow. Analysis of cross flow filtration is similar to that for ultrafiltration. The equipment which could be used here is available for various scales and application is a question of adaptation rather than actual design. The simplified model put forwarded in earlier section[33] is also applicable here.

10.2.6 Electrical Field

The methods which used electrical field in molecular seperation are the following.

(a) *Isoelectric focusing* — This is limited to a laboratory scale primarily due to the problem of pH gradient instability on a large scale.[37]

(b) *Electrophoresis* — This too is limited to a laboratory scale. The problems here are the high generation of heat due to the electric current and the complicated equipment which will be required for separation of a mixtrure of enzymes on a large scale.

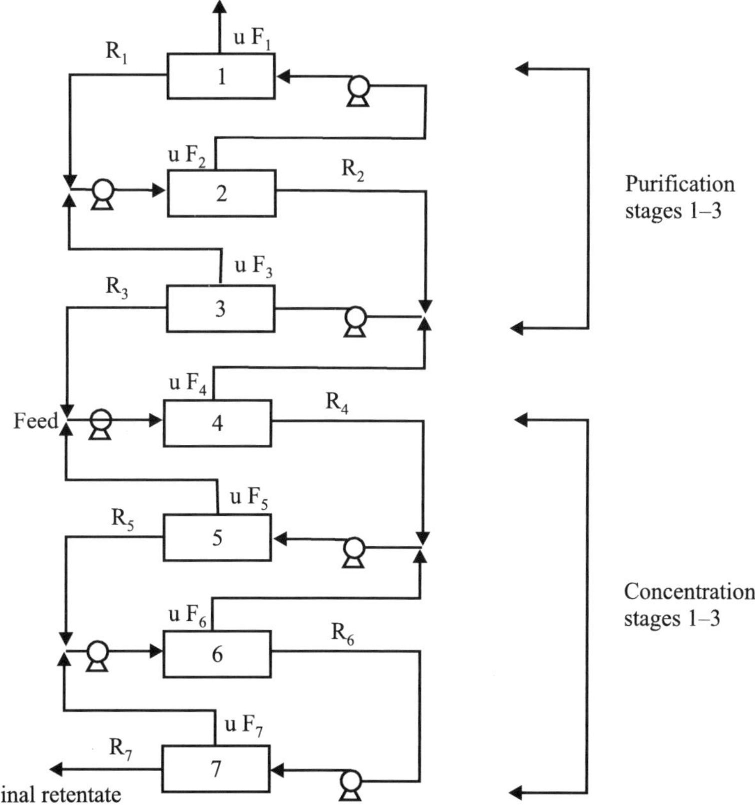

Fig 10.9 Cascade multistage separation for partially rejected solute

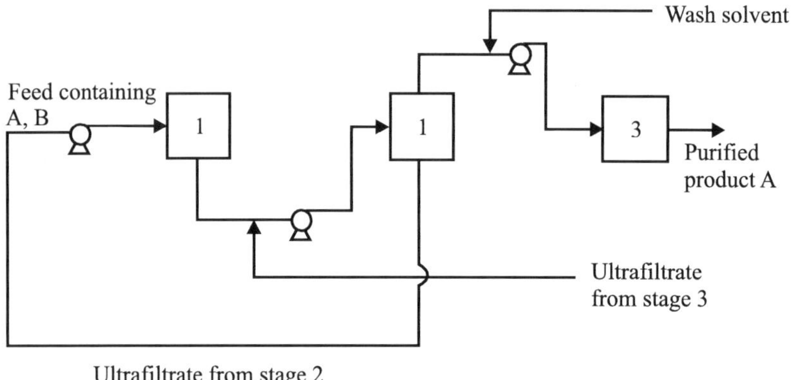

Fig 10.10 Continuous counter current ultrafiltration

10.2.7 Centrifugation

The use of centrifuges is somewhat limited on a large scale because:

(i) Refrigeration costs are quite high.

(ii) As the size is increased the cost of the equipment is very high due to the cost of fabrication.

The only system which may be feasible would be a battery of continuous centrifuges connected to the same outlet manifold. The following equation is applicable to scaleup:[36,37]

$$Q = \frac{Y\,(D_P^2)\,w^2\,(\rho_p - \rho_L)\left(r_1^2 - r_0^2\right)}{36\,(r_1 - r_0)^2\,\mu} \qquad (10.17)$$

where Q – Allowable flow rate
Y – Length of bowl
w – Angular rotational speed
r_1, r_0 – Outside and inside radii of bowl
D_p – Particle diameter
μ – Viscosity of suspending liquid
ρ_L’ ρ_p – Density of liquid and particle respectively
F_s – Correction factor for particle interactions

10.2.8 Counter Current Distribution

This method involves the separation of the components of the mixture by treatment with a solvent in which one or more of the solvents is preferably soluble. The following problems must be considered in the scale up of this method:

(i) Enzymes are unstable when subjected to mechanical agitation in a two-phase liquid system at room temperature. This may be due to the tendency for denaturation to occur at the very large liquid-liquid interface.

(ii) Controlled low temperatures may be required and the solvents used must be suitable for low temperature operation.
(iii) Foaming would have to be minimised.

The equipment required for this technique is similar to that used in liquid-liquid extraction,[38] and scale up would involve similar mass transfer equations.

10.2.9 Foam Separation[39-44]

1. General

This is a method of separation the components of a solution by utilizing differences in surface activity. The principle underlying this process is that enzymes partition themselves between the bulk and the surface region of an aqueous system. However, when two or more enzymes are present in the same solution, then the concentration ratio in the foam will be different from that of the bulk. This is as a result of different adsorptions of the components present.

The following factors are important for scale up here[39,40]:

(i) *Enzyme Concentration :* The enrichment ratio increases with decreasing concentration of protein in the bulk solution. In a batch process, as the concentration of the enzyme preparation is increased, a monolayer forms resulting in decreased surface tension and the presence of a surface excess. As the foam separation continues, the concentration of the enzyme in the bulk solution decreases until there is insufficient protein for stable cell formation. It is important to operate at a low concentration to get a high enrichment ratio but a concentration high enough to produce foaming.
(ii) *Flow Rate :* Enrichment ratio increases with decreasing gas flow rate, down to a limiting flow rate where the gas bubbles arive too infrequently at the top of the solution for a foam to form. The bubbles must have adequate residence time for solute adsorption.
(iii) *Foam Height :* The higher the foam column is allowed to rise before foam is removed to give a foam, the greater will be the enrichment due to drainage and/or coalescence of the surface excess layers comprising the foam.
(iv) *Environmental Factors :* Enzymes are most susceptible to foaming at pH values near the iso-electric point. Temperature is not significant within the normal ambient range.
(v) *Denaturation :* The risk of denaturation is reduced by using an inert gas to produce foam, by avoiding mechanical agitation and by using a once through process rather than a recycle one. The use of an inert gas may affect process economics significantly.

Table 10.5 gives an idea of purification of catalase and amylase by this method.

Table 10.5 Foam separation of catalase and amylase

Foaming Agent	*Recovery %*	
	Catalase	*Amylase*
10% $(NH_4)_2SO_4$	84.5	94.5
50% $(NH_4)_2SO_4$	78.2	99.0

2. Equipment

The different systems that could be used for large scale operation are given in Fig. 10.11.

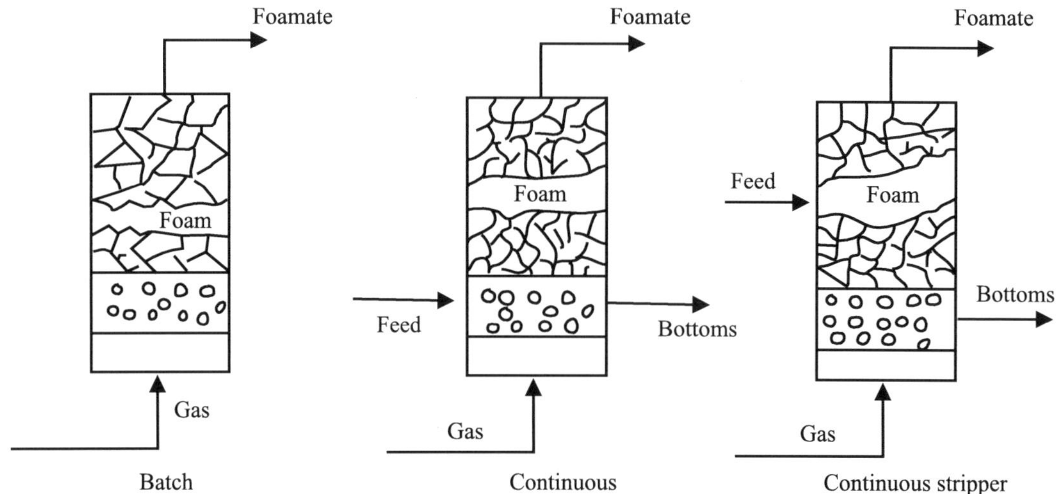

Fig. 10.11 Various modes for large scale foam fractionation

The following equations are applicable for steady state flow in a continuous flow stripper:
Tall column

$$C_Q = C_F + \frac{GS\,\Gamma_W}{Q} \tag{10.18}$$

$$C_W = C_F - \frac{GS\,\Gamma_F}{Q} \tag{10.19}$$

$$C_D = C_F + \frac{GS\,\Gamma_F}{D} \tag{10.20}$$

where C_F, C_W, C_Q – Concentration of enzyme to be separated in the feed stream and foamate.
Γ_W – Surface excess in equilibrium with C_W
S – Surface to volume ratio for a bubble (for a sphere S = 6/d)
G, F, Q – Volumetric flow rates of gas, feed and bottoms
D – Volumetric flow rate at which net foamate is removed.

Scale up of this equipment could produce channelling or significant deviation from plug flow of the foam. This could be minimized by using a low L/D ratio or lowering the liquid and gas flow rates.[41]

10.3 NEWER METHODS

10.3.1 Cross Filtration and Cassette Separation[45-59]

1. Introduction

In recent years many novel purification processes have been developed. A few of them are based on the interaction between complementary biomolecules. This basis was adapted to circumvent the difficulties encountered in conventional affinity based separations. Biomolecule separation by ligand binder complexing has been termed affinity cross flow filtration. Many novel bioproducts obtained through upstream bioprocessing of recombinant biocells are often unstable. Presence of other similar materials favours this instability further. In order to overcome many of these problems impressive progress has been achieved by combining affinity interactions and membrane separation and exploiting the natural affinity displayed between biochemicals and their complementary ligands.

2. Basic principle

As mentioned above it is a combination of affinity interaction and membrane separation. In this method the product to be separated (binder) when present in a crude mixture, will pass through the membrane. The membrane, however, will retain the binder when it crosslinks to a very high molecular weight ligand (macroligand). The unbound components pass through the membrane. From the ligand-binder complex the binder is separated by desorbing it from the ligand using suitable eluant. The isolated product (binder) is collected and macroligand is recycled through reconditioning.

3. Operation

In separating product from a homogenate if it contains no particulate matter, the crude fluid batch of the product (binder) is mixed with the ligand to allow affinity binding to occur. But for continuous purification of material from a bioreactor the crude fluid and the macroligand are delivered separately to either side of a suitable molecular weight cut off membrane. The retention/binding occurs when the product to be purified passes through the membrane. Like in other affinity methods selection of suitable element and elution procedure is important to keep conditions favourable for the product and the membrane. Thus the idealized concept (Fig. 10.12) of affinity cross flow filtration include, (A) separation of impurities and (B) elution of product from ligand binder complexes. Considering gel polarization model one can make a solute mass balance over a thin volume slice at the memberane solution interface for a batch or cross flow continuous cell at any position.

4. Theoretical base

Based on gel polarization model (GPM) one can write

Mass flux to interface = Mass flux away from interface.

This in mathematical terms

$$V_w C = D \frac{dc}{dr} + V_w C_P \tag{10.21}$$

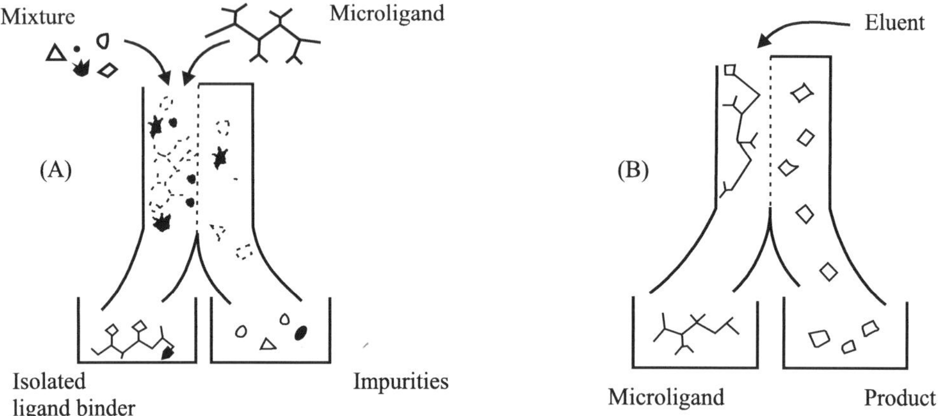

Fig. 10.12 Idealized concept of affinity cross flow filtration

Rearrangement and integration between mass boundary layer thickness δ provides

$$V_w = \frac{D}{\delta} \ln \frac{C_w - C_P}{C_b - C_P} \tag{10.22}$$

Putting $R = 1 - \frac{C_P}{C_w}$ one may obtain

$$\frac{C_w}{C_b} = \frac{1}{R + (1 - R)\, e\,(V_w\, \delta/D)}\; e\,(V_w \delta/D) \tag{10.23}$$

For $C_P = 0$, R = 1, the GPM

$$V_w = \left\{\frac{D}{\delta}\right\} \ln \frac{C_w}{C_b} \tag{10.24}$$

or

$$\frac{V_w}{D} = \frac{1}{\delta} \ln \frac{C_w}{C_b} = Pe_{w'} \tag{10.25}$$

Since, *D/δ* = *K*, film mass transfer coefficient

$$\frac{V_w}{K} = \ln \frac{C_w}{C_b} = Pe_{w'} \tag{10.26}$$

So it depends on flow characteristics of the water, as value of K is laminar or turbulent flow dependent. Considering combined affinity interaction mediated membrane separation to be tubular cross flow filtration as shown in Fig. 10.13 the following flow characteristics based equations are applicable for laminar flow

$$Sh = 1.295\ (R/L\ .\ ReS_C)^{1/3} \tag{10.27}$$

and,

$$k = 0.816\ (r/L\ D^2)^{1/3} \tag{10.28}$$

where r = U/R = U_{max} /2R, L = flow path length

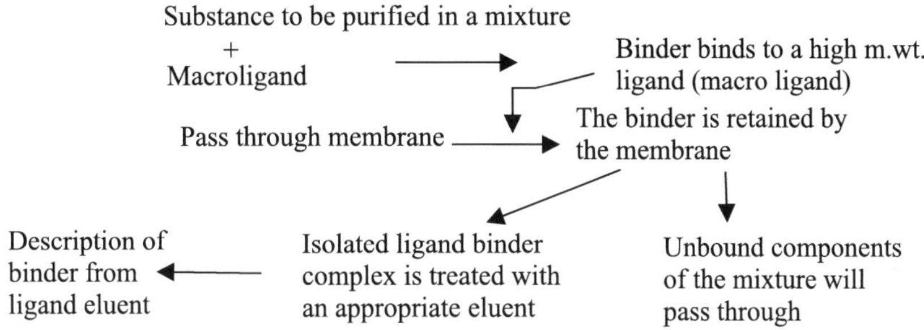

Fig. 10.13 Operation principle flow diagram

This method of separation is bound by certain limitations like the following:

- limited by the availability of suitable adsorbents.
- in case of a particle boundligand, there is a limit to the amount of binder that can be bound.
- in case of viscous liquids flow characteristics may pose difficulty.

For turbulent flow

$$Sh = 0.023\ Re^{\alpha} S_C\, \beta$$

$\alpha_{theor} = 0.83$ $\alpha_{experi} = 0.875$

$\beta_{theor} = 0.33$ $\beta_{experi} = 0.25$

Significances of Equations : The hydrodynamic diagnositics of these equations indicate three significant and useful results. These are:

1. The flux, V_w is proportional to In c_b^{-1} (Eq. 10.24)
2. The flux, V_w is invariant with applied pressure
3. The flux, V_w is proportional to the average axial velocity *U* to the 0.33 power for laminar flow and to the 0.83 power for turbulent flow.

Microfiltration and ultrafiltration membranes have made use of cross flow filtration principles.

5. Modern cassette filtration

The principle of modern cassette filtration using membrane advantage has been depicted in Fig. 10.14. The uses of this system and the advantages claimed are given in Table 10.6 and 10.7. Typical cassette filter performance and membrane applications are provided in Tables 10.8 and 10.9 respectively. The desirable characteristics of the semipermeable membrane include the following:

Table 10. 6 Uses of membrane packet cassette filtration system

- Protein concentration
- Virus and bacteriophage concentration
- Cell harvesting
- RBC ghost processing
- Serum dialysis
- Depyrogenation
- Continuous culture fermentation
- Fractionation of biological components

Table. 10.7 Advantages claimed

- Time saving
- Exceptionally high recovery
- High starting vol.
- Easy to instal, maintain & use
- Resuable filters
- Safe operation
- Unsurpassed versatility

Table 10.8 Typical cassette filter performance

Application	*Process Vol.*	*Sonen Factor*	*Time*
Urine concn.	101	20x	60 min
Interferon (affinity elution)	51	20x	30 min
Bacteriophage	101	100x	45 min
Mammalian virus	201	100x	2 Hrs
E. coli (109/ml)	201	20x	20 min
Serum dialysis (l)	51	NA	20 min

Based on 5 ft^2 membrane.

Table 10.9 Typical membrane type applications

	Membrane Type	*Porosity*	*Uses*
a.	Ultra		
	Cellulose polymeric	1000 MW	Desalting or concentration of peptide
	Polysulfone	10,000 MW	Concentration of enzymes, proteins Depyrogenation of solutions, purification of hormones.
	Cellulosic polymer	1,000,000 MW	Concentration of virus from egg albumin
b.	Micro		
	Cellulose acetate	0.2m	Cell harvesting
	Fluorocarbon Polymer	0.5 m	Clarification of interferon etc.
	Nitrocellulose	0.22 m	Cell harvesting
	Nitrocellulose	0.45	Cell harvesting
	Nitrocellulose	1.2	Cell especially large cells

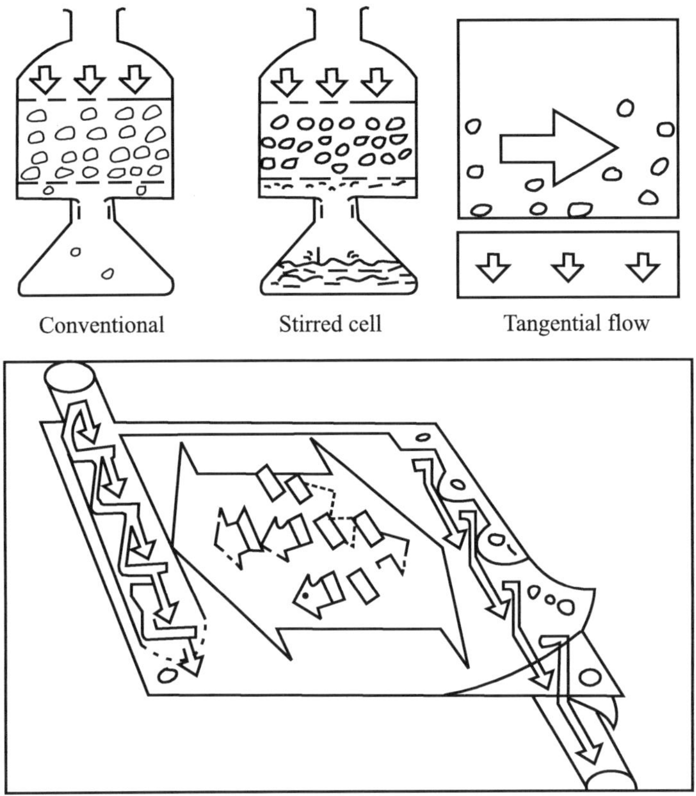

Fig 10.14 Two membrane packet cassette

- High hydraulic permeability of solvent (water)
- Sharp molecular cut off
- Good mechanical durability and chemical and thermal stability
- High fouling resistance, easy cleaning and sterilization
- Long life

10.3.2 Dispersive Separations[15-17]

1. Introduction

In separation and purification of materials from mixture dispersive systems likes sol-gel or biosol-biogel systems having characteristics as shown below has been useful.

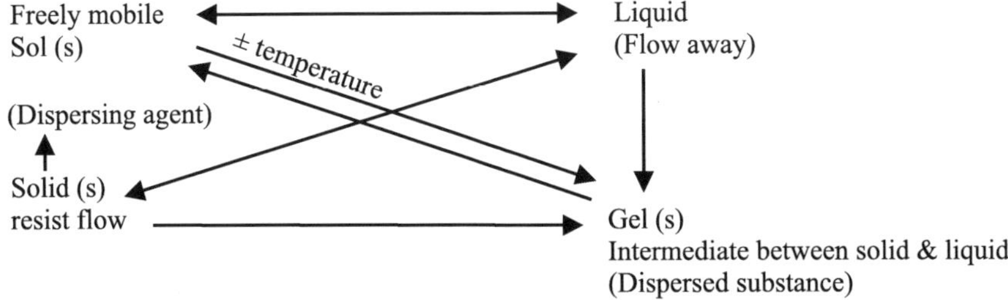

Sol-gel or biosol-biogel processing systems have been used significantly in biomolecule separations from mixture. The dispersions like sol-gel can be of different nature as shown below.

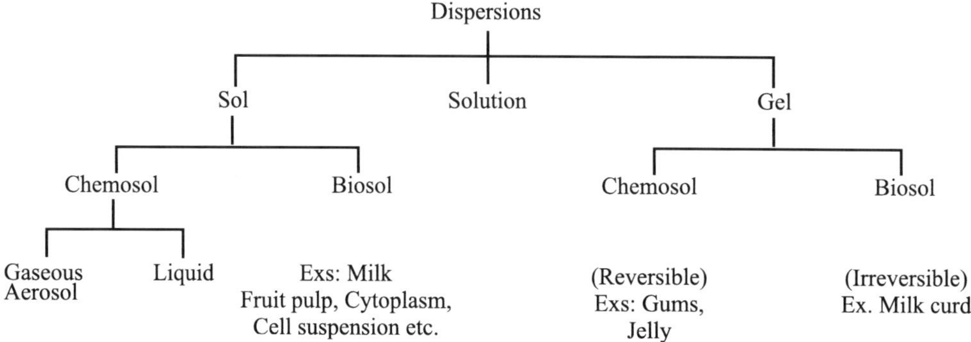

In dispersive separation systems like gel filtration the dispersed substance has three dimensional network of linear macromolecules. The macromolecules are held together at junction points by either secondary valence force (H-bonds, dipole-dipole interactions etc.) or primary valence forces (ionic or covalent). The dispersing agent used is distributed throughout the pores in the network. The reason of using gel in dispersive seperations are the following.

1. Small molecules can permeate the solvent in the gel phase.
2. Large molecules are partly or completely excluded from the gel phase by macromolecular network.
3. The diffusion rates of large molecules are reduced more in the gel than the diffusion rates of small molecules.

2. *Fundamental theory*

(i) Forewords : In dispersive system seperation results when smaller soluble molecules are more retarded in their passage through a gel filtration column. The reason behind this is that smaller soluble molecules have the ability to penetrate the stationary phase (gel) more effectively than larger molecules depending on many parameters. These parameters are important in gel filtration column design. Major considerations for gel column design are (a) gel volume and elution volume, (b) zone broadening (c) gel types and (d) gel stability.

(ii) Gel and Elution Volume : In ascertaining gel bed volume (V_t) one may consider the following.

$$V_t = f\ [\text{volume of gel particles + Volume of surrounding interstitial solvent in the matrix}] \tag{10.29}$$

Actually

$$V_t = V_0 + V_i + V_m \tag{10.30}$$

V_0 = Outer volume (volume of solvent between gel particles)

V_i = Inner volume (volume of solvent imbibed in gel)

V_m = Volume of gel matrix

In this relation V_0 is measured by measuring the elution volume (V_e) of a high molecular weight substance that is completely excluded from the gel particles. The value of V_i can not be measured directly. It is estimated as zero gels (i.e. gels from which all solvent has been removed).

$$V_i = \frac{G \cdot S_r}{\rho_L} \tag{10.31}$$

In this correlation G is dry weight of gel in column, S_r is the solvent regain factor defined as the ratio of gram of solvent imbibed to gram of dry gel forming material and ρ_L is density of solvent. In case G is unknown

$$V_i = \frac{Sr\,\rho_G\,(V_t - V_0)}{\rho_L\left(\dfrac{S_r}{\rho_L} + 1\right)} \tag{10.32}$$

where ρ_G is the density of swollen (wet) gel. The correlation between V_e, V_0 and V_i is given by

$$V_e = V_0 + K_d\,V_i \tag{10.33}$$

where K_d is the distribution coefficient which provides a measure of the degree of penetration of the gel by solute. Depending on the magnitude of K_d the following cases may arise.

Case I. $K_d = 0$, for large solute molecules giving, $V_e = V_0$

Case II. $K_d = 1$, for small solute molecules giving, $V_e = V_0 + V_i$

It indicates that in such a case all the gel phase is accessible.

Case III. $0 > K_d < 1$, for molecules of intermediate size which are partly excluded giving, $V_e = f$ (size of molecules).

Two types of deviations from ideal may appear.

Type 1: Even small solutes are eluted with $0 < K_d < 1$, because (a) some solvent solvates the gel matrix. (b) solvated solvent is not available to solute.

Type 2: Occurrence of adsorption when $K_d > 1$. Aromatic compounds in organic solvents often adsorb some what on styrene-divinyl benzene gels. This property has been utilized to seperate aminoacid on sephadex G[10].

Estimation of K_d: For obtaining the value of K_d one may have the following parametric correlation.

$$K_d = \frac{V_0'}{V_i}\left[\frac{C_{orig} - C_{sup}}{C_{sup}}\right] \tag{10.34}$$

in which V_0' is volume of solution, V_i is equilibrium swollen gel volume, C_{orig} is original concentration of solute and C_{sup} is concentration of supernatant. Since V_i is not directly measurable K_d is measured as K_{av} as below.

$$K_{av} = \frac{V_e - V_0}{V_i - V_0} \tag{10.35}$$

(iii) Zone Broadening: This influences separation efficiency and has direct bearing on column height design. Zone broadening occurs due to the following causes:

- Molecular diffusion and fluid mixing in axial direction.
- Distribution of solute molecules between the gel and mobile phases.
- Nonequillibrium between two phases.
- Irregular flow pattern in the column.

Computation of number of theoretical plates (N) provides an index of zone broadening and is correlated to theoritical plate height (H) by the following relations.

$$N = \left(\frac{V_e}{\sigma}\right)^2 = \left(\frac{4V_e}{W}\right)^2 \tag{10.36}$$

considering column length (L) is divided into N number of theoretical plates, each plate having a height H one may write

$$H = \frac{L}{N} \tag{10.37}$$

In the above relations, σ is the standard deviation of elution curve, and W is the base line width between lines drawn tangent to inflection points in elution curves.

Zone broadening effect limits the number of components that can be seperated by gel filtration. Seperable maximum number of components in gel filtration may be given by the following equation.

$$M_e = 1 + 0.2\ N^{1/2} \tag{10.38}$$

In gel filtration since gels are compressible the pressure drop ΔP across the bed becomes a function of flow rate. It has been observed that above a certain threshold flow rate irreversible deformation of gel occur reducing the flow rate.

(iv) Gel Types: In gel filtration mainly two types of gels have been useful. These are elastic and non-elastic types.

In elastic gel partial dehydration leads to the formation of an elastic solid from which the original solution may be readily regenerated by the addition of water and warming if necessary. Gelatin gel, milk gel, alginate gel, pectin gel, starch gel, agar gel, dextran gels are few examples of elastic gel types.

Non elastic gels on drying become glossy or fail to powder and lose elasticity. The solution can not be obtained by mere addition of water to the dry solid. Silica gel and some polyacrylamide gels are examples of this type.

(v) Gel Stability: Depending on the nature and type sol-gel system transformations can be reversible or irreversible under given conditions. Major factors influencing gel stability may be similar to those involved in gel broadening. These factors, through zone broadening, cause ultimate collapsing of gels.

3. Application areas

Dispersive seperation process is widely used in biotechnology. Examples are (a) milk (sol) to curd (gel) transformation by *Lactobacillus* species. (b) fruit juice/pulp (sol) to Jelly/Jam/Marmatade transformation, (a) starch suspension to starch gel formation by thermal processing which is used in food industries and in many others.

10.3.3 Membrane Separations [48, 52-59]

Applying the membrane advantage many commercial separations are being solved by membrance processes. When a solvent and a solute is transported through a semipermeable membrane it is governed by certain mechanisms. In fabricated *in vitro* membranes the followed mechanisms include: osmosis/dialysis, reverse osmosis (R_0), ultrafiltration (UF), nanofiltration (NF), electrodialysis (ED), pervaporation (PV), micro and cross filtration and gas permeation. For advantageous applications in biological recovery processes membranes have been designed to follow the above mechanism types. For examples, UF and R_0 membranes have been found to be very suitable for clarification, concentration and purification of fruit juices, milk and whey concentration, purification of enzymes, proteins and macromolecules.

The membranes which are used in processing for seperation can be hard and soft types. Hard membranes are permeable to water but pass only negligible quantity of other constituents. Soft membranes on the other hand allow selected solutes to pass through with the water. For concentration of food or some biological materials hard membranes have been used. Fruit juices are concentrated while retaining their natural aroma and fresh flavour. Egg white can be concentrated without denaturing the protein or damaging its functional properties.

Purification or fractionation application in food industries use softer membranes. The most widely studied application of this type, processing of cheese wheys had led to the first commercial scale operation of R_0 in food processing.

Whey by product of cheese and cottage cheese making is a serious waste disposal problem in its unprocessed form. By using membranes permeable to water and small solute molecules it can be separated into two concentrated fractions, one rich in protein and the other rich in food grade lactose, while substantially reducing lactic acid and ash content of the protein rich fraction.

The selectivity of membranes of course, makes the separation possible. Membranes can be manufactured to possess greater or lesser selectivity characterized by separation factor. The degree of separation which may be obtained with any particular membrane separation process is indicated by the separation factor, α_{w-s}, defined as

$$\alpha_{w-s} = \frac{C_{S_1} \cdot C_{W_2}}{C_{S_2} \cdot C_{W_1}} = \frac{N_w \cdot C_{W_1}}{N_s \rho_w} \tag{10.39}$$

or

$$\alpha_{w-s} = \frac{K_w (\Delta P - \Delta\pi)}{\rho_w K_s} \tag{10.40}$$

In these relations C_{S_1} and C_{S_2} are solute concentrations across two sides of the membrane, N_w and N_s are water and solute flux across the membrane (in Moles/unit area), K_w and K_s are empirical constants depending on membrane structure and the nature of the salt, ΔP is the total pressure drop across the membrane, $\Delta\pi$ is partial pressure drop across the membrane.

10.3.4 Adsorptive Separations[43-50]

Adsorptive columns packed with uncharged adsorbents (e.g. hydrophobic copolymers) have been used for specific separations such as isolation of trace levels of organics (e.g. humic and fulric acids) present in waters. Adsorption on a non-polar substrate (e.g. Sep Pak® cartridge which contain a silica base material coated with a C_{18} hydrocarbon) have been carried out for organic materials. Adsorbed substances are retrained through elution with solvents in

a. Open column Adsorption Liquid Chromatography
b. HPLC (High Performance Adsorption Liquid Chromatography)
c. Adsorbent Extraction: This is very similar to HPLC in that it is based on the same separation processes and uses similar stationary phases.

Algae immobilized onto controlled pore glass may serve as adsorbent extractor. The algae cell wall may act as a selective adsorptive seperator. Likewise the method for removing heavy metals from industrial waste water using fungi provides a good example of adsorptive-absorptive capacity of bioseparation. It has been claimed that fungus had higher separation capacity and was more economical than other microbial separation processes.[51]

Beside the above, in more recent years many proteins or enzyme material are being attempted to be separated from hospital wastes like placental fluid using adsorptive bubble or foam separation techniques.[43] This technique takes advantage of the tendency of surface active solutes to collect at the interface between solution and inert gas. Thus surface adsorptive separation phenomena is the basis for bubble separation. When a solution contains more than one solute preferential adsorption must occur if these components are to be fractionated by adsorptive bubble separation process. A classification of various adsorptive bubble separation methods are given in Fig 10.15. The separation efficiency of proteins by this method is influenced by several factors like concentration of enzyme in the fluid, inert gas flow rate, bubble foam bed height, environmental conditions of separations e.g. pH, temperature and denaturation character of the proteins.

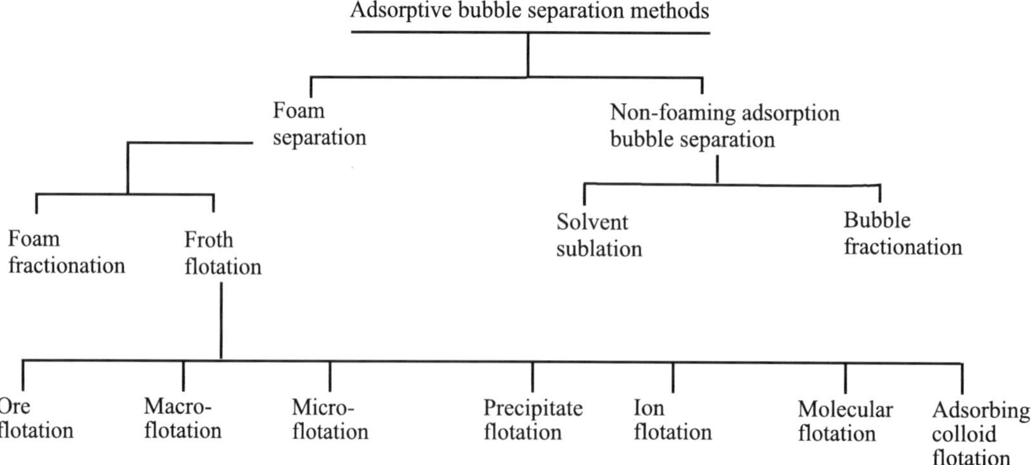

Fig. 10.15 Classification scheme for the various adsorptive bubble separation methods

10.3.5 HPLC Column design factors

The performance/functioning of a HPLC column will depend on many extrinsic and intrinsic factors of its design. These involved factors are tabulated in Table.

Item No.	*Design factors*	*Operational factors*
1.	Column number $N = 16\left(\frac{t_R}{w}\right)^2$ or $N = 5{,}54\left(\frac{t_R}{w_{0.5}}\right)^2$	1. $K = \left(\frac{V_R - V_M}{V_M}\right) = \left(\frac{t_R - t_M}{t_M}\right)$ or $k = \frac{\text{mass of sample in stationary phase}}{\text{mass of sample in mobile phase}}$
2.	Plate height $H = \frac{L}{N}$	2. Column pressure resistance $\Delta p = \frac{u \cdot \eta \cdot L \cdot \phi}{dp^2}$
3.	Reduced place height $h = \frac{H}{dp}$	3. Capillary pressure resistance $\Delta p = \frac{(F \cdot 8 \cdot L \cdot \eta)}{\pi r^4}$
4.	Linear velocity $u = \frac{L}{t_m}$	4. Up scaling/Downscaling $\frac{F_{analyt}}{F_{prep.}} = \frac{m_{analyt}}{m_{prep.}} = \frac{d^2_{analyt}}{d^2_{prep.}}$
5.	Hold up time $t_m = \frac{V_M}{F_C}$	
6.	Total retention time $t_R = \frac{V_R}{F_C}$	
7.	Linear vel. $u = \frac{L}{t_M}$	
8.	Peak resolution $R_S = \frac{2\left(t_{R_2} - t_{R_1}\right)}{\left(W_{0.5_1} - W_{0.5_2}\right)}$	

The nomenclatures of the parameters in these factors are as given below:

- $d_{analyt.}$, – ID analyt. col., $d_{prep.}$ – ID prep. column, dp – particle size diameter.
- F – flow, $F_{analyt.}$ – flow analyt.,

  F_C – flow volume, $F_{prep.}$ – flow prep.

  H – plate height, h – red. p. height

  K – retention factor

L – column length, $m_{analyt.}$ – analyt. mass

$m_{prep.}$ – prep. mass, N – plate number/count

R_S – peak resolution, t_M – hold up time

t_{R_1} – total retention time 1st. peak

t_{R_2} – total retention time 2nd. peak

u – linear vel

V_M – hold up volume, V_R – retention volume

W – peak width, $W_{0.5}$ – peak width at half height

$W_{0.5_1}$ – peak width at $\frac{1}{2}$ height 1st peak

$W_{0.5_2}$ – peak width at $\frac{1}{2}$ height 2nd peak

η – viscosity,

ϕ – specific column resistance

Δp – pressure drop resistance

10.4 REFERENCES

1. Dunnill, P. and M.D. Lilly, "Continuous Enzyme Isolation", *Biotechnol. & Bioeng. Symp.* No. 3, pp 97, 1972.
2. Grieves, R.B. *et al., New Developments in Separation Methods*, (Grushka, I. ed), Marcel Dekker Inc., N.Y., 1976.
3. Schoen, H.M. (ed.), *New Chemical Engineering Separation Techniques*, Interscience Publishers, John Wiley and Sons, N.Y., 1962.
4. Morris, C.J. and P. Morris, *Separation Methods in Biochemistry*, John Wiley and Sons, N.Y., 1976.
5. Atkinson, A., "The Purification of Microbial Enzymes", *Proc. Biochem.* pp 9, 1973.
6. Dunnill, P. and M.D. Lilly, *Protein Extraction and Recovery from Microbial Cells—Single Cell Protein II,* pp. 179, (Tannenbaum, S.R., Wang, D.I.C., ed), MIT Press, Cambridge, Mass., USA, 1975.
7. Dunnill, P. "The Recovery of Intracellular Products", *Proc. IV Int. Ferm, Symp.—Ferment. Technol. Today*, pp 187, 1974.
8. Brookman, J.S. "Mechanism of Cell Disintegration in a High Pressure Homogenizer", *Biotechnol. & Bioeng.*, Vol. 16, pp 261, 1974.
9. Mogren, H. *et al.* "Mechanical Disintegration of Microorganisms in an Industrial Homogenizer", *Biotechnol. & Bioeng.*, Vol. 16, pp 261, 1974.
10. Brookman, J.S. "An Extreme Pressure Pump for Continuous Cell disintegration", *Biotechnol & Bioeng.*, Vol. 15, pp 693, 1973.
11. Jakoby, W. (ed.), *Methods in Enzymology*, Vol. 22, Academic Press, N.Y. USA.
12. Leninger, A.L., *Biochemistry*, Worth Publishers Inc., New York, USA, 2nd. ed., 1975.
13. Webb, E.C. and M. Dixon, "Enzyme Fractionation by Salting Out: A Theoretical Note", *Adv. Prot. Chem., 16*, pp 197, 1961.
14. Foster, P.R. *et al.,* "Salting Out of Enzymes with Ammonium Sulphate", *Biotechnol. & Bioeng.*, Vol. 13, pp 713, 1971.
15. Dubey, A.K., S.N. Mukhopadhyay and R. Thukral, "Recovery Purification and Variables of Activity of Native *Bam H1*", *Indian Chem. Engr.*, pp 37(4), 169-175, 1995

16. Charm, S.E. *et al.,* "Scaling up of Elution Gel-Filtration Chromatography", *Anal. Biochem.* 30, pp 1, 1969.
17. Mashelkar, R.A. *Intelligent Gels,* Jawaharlal Nehru Birth Centenary Lecture, IIT Delhi, 1995-1996.
18. Coulson, J.M. *et al., Chemical Engineering*, Volume 2, Pergamon Press, Oxford, U.K., 1962.
19. Brown, P.R. *High Pressure Liquid Chromatography—Biochemical and Biomedical Applications*, Academic Press, New York, USA, 1973.
20. Hamilton, P.B. *et al.,* "Ion-Exchange Chromatography of Amino Acids—Analysis of Diffusion (Mass Transfer) Mechanisms", *Anal. Chem.*, 32(13), pp 1782, 1960.
21. Giddings, J.C., "The Role of Lateral Diffusion as a Rate Controlling Mechanisms in Chromatography", *Jour. of Chromatogr.* 5, pp 46, 1961.
22. Fox, J.B. *et al.,* "Continuous Chromatography Apparatus—I, II, III", *Jour. of Chromatography*, 43, pp. 48, 55, 61, 1969.
23. Ono, H. *et al.*, "Process Design for Separating Nucleoside by a Counter Current Ion—Exchange Process", *Ferment. Technol. Today, Proc. of 4th. Int. Ferm. Symp.*, Kyoto, Japan, ed. Terui, G., pp 230, 1972.
24. Michaels, A.S. "New Separation Technique for CPI", *Chem. Eng. Prog.*, 64(12), pp 31, Dec. 1968.
25. Blatt, W.F. *et al.*, "Solute Polarization and Cake Formation in Membrane Ultrafiltration", *Membrane: Science and Technology*, pp. 47, (Flinn, J.E., ed.), Plenum Press, N.Y., 1970.
26. Kozenski, A.A. *et al.,* "Protein Ultrafiltration: A General Example of Boundary Layer Filtration", *AICHE Jour.*, 18(5), pp 1030, Sept. 1972.
27. Goldsmith, R.L. "Macromolecular Filtration with Microporous Membranes", *Ind. Eng. Chem. Fund.*, 10(1), pp 113, 1971.
28. Wang, D.I.C. *et al.*, "Recovery of Biological Materials through Ultrafiltration", *Biotechnol. & Bioeng.*, Vol 11, pp. 987, 1969.
29. Wang, D.I.C. *et al.,* "Enzyme and Bacteriophage Concentration by Membrane Filtration", *Anal. Biochem.*, 26, pp 277, 1968.
30. Charm, S.E. *et al.*, "Comparison of Ultrafiltration Systems for the Concentration of Biologicals", *Biotechnol. & Bioeng.*, Vol 13, pp. 185, 1971.
31. Poter, M.C. "Applications of Membranes to Enzyme Isolation and Purification", *Enzyme Engineering*, pp 115, (Wingard, L. ed.), Intersci. Publishers, John Wiley and Sons, N.Y., U.S.A., 1972.
32. McCabe, W.L. and Smith, J.C., *Unit Operations of Chemical Engineering*, McGraw Hill, N. Y., USA, 1956.
33. Hancher, C. W. *et al.*, "Evaluation of Ultrafiltration Membranes with Biological Macromolecules", *Biotechnol, & Bioeng.*, Vol. 15, pp 677, 1973.
34. Bailey, P.A., "Ultrafiltration—The Current State of the Art", *Filtration & Separation*, pp 213, 1977.
35. Balakrishnan, M, G.P. Agarwal and C.L. Cooney. J., *Membrane Science*., pp 85, 111-128, 1993.
36. Li, N., ed. *Recent Developments in Separation Science* Vol. 2, CRC Press, USA, 1972.
37. Catsimpoolas, N. ed., *Methods of Protein Separation*, pp 93, Vol. 1, Plenum Press, N. Y. USA, 1975.
39. Charm, S.E. *et al.*, "The Separation and Purification of Enzymes Through Foaming", *Anal. Biochem.*, 15, pp 202, 1966.
40. Wiseman, A. ed., *Topics in Enzyme and Fermentation Biotechnology-1*, pp 43, Halstead Press, John Wiley and Sons, 1977.
41. Lemlich, R. "Adsubble Methods", *Recent Develop. in Sep. Sci.*—Vol. 1, pp 113, (Li, N.N., ed.), CRC Press, Ohio, USA, 1972.
42. Gray P. *et al.*, "The Continuous Flow Isolation of Enzymes", *Proc, IV Int. Ferm. Technol. Today,* pp 347, 1974.
43. Sen. K. *Ph.D. Thesis*, Jadavpur University, Calcutta, 1991.
44. Wilson, D.J. andA.N. Clarke, "Bubble Foam Separations—Waste Treatment", *Handbook of*

Seperation Process Technology., pp 806-825, (R.W. Rousseau ed.), John Wiley & Sons, New York, 1987.

45. Ladish, M.R. "Separation by Sorption", *Advanced Biochemical Engineering*, pp. 219-237, (G. Belfort and H.R. Bungay eds.), John Wiley. & Sons., New York, 1987.
46. Bell, G. and R.B. Cousins, "Membrane Separation Processes", *Engineering Processes for Bioseparations,* pp. 135-1965, Chapter 6, (L.R. Weatherly ed.), Butterworth/Heinemann, Oxford, 1994.
47. Mattiason, B. and O. Hoist., *Extractive Bioconversions–Bioprocess Technology*, Vol. 2, Marcel Dekker, *Extractive Membrane Reactors and Ethanol Removal from a Bioreactor by Per Vaporation,* New York, 1991.
48. Cheryan, M. *Ultrafiltration Handbook*, Technomic.
49. Weatherley, L.R., "Near Critical Fluid Extraction for Biological and Food Product", *Engineering Processes for Bioseparations*, pp 233-257, (L.R. Weatherly ed.) Butterworth/Heinemann, Oxford, 1994.
50. Chisti, Y. and M. Moo Young, "Separations Techniques in Industrial Bioprocessing", *Bioproducts Processing. Technologies for the Tropics*., (M.A. Hazhim ed.), *ICHME Sympo. Sr: No.* 137, pp 135-146, Rugby, UK, 1994.
51. Oliver, C. *Current Biotechnol, Abstracts* Issue 5, No.2297, pp 2304, May 1987.
52. Wang, D.I.C. and A.E. Humphrey, "Biochemical Engineering", *Chemical Engg.* pp 108-120, Dec. 15, 1969.
53. Ghose, T.K. and J.A. Kostic, "A Model for Continuous Enzymatic Saccharification of Cellulase with Simultaneous Removal of Glucose Syrup", *Biotechnol. Bioengg*., pp 12, 921-46, 1970.
54. Mukhopadhyay, S.N., "An Overview of Taking Membrane Advantages in Food and Fermentation Process Biotechnology Industries", *Abstracts: Book of National Seminar on Membranes in Chemical and Biochemical Industries,* pp 45-46, 1996, I.I.T. Delhi; "Modern Concepts and Multifacet Role of Membranes in Biosystems and Bioprocessing", *Lecture Notes of the Course Membranes and its Applications*, pp 181-185, IIT Delhi, Feb. 13-15, 1996.
56. Sirkar, K.K. "Membrane Separations: Newer Concepts and Applications for Food Industry", *Bioseperation Processes in Foods,* (Singh. R.K. and S.S.H. Rizvi eds.), Marcel Dekkar, New York, 1995.
57. Sirkar, K.K. "Membrane Separation Technologies: Current Development and Future Opportunities", Key Note Lecture in XIV *National Membrane Soc. Sympo.*, IIT Delhi, 1996.
58. Teslik, S. and K.K. Sirkar, Paper Presented at the *182nd ACS National Meeting*, New York, Aug. pp 23-28, 1981.
59. Rousseau, R. W. ed., *Hand Book of Separation Process Technology*, Wiley Inter Sci. Pub., John Wiley & Sons, New York, 1987.
60. R. Hatti-Kanl and Bo Mattiasson. Isolation and Purification of Proteins, Marcel Dekker, Inc., New York, 2003.
61. R. Giovannini and R. Freitag, Biotechnol. Bioeng., 73, 522-529, 2001.
62. S. Ghose, G.M. Forde and N.K.H. Slater; Affinity Adsorption of Plasmid DNA, Biotechnol. Prog, 20, 841-850, 2004.
63. Labor Praxis, LP, April 2006, Special p 35.

Chapter

11

TREATMENT BIOTECHNOLOGY OF LIQUID WASTES AND WATER

11.1 INTRODUCTION

In recent years the more common waste water treatment relies on its treatment process biotechnology. In biological treatment procedure concentrated masses of microorganisms break-down organic pollutant matter, resulting in the stabilization of putrifiable wastes or refuses. These microorganisms are broadly grouped as aerobic or oxic, facultative, and anaerobic or anoxic. In brief the characteristics of these microorganisms are as below.[1,2]

(i) Oxic microorganisms need molecular oxygen for metabolism.
(ii) Faculative microorganisms may function in either oxic or anoxic conditions.
(iii) Anoxic microorganisms derive energy from organic molecules and function in the absence of oxygen.

Heterotrophic microorganisms are usually prominent species in mixed treatment process biotechnology. These microorganisms need an organic carbon source for both energy and cell mass synthesis. Autotrophic microorganisms in contrast, use an inorganic carbon source, such as CO_2 or carbonate. This type of microrganisms derive energy from the oxidation of inorganic compounds like nitrogen or sulfur (chemosynthetic) or from solar energy (photosynthetic).

11.2 GENERAL CONCERNS AND PRINCIPLES

11.2.1 Forewords and Parameters Definition

Basically the treatment bioprocessing involves either of two mechanisms to accumulate and store the biomass. The first is a flocculated suspension of biological growth called activated sludge, which is mixed with the waste waters. In the second, a biological film is fixed to an inert surface support medium on which the waste waters pass over. The applied process biotechnology in the past therefore has comprised mostly three systems. These are, (a) the activated sludge process (ASP), (b) the trickling filter (a fixed film process, FFP) and (c) the anaerobic digestion (AD) of waste organic materials.

The purpose of treatment of waste waters or liquid wastes is to avoid possible fates of disposal of untreated one. These fates as shown in Fig. 11.1 indicate the cause of happening of hazards depending on the liquid waste origin (Fig. 11.2). So the purposes of treatment and undesirable materials to be removed from waste water are many as are evident from Table 11.1 and Table 11.2.

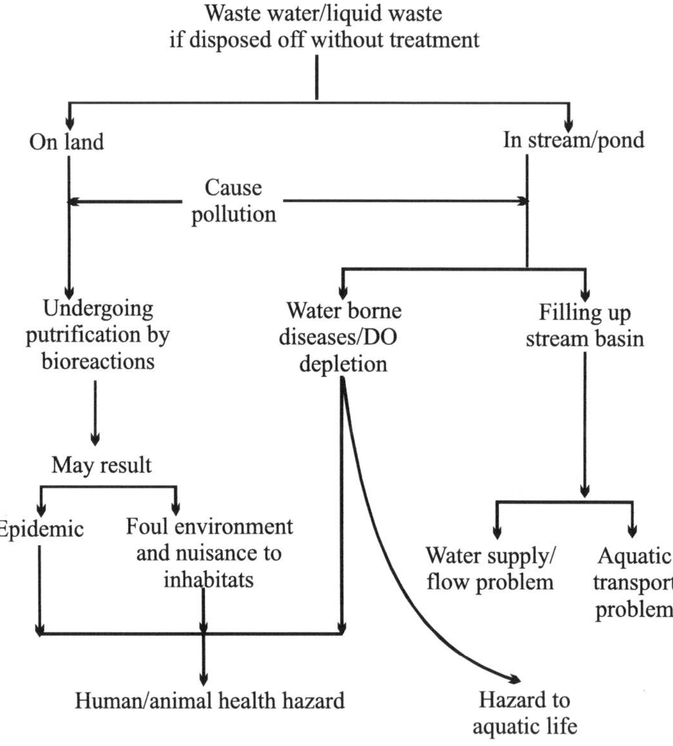

Fig. 11.1 Possible fate of disposal of untreated waste water or liquid waste

Table 11.1 Purposes of biological treatment

- For reducing existing pollutants
- For water reuse by preventing injury to receiving waters.
- For by product recovery.
- For taking care of pollution discharge increase due to plant expansion and production increase.
- For taking care of society considering plant location.

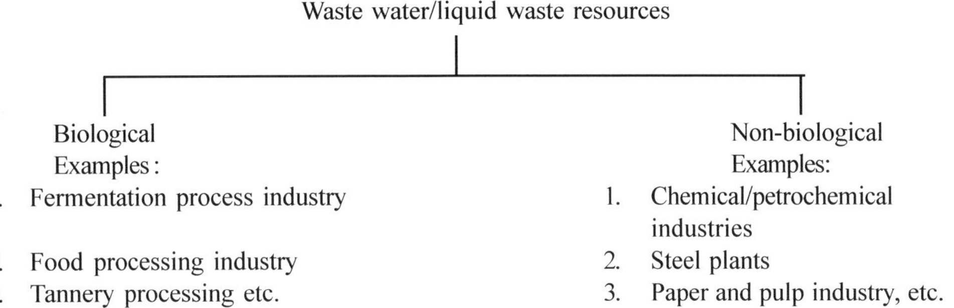

Fig. 11.2 Waste water resources types

Table 11.2 Type of undesirable materials to be removed

- Soluble organics causing dissolved oxygen (DO) depletion in receptackle.
- Suspended solids.
- Trace organics like phenols causing bad taste in drinking water.
- Heavy metals, cyanides and toxic organics.
- Colour and turbidity nitrogenous and phosphorous compounds.
- Refractory materials.
- Oil and volatile materials.
- Radioactive component etc.

In more recent years advances in treatment process biotechnology have primarily involved improvements in the basic biotechnology, innovations, broadening of the application of the process, and an advancement in the design, analysis and operational procedures.

In treatment bioprocessing microbial cell populations may be specifically adapted to certain compounds and successfully achieve biooxidation. Examples of such compounds are many. Phenol, cyanide, polyphenols, thiocyanates are few examples. Most organic materials present in industrial wastes are amenable to biooxidation implying thereby that they are amenable to biological treatment. When a specific toxic or inhibitory waste streams are present in the total stream, successful biological treatment is hampered. In such cases proper biological waste water treatment design procedures for complex industrial wastes is essential. It should include characterization of various waste streams contributing to over-all flow e.g. river or other flowing system. The most important characterization parameters include biochemical oxygen demand (BOD) and chemical oxygen demand (COD). The two parameters in turn are usually found to be related to each other by a simple correlation.

11.2.2 Biochemical Oxygen Demand

1. General considerations [3,4]

Biochemical oxygen demand (BOD) is usually defined as the amount of oxygen required by bacteria while stabilizing decomposable organic matter under aerobic conditions. The BOD test is essentially a bioassay procedure involving the measurment of oxygen consumed by living organisms (mainly bacteria) while utilising the organic matter present in a waste. This test is widely used to determine the pollution strength of sewages and industrial wastes in terms of the oxygen that they will require if discharged into natural water courses in which aerobic condition exists. Biological degradation of organic matter under natural conditions is brought about by a diverse group of organisms that carry the oxidation essentially to completion, i.e., almost entirely to carbon dioxide and water. Therefore, it is important that mixed group of organisms, commonly called 'seed' be present in the test. The rate at which the reactions proceed is governed to a major extent by population numbers and temperature. Temperature effects are held constant by performing the test at 20°C. Theoretically, an infinite time is required for complete biological oxidation of organic matter but for all practical purposes, the reaction may be considered complete in 20 days. However a 20-day period is too long to wait for results in most instances. It has been found by experience that a reasonably large percentage of the total BOD is exerted in 5 days; consequently the test has been developed on the basis of a 5-day incubation period.

2. The nature of BOD reaction

Studies of the kinetics of BOD reactions have established that they resemble unimolecular reactions or first order in character, or in reality the rate of the reaction is proportional to the amount of oxidisable organic matter remaining at any time.

$$\frac{d_L}{d_t} = -\,KL \tag{11.1}$$

Where, L = organic matter remaining i.e., organic matter to be oxidized.

$$\int_{L_a}^{L_t} dL/L = -\,K \int_0^t \text{ or, } \log_e L_t/L_a = -\,kt \text{ or, } L_t/L_a = e^{-Kt}$$

or $$L_t/L_a = 10^{-kt}, \text{ where } k = 0.4343\ K$$

so, $$y = L_a - L_t = L_a\,(1 - L_t/L_a) = L_a\,(1 - e^{-Kt}) \text{ or } L_a\,(1 - 10^{-kt}) \tag{11.2}$$

where, y = BOD at any time t; L_a = ultimate BOD

3. Phases of BOD curve

A typical BOD curve is shown in Fig. 11.3. The curve shows two distinct phases. The 'seed' which is derived from soil or domestic sewage, contain large numbers of saprophytic bacteria that utilize carbonaceous matter present in the samples. In addition they normally contain autotrophic bacteria particularly nitrifying bacteria, which are capable of oxidizing non-carbonaceous matter. The nitrifying bacteria are usually present in relatively small numbers in unaerated domestic sewage and, fortunately, their reproduction rate at 20°C is such that their populations do not become sufficiently large to exert an appreciable demand for oxygen until about 8 or 10 days have elapsed in the regular BOD test. Once the organisms become estabilished, they oxidize nitrogen in the form of ammonia to nitrite and nitrate by using oxygen.

$$2NH_3 + 3O_2 \xrightarrow[\text{bacteria}]{\text{Nitrite forming}} 2NO_2^- + 2H^+ + 2H_2O$$

$$2NO_2^- + O_2 + 2H^+ \xrightarrow[\text{bacteria}]{\text{Nitrite forming}} 2NO_3^- + 2H^+$$

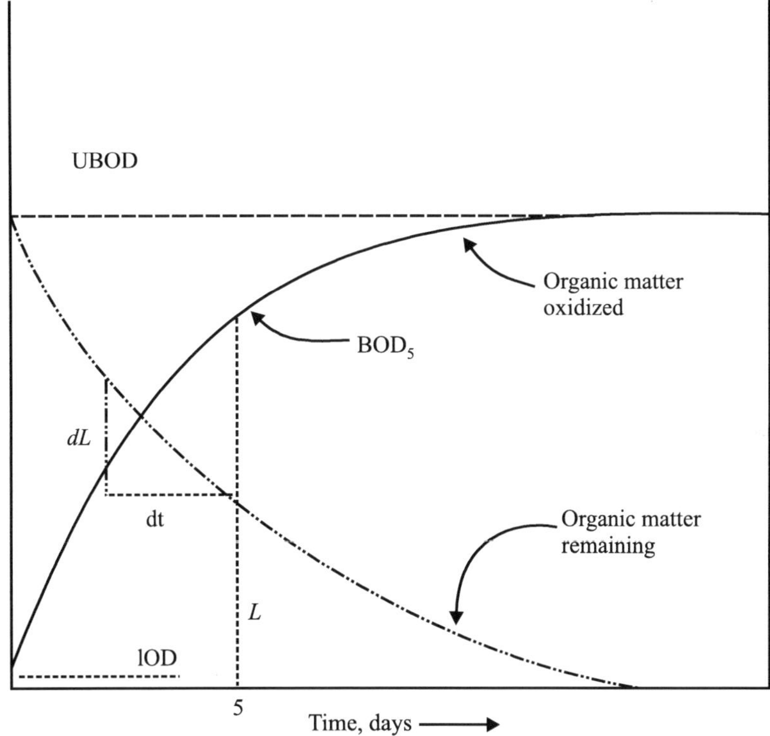

Fig. 11.3 BOD reaction profile

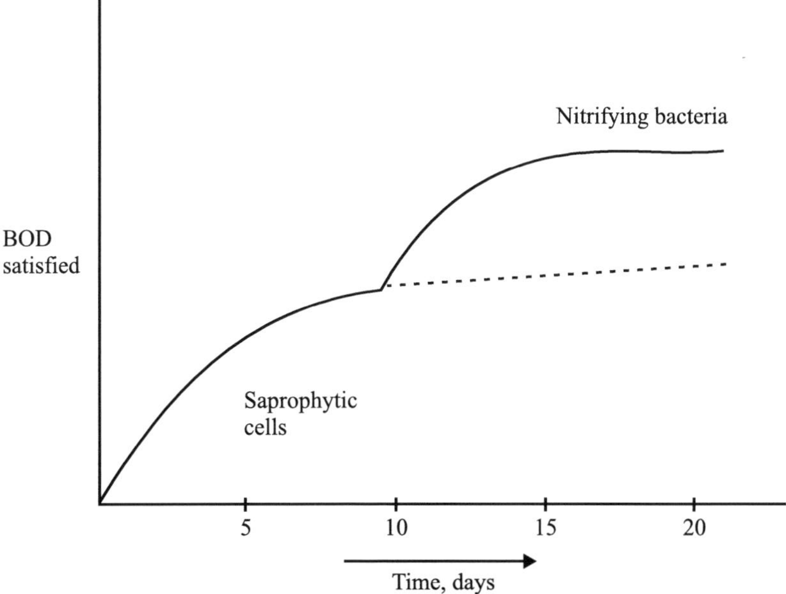

Fig. 11.4 BOD curve

The interference caused by nitrifying organisms makes the actual measurements of total carbonaceous BOD impossible unless provision is made to eliminate them. It was a major reason for selecting a 5-day incubation period for the regular BOD test.

In case where the effluent is from biological treatment units, such as trickling filters and activated sludges, it often contains populations of nitrifying organisms sufficient to utilize significant amounts of oxygen during the regular 5-day incubation period. It is important to know the amount of residual carbonaceous BOD in such cases in order to be able to measure plant efficiency. The action of nitrifying bacteria can be arrested by the use of specific inhibiting agents such as methylene blue, or the microbial populations can be made absent from the samples by sterilization.

4. Evaluation of the values of K and L_a

Formulation of the first-stage BOD of waste water as a first order reaction yields the following equations

$$dy/dt = K\,(L_a - y) \text{ or } \int_{y_0}^{L_a} dy/(L_a - y) = K \int_0^t dt$$

or
$$\log_e \frac{L_a - y_t}{L_a - y_0} = -K_t \quad \text{or} \quad \frac{L_a - y_t}{L_a - y_0} = e^{-kt} \text{ or } 10^{-kt} \qquad (11.3)$$

Rearranging,
$$1 - \frac{L_a - y_t}{L_a - y_0} = 1 - 10^k \quad \text{or, } y_t - y_0 = (L_a - y_0)\,(1 - 10^{kt})$$

or,
$$y_t = (L_a - y_0)\,(1 - 10^{-kt}) + y_0 \qquad (11.4)$$

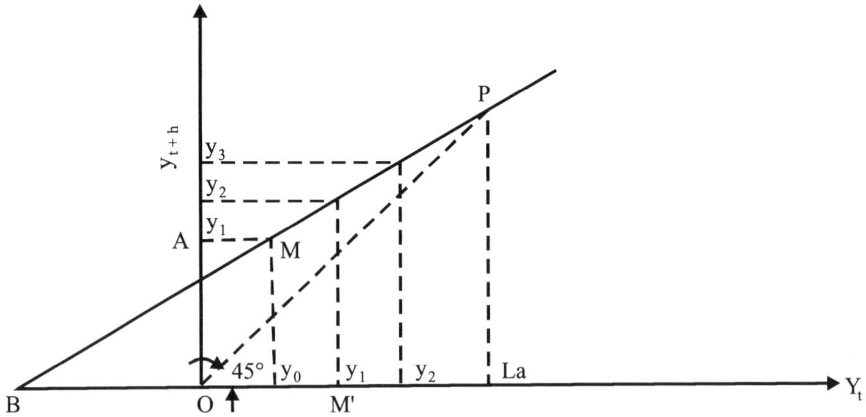

Fig. 11.5 Graphical evaluation of L_a and k

similarly,
$$\begin{aligned} y_{t+h} &= (L_a - y_0)\,(1 - 10^{-k\,(t+h)}) + y_0 \\ &= L_a - (L_a - y_0)\,10^{-k\,(t+h)} \\ &= L_a - (L_a - y_0)\,10^{-kh} + (L_a - y_0)\,10^{-kh} - (L_a - y_0)\,10^{-k\,(t+h)} \\ &= L_a - L_a\,10^{-th} + \{(L_a - y_0)\,(1 - 10^{-kt}) + y_0\}\,10^{-kh} \end{aligned}$$

$$= L_a - L_a\, 10^{-kh} + y_t\, 10^{-kh}$$

$$y_{t+h} = L_a(1 - 10^{-kh}) + 10^{-kh}\; y_t \qquad (11.5)$$

If y_{t+h} is plotted as the ordinate against y_t as the abscissa, the value of the intercept on the ordinate at $y_t = 0$ of a straight line fitted either by eye estimation or by the method of least squares is

$$L_a(1 - 10^{-kh})$$

and the intercept on x-axis, i.e. when $y_{t+h} = 0$, is

$$L_a(1 - 10^{-kh})/10^{-kh}$$

$$OA = L_a(1 - 10^{-kh});\ OB = L_a(1 - 10^{-kh}) / 0^{-kh}$$

Slope of the line = OA/OB = 10^{-kh} and if h = 1,

$$k = \log_{10} \frac{OB}{OA}$$

Graphical evaluation of L_a: At P, $y_t = y_{t+h}$ and thus in equation (11.3) $y_t - 10^{-k} \cdot y_t = L_a(1 - 10^{-kh})$ or, $y_t = L_a$

Hence, the particular value of y_t at the point P is L_a.

Eavaluation of y_0: Plot y_1 on y-axis and draw a horizontal line to cut the BOD line at M. Drop a perpendicular from *M* on *y*-axis *and it meets y*-axis at M'. OM' = y_0.

Alternatively, equation (11.2) may be used after evaluating L_a, K and it writes as

$$y_1 = (L_a - y_0)(1 - 10^{-k}) + y_0 \qquad (11.6)$$

or

$$10^{-k} \cdot y_0 = y_1 - L_a(1 - 10^{-k})$$

or

$$y_0 = (y_1 - OA)\quad 10^{k} \qquad (11.7)$$

11.2.3 Chemical Oxygen Demand (COD)

The amount of oxygen required to oxidize waste water component by purely chemical reaction under specified condition has been termend chemical oxygen demand.

11.2.4 BOD-COD Correlation

From the above discussions and definitions, the BOD measures waste which are biologically oxidizable and COD measures organic and inorganic wastes which are chemically oxidizable. Usually COD is greater than BOD. All wastes whether organic or inorganic will have a percentage of following component.

(a) (i) Biochemically oxidizable part (BO)
    (ii) Not biochemically oxidizable part (NBO)

(b) (i) Chemically oxidizable part (CO)
    (ii) Not chemically oxidizable part (NCO)

One may represent mathematically,

$$I = \text{Inorganic} = I_{CO} + I_{NCO} = I_{BO} + I_{NBO}$$

$$O = \text{Organic} = O_{CO} + O_{NCO} = O_{BO} + O_{NBO}$$

Now,

$$COD = I_{CO} + O_{CO} = (I_{CO} + O_{BO}) + (O_{NBO} - O_{NCO})$$

$$BOD = O_{BO} + I_{BO} = (O_{BO} + I_{CO}) + (I_{NCO} - I_{NBO})$$

$\therefore$

$$COD - BOD = (O_{NBO} - O_{NCO}) - (I_{NCO} - I_{NBO})$$

It shows that

$$COD > BOD \text{ if } (O_{NBO} - O_{NCO}) > (I_{NCO} - I_{NBO})$$

In other words,

$$COD > BOD \text{ if } (O_{NBO} + I_{NBO}) > (I_{NCO} + O_{NCO})$$

or if,

waste components resistant to biochemical oxidation > waste components resistant to chemical oxidation.

11.2.5 Other Indices

In literature besides BOD and COD various other indices have been used for measuring strength of waste and waste waters. In brief their definitions are given below.

Total Oxygen Demand (TOD): It is the stoichiometric amount of oxygen required to oxidize completely a substance to products like CO_2, H_2O, HNO_3, H_3PO_4, H_2SO_4 etc.

Ultimate Biological Oxygen Demand (UBOD) : The total BOD measured over an incubation period long enough for the reaction to reach virtual completion.

Immediate Oxygen Demand (IOD): The amount of oxygen utilized by a waste or waste water sample immediately (within 15 minutes) upon being mixed with air saturated distilled water.

11.2.6 Correlation of BOD with Other Indices

From the time profile of BOD as shown in Fig. 11.3 the distinction between the indices are clear. It has been shown that

$$y_5 = BOD_5 = (UBOD - IOD)(1 - K^t) \quad (11.8)$$

Where K is rate constant = 0.794 and t is time in days. So,

$$y_5 = BOD_5 = (UBOD - IOD)(1 - 0.794^5)$$

or

$$y_5 = BOD_5 = 0.68 (UBOD - IOD) \quad (11.9)$$

11.2.7 Determination of Indices (API Method)

BOD_5: Sample is diluted with distilled water (standard), seeded with bacteria and then incubated at 68°F (20°C) for 5 days. The decrease in oxygen content between original sample and incubated sample gives $BOD_{5\,(20°C)}$. COD: Sample is digested for 2 hours at 290°F with H_2SO_4 and excess $K_2Cr_2O_7$. The consumption of $K_2Cr_2O_7$ is the 2 hr COD. It is also expressed as 4 hr $KMnO_4$ value of COD.

IOD: The sample waste water is diluted with aserated distilled water and allowed to stand for 15 minutes. The dissolved oxygen (DO) content is determined for the diluted mixture. The oxygen consumed is obtained from the difference between the oxygen added with the distilled water and that remaining in the diluted mixture at the end of 15 minutes reaction period.

11.3 TREATMENT BIOTECHNOLOGY FOR WASTE WATERS

11.3.1 Brewery and Distillery Effluents [6-10]

Breweries and distilleries produce huge quantity of liquid effluents originated from different sections of the industrial processing. These effluents are highly pollutants bearing in terms of BOD and COD loadings.

1. Origin of wastes

The malting process produces two major wastes: those arising from the steep tank after grain has been removed, and those remaining in the germinating drum after the grain malt has been removed. Brewery wastes are composed mainly of liquor pressed from the wet grain, liquor from yeast recovery, and wash water from the various sections. After the distillation of the alcohol process, a residue remains which is generally referred to as 'distillery slops', 'beer slops', or 'still bottoms.'

There are several sources of wastes in a distillery. Of major concerns are the 'dealcoholized' still residue and evaporator condensate, when the stillage is evaporated. Minor wastes include redistillation residue and equipment washes.

In the manufacture of compressed yeast seed, yeast is planted in a nutrient solution and allowed to grow under aerobic conditions until maximum cell multiplication is attained. The yeast is then separated from the spent nutrient solution, compressed, and finally packaged. The yeast plant effluent consists of: (1) filter residues resulting from the preparation of the nutrient solutions, (2) spent nutrients, (3) wash waters, (4) filter press effluents, and (5) cooling and condenser waters (Tables 11.3 and 11.5).

2. Plant lay-out

Wastes emanate from the malting, brewing and washing operations, as shown in the Fig. 11.6. In the brewing operation malt is prepared in the mash tun at elevated temperature with water containing calcium and phosphate salts. After the malting operation, the mash is discharged to a screen filter (lanter tub) from which the spent grains are removed to a hopper and trucked away. The malt liquor is then discharged to the kettle to which the hops are added. Following heating in the kettle, the mixture is sent to a filter (hop jack) for removal of spent hops. The filtered mixture is pumped to a settling (hot wort) tank, then cooled and sent to storage (cold wort tank). The wort from storage is filtered through diatomaceous earth and passed to the fermentation tank. Yeast is added to the fermentation tank, in which a temperature of 61-70°F is maintained. After fermentation the beer is removed to warm storage. The beer from warm storage is carbonated

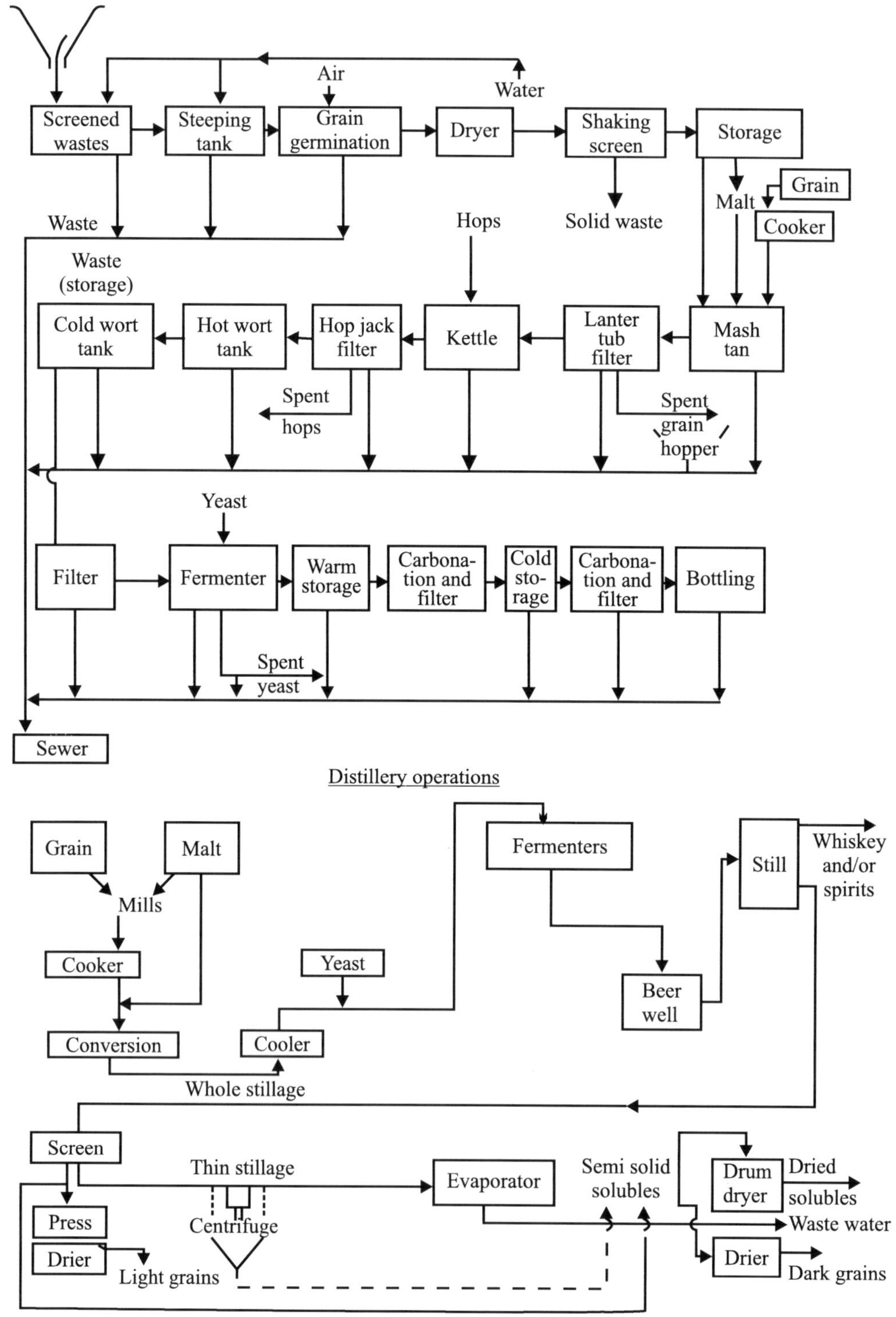

Fig. 11.6 Pockets of waste water generation in brewery and distillery

and filtered through diatomaceous earth and sent to cold storage. Carbonation and filtration follow and the beer is then bottled.

3. Waste water characteristics

Malt wastes

Plant capacity	6996 bushels of barley/day.
Suspended solids	72 mg/*l*
5-day BOD (20°C)	390 mg/*l*
Water consumption	75 gallons/bushel.

The solids are mainly orgainc and high in nitrogen, indicating considerable proteinous material. A major portion of the solids was in solution, as indicated by the low suspended solids content.

Yeast wastes consist primarily of the spent nutrient (although only 20 per cent of the wastes by volume, they account for 75 to 80 per cent of the total BOD). They are brown, have a typical odour of yeast, and are highly hygroscopic. The solids are almost entirely dissoved and colloidal; the suspended solids content is seldom above 200 mg/*l*. The composition of this waste is given in Table 11.6. Characteristics are given in Table 11.7.

Table 11.3 A summary of individual waste from a typical Bourbon distillery

Source of Waste	*Volume, Gallon*	*Suspended solids Total mg/l*	*mg/l*	*pH*	*BOD mg/l*	*Pop. Equiv.*
Cooker condensate	54,000	7	6	7.2	5.4	14
Cooker wash water	2,750	–	–	–	1,370	185
Redistillation residues	1,000	–	–	7.7	1,700	84
Floor and equipment wash	–	–	–	–	–	227
Evaporation Condensate	29,490	35	30	4.5	375	540
Thick slop to Feed house	35,235	50,000	48,000	4.3	20,000	35,300

Table 11.4 Composition of some 'distillery slops'. All the slops have an acid reaction, and contain from about 2 to 7 per cent total solids concentration.

Item	*Spirit Type*	*Bourbon Type*	*Molasses*	*Apple Brandy*
pH	4.1	4.2	4.5	3.8
Total solids, mg/*l*	24,345	37,388	71,053	18,866
Suspended solids, mg/*l*	24,800	17,900	40	50
BOD, mg/*l*	34,100	26,000	28,700	21,000
Total volatile Solids, mg/*l*	43,300	34,226	55,608	16,948

Table 11.5 The solids concentration and BOD content of fermentation wastes

Fermentation waste	*Solids, %*	*BOD, mg/l*
Brewery-press liquor	3	10,000–25,000
Yeast plant	1 – 3	7,000 – 14,000
Industrial alcohol	5	22,000
Distillery slops	4.5-6	15,000–20,000

Table 11.6 Composition of the yeast waste

Characteristics	*Concentration or Value*
Total solids, mg/*l*	10,000 – 20,000
Suspended solids, mg/*l*	50 – 200
Volatile solids, mg/*l*	7,000 – 15,000
Total nitrogen, mg/*l*	800 – 900
Organic nitrogen mg/*l*	500 – 700
Total carbon, mg./*l*	3,800 – 5,500
Organic carbon, mg/*l*	3,700 – 5,500
BOD, mg/*l*	2,000 – 2,500
Sulphate, as mg/*l* SO_4	2,000 – 2,500
Phosphate, as mg/*l* P_2O_5	20 – 140
pH	4.5 – 6.5

Table 11.7 The average characteristics of a fermentation process-plant waste

Characteristics	*Concentration or Value*
5– day BOD (20°C), mg/*l*	4,500
pH	6 – 7
Total solids, mg/*l*	10,000
Settleable suspended solids, mg/*l*	25

4. Distillery effluent in biogas generation [6-14]

(i) *General Considerations* : India has more than 160 molasses based distilleries. About 900 million liters of distillery effluent are generated annually by them. It is one of the most polluting and environmentally unacceptable organic liquid wastes which cause health hazard to the people in the surrounding locality.[10] The major sources of liquid waste water for molasses based distillaries are: (a) process waste stream like spent wash and digester sludge. and (b) non-process waste stream like cooling water, boiler blow down water etc. Government stringent regulations as well as mass health considerations have made it a compulsion to treat this hazardous effluent using efficient process tenchnology such as anaerobic digestion for production of biogas and abating pollution. Many biogas installations from distillery waste based on Indian Technology are now in operation in India. A number of technologies from various countries such as U.K.,

USA, France, Belgium, Thailand, Canada, Switzerland and Italy have established collaboration with various Indian distilleries for biogas generation from their effluent (Tables 11.8 and 11.9). Also, in about three cases the plants are yet to be commissioned and some are in the process of being commissioned. Table 11.8 gives a list of biogas installations from distillery waste based on Indian technologies and foreign

Table 11.8 Biogas installations for distillery effluent in India using Indian technological knowhow

Location of Distillery	*Process Installtion Informatic*
DCM Sugar Works, Daurala, UP	Biphasic process Installation capacity 100 m^3/d
Liquor (India) Pvt. Ltd., Hyderabad	BERC, IIT Delhi process based pilot demostration Unit (15 m^3 of effluent per day) Biphasic process/immobilized cell continuous process Distillery effluent BOD - 50,0 to 60,000 ppm BOD reduction % – 90 in 3 days
Polychem distillery, Nira, Maharashtra	Biphasic anaerobic contact process 25 m^3/d treatment capacity Energy output to input ration = 17.3
Pungam, Gujarat	Effluent spent wash from 3000 *l*/d alcohol unit BOD = 50,000 ppm Gas production 35-40 m^3/m^3 spent wash BOD removal = 90% Methane % = 55-65
KCP Ltd. Sugar Factory, Vuyyum, AP	Two digesters of total capacity 20,000 *l*/h Treated

Table 11.9 List of Indian distillery installations with overseas collaboration for biogas production from their effluents.

	Distilleries	*Overseas Collaborator*
1.	Shakti Sugar Ltd., Coimbatore	Society General Pour Techniques Noovless, France B.S. Sinoglen, Italy
2.	Kolhapur Sugar Mills Ltd., Maharashtra	B.S. Sinoglen - Italy
3.	Dharmasi Morarji Chemical Co. Ltd., Bombay	Larson International Inc., USA
4.	Shaw Wallace and Co., Calcutta	Aqua Technor Co. Ltd., Bangkok (Thailand)
5.	Ashok Organic Industries Ltd., Bombay	-do-
6.	Rqampur Distillery and Chem-Co. Ltd., Delhi	-do-
7.	McDowell and CO. Ltd., Madras.	-do-
8.	Ajudhya Distillery, Vizak.	AD1-BVF, Canada
9.	Mohan Meakins, UP	Degremont, France
10.	Vam Organic Chem. Ltd. Gajraula, UP	Biotim, Belgium
11.	Modi	Sulzers, Switzerland
12.	Rajpur and Haryana Plant	PAQUE, Holland

Table 11.10 Comparison of technical knowhow of methane generation from distillery effluent anaerobic digestion of three technologies (Data 1987)

Know-how Item	*Distilleries*		
	Vam Organic Chemicals Ltd. (VOCL)	*Rampur Distillery and Chem. Co.*	*Ajudhya Distillery*
1. Capital investment for creation (Rs. in Lacs/m^3 effluent digestion/treatment)	225.4 Lacs	195.0 Lacs	120
2. Operational cost (")	–	–	–
3. Reduction of BOD (%)	88-90	85-90	90
4. Reduction of COD (%)	60	65-67	70
5. Biogas generation (nm^3/m^3 spent wash)	25	30	30
6. Methane content in biogas (%)	60-65	60	55
7. Calorific value of biogas (k. cal/m^3)	4700	5000	4600
8. Other gases present (%) CO_2 H_2S	– –	38 2	– –
9. Process stabilization period (months)	–		–
10. Waste flow installed capacity (m^3/day)	8	6	8
11. Power requirement for running the unit (KWH/nm^3 gas)	approx. 0.25	approx. 0.3	–
12. Generation and its frequency (months)	–	" 0.5	–
13. Chemical cost	–	" 0.10	–
14. Total running cost (Rs. m^3/gas)	–	–	–
15. Year of installation	–	–	–
16. Project implementation period (months)	–	12	–
17. Coal equivalent (MT/d)	24.02	–	–

collaboration technologies on the basis of available data. Table 11.10 provides comparative results claimed by the various technology suppliers. Some of them have claimed biogas generation from 30-35 m^3 per m^3 of spent wash of methane content 70% which, seems to be on the high side. Anaerobic digestion of concentrated industrial effluents from sugar mills, distilleries, breweries, paper and pulp mills, dairies, canneries, animal breeding etc. under properly controlled/regulated conditions generates large amount of methane/biogas. It is an ideal fuel for boilers and for generating electricity or for consumption of energy in rural India. Its need for alternate energy supplies for rural development and rural environmental protection is increasingly apparent. The present energy generating system in rural parts of developing countries like India depend largely on local resources like fire wood, straw or dung cake for burning. The smoke of these fuels create unhealthy conditions to villagers. In order to solve this problem to a great extent and to meet the energy demand of villagers use of biogas as a clean fuel has been recommended. So biogas concept has drawn extensive attention and importance all over the globe including India. Typical distillery effluent raw material specification is shown in Table 11.11.

Table 11.11 Distillery effluent raw material specifications as used in BIOTIM-NV-VOCL process technology

Parameter	*Unit*	*Specifications*
Effluent colour		Brown
specific gravity at 20°C		1.05
Temperature from distillery source	°C	85
Temperature after cooling	°C`	40
BOD total	ppm	44750
BOD soluble	”	42500
COD total	”	95400
COD soluble	”	90490
TSS	”	2120
TDS	”	92220
TS	”	94340
Kjeldahl N_2	”	120
Orthophosphate as ‘P’	”	19.5
pH	”	4.15
Alkalinity as $CaCO_3$	”	Nil
Volatile as HAC	”	2184
Sulphate as SO_4	”	4400
Chloride as Cl	”	6320
Sulphide as S	”	40
Potassium as K_2O	”	10680
Calcium as CaO	”	2350
Ash	”	29190
Fe	”	1.16

It is the volatile portion of solids that provides the food for the microorganisms in anaerobic digestion system. Actually the process involves two phases from bacteriological stand point. In the first phase anaerobic acidogenic bacteria breakdown the organic fractions of the solids generating volatile organic fatty acids in the digester. These acids next become the substrate for methane producing bacteria. Total reduction (100%) of original volatile matter in the sludge is virtually nonachievable. In practice the volatile solids (VS) in the raw distillery sludge are reduced by 40 to 70%.

In order to make the distillery effluent treatment plants economically viable one has to keep in mind that the process should provide maximum methane formation (of course without compromising the quality or life of the particular system adopted). For obtaining maximum CH_4

economically every single distillery effluent treatment process has to adopt 'Anaerobic Digestion' biotechology. It can be mesophilic' or 'thermophilic' depending on the temperature of performance of the digester. From a comparative view point one can observe that out of several overseas technologies only one has adopted thermophilic anaerobic digestion technology of M/S Aquatech (Thailand) which is located at the Rampur Distillery and Chemical Co. Ltd. The biogas generation has been claimed to be 29 m^3 per m^3 of spent wash. The methane content is 55% and thus the calorific value is 4700 k. cal/m^3. Although there are a few advantages in choosing thermophilic anaerobic digestion but the disadvantages are many. It is learnt that the same technology used at the Ashok Organic Plant has not yet yielded very satisfactory results. Indian climatic conditions are such that 'mesophilic' digestion is very well suited in most parts of the country. Moreover the 'mesophilic' temperature range (35-40°C) is more conducive and operationally easier to methane bacteria. Not only that since the source of the distillary effluent contains lot of important materials suitable as a biofertilizer many investigators have tried to look into the possibility of using the sludge of the biogas digaster as a source of biomanure as well as animal feed. Necessity of having a thorough study on the details of the anaerobic digestion biotechnology is therefore obvious.

(ii) Theoretical Considerations:

A. Molasses resources and distillery

Molasses is the syrup that is left after the recovery of crystalline sugar from the concentrated juice of sugar cane. Depending on processing of sugar cane juice two kinds of molasses have been reported in the literature. They are 'Blackstrap molasses' and 'High test molasses.' Blackstrap molasses has been used principally in industrial alcohol production in distilleries. It usually contains 48 to 55% of sugars mainly sucrose. However, 'High test molasses' has also been used for ethanol manufacture. It is an evaporated juice but most of it remains in inverted sugar form as a result of acid hydrolysis. This type of molasses is usually high in sugar content. Occasionally it may contain as high as 78 per cent sugar. In India 'blackstrap molasses' has been widely used for industrial alcohol production.

The industrial process adopted by the distilleries consists of fermenting the diluted molasses with yeast and distilling the alcohol produced in distillation columns by passing a counter current of steam while allowing the fermented mash to come down the tall column. Only about 10 per cent of the molasses is utilised in the process and the major remaining liquid part comes out as effluent in the process. This liquid effluent consists of spent wash and yeast waste sludge and floor washings. Yeast waste sludge is separated out and dried and used as animal feed. After removal of yeast the liquid effluent is called distillery effluent and has been used as substrate for long time in anaerobic digester for its treatment and disposal.

B. Basic biogas technology concept

Biogas production from available liquid waste resources from distillery effluent through anaerobic digestion for biomethanation is an era old concept. An idea of daily availability of distillery effluent has been given in literature. As this effluent discharged by an alcohol/distillery industry is environmentally most polluting containing unacceptable organic waste in terms of COD (approx.

80,000 to 1,00,000 ppm) and BOD (approx, 40,000 to 55,000 ppm) loading its proper disposal retrieving benefit to maximum extent is essential. Anaerobic digestion for management and disposal of distillery effluent both in terms of utilization and protection of environmental pollution has been critically analysed by engineers taking into consideration the general properties of distillery effluent as given in the Table 11.12. Basic biogas technology comprises therefore, the bioconversion of carbonaceous material into volatile organic acids by acid forming bacteria in absence of air, subsequently bioconversion of volatile organic acids by methane bacteria in absence of air into methane.

C. Thermodynamic basis of quantitative analysis

As can be seen from Table. 11.12 that the major component in distillery effluent is carbonaceous organic matter responsible for anaerobic biomethanation. The stoichiometry of hydrolytic methanization of carbonaceous component has been preliminarily based on a very simple chemical equation. However, in this simple chemical stoichiometry chemically bound nitrogen has not been considered. But nitrogen negatively affects the course of anaerobic digestion. As sometimes the content of bound nitrogen in distillery effluent may be appreciable and variable, its rise brings about a drop in the methane yield coefficient $Y_{(CH_4/s)}$. In that case the above referred simple chemical balance need to be modified by the nitrogen and other negatively affecting elements like sulfur present. The overall hydrolytic energy retrieval stoichiometry need to be considered accordingly. From the knowledge of electron participation in anaerobic digestion of distillery effluent and considering the general formula of distillery effluent substrate containing nitrogen and sulfur, it is theoretically possible to measure degree of bioreducibility of this substrate. It implies that due to the presence of elements like N, S etc. as acceptors of electrons in anaerobic digestion redox reaction has a negative effect. Accordingly higher levels of nitrogen, sulfur and other similar elements which may act as electron donors or acceptors in anaerobic digestion influence on biomethanation. In most developing countries like India where sugar based industries produce large amounts of molasses it will be highly desirable to recycle the molasses for biomethanation through anaerobic digestion to replace its coal/furnace oil requirement as well as to prevent pollution of the locality. On the basis of theoretical and investigational informations various basic biotechnological process engineering designs have been developed in many countries. A comparative design figures of them are given in Table 11.10. In order to determine these basic biotechnological parameters of anaerobic digestion, elemental analysis of the resource substrate is very essential. It yields the empirical substrate formula referred to 1C atom and values of substrates reducibility degree (v_s) and yield coefficient (Y_s). These values then aid in determining the $Y_{(CH_4/s)}$ theoretical, COD theoretical and per cent methane. Also, the content of v_s, yield coefficient, Y_{exp} and COD are determined by experiments. If the substrate composition is unknown the value of Y_s for a given biomass can bc determined from the experimental COD and v_s from the content of CH_4 in the biogas. Measurement of these quantities during the course of digestion makes it possible to characterise semiquantitatively the course of individual phases of the digestion process. Using Y_{exp} and Y_{theo} values it is possible to calculate the actual biotechnological efficiency (η from the values of Y_s determinedes % CH_4 in the biogas and from v_s assessed by means of COD value, the theoretical amount of heat, Q yields by combustion of CH_4 from anaerobic digestion can be determined. From the known

Table 11.12 Properties of molasses based distillery effluent

Properties of Distillery Effluent	*Unit*	*From Resource Molasses*	
		Black Strap	*Hightest*
COD	ppm	70,000-90,000	80,000-1,00,000
BOD	"	50,000-60,000	40,000-50,000
TS	"	80,000-85,000	60,000-90,000
VS	"	–	45,000-65,000
Carbon	"	–	Approx. 25,000
Ash	"	25,000	Approx. 12,000
Nitrogen	"	900	1,200
Vitamin	–	High	High
pH	–	4.5-5.0	4.5-5.5

calorific value of coal it will now be possible to determine the coal/furnace equivalent of the heat obtainable from biogas. Thus the amount of coal that can be replaced by the generated biogas may be calculated.

The engineering analysis of mass and energy balance made it therefore, possible to evaluate the efficiency of different biotechnology process devices for distillery effluent digestion in biogas production.

D. Kinetic considerations

Based on reaction rates of distillery effluent it is necessary to analyse the kinetics of anaerobic digestion. It is helpful to know the key factors affecting efficiency and stability of digestion in which solids residence time is important.

Importance of residence time: One of the key factors for bacteria growth is residence time. To ensure efficient bioconversion of organic matter to methane and carbon dioxide, the population of bacteria in the digester must be of sufficient quality and concentration. Also they must have adequate active residence time to allow substrate metabolism and to prevent depletion of bacteria. For the designer and operator this means providing sufficient reactor volume for a given operating condition which directly affects technology cost. The use of residence time specifically biological solids residence time (SRT), as the most important design factor is a concept that provides information on how changes in operating conditions affect performance of the technology and its reliability. Operationally SRT has been defined as the mass of solids contained in the digester divided by the mass of solids discharged from the system per day. Depending on the operational performance efficiency various technologies have different residence times for distillery effluent. The relationship between volatile solids loading rate (VSLR) and hydraulic retention time (HRT) is important. This relationship is dependent on influent COD and/or BOD concentration. SRT is now recognized as the most important kinetic parameter for anaerobic digester design and operation because it more accurately defines the relationship between the bacterial system and digester operating conditions as evidenced by several reports. Also, at a suitable SRT the required

HRT can be very low. Thus an efficient anaerobic digestion (AD) would involve relatively small and very economic digester. It is not desirable to design and operate anaerobic digester near maximum specific growth rate for any extended period of time. Engineers should select the proper design SRT to accomplish a given treatment efficiency with more reliability and large values of SRT. In suspended growth digesters a large digester volume is required or else provisions for biomass recycle would be needed. In that case SRT is controlled by purposely removing solids. Process designs such as upflow anaerobic sludge blanket process and anaerobic baffled digester all inherently provide high values of SRT at low HRT.

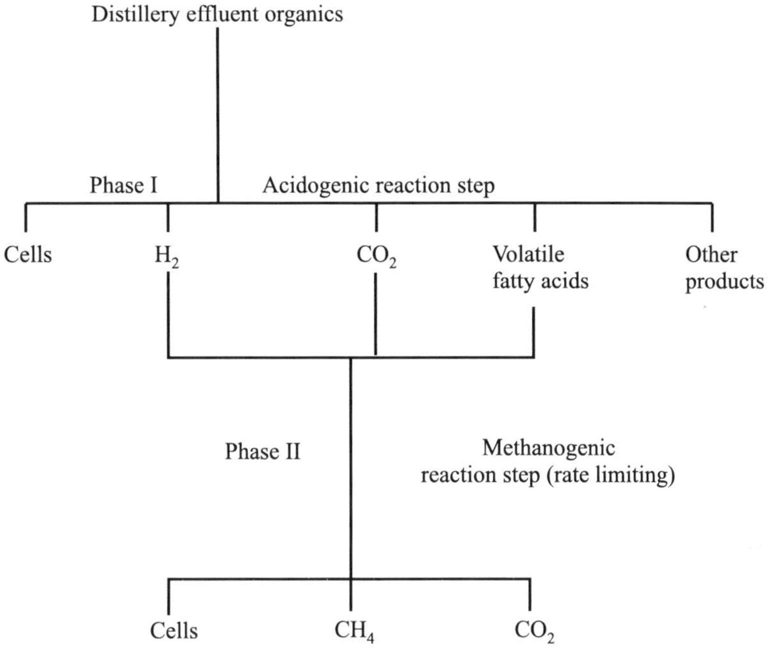

Fig. 11.7 Simple schematic of two phase digestion (anaerobic)

E. Rate limiting step

A simplified schematic representation of the biphasic distillery effluent bioconversion reaction phases is shown in the figure Fig. 11.7.

In phase I reaction kinetics organic materials of distillery effluent are broken down to organic acids, mainly acetic, propionic and butyric acids by saprophytic acidogenic becteria and their enzymes. The principal acidogenic microbial flora consits of *Acetobacter* and *Propionibacterium* sp. Nearly 3000 - 5000 ppm of volatile acids are produced at this reaction phase. Kinetically in Phase II bioconversion of acids mainly to methane and carbon dioxide takes place by methanogenic bacteria principal flora being *Methanobacterium* sp., *Clostridium* sp. and *Desulfovibrio* sp. Among these biphasic reactions, the second phase becomes rate limiting in anaerobic digestion of distillery effluent. However, although it is depeneding on the nature of organic substrate the rate limiting step may change for different effluent substrates. For example, hydrolysis of complex organics becomes rate limiting during anaerobic digestion of waste where activated sludge kinetic illustration of above biphasic reactions have been described by simple kinetic breakdown of fatty acids using standard Monod's expression. Many other factors like temperature, pH, mixing, toxicity etc. have been found to exert influence on the digestion kinetics.

(iii) Other Factors Affecting System Design and Performance : The usefulness of kinetic considerations has been demonstrated through the relationships of the effect of SRT, temperature, mixing, toxicity and a few other characteristics on anaerobic digestion efficiency. Reduction of BOD, COD and VS in anaerobic digestion greatly depend on the bacteria grown during digestion process. McCarty[11] accounted the contribution of grown bacteria to reduce organic loading and noticed larger values of SRT minimized the concentration of produced bacteria in the effluent.

A. Effect of temperature

It has been often noticed that thermophilic methanation process is less stable than a mesophilic one. In thermophilic processing temperature regime (50°C - 60°C) irregularities in loading rates did cause severe damage to thermophilic digestion. It has been reported that when the loading rate in mesophilic (35°C - 40°C) and thermophilic digesters was doubled by the reduction of HRT half gas production increased immediately by a factor of two. It has also been reported that when temperature was lowered or increassed for short (2hrs.) or long (18 hrs. or 4 day) periods the changes of daily biogas production was not very significant. Report is also available that a decrease in the digestion temperature by 3°C for 4 days or by 10°C for only 2 hrs. had no or little transient effect on the biogas production of mesophilic and thermophilic digestion system. Lowering digester temperature to 18°C for 8 hrs. however could show reduction in gas productivity by 50% in mesophilic and thermophilic digesters. The sensitivity of methanogenic bacteria to alterations in temperature, compared with other microorganisms in the digester is well known. The anaerobic digestion process has been examined to be unsuitable for dilute effluents at a low temperature. The efficiency of conversion of carbonaceous substrate, cell growth being dependent on temperature, the maximum bioconversion product yield is expected to occur at a temperature near to maximum specific growth. So majority of distillery industries which generate significant quantities of waste heat as a component of their effluent system have utilized to maintain mesophilic temperature in their process design taking the advantage of the waste energy.

B. Effect of gas recycling and mixing

In several units of distillery effluent management by anaerobic digestion gas recycling and mixing is used and recommended. One of the reasons of this is to provide adequate mixing of the digester content to prevent sludge accretion/stratification. It helps efficient uilization of the entire digester volume and uniformity of temperature. Also, it disperses metabolic end products and any local over-accumulation of toxic material and to maintain intimate contact between substrate, bacteria and bacterial enzymes. In short, adequate mixing provides uniformity in digestion which is one of the ways to achieve a good digestion. Inefficient mixing on the other hand effects on process kinetics manifesting the decrease in effective reduction leading the digestion towards instability and failure causing reduction in gas productivity. In combination with temperature gradient due to inefficient mixing these reductions can be devastating.

Adequate mixing is most critical if digesters are to operate as designed. In this regard efficient gas recycling is of great help providing advantages of better control of scum collection at the top of the reactor sludge collection and removal of the bottom of the digester and additional mixing from natural gas evolution by convection currents.

Also recycling of anaerobic digestion product gases through the digestion mixed culture was expected to increase methane products because of additional methane fermentation from increased reduction of carbon dioxide. The sweeping action of the recycled gas was expected to accelerate removal of the gaseous products surrounding the microorganisms thereby minimizing any product repression. From the experience of gas recycle it could be seen that as the gas recycle ratio is increased to an optimum level the opportunity of carbon dioxide reduction and sweeping of the gaseous digestion products out of the digester increases thereby stimulating methane production. However, as the gas recycling ratio is increased further the culture is increasingly saturated with gaseous end products thereby tending to repress or inhibit additional methane production. The inhibitory effect of increasing gas recycle on methane production equal each other at the optimum gas recycle ratio which maximizes methane yield. Such participation of carbon dioxide in reductive pathways for additional methane has been demonstrated more recently. It has been shown that nearly 18% of excess methane production was originated by CO_2 reduction reaction.

C. pH profile and pH effect

In conventional anaerobic digestion of carbonaceous distillery effluent at the beginning of the acidogenic phase (phase I) the pH drops due to formation of organic acids. Later these acids are broken down and pH rises. This rise starts after 2 to 3 days of digestion and rises continuously till neutrality reaches to about 6.9 to 7.2 in about 10 to 15 days in batch digestion system. During this period (Phase-II) there is a rapid increase in methane production with corresponding decrease in volatile acids. In a classical study of digestion the initial pH was nearly 5.8. It decreases linearly due to volatile acid formation to 5 in 3 days after which it again incresed due to consumption of V A as substrate releasing NH_3 by deamination of amino acids, which favours the growth of methanogenic bacteria. This increase occured continuously till 11 to 12th day after that it was almost constant, total acidity increased up to first three days then it continuously decreased, total v.s. was also continuously decreased throughout the process. The methanogenic bacteria have a limited pH range around maturity while the acidogenic bacteria exhibit intolerance of low pH values. Moreover, propionate, a volatile fatty acid and infact other transient may be toxic to the bacteria assimilating hydrogen in methane production as shown in the figure of rate limiting step.

In a phase separated system, however, lower pH values may be possible in acidogenic phase where these may be advantageous to the associated microorganisms.

D. Effect of toxicity

In anaerobic digestion of distillery effluent toxic substances can be present in the influent sludge as well as in the course of digestion. These toxic substances effect on anaerobic digestion to alter kinetics of organic (COD/BOD) matter degradation. The extent/magnitude of the toxicity depends on the nature and concentartion of the toxic material. In such conditions SRT will play significant role in process performance in order to minimize the adverse effects of toxicity on methanogenic microbial activity. Therefore, presence of propionic or transient toxic substances temporarily or permanently alters the kinetics of anaerobic digestion. In case of presence of the inhibitory substance like formaldehyde to the extent of 100 ppm in distillery effluent has been demonstrated to cause an approximately 14% decrese in BOD removal efficiency at a SRT of 15 days and a 54% decrease in BOD removal efficiency at a SRT of 10 days. Likewise transient toxic materials like accumulation to high propionic acid in the digester requires to control SRT in methanogenic phase. Proper control of SRT also maximizes acclimation to toxicity.

E. Oxygen participation necessary or unnecessary?

Apparently oxygen plays important role by its presence at high tension. At high oxygen anaerobic digestion is impaired. Most probably because at high oxygen tension microbial metabolism of the flora begin to shift from anaerobic to aerobic and less methane is produced with a corresponding increase in cell biomass. It appears that as optimal concentration of cell mass is required in anaerobic digestion trace amount of oxygen are required for biomass level maintanance. Air bubbling for this need is not desired as this oxygen demand is met by the nascent oxygen participation generated by cleavage of oxygen containing unsaturated materials in the digester. However, detailed analysis of this substitution of oxygen by oxygen containing compounds is scanty.

(iv) Survery Analysis of Three Distillery Effluent Treatment Process Technology : A survey has been conducted by the appointed consultant of three distilleries which are using imported technologies. These three distilleries are, (1) Vam Organic Chemicals Pvt. Ltd. utilizing BIOTIM Process of Belgium, (2) Rampur Distillery and Chemical Co. Ltd. using M/S AQUATECH Process, Thailand, and (3) Ajudhya Distillery—using ADI-BVF Process of Canada. Their comparative data has been provided in Table 11.10.

The operational differences of these technologies arise because of the difference in knowhow. A comparative basic difference of these three technological knowhow in terms of cost, efficiency and few other technological parameters is presented in Table 11.10 as per data made available and approximated.

A. BIOTIM-NV- VOCL process technology

This overseas technology supplied by BIOTIM-NV to VOCL is microbial system mediated anaerobic process. The process consists mainly of two microbial reaction stages/phases. The first digester has been called biological conditioning and control reactor (BCCR). In this bioreactor buffering and anaerobic hydrolytic reactions are carried out. The second digester has been called Methane Upflow Reactor (MUR) or Upflow Anaerobic Sludge Blanket Reactor (UASBR). In this reactor anaerobic methane generation reaction is carried out. This process technology has been stated to have designed for installed capacity of 650 m^3/day of distillery effluent to produce treated distillery effluent of BOD 100 mg/l and biogas 5.73 nm^3 per annum on 300 working days and 3 shifts basis.

The essential features of this process as stated consists of receiving the distillery effluent at 85°C and cooling it to 40°C by plate heat exchanger. This raw material specification is given in Table 11.11. Next phosphoric acid is added to it as a nutrient. The addition of caustic soda is only required during the phase start-up. This effluent with required amount of nutrient enters the BCCR and completely mixed by agitators. In this bioreactor the acidogenic bacteria break the complex organic carbonaceous molecules into simpler molecules of volatile organic acids suitable and susceptible to biomethanation reaction. This conditioned effluent from BCCR is desludged in parallel plate separator (PPS) and part of the sludge is recycled to BCCR. The liquid effluent from PPS is mixed with requisite chemical to adjust pH adequate for methane formation reaction and pumped to MUR through the distribution system at the bottom of the reactor. In MUR the methanogenic bacteria act on smaller molecules of volatile organic acids to produce methane containing biogas. Clear treated effluent overflows to the effluent holding tank. Part of this treated effluent is recycled and the rest is sent to the secondary treatment system for further treatment. Biogas is sent to captive boiler with the help of a blower for use as fuel replacing furnace oil. Excess gas if any may be flaired. Utilities consumption for treatment of 680 m^3/day of distillery effluent has been stated to be as follows: caustic soda only during start up, H_3PO_4- 60 kg/day, cooling water 60 m^3/h (circulating) and Power-1050 KWH/day. Why BIOTIM N V Technology has been selected by VOCL ? After thorough investigation of similar treatment processes for distillery effluent VOCL observed and stated that the two stage reaction system of BIOTIM is very efficient in BOD reduction and biogas production. It is also claimed to be capable of adjusting to variations in operating conditions. Also it is claimed that this technology has the following salient features:

- Two stage digestion system for rigid control of microbiological reaction with minimum packing.
- Lower capital investment because of lower packed volume.
- Special design feature of packing dominates clogging of foaming.
- Reduction of BOD and COD to the extent of 80% and 70% respectively.

B. AQUA TECHNO-RDCL process technology

RDCL's Envisaged Scheme: RDCL has envisaged for treatment of 1000 m^3/day spent wash effluent from the cane-molasses based distillery having BOD level of 40,0000 to 50,000 ppm to generate 3000 m^3/day biogas rich in methane having calorific value of 5000/5500 k. cal/m^3 which can be used for generation of heat/power by adapting the anaerobic digestion technology of M/s AQUA TECHNO, Bangkok. RDCL also envisages to utilize methane generated from degradation of spent wash for replacing its furnace oil requirements in its SSP granulation plant, as a fuel in its boiler and partly for generation of power.

Process Biotechnology: The process involves anaerobic digestion of the dilute distillery effluents with constant agitation in presence of limited supply of air. The methane gas generated during the digestion process is scrubbed and stored in gas holders. The spent wash has been envisaged to pass through trickling filter for deodourising and discharged in the channel for dilution. The treated sludge from the tank has been planned to be sun dried and used as filler/fertiliser.

C. Analysis of the comparative data of the three technologies

The digestion of distillery spent wash/molasses slop was studied nearly fifty years ago. This and other studies used conventional stirred tank digesters resulting in SRT exceeding a week.

Typical degradation was seldom higher than 3.5 m^3. m^{-3}.d^{-1}. Even by the use of anaerobic contact processes the anaerobic digestion of distillery effluent could not be improved to any great extent. HRT and hence reactor volumes were nearly the same order of magnitude. The application of the UASB/MUR to diluted molasses based distillery effluent as used by Vam Organic Chemical Ltd. (VOCL) and to other process technology is restricted to low or medium strength effluents while initial concentration of distillery effluent COD may be as high as 100 to 120 gsl^{-1}. Therefore suitability of such effluent digestion process technology in sludge bed digester still remain under scope of constraint.

(v) A Typical Process Design Information

A. Process data

Distillery capacity	:	60-65 kilo litre day^{-1}
Effluent flow	:	880-900 M^3/day
COD of effluent	:	100,000 mg/*l*
BOD of effluent	:	45,000 "
COD Load	:	88-90 MT/day
Loading rate	:	12.5-14 kg M^3/day
COD reduction	:	60-65%
BOD reduction	:	88-90%
BOD of treated effluent	:	4000-5000 mg/*l*
COD of treated effluent	:	35,000-40,000 mg/*l*
Temperature of effluent	:	75-85°C
Temp. of treated effluent	:	35-38°C
TSS of distillery effluent	:	4,200 ppm
TSS of treated distillery effluent	:	2,700 ppm
pH of distillery effluent	:	4.3
pH of treated distillery effluent	:	7-8

B. Process outline of methane upflow reactor (MUR)

Distillery effluent is first conditioned by increasing its pH with additon of lime and chemicals (nutrients) and then if necessary cooled to 40-45°C. The conditioned effluent is fed to first stages reactor BCCR where degradation of organic matter in the effluent into volatile fatty acids (VFA) take place by liquefying and acidogenic microbial flora (bacteria). Effluent of BCCR is passed through pps (parallel plate seperator) and seperated sludge is recycled back to BCCR. Effluent from pps is fed to the two MUR where VFA are converted into methane gas by methanogenic bacteria. Effluent of MUR is passed through cross flow pps and goes to secondary treatment.

C. Process operating cost

Chemicals	Rs 2832/day
Power	Rs 2835/day
Total	Rs 5667/day

D. Process economics data

Biogas/spent wash	30 NM^3/M^3
Total biogas	26000-27000 NM^3/day
Methane content	60%
Calorific value of biogas	5400 k cal/m^3
Calorific value of coal	4200 k cal/kg
Coal equivalent to biogas	33280-34560 kg/day
Saving of coal @ Rs 1000/MT	33280-34560 kg/day
Operating cost	Rs 5667/day
Net-Annual saving for 300 days working	Rs 82.83-Rs 86.67 Lakhs.

11.3.2 Coal Processing Effluent Water [15-17]

1. Forewords

The present energy generating system in rural and most industial areas in India is coal. Coal has been expected still to be an alternative energy source in place of oil. About 7308 million tons of coal reserves was confirmed in 1986 and is omnipresent in many countries. The smoke of coal combustion like biomass burning in rural areas creates an unhealthy environment to local dwellers. Also, coal has the problem of handling and SO_2 produced by its combustion leads to acid rain[12-16].

Many coal based industries like steel, fertiliser, carbon black etc. are in operation in Eastern India particularly in Durgapur industrial belt of West Bengal. Also the petroleum refinery at Haldia has constituted another dimension to the industrial development of Eastern India. All of these industries generate large volumes of wastes/residues and waste waters. These wastes and waste wasters are vulnerable to cause pollution hazards in the locality or local portable/ usable water. They need adequate processing for pollution abatement prior to their recycling or disposal. If they are disposed of without giving adequate treatment/care they are likely to create environmental pollution either by putrifaction or by biodegradation. Liquid waste effluents discharged from these industries ranges between 0.03 to 0.4 M^3/ton of coal processed. Characters of these waste waters/liquid effluents are toxic in terms of pH, colour, dissolved solids, phenol, free ammonia, thiocyanate, cyanides, sulfide, BOD, COD, etc.

2. Hazardous components and toxicity

The major toxic components in the liquid effluent of these industries are phenol, cyanides, thiocyanates etc. Toxicity features of few of them are presented in Table 11.13. When humans unknowingly consume water polluted with phenol they have been reported to become ill due to diarrhoea, mouth sore, dark urine and burning mouth. The toxic effects of phenol may not be so acute with regard to human being but its presence in traces in potable water is objectionable, simply because upon chlorination it forms chlorophenols, which impart unpleasant taste. Also the basic phenolic compounds are reported to be carcinogenic in nature. Phenol toxicity to fish life has been recognised as early as 1928. When 8" carps were exposed to phenol concentration of 400 mg/*l* within 1 hr they have been killed.

Table 11.13 Coal processing industrial effluent resources and toxicity

Component	*Nature/ Symptom of Toxicity*	*Toxicity Level*
Phenols	A. Towards human (a) Diarrhoea (b) Mouth sores (c) Dark urine (d) Burning mouth etc B. In potable water (a) Unplesant taste (b) Harmful to aquatic ($0.03 \text{ mg } l^{-1}$) life like fish	In traces ($0.001 \text{ mg } l^{-1}$)
CN^-	(a) Inhibits cytochrome oxidase action and makes tissue cells unable to use O_2 (b) Paralyse the respiratory centre of brain cells	0.009 mg per kg body wt.
SCN	Dizziness, skin eruption, running nose, vomitting, nausea, thyroid problem, disorder of nervous system	$0.015 \text{ mg } l^{-1}$

Cyanide is an extremely toxic substance. In mammalian systems hydrocyanic acid prevents the process of oxidation in the tissue cells. It paralyses the respiratory centre of the brain cells. The lethal effect of cyanide ions is due to the inability of the tissue cells to utilize oxygen. Cyanide is known to be an inhibitor at the terminal oxidation of the cytochrome (cytochrome oxydase). Cyanide forms a stable complex with cytochrome oxidase. This complexion results in loss of the enzyme activity resulting in death. Hydrocyanic acid is toxic at 0.3 mg/*l* of the air inhaled. The lethal dose of the toxicant is 1.0 mg/kg body weight. The fatal dose for animals is 9.0 mg/kg body weight. Fish has high sensitivity to cyanide. Minnows, catfish and carps behaved sick at a concentration of 0.3 mg/*l*. Pottassium cyanide at concentrations between 0.03 to 0.12 mg/*l* has killing effect on gold fish when exposed to the toxicant for 3-4 days. In flowing water, containing cyanide above 0.03 mg/*l* cent per cent chance of survival of white carps is uncertain.

Thiocyanate at concentrations above 15 mg/100 ml of blood is critically dangerous. Chronic adsorption of thiocyanate may cause dizziness, skin eruptions, running nose, vomiting, nausea and mild to severe disturbances of the nervous system. Thiocyanate containing water upon chlorination or irradiation releases the cyanide by splitting the sulphur moiety. It inhibits the adsorption of iodine by thyroid gland. Ammonium thiocyanate is reported to have lethal effect on average spotted shellfish at 280-300 mg/*l* while goldfish exposed to 1600 mg/*l* concentration has been reported killed in 24 hours.

Free ammonia has been found to be toxic to fish life even at concentration level upto 2.8 mg/*l*. The toxicity of ammonia is due to the unionized ammonium ion concentration which increased in solution with increase in pH.

Waste water from the coal carbonization industries, when it is fresh, has a straw yellow colour. The colour is intensified upon storage and exposure to atmospheric conditions and aeration. Several explanations have been given for the development of this colour. The catechol present in the waste under alkaline conditions oxidized catechol. The wastes contain iron which can also form colouring complex with thiocyanates, cyanides etc to impart colour to the waste. The chemistry of the colour development is yet unknown. However, the colour development during exposure to air and light has been shown to exhibit toxicity of algal population above 600 units.

Very little information is available with reference to the sulphide content in the coal carbonization effluents except that in the case of LTC process it is between 67-74 mg/*l*.

Soluble sulphide in water react with hydrogen ion concentration to form HS or H_2S. The toxicity of sulphide is derived from the H_2S rather than the sulphide ion. The lethal concentration of sulphide for fish life is reported to be between 0.032 and 0.355 mg/*l*.

The BOD to COD ratio of the wastes from different coal carbonization processes works out to be between 0.5 to 0.9 indicating that it is amenable for biological treatment. Several attempts have been made to treat the waste after dilution with domestic sewage.

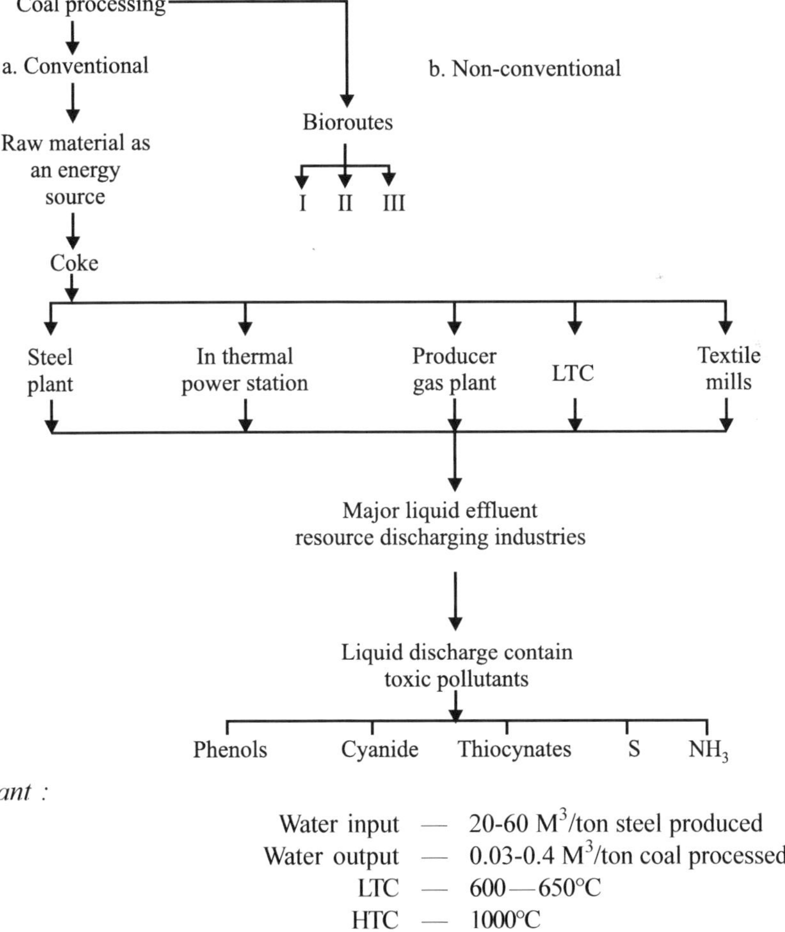

Fig. 11.7 Major liquid effluent origins in coal processing routes (a) conventional (b) non-conventional

3. Major liquid effluents origin in coal processing routes

Both conventional and non-conventional coal processing routes have been provided by scientists and technologists (Fig. 11.7 and Fig. 11.8). Conventionally coal has been processed as a raw material for energy source and to produce coke for many industries. In recent years its non-conventional bio-processing routes have also been known (Fig.11.8).

In both routes the need of coal processing has been to serve the following purposes:

(a) Produce low sulfur coal

(b) Reduce smoke generation

(c) Reduce air pollution

(d) Reduce health hazard

(e) Reduce COD/BOD

(f) Higher heat generation from coal and

(g) Obtaining possible useful metabolites/chemicals.

(i) Conventional : Conventional route of coal processing is shown in Fig. 11.7. However, conventional processing of coal is expensive. For partial reduction of the expense possibility of unconventional microbial biodegradability of pollution generating liquid effluents has been shown.[15] Biodespiritization of coal by microbial processing is one such approaches. Bioliquefaction and biodesulfurization of coal are other approach. It is necessary to identify potential microbial strains for such purposes. However, microbial processing of coal for bioremediation of hazards is associated with both merits and demerits (Table 11.14). A comparative process conditions of both routes are given in Table 11.15.

Table 11.14 Microbial bioprocessing of coal and coal processing effluents

Merits	*Demerits*
Less energy intensive	Slow process
Less capital intensive	In most systems undefined cell population
Less costly	Control and regulation difficult

(ii) Non-conventional : Bioremediation

1. Aspects of bioremediation

(i) Potential Microbial Strains : Non-conventional bioremediation routes make use of potential activity of microbial strains in degradation of pollution generating components in coal and coal effluents.

Some eubacteria and archaebacteria have been found to be highly potential in bioprocessing of coal for bioremediation. These microorganisms accelerate the oxidation of pyrite producing ferric sulfate and sulfuric acid. Few potential microbial strains of coal bioprocessing are given in Table 11.16.

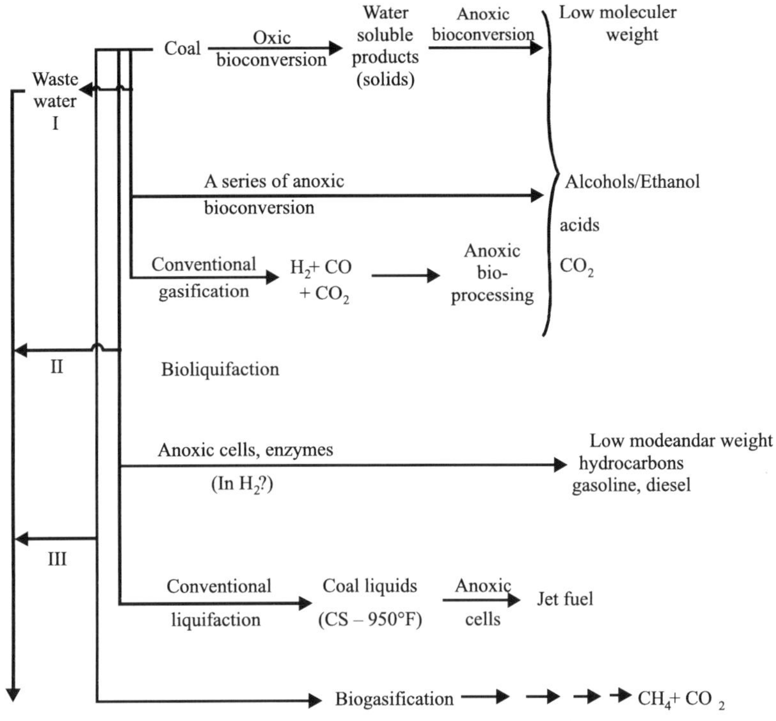

Fig 11.8 Non-conventional routes of bioprocessing of coal to liquid and gaseous fuels and chemicals

Table 11.15 Conventional vis-a-vis non-conventional processing of coal

Conversion Parameters	*Thermal/Chemical Processing*			*Bioprocessing*		
	Gasification	*Liquifaction*	*Desulfu-rization*	*Depyri-tization*	*Bio-liqui-faction*	*De-sulfurization*
Temp (°C)	700	400	375	30-35	30-35	30-35
Pressure (PSIG)	1000	2000	—	lab	lab	lab
Catalyst treatment	—	+	Molten caustic	Microbes	Microbes	Microbes
Reaction/Product				*	**	***

* $4FeS_2 + 15O_2 + 2H_2O \xrightarrow[\text{ferroxidants}]{\text{Thiobacillus}} 2\,(Fe)_2\,(SO_4)_3 + 2H_2SO_4$

** Acids, Low molecular weight alcohols and CO_2

*** Organic sulfur (C-S) removal (controversial pyrite sulfur)

Table 11.16 Examples of potential microbial strains for biodepyritization of coal by microbial leaching

1. Eubacteria
   Thiobacillus thiooxidans
   (oxidizes only sulfur)
   Thiobacillus ferroxidans
   Leptospirillum ferroxidans
   Putida fluorescence
   Acidianus brierleyi
   Pseudomonas alcaligens etc.
2. Archaebacteria
   Sulfolobus acidocaldarins
3. Yeast
   Candida tropicalis
   Debromyces globosus
   Pichia sp.
   Trichosporon cuteneum
4. Fungi
   Aspergillus sp.
   Penicillium sp.
   Neurospora sp.

Table 11.17 Features of biodepyritization design strategies

Design Strategies	*Mode/Parameters*	*Features*
Heap/Percolation	recycle: 1hr	Simple & inexpensive
Leaching	duration	Long residence times
	run off-mode, lump coal	Indigenous
		Cell population use
Tank bioreactor	length - 8'	More complicated operation
Operation	depth - 20"	Shorter residence times
	1/2 angle of base - 30°	
	Slurry volume - 120 *l*	
	baffles	
Other possible designs	Lagoon	Inclination to horizontal
	Slurry pipe line bioreactor	

(iii) Biodepyritization Strategies[20,21] : As in Table 11.17 biodepyritization strategy may vary depending on conditions. In heap or percolation bioleaching the actual composition of microbial population is still not clearly known. The disadvantage of this method is long time required for desulfurization. However, its advantage envisaged is that thermophilic operation (50-60°C) possibly accelerate rates at elevated temperatures.

Treatment without dilution with domestic waste has also been reported but by supplimentation with phosphorus. The influent phenolic concentration has been found to influence the aeration period. Pilot plant studies have showed that the waste water from steel mills (coke ovens) could be treated in aerobic activated sludge plants with an organic loading of 0.716 lb/lb of sludge/per day. Ammonia concentration above 4000 mg/*l* is reported to inhibit severely the biological activity of the sludge. Apart from ammonia, thiocyanate, cyanide, sulphide oxidized polyhydric phenols, calcium and chlorides also affect the biological process. Biological treatment of coal carbonization waste is widely practised in Britain independently because in most cases, discharge municipal sewage is not available for making enough dilution.

Waste water containing phenols, cyanides, thiocyanates and ammonia is amenable for biological degradation, there are many inherent factors in bioremediation by biodegradation of organic pollutants of coal. These factors and their consequences are listed in Table 11.18 to 11.20.

(iii) Fundamentals of Bioremediation : Phenolytic microorganisms may belong to bacteria, archaebacteria, yeast and fungi. The metabolism of the aromatic ring can take place under anoxic as well as aerobic condition. Considerable amount of information is available on the oxic metabolism of aromatic compounds. Biologically phenol forms catechol. The enzymes involved in biological pathways are hydroxylases, oxygenases, dehydrogenases and aldolases. These enzymes are subjected to feed back inhibition. The substrate itself act as substrate inhibitor to the whole cells.

Table 11.18 Chemical and environmental factors influencing biodegradability of organic pollutants for bioremediation

(a)	*Structural Factors*	*Consequences*
1.	M. wt. or size	Limited active transplant
2.	Polymeric nature	Extracellular metabolism required
3.	Aromaticity	O_2 requiring enzymes
4.	Halogen substitution	Lack of dehalogenating enzymes
5.	Solubility	Competitive partitioning
6.	Toxicity	Enzyme inhibition cell damage
7.	Xenobiotic origin	Evolution of new degradative pathways
(b)	*Environmental Factors*	*Consequences*
1.	Dissolved oxygen requiring	O_2 sensitive & oxy enzymes
2.	Temperature	Mesophillic temperature optimum
3.	pH	Narrow pH optimum
4.	Dissolved carbon	Organic/pollutant complexes concentration dependent growth
5.	Particulates, surfaces	Competition for substrate
6.	Light	Photochemical enhancement
7.	Nutrient & trace elements	Limitation on growth & enzymes synthesis

Table 11.19 Biological factors influencing the biodegradation of organic pollutants for bioremediation

Biological Factors	*Consequences*
Enzyme ubiquity	Low frequency of degradation species
Enzyme specificity	Analogous substrates not metabolized Reacclimation
Plasmid encoded enzymes	Low frequency of degradation species Instability
Enzymes regulation	Repression of catabolic enzyme synthesis Required acclimation or induction
Competition	Extinction of low density populations
Habitat selection	Lack of establishment of degradative populations
Population regulation	Low population density of degradative organisms

Table 11.20 Factors influencing the analysis of the kinetics and extent of biodegradation for bioremediation

	Experimental Factors	*Problems Encountered*
(*a*)	Analytical method substrate disappearance	Competing abiotic processes
	Biotransformation	Complex analysis
	Mineralization	Incomplete biochemical pathways
	Scale up/down	Comparability among ractor designs
(b)	Feed stock complexity chemically/biologically undefined complex waste waters	Poor simulation and predictability difficult in interpretation

In bioremediation biological oxidation may occur by the different routes:

(i) Removal of electrons by transformation of metallic form of ferrous iron to ferric
(ii) Removal of hydrogen as in the case of alcohol to acetaldehyde and,
(iii) Addition of oxygen as in the case of oxidation of carbon to carbon-dioxide.

The participation of oxygen in the reactions is that of the electron from the terminal oxidation stage. Oxygen is required in certain other enzymatic reactions. The steps in the biochemical transformation of the aromatic involve the introduction of molecular oxygen. One atom of oxygen is inserted into the substrate and the other atom of the molecule is reduced to water as given below:

$$RH + O_2 + 2\,(H) \longrightarrow ROH + H_2O$$

Here RH represents the aromatic molecule. The aromatic ring is attacked by the enzyme "oxygenase". For ring fission both atoms of one molecule of oxygen are incorporated into the hydroxylated ring. In the oxidation of a simple aromatic molecule, in addition to the electron transport chain reaction, molecular oxygen is also required for the opening of the aromatic ring.

A variety of microorganisms have been found to metabolize cyanide and phenolic compounds. Most of them have metabolic pathways leading to the formation of aminoacids.

(iv) *Bioprocess Engineering Analysis*[14, 18, 20-23] : The scheme of detoxification of phenolic waste water at pilot plant level bioremediation is shown in Fig. 11.9 in which *Candida tropicalis* was used. Inoculum need in the process was developed as described in Fig. 11.10. Considering the schematic diagram of Fig. 11.9 and operation of completely mixed ASP system, the material balance of the substrate detoxification is given by:

$$V.\ dX/dt = Q_iX_i - \{Q_wX_w + (Q_i - Q_w)\ X_e\} + V.\ r' \qquad (11.10)$$

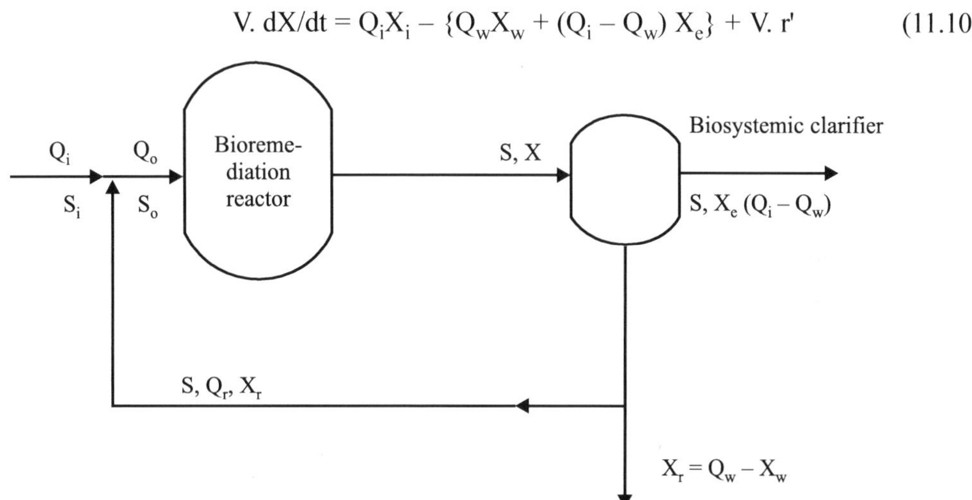

Fig. 11.9 Schematic of bioremediation

In Fig. 11.9 the symbols used are as given below

X_e, X, X_w, X_r = MLSS (mg/*l*) in bioreactor, effluent suspended solid, recycle suspended solids
Q_i, Q_r, Q_w = Flow rates (*l*/hr), in influent, recycle, wastage
S_e, S = Substrate concentration (mg/*l*) influent and in the bioreactor
t = Hydraulic detention time (hr)
θ_c = Mean cell residence time (hr)
K = System rate constant
K_s = Substrate concentration at half of μ_{max}
V = ASP reactor volume (*l*)
Y = Yield coefficient
μ_m = Maximum sp. growth rate (hr^{-1})
k_d = Biological decay rate constant (hr^{-1})
k = Maximum substrate utilization rate (d^{-1})

From equation 11.10

$$V.\ r' = (Q_w\ X_w) + (Q_1 - Q_w)\ X_e \qquad (11.11)$$

where

$$r' = \frac{\mu_m\ XS}{K_s + S} - K_d\ X \qquad (11.12)$$

On dividing by VX, equation obtained is

$$Vr'/VX = (Q_w X_w) + (Q_i - Q_w) X_e/VX = 1/\theta_C \quad (11.13)$$

On simplifying it reduces to $1/\theta_C = Y.U - K_d$ (11.14)

By plotting $1/\theta_C$ against U (phenol utilization rate) values for Y and K_d can be otained. The growth or microorganisms occur by the utilization of the substrate according to equation 11.14

$$[(\mu_m - X_s)(K_s + S)] V = YQ_0 (S_0 - S) \quad (11.15)$$

or

$$k (S/K_s + S) = (S_0 - S)/\theta X \quad (11.16)$$

where $\mu_m = kY$

By rearranging equation 11.16 equation 11.17 can be obtained

$$\theta X/(S_0 - S) = [K_S / k] [1/S] + 1/k \quad (11.17)$$

and by plotting l/S against $\theta X/(S_0 - S)$ values for k and K_S can be obtained. Also since oxygen plays important role in biosystems[14] the oxygen utilization in the system can be obtained by mass balance in the following way[14]

Net oxygen consumed = Oxygen utilised for substrate oxidation + Oxygen utilized for respiration (11.18)

So, kg O_2 utilized/day = a' kg O_2 utilized for substrate oxidized + b' kg O_2 utilized for respiration (11.19)

The plot, kg. substrate removed/day against kgO_2 utilized/day can give values of a' and b'.

(v) Bioremediation Reactor Studies [14, 21-23] : In recent years considerable increase in the environmental impact of waste waters/liquors from coal processing systems is evident. This is arising from the coal gasification and liquifaction processes which are still under development. Among the compounds that are the greatest biohazardous in coal derived waste liquors as discussed in preceeding sections are phenols thiocyanates, ammonia and cyanides. Bioremediation by simply eleminating low level of phenol from waste waters through phenol fermentation has been used most frequently.

The general strategy to bioremediation of waste liquors is the application of highly evolved symbiotic populations of microbial flora (aerobic or anaerobic) in a classic reactor design so that all hazardous polluting compounds are degraded in the process.

For a long time the basic reactor design continued to be the simple activated sludge aeration vessel as used in ASP followed by a clarifier. Many investigators have made systematic studies to ascertain the optimum operation parameters for the activated sludge in a continuous stirred tank bioreactor (CSTBR). Techniques of determining limiting reactants, minimum retention time for biodegradation of limiting reactants and understanding of the relative inhibiting effects of various compounds upon other compound degradation rates for different feed rates and concentrations in three different conventional reactor configurational modes CSTBR, a three phase (FBBR) was interesting. It could elucidate relative merits of each bioreactor for accomplishing bioremediation in terms of degradation of a given daily discharge of phenol bearing waste water having common synthetic feed composition. In all bioreactors the general equation used in comparison of degradation rates (DR) was as given below.

$$DR = \frac{Q_L (C_i - C)}{V_R}$$

In which Q_L is the volumetric flow rate. V_R is the volume of the reactor and C_i and C are concentrations of phenol in inlet and at any time.

Typical experimental results using active symbiotic bacterial population could indicate[23-25] that if the volumes of the bioreactors were about equal, the CSTBR could treat 2 V_R (volume/day), the PBBR 5.0 V_R and the FBBR 8V_R (undiluted volumes). These informations provided preliminary indication on the suitability of FBBR in the effective bioremediation of phenolic hazards from coal processing liquid effluents.

More recent study on phenol fermentation in a small continuous STR bioreactor using pure culture of *Pseudomonas putida* strain (ATCC 17484) could develop rate equations of phenol biodegradation, the rate of intermediate inhibitor accumulation or degradation and the rate of cell biomass production. The phenol biodegradation rate constant for pure culture system was about 0.4-1.2 while in mixed sludge culture system k_{phe} was about $1.9 \times 10^{-2} \pm 8.8 \times 10^{-3}$. In sludge it is determined using acridine orange direct counting (AODC) procedure.[26, 27]

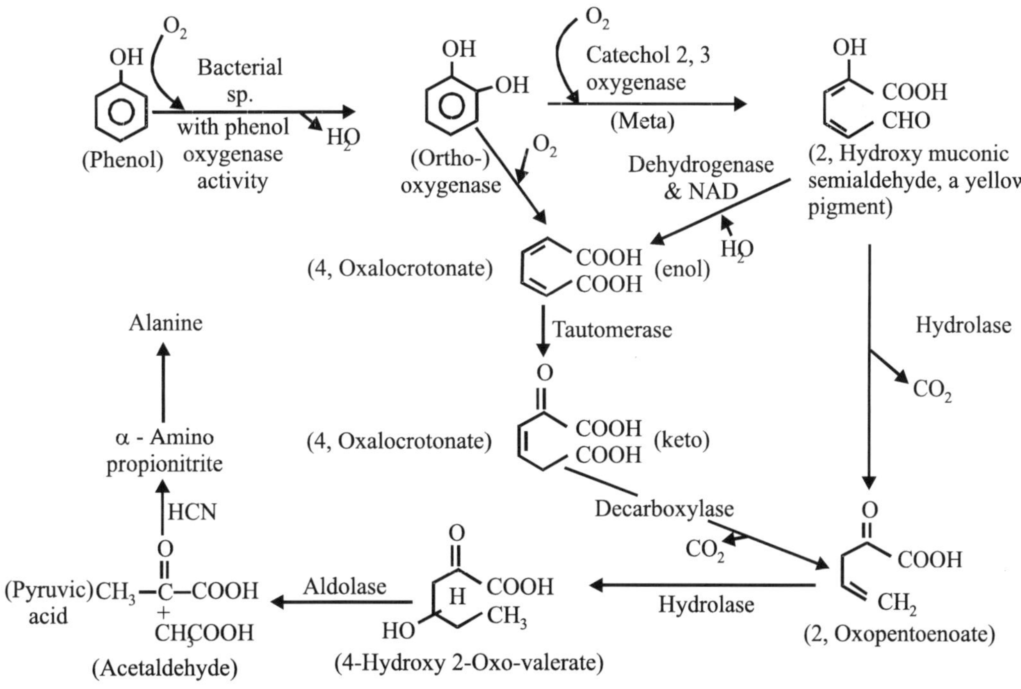

Fig. 11.11 Bioremediation of phenolics in coal processing effluents

(vi) Useful Chemicals from Bioremediation Pathways :

A. Meta-ortho pathway:

Coal bioprocessing and bioremediation of coal processing effluents produce several important metabolites by transforming hazardous components of coal. One example is the formation of useful amino acids through meta-ortho bioremediation pathway[14,17] (Fig. 11.11).

In this pathway 2, hydroxymuconic semialdehyde has been stated to be an important intermediate.[17] However, in terms of its usefulness it has not been characterised as yet.

B. Organic sulfur removal pathway

Bioremediation for microbial desulfurization of coal is to remove sulfur cleaving C–S bonds in model compound. It resembles coal organic sulfur. Dibenzothiophene (DBT) has been used most extensively as model compound. This process causes liberation of sulfate without oxidation or degradation or organic carbon matrix. A possible pathway of this sulfur removing bioremediation involves steps as available elsewhere. At international level lot of research is in progress for cloning of responsible genes for this pathway for more efficient desulfurization and ability to transfer such genes to other organisms in order to develop potential technologically redesigned cells.

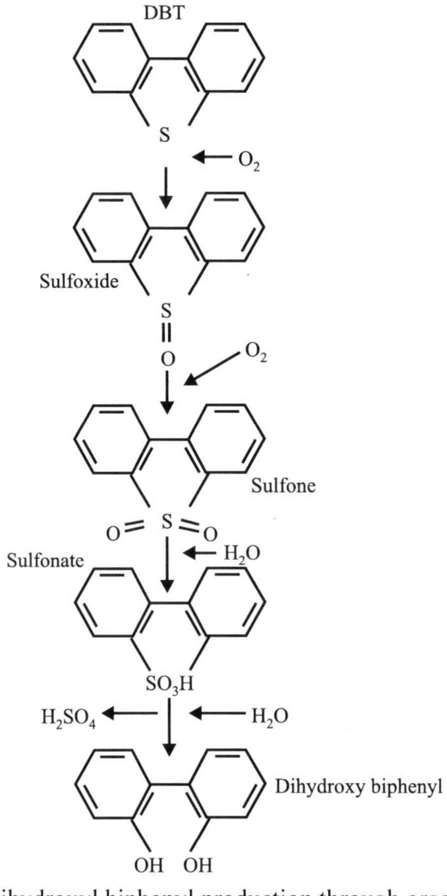

Fig. 11.12 Possibility of dihydroxyl biphenyl production through organic sulfur removal pathway of bioremediation

11.3.3 Food Processing Effluent Waters

1. Forewords

Food industries like canning, sugar mill, rice mill, distilleries, live stock and meat processing dairy industries, fruit and vegetable processing etc. generate a big quantum of by-products as waste and waste water. Since food processing plant waste waters may contain a variety of materials their compositions and contamination loads vary greatly. However, on the whole food plant waste waters can be broadly classified according to the nature of their impurities and pollution strength, which determines what treatment method, may be appropriate/suitable.[28-34]

In food plant waste water materials present may vary from coarse floating or sinking solids to colloidal particles. Also, beyond this size limit there are substances in true solution. Water insoluble liquids like oils, fats and solvents may be present also. The impurities present in all these materials are of either chemical or of biological nature. Besides hazardous metallic contaminants water and waste waters usually contain organic nitrogenous material. In waste water purification microbial nitrogen rich carbon poor (or low C/N ratio) environments of denitrification process may serve as key to clean water. When C/N ratio is high causing short circuiting nitrogen cycle the objective of waste water treatment is defeated.

2. Treatment of waste and waste water from food industries

Nearly all thermal processes in food industries use steam for various operations. For example, in the canning of food exhausting, blanching and sterilization/pasteurization are the major operations involving utilization of steam. The range of steam requirement in these operations is given in Table 11.21. To meet this requirement steam is produced in a boiler to maintain a line pressure of 100-125 psi. Steam production, flow and consumption is expressed in terms of boiler horse power (1 boiler horse power = 7200 k cals/hr). For a process lasting an hour a total of approximately 300 *l*bs of steam of 8.7 boil horse power per hour is consumed. It corresponds to energy requirement of about. 6.5 × 104 k cals/hr. A part of this energy can be recovered from the generated refuse waste of the food industry through its anaerobic bioconversion in biogas plant into methane. Essentially a single stage biogas plant consists of two units. First, a digester with an inlet into which the waste materials are introduced in the form of slurry. In the digester bioconversion of refuse waste is carried out at 35-40°C. The second unit is a gas holder to collect biogas containing 60-65% methane as combustible component the rest being mostly CO_2. In a typical anaerobic digestion process to generate biogas in the digester the complex organic waste food materials are degraded in a sequence of two steps mediated by two different types

Table 11.21 Major operations for steam requirement in canning of foods

Unit Operation	*Steam Requirement*		*Av. Energy Reqirement (Boiler H.P.)*
	Peak Demand (lbs/hr.)	*Operations Demand (lbs/hr.)*	
Exhausting (4' × 20' size)	500	500	8.7
Blanching (real)	2000	100-200	
Autoclaving (1" steam inlet)	2500	100-200	

Table 11.22 A few important sources of food wastes (in north India)

Source	*Computed daily Availability(kg)*	*Energy Equiv.*	
Fruits and vegetables processing wastes	7.5×10^4	1768	$\frac{\text{k cals}}{\text{kg waste}}$
Dairy and meat processing shed wastes (Dung)	4.0×10^8	1128	"
Fisheries	3.0×10^5	1344	"
Rice mills (husk)	30.0×10^6	975	"
Sugar mills (basasse)	15.0×10^6	784	"
Distilleries	15.0×10^6	720	"

of mixed microbial flora. In the first liquefaction and acidification step acidogens like acetic acid bacteria play role for nearly seven to ten days. Liquefied acidic materials are acted upon by methane forming organisms in the second step and digestion is completed by another five to eight days. Improvements of this basic process biotechnology of biogas generation from food wastes have been made and thereby digestion time has been reduced simultaneously methane productivity has also been increased to a great extent. A list of computed daily availability of biogas from food waste and its energy equivalent is given in Table 11.22. Although these waste resources are exploitable but it appears that these important resources have not been exploited for small scale bioconversion into methane.[29,32]

The waste water from food processing industries like dairy use the principle of permeability of membranes in whey seperation and treatments.[33, 34] Also for purification and fractionation as well as in waste disposal and by product recovery from waste liquid effluents membrane processing has been very useful. Membrane treatments primarily provided major advantage in retaining natural aroma and fresh flavour. That is why in treatment of fruit juices and other beverages membranes have been favoured extensively. In beer and alcohol distilleries clarification and removal of yeast by microfiltration (MF) is now in practice.[35]

11.3.4 Tannery Effluent Waters[36-41]

1. Forewords

Tannery effluents are generated in various steps in producing leather from raw skins and hides. After deskining and setting tanning objectives various process steps which are involved in the manufacture of finished leather include, curing, soaking, liming, dehairing/unhairing, bating, oiling, pickling, dying and finishing. Many chemicals are used in these processing steps. Among the chemicals used chlorides, sodium carbonates, ammonia, calcium and sodium dichromates, sulphuric acid etc are the major ones. In finishing step organic dyes are employed. It has been estimated that per kilogram of finished leather nearly 35 liter of effluent water is generated. This waste water needs adequate treatment before disposal because untreated tannery waste waters corrode sewer lines, cause ground and surface water pollution and imparts odor problems. For abatement of these adverse effects tannery effluents must be treated to safegaurd the receiving bodies/sink and surface and ground water sources. As shown in Fig. 11.13 animal skin has several layers. Among these layers only inner corium layer is useful in leather making. The corium is made up of collagen (C_{102} H_{149} N_{31} O_{38}). The objectives and processes in tanning indicating waste water resources are described below.

2. Objectives of tanning

- To strip off two outer layer from the skin to subject the corium to the action of tanning agents.
- When subjected to the action of tanning agents it undergoes a transformation and becomes insoluble in water, tough and flexible as a highly durable leather.

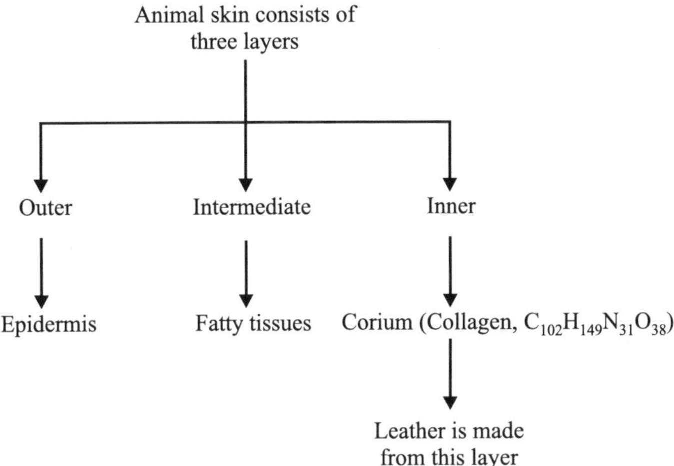

Fig. 11.13 Layers of animal skin

3. Processes in tanning and waste water resources

(i) Curing:

All Skins

Covered with numerous bacteria.

When an animal is alive, these bacteria have little effect on the skin.

Slaughtered or dies

Proteolytic bacteria quickly attack the skin and reduce its value and utility by damage.

Damage prevention

Skin is cured with salt or by drying in air and a combination of both.

It removes

Free water from skin, reduces bacterial growth $\longrightarrow$ Waste water.

(ii) Beem House Processing:

A. Soaking

Raw salted hides pitting/in rotating drum

Waste water discharge (5 *l* effluent/kg raw hide) ←——— Soaked in water for 16-24 hrs. to remove blood, dirt, free salt (with frequent change of water)

B. Liming

Intermittent lime effluent (5 *l*/kg raw hide) ←——— Soaked hide liming pit for 21-48 hrs. for swelling the skin loosening the hairs

C. Unhairing & fleshing process

After liming machining by knife bearing rollers hairs & fleshings are removed

Waste water ←——— from the hides

D. Bating process

Unhaired hide treated in a culture of proteolytic enzymes bath pancreatic or trypsin + NH_4 –salts like $(NH_4)_2$ (SO_4)

bating for 5-6 hrs ↓

Waste water ←——— Removal of lime & hydrolyse by some undesirable proteins from leather

Leather

E. Tanyard processing

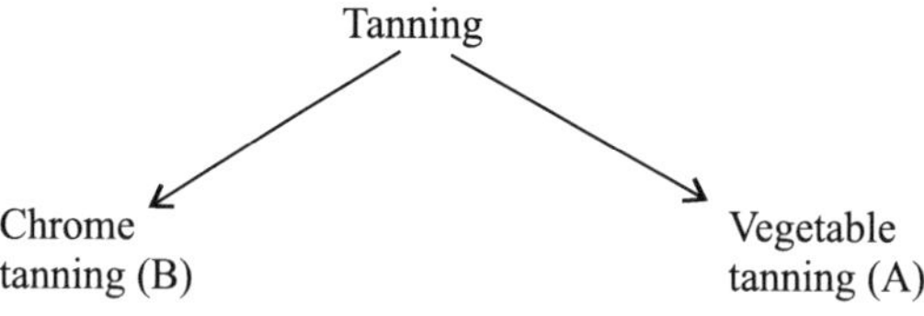

(a) Vegetable Tanning

Bated hides — Placed in contact with solutions of tanning extracts (3-6 weeks)

Effluent water (characteristics in Table 11.23) 3.6 *l*/kg hide

(b) Chrome Tanning

Requires preconditioning by treatment with a solution of H_2SO_4 & NaCl for few hours—pickling process

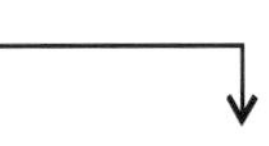

Basic chrome sulfate solution

Waste water characteristics in Table 11.23 ←——— Treatment for 6 hrs. in a rotating drum

Kept in piles for 24 hrs. for further fixation/absorption of chromium

F. Fat liquoring and dyeing

Tanned leather is treated with emulsion of sulphonated castor oil or dyed with different colours to produce finished leather and generating waste water (characteristics in Table 11.23).

However, the waste waters from various steps having nature as given in Table 11.23 when reaches the treatment plant the tannery composite waste water characteristics become as given in Table 11.23 and biological composition of settled and filtered composite tannery waste shows value, as in tables, 11.24 to 11.26.

Table 11.23 Characteristics of step generated tannery effluents

Parameters		*Vegetable Tanning*	*Chrome Tanning*	*Finishing Units*
pH		5.7-11.5	7.5-10.0	5.8
Total dissolved salts (TDS)	(mg/*l*)	1,680-26,250	9,000-20,000	4,400
Suspended solids	(mg/*l*)	160-6,200	1,250-6,000	300
Cl'	(mg/*l*)	500-7,100	1,900-26,200	600
SO_4''	(mg/*l*)	80-2020	–	2040
COD	(mg/*l*)	1000-103,00	5100-7200	276
$BOD_{5(20°)}$	(mg/*l*)	455-4682	2318-3273	126

Table 11.24 Tannery composite waste water characters[36-39]

pH	7-10.4	
D. VS	2700-4400	mg/*l*
TDS Soluble	15000-35000	”
COD Soluble	2700-5000	”
BOD_5	1400-2500	”
TKN	200-270	”
T.P as PO_4''	3-22	”

Table 11.25 Tanning step originated waste water nature

Source Step	*Nature*
Soaking	Olive green in colour, contain dirt, dung, blood, hairs & salt highly putrescible & has obnoxious smell.
Liming	Highly alkaline, one of the heaviest of waste fractions in terms of S.S. & BOD.
Unhairing & fleshing	Hairy, fatty & fleshy particles in suspension.
Spent bating & deliming liquors	Contain significant conc. of dissolved organics & has high BOD.
Spent vegetable tan liquor	Probably the strongest fraction in the composite tannery effluent. It is acidic in nature and has a high BOD & persistent colour which is difficult to remove by chemical & biological treatment.
Spent chrome	It is also highly acidic and greenish in colour. It contains a high conc. of chromium & salt which render the effluent highly acidic toxic. The BOD value is generally low because of the presence of chromium in it.
Fat liquering & dyeing operation	Colours and oil emulsions.

Table 11.26 Biological composition of settled and filtered composite tannery waste

Item	*concentration mg/l*
Dissolved protein	1000-1700
Volatile fatty acids as HAC	200-500
Ether solubles	80-140
Tannin as tannic acid	530-900

4. Treatment methods of effluent waters

Wastewater from tanning industry can be treated in the following steps: Segregation, Primary treatment, and Secondary treatment.

(i) Primary Treatments : The immense difficulty felt with tannery effluent is its ever changing composition and flow rate. Therefore, to have a proper control on effluent treatment, the different types of operational discharge are stored in a storage tank for a period of about 12 hours to equalize and to facilitate neutralization of acid and alkali waste.

The removal of suspended solids further can be facilitated by the use of coagulants like alum, ferric chloride, sulphuric acid, etc. Flocculation with ferrous sulphate and polyelectrolyte combination of tannery effluents is significant in lowering of (i) total solids (ii) BOD (iii) sulphide content (<5 ppm).

In general some initial pretreatment processes are carried out to facilitate the overall treatment system. These can be highlighted as follows:

A. Segregation

Effluents from different tannery operation are highly varying in nature in pollution load. Therefore, the wastewater from such an operation which contribute to a great extent to the pollution load should be treated separately to reduce the intensity of pollution. It is better to segregate soaking effluent containing a very high quantity of chloride. The segregated effluent from soaking operation can be evaporated in a solar evaporation pan.

B. Removal of sulphide

The suspended matter like lime, hair, fleshings, etc., can be removed along with toxic trivalent chromium by simple mixing and sedimentation which can reduce about 70-80% suspended solids and about 30-40% BOD of the tanning waste. But before doing so, it is advisable to go for removing sulphide from the lime liquor first, otherwise the sulphide removal after mixing acidic and alkaline effluent will need to ventilate with considerably greater volume of effluent.

C. Recovery of chromium

Large amount of chromium chemicals are used in the process. Fortunately, however, most of the chromium used is of trivalent nature. Hence its removal or recovery system is relatively simple. There are two types of simple possibilities of recovery of chromium for its reuse. The first one is the simple filtration of chrome tannage effluent to remove the hide fibres and use the liquor for the initial mild pretannage in the subsequent batches. This helps in reducing the discharge load of chromium in the effluent.

The second process involves precipitation of chromium after collecting the effluent from chrome tannage seperately by means of alkalis. The chromium hydroxide precipitate can be redissolved by sulfuric acid and mixed with sodium sulfate to produce a tan liquor for use in the next tanning batch. The recovery of hydroxide may be made with filter press or centrifuge.

D. Removal of suspended solids

Tannery effluent and the large suspended solids content are very synonymous. As already said, the suspended solid consists of lime, lumps of '*stringy*' flesh and hair. These small lumps can be easily removed by screening.

(i) Secondary Treatment Processes : Normally an aerobic process is used to reduce the organic content of the effluent i.e., BOD and COD. However, because of the high values of these components the energy consumption in the process which is necessary for the supply of oxygen required for the oxidation of the organic components is quite high. Presently a combination of anaerobic and aerobic method is favoured. This involves passing the effluent through an anaerobic filter followed by the aerobic process. Aerobic process may be chosen by anyone among the many systems being used as outlined briefly in the following sections.

A. Attached growth process

Trickling filter is one type of attached growth process. Here the microorganisms grow firmly attached to solid support while the waste water flows through the packed bed of solid support. In this way, microbial growth continues due to the sprinkling of waste water on to the filter bed thereby forming bacterial slime augmenting day by day creating ultimately such a situation when the inner layer is deprived of oxygen weakening the attachment with the filter bed allowing a part of the slime to slough off. Most of the BOD is removed and the residual solids are settled out in the form of stabilized sludge.

(a) Merits and Properties of Plastic Media

The basic process has been modified to enrich the performance of such a filter. The greatest change from the basic pattern is the use of plastic media in place of crust rocks. Trickling filter with plastic media weighs much less thereby the bed depth can be increased utilizing a minimum land area. Plastic packing is of greater specific surface enabling a high strength liquor treatment with higher efficiency due to high voidage and here lies the marked difference with mineral media. Another reason for the replacement of mineral rocks is the high building costs of deep packed mineral beds. Their merit is also in removing more BOD and greater open structure facilitating air circulation throughout the bed depth. They do also satisfy the already existing quantities of mineral rocks surpassing the merits of the latter. Moreover, the bacterial slimes produced in plastic media is biologically similar to that on the other one. No objectionable report on the settleability of the sludge from such a media is yet available. With the decrease of specific surface, the phase separation decreases. It is known as low-age sludge or, in the other sense, these are not stabilized.

(b) Rotary Biological Contactors

It is a novel modification to the traditional bio-oxidation techniques to achieve a high operational performance by retaining a high concentration of the active biological solid in the oxidation zone for a long period of time. In this process a series of flat circular plastic plates are arranged to rotate on an axis in such a way as to submerge it partially. Bacterial food is produced in the immersed section whereas the outer zone acts as a source of oxygen. This system is more reliable in operation than the other one. Nowadays an extended form of rotary biological contactors is employed in a perforated rotating drum packed with random plastic packings.

B. Suspended growth process

(a) Activated Sludge Process

This process is a fundamental suspended growth process, accounts for most of the biological purification in sewage treatment plant because of its less working area than the trickling filter process. The basic principle of this operation is the microbial growth in an aerated system containing bio-degradable organic food. The microorganisms grow and form flocs mixed with some organic and inorganics. When aeration is stopped after the consumption of food the mixed flocs will aggregate and settle down leaving a clear supernatant of low BOD and suspended matter.

(b) Usefulness of Combined Treatment of Tannery Effluent and Settled Sewage

Tannery effluent after primary treatment is better to mix with sewage. It acts as a dilution to the concentration of tannery effluent with respect to the presence of toxic substances like Cr III as well as some bactericide used as preservative in leather processing. These substances used in tannery and present in wastewater might be inhibitory to treatment in an industrial biological treatment plant but dilution with sewage decreases their hindrance. The activated sludge process otherwise is too easily upset by the toxic substances present in the undiluted tannery effluent.

That is why, the activated sludge plant is very unlikely to be suitable for such effluent treatment. The large volume of biological solids present either as bacterial slime in trickling filter or as activated sludge in such a treatment process helps also to absorb such toxic substances alongwith certain other organic and inorganics to the extent of 0.5% of the dry weight of fresh sludge thereby reducing the accentuating mark of such materials potent of adverse effects present in industrial pollutants. Obviously, the pollutants this way change their form of pollution, namely from liquid to solid creating the problem of the sludge disposal. Tannery wastewater contains biodegradable organic matter but it is a necessary fact that the tannery discharges do not contain all the nutrients needed for biological growth in the required ratio, that is BOD : N : P = 100 : 5 : 1.

11.4 POTABLE WATER TREATMENT BIOTECHNOLOGY[42-54]

11.4.1 Introduction

Amount of natural water resources for drinking like ground waters are in general, relatively pure and free from bacteria and other contaminants because of the filtering action of the earth (Table 11.27 and 11.28).

Table 11.27 Water uniqueness and resources

	Uniqueness	*Water Resources Categories*
1.	Prime natural resource	Rain water
2.	Essential for life survival	Surface water
3.	In water/hydrological cycle, total amount of water is constant.	Stored water
4.	It can neither be increased nor diminished.	Ground water
5.	Essential for process industry	Waste or polluted water

This removes all the bacteria and also any suspended particles and organic materials. Deep wells contain usually fewer microorganisms than water from shallow wells. It is due to the deeper layers of filtering material. Water resoures receive microbial load, organic nitrogen and other polluting factors from soil, air, sewerage, organic wastes, dead plants and animals, process industry effluents, municipal sewage etc. Thus to define the purity of water standard specifications have been used by different nations for safeness of their usability. The important specifying factors and their approximate parametric standard limits have, therefore, been listed (Table 11.29).[40-48]

However, ground water is replenished/recharged by hydrological/water cycle. This replenishment may be due to rainfall, less evapotranspiration and surface run off.

Drinking water supplies in almost all urban metropolitan cities in our country have been known to contain pollutants. This is primarily because of either sewerage is absent or partial. In such situations microbial pollutants may predominate sometimes and pose a major health hazard. Not only that relatively minor pollutants relate to leaking sewers. In developed countries as well as in mountaneous health resorts and industrialized areas road deicing and other urban processes also cause pollution in ground water supplies.

Table 11.28 Comparative information on fresh water withdrawal in India vis-a-vis worldwide and in a modernized region (D-Domestic, I-Industry, A-Agriculture)

Place/Country	*Approximate Annual Withdrawal*		*Sectoral (%)*		
	% of Water Resources	*Per Capita* (m^3)	*D*	*I*	*A*
India	18-20	612	3-5	4-8	93-87
Worldwide	8660	8	23	69	
Northern and central America	10	1692	942	49	

Many of the organic contaminants are very site specific. In some urban metropolitan cities in our country two groups of compounds may also be detected in water supplies time to time. These are chlorinated hydrocarbon solvents and aromatic compounds arising from petroleum fraction present in water during chlorination disinfection.

Industrial organic chemicals in ground water may arise from the same source that create contaminated land e.g. industrial premises, fuel storage, transport and pipe-line spillages. Also water resources become polluted and contaminated by sewerage discharge and human excrement. Effluent loads discharged into the natural streams or stored water receptacles at various disposal points cause the water resource polluted. The major effluent load discharging systems may emanate from process industries.

Pollution by sewage or by human excrement may be greatest danger associated with drinking water. These pollution contributors are usually carriers of such infectious diseases such as typhoid fever, dysentery or jaundice. In such cases water contains living microorganisms or viruses which cause the disease thereby causing health hazard. Faecal pollution organisms like *E. coli, Streptococci sp.* are common resulting exertion of $BOD_{5(20°C)}$ and COD values in potable water as well. (Table 11.29) Possibility of fire hazards by oil spills in supra-national long oceanic avenues and its prevention scope by technologically redesigned microorganisms has been shown in literature.[44]

11.4.2 Purification for Environment and Hazard Protection

1. By Bioprocessing

For maintaining purity of municipal/corporation water supplies its chlorination is highly effective in purification of water from microbial contamination thereby preventing spread of infectious diseases. Not only municipal/corporation water supplies but also other water supplies must pass through a series of purification steps before pipe line supply to make it safe for either human consumption or for process industry and agriculture requirements. In some cases, however, the water resource may be sufficiently pure to require only treatment with a disinfectant like chlorine, chlorocresol etc. depending on the quality of treatment desired and the purpose. In many instances the condition of water resource is such as to require normally three stages of primary purifications namely, sedimentation, filtration followed by disinfection. However, in recycling of used water in industries or for their disposal in natural water ways stringent treatment methods are needed to make waste water/liquid effluent safe for recycling, for aquatic life and prevention of water basin filling up by metallic or other solids. Reference is therefore made to water resources and the danger of their pollution.

Table 11.29 Important pollution specifying factors and their approximate usability specifications in water for different purposes

Pollution Factors	*Approximate Usability Specifications of Water for the Purpose of*		
	Drinking	*Process Industry*	*Irrigated Agriculture*
Physical appearance	Clear, Colourless	Clear, Colourless	Preferably Colourless
Odour	Nil	Nil	Nil
pH	7.0	6.9	5.5-9.0
Chemicals (ppm)	500	–	2000
Chloride as Cl'	200	–	600
Sulphate	200	–	1000
Nitrate	40-50	–	1000
Phenol	0.002	1.0	1.0
Lead	Nil	Nil	Nil
Arsenic	0.005	–	–
Oil & grease	0.3	1.0	1.0
BOD_5(20°C) (ppm)	4.5-5.0	4.5-0	6-7
COD (ppm)	7-8.5	–	–

(i) Oxic Bacterial Process Biotechnology : It is well reorganized that there are limits to the self purifying ability of a natural body of water. This limit pertains to both capacity and the speed of self purification. In recent industrialized societies necessity of development of rapid man-made water purification has become obvious.

In a more recent process a mix of various strains of bacteria has been used to assimilate organic matter natural as well as man-made consuming oxygen and producing chiefly CO_2 and H_2O.

The technological success greatly depends on the type of water and apollutants, their amount and concentration, the consistency of these determinants and last but not the least, on the speed of bacterial assimilation and the presence of inhibitory ingredients. Many process biotechnology have been developed in laboratories and pilot plants. Their operational reliability is of utmost importance, both in order to ensure continuous supply and necessary quality of treated clean after the purification process. Oxic biological nitrification of organic present in polluted water is also one of the major concerns in this bioprocessing to avoid eutrophication.

(ii) Anoxic Bacterial Process Biotechnology : Many microbes not only survive but even grow rapidly when starved of oxygen. For survival these microbes avail gene machines which encode enzymes essential for anoxic growth. The most successful bacterial groups can use nitrate as a substitute for oxygen/air. In anoxic stage of water purification/treatment less energy is derived from nitrate reduction than from conventional cell respiration, so genes, for nitrate reduction are

activated only when nitrate is present but oxygen is unavailable. However, the product of nitrate reduction is very toxic. Actually, nitrate respiring bacteria in water purification does make provision for removal of nitrate, so formed.

(iii) Integrated Oxic-Anoxic Process Biotechnology : Consideration: In the water purification bacterial nitrogen metabolism is an important key to clean water. Bacterial metabolism of three molecular species: ammonia, nitrate and nitrogen, dominates the oxic-anoxic integrated biological nitrogen cycle. In oxic biotechnology nitrification plays major role while denitrification fixation governs anoxibiosis in the process biotechnology. A striking balance between oxic-anoxic bioprocessing and water pollution is important so that the objective of waste water purification is not defeated.

(iv) Oxic-Anoxic Design Scheme : In order to overcome the problem of eutrophication in waste water purification nitrogen content in water must be removed otherwise, it will cause BOD increase. The removal of nitrogen from waste/water can be done by appropriate schemes of oxic-anoxic design systems for nitrification/ denitrification. Operational characteristics of three schemes for designs of nitrification and denitrification have been described below (Fig. 11.15).

Scheme 1: This scheme depends upon the endogenous respiration of the activated sludge to achieve denitrification.

Scheme 2: Here a portion of the influent waste water is by-passed to the denitrification tank to provide food for the facultative organisms thereby increasing the respiration rate and hence the denitrification rate.

Scheme 3: It uses an influent waste water which is nitrogen deficient as a food source for denitrifying organisms. The waste water should contain a readily available carbon source.

(v) Relative Advantages and Disadvantages of the Schemes : In scheme 1 while the bioprocessing achieves a low nitrogen effluent, the slow rate of denitrification under endogenous respiration conditions results in a large denitrification tank. In scheme 2 while some reduces the required size of the denitrification tank it has the disadvantage of increasing the unoxidized nitrogen in the treated effluent and in most cases increasing the effluent BOD. While scheme 2 practice will not contribute nitrogen to the effluent, careful controlled operation is required to avoid increasing the effluent BOD. Experimental results and experience indicated that economic use of this process scheme necessitates increasing the respiration rate and hence denitrification rate in denitrifying unit. It is also required for only carbonaceous BOD removal. If higher O_2 level is maintained in the aeration tank for maximum nitrification rate, the power requirement will be about two and half times that required for conventional activated sludge process operation.

(vi) Acceleration of Denitrification : Biodenitrification for removal of nitrate and nitrite could be accelerated by a using appropriate amount of methanol. Based on stoichiometric equations of biodenitrification it could be computed that 1 mole NO_3 is equivalent to 5/6 mole methanol. When the waste water which is to be treated contains dissolved oxygen (DO) it needs to be removed

before denitrification step. This has been accomplished by adding extra amount of methanol. From these considerations the total amount of methanol (C_m) requirement could be computed by the following relation:

$$C_m = 2.47\ N_0 + 1.53\ N_i + 0.87\ DO$$

Here N_0 is the initial nitrate, N_i is the initial nitrite and DO is the initial dissolved oxygen concentration.

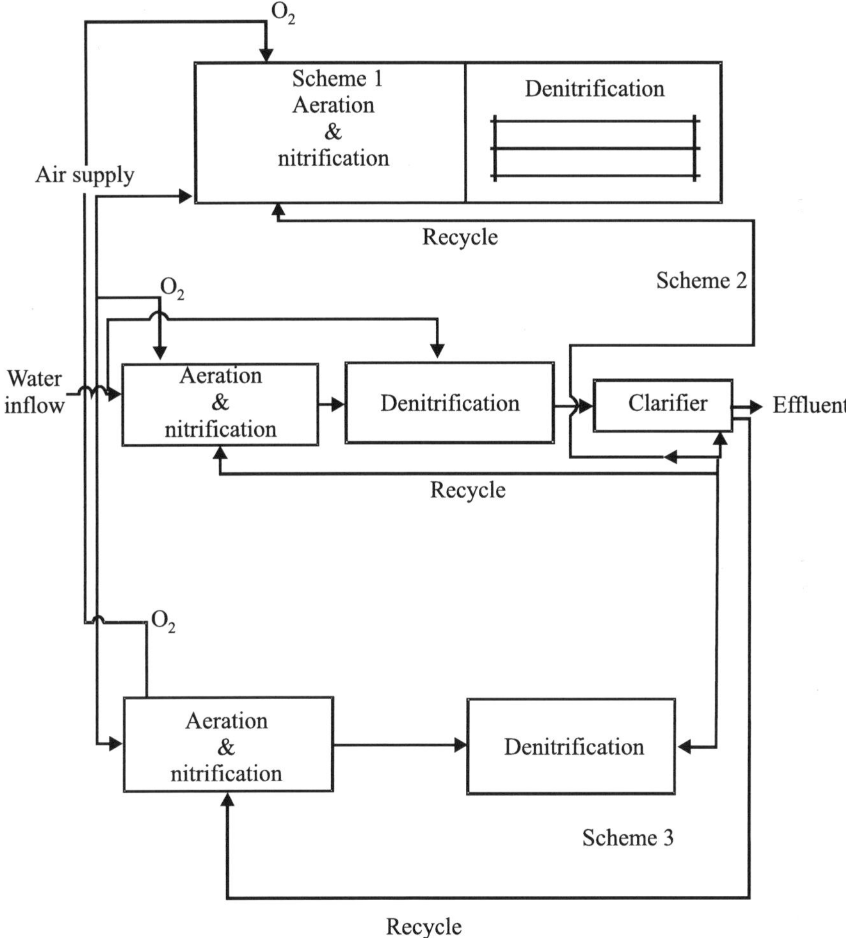

Fig. 11.15

2. Chlorine disinfection and biohazard

Purification of drinking water by chlorine disinfection is an age old process. It is very effective in killing hazardous microorganisms in potable water. However, biomolecular design engineeing concerns of water chlorination hazard are being known in more recent years.

Overchlorination in water is hazardous to human health. The relationship between the concentration of available chlorine and the time taken to kill the organisms in water is exponential i.e.

$$c^n t = \text{constant (k)} \tag{11.20}$$

It has been stated that in human lymphocytes, chlorinated humic substances produced DNA strand cleavage but only at a concentration that caused cytotoxicity.

11.5 TREATMENT BIOTECHNOLOGY OF GENETICALLY ENGINEERED CELL PROCESSING EFFLUENTS

These types of wastes are usually radionuclide containing or nuclear. These waste streams have been given significant attention recently by the research community. Also, working with pathogens or genetically engineered cells/microorganisms demands besides biosafety, corrolary of biocontamination, combination of good micorobiological processing techniques and facility design to take care of these hazardous cell processing effluents. Effluent discharges to air, water and soil must be done in accordance with environmental regulation.

In more recent years treatment techniques are being used to reduce human exposure to the toxic/hazardous and infectious components of genetically engineered cell processing effluents. The most commonly used techniques include internal segregation, containment and irradiation. Other common treatment techniques include grinding, shredding and disinfection e.g. autoclaving and chemical treatment followed by land fillings[55]. However, incineration destroys the broadest pathogenic wastes and is an appropriate alternative to burial of these pathogenic effluents.[55] Use of mutation of genetically engineered cells in the effluent may be an alternative approach to their treatment to reduce these hazardous effluents.[56] It has also been suggested that when viable recombinant DNA (rDNA) organisms are contained in bioprocessing wastes, the wastes must be treated by sterilization or decontaminated, before being discharged to the sewer or waste treatment system as per the requirement of NIH guidelines.[57] Continuous sterilization systems associated with BLI-LS facilities is useful. BLI-LS stands for “Biosafety Level I, Large Scale”.

11.6 REFERENCES

1. Rich, L.G., “Biological Phenomena”, *Environmental System Engineering*, pp 70-98, ISE, McGraw Hill Kogakusha Ltd., 1973.
2. Bradshow, A.D. R. Sherwood and F. Warner, *The Treatment and Handling of Wastes,* Chapman and Hall for the Royal Society, London, New York, 1992.
3. Metcalf & Eddy, Inc., *Waste Water Engineering* 3rd edn., McGraw Hill, New York, 1991.
4. Fujmoto, Y. *Graphical Use of First Stage BOD Equation,* pp 36, 69, J.W.P.C.F., 1964.
5. Eckenfelder, W.W. and D.J. O′Connor, *Biological Waste Treatment*, Pergamon Press, 1961.
6. Braun, R. and S. Huss, “Anaerobic Digestion of Distillary Effluents”, *Process. Biogas*., July-Aug 25-27, 1982.
7. Ghose, T.K. and S.N. Mukhopadhyay, “Some Basic Engineering Considerations to Maximize Bioenergy Production”, *ICE*, 18 (4), pp 12-16, 1976.
8. Mukhopadhyay, S.N. and T.K. Ghose, “Integration of Bioconversion, Environment and Genetic Engineering in Bioenergy System”, pp 260-63, *Proc. BESI Conf.* (O.P. Vimal ed.), 1985.
9. Moletta, R.D. Verrier and G. Albagnae, “Dynamic Modelling of Anaerobic Digestion”, *Waters Res*. 20 (4), pp 427-34, 1986.

10. Ghosh, P. and T.K. Ghose, "Distillary Effluent Treatment Technological Options", *Biotechnology and Bioprocess Engineering,* pp 605-613, United India Press, New Delhi, 1985.
11. McCarty, P.L., "The Methane Fermentation", *Principles and Applications of Aquatic Microbiology,* (H. Heukeiekian and N. Dondero eds.), Chapter 16, John Wiley, New York, 1964.
12. Bootille, A.L., *Acid Rain: How Great a Menace*? National Geographic (Nov.) pp 652-82, 1981.
13. Mukhopadhyay, S.N., N.K. Nigam, and T.K. Ghose, "Production of Methane in Biogas from Indegenous Resources", *Proc. Annual Meeting, IIChE*, pp II 8.5.1-5.12., IIT Bombay, 1979.
14. *NEERI Final Report*, "Detoxification of Phenol and Cyamide Bearing Industrial Wastes", Dept. of Energy, IIT, New Delhi. 1982.
15. Parekh, B.K., W.F. Scotts, and J.G. Groppo, "Column Flotation Studies of Ultrafine Coals," *Processing and Utilization of High Sulfur Coals* II, pp. 197-208, (Markuszewiski. R. and Wheelock, T.D. ed.), Elsevier Science Pub., Amsterdam, 1990
16. Yoon R.H., G.T. Adel, G.H. Luttrell, M.J. Mankosa, and A.J. Weber., "Microbubble Floatation of Fine Particles", (Y.A. Attia, B.M. Moudgell and S. Chander eds.), *Interfacial Phenomena in Biotechnology and Material Processing*, pp 363-74, Elsevier Sci. Pub.Amsterdam., 1988.
17. Li. J. and A.E. Humphrey, "Kinetics and Fluormetric Behavior of Aphenol Fermentation", *Bioprocess Engineering: The First Generation*, pp 190-206, (Ghose, T.K. ed.), Chichester Ellis Horwood Ltd., 1989.
18. Ohmura, N. and H. Saiki, "Desulfurization of Coal by Microbial Column Floatation", *Biotechnol and Bioeng*., pp 44, 125-131, 1994.
19. Sayler. G.S., A., Breen, J.W: Blackburn and O. Yagi, "Predictive Assessment of Priority Pollutant Biooxidation Kinetics in Activated Sluge", *Environ. Prog.* 3 (3), pp 153-63, 1984.
20. Chandra. D. P. Ray, A.K. Mishra. N.K. and S.G., Choudhury, "Removal of Surface Coal by Thiobacillus ferroxidans and by Mixed Bacteria Present in Coal", *Fuel,* pp 59. 249, 1980.
21. Kilburn II, J.J. and J. Jackowski, "Biodesulfurisation of Water Soluble Coal Derived Material by *Rhodococcus Rhodochrous*", *IGT,* 58, 40-9, pp 1107, 1992.
22. Mukhopadhyay, S.N. and D.K. Das, *Oxygen Responses Reactivities and Measurements in Biosystems*, pp. 82-85, Boca Raton, Florida, CRC Press, 1994.
23. Holladay, D. W., D.D. Hancher, D.D. Chilcate, "Biodegradation of Phenolic Waste Liquors in Stirred Tank, Columnar and Fludized Bed Bioreactors", *AICHE, Symp. Series*, 74, (172), pp 241-52, 1978.
24. Catchpole, J.R. and R.L. Cooper, *Water Res*., 7.1137, 1973.
25. Atkinson. B., *Biochemical Reactors*, Pion Press, 1974.
26. Hobbie. J.E., et al., "Use of Nucleopors Counting Bacteria by Fluoroscence Microscopy", *Appl. Environ. Microbiol*., pp 33, 1225, 1977.
27. "Operation of Municipal Waste Water Treatment Plants", Fifth edn., Water Environment Federation, *Mannual of Practice*, MOP 11, Vo12, 1996.
28. Mukhopadhyay, S.N. and K. Das, "Retrieval of Bioenergy from Agrobased Food Wastes as a Service to Rural Food Industries", *Proc. AFST Seminar,* pp 55-57, Small Scale Food Industry for Rural India.
29. Potter, N.N. and J.H. Hotchkins, "Food Processing and the Environment", *Food Science*, Chapter 22, Chapman and Hall, New York, 1995.

30. Mukhopadhyay, S.N., "Water Resources, Pollution and Purification for Environment and Hazard Protection", *Environment and Development of Process Industries*, pp 189-200, INAE, New Delhi, 1995
31. Ghosh, S. and D.L. Klass *Process Biochem,* 13 (4), pp 15, 1978.
32. Ghose, T.K *Fuels from Biomass*—Status Report on Some Tasks and Coordination Submitted to National Isteering Committee, DST, GOI, 1978.
33. Mukhopadhyay, S.N., "An Overview of Taking Advantage of Membranes in Food and Fermentation Biotechnology Industries", Extended Abstracts Book of *XIV National Symposium on Membranes in Chemical and Biochemical Industries,* pp. 45-46, Feb. 16 & 17, 1996.
34. Mukhopadhyay, S.N., "Modern Concepts and Multifacet Role of Membranes in Biosystems and Bioprocessing", Lecture Notes of Membranes and its Applications, pp 181-185, Short Course Sponsored by FITT, I.I.T. Delhi, Feb 13-15, 1996.
35. M. Chareyan, "Membrane Technology: Principles and Selected Applications", *Ibid.*, pp. 10-16.
36. Chakraborty, R.N., *Ph. D. Thesis*, Jadavpur Univ., 1974.
37. Chakraborty, R.N., "Some Aspects of Treatment and Disposal of Tannery Wastes", *Treatment and Disposal of Tannery and Slaughter House Waste*, pp 35-41, (V.S. Krishnamurthy, C.A. Sastry and T.R. Bhaskaran eds.), CLRI, Madras, 1972.
38. Basu S.K. and R.N. Chakraborty, "Effluent Treatment in Leather Processing Industries", *Ind. J. Env. Poll.* 9 (12), pp 904-908, 1989.
39. Basu, S.K. and R.N. Chakraborty, "Effluent Treatment in Leather Processing Industries", Part II, *Ind. J. Env. Poll.* 10, (9), pp 661-65, 1990.
40. Guha, B.K., *Biological Treatment of Tannery Effluents* Course Leature in Newfrontiers in Bioprocess Engineering, Dept. of Biochemical Engineering and Biotechnology, I.I.T. Delhi, Sponsored by DBT, GOI, 1993.
41. Robinson, D.G. J.E. White and A.J. Callier, *Chem. Engg.*, pp 110-114, April 1997.
42. Choudhury, N., Keynote Lecture on Water Management, The National *Concerns, Challenges for Survival* Organized by J.U. Alumni Association at India International Centre, July 30,1994.
43. Krishna, J., "Water Management Perspectives: Problems and Policy Issues", *INAE Pub.*, 1990.
44. Chakraborty, A.M. and J.F. Brown. Jr., *Genetic Engineering,* pp. M 185, (A.M. Chakraborty, ed.), CRC Press, 1978.
45. Chipman, J.K. *Biotechnology News*, 1993.
46. Shah, D.B, L. T. Novak, P.M. Schierholz G.A. Coulumana, "Water Treatment: Chemical Engineering Methods in Action", *AICHE Sympo. Series* 71 (151), pp 360-366, 1975.
47. Koch, O., "The Chemical Industry in the Eighties", *Env. & Ind.* Spl. Issue No. 3, pp 26-32, 1982.
48. Mukhopadhyay, S.N., "The Dimension of Biotechnology in Transportation System Studies", *Proc. Transp. System Analysis & Policy Studies,* pp. 350-54, (P.S. Satsangi and A.L. Agarwal, eds.), Tata McGraw Hill, New Delhi, 1987.
49. *World Resources,* 1990-1991.
50. Roy, T.K., *Personal Communication*, 1995
51. *WHO International Standard for Drinking Water,* 2nd edn., Geneva, W.H.O, 1963.
52. Kantawala, D., "Abatement of Water Pollution", *Chemical Technology for Better Environment,* pp 76-115, (T.K. Roy ed), INAE, Allied Publishers Ltd, New Delhi, 1998.

53. Mukhopadhyay, S.N. and R.K. Baisya, "Role of Water Composition in Relation to Food Biotechnology", *Proc. AP. Biochem* C' 97, pp 354-1357, (Z. Y. Shen, F. Ouyang, J. T. Yu and Z.A. Cao eds.), Tsinghua Univ. Press, Beijing, 1997.
54. Mukhopadhyay, S.N. and P. Mukhopadhyay, "Water: Properties, Pollution and Management in the developing world", Ecological Engineering Approach, Univ. of Kalyani, Kolkata and I.E.E. Society, Switzerland Pub., B.B. Jana, R.D. Banerjee, B. Guterstam and J. H. Heebs (eds) 2000, pp 551-557.
55. Anonymous, "Air Waste", pp 44 (10), 1176-9, 1994.
56. Gomperts E.D. S.K. Courter, M.D. Lyaes and D.A. Baker, *Developments in Biological Standardization*, pp 83, 111-117, 1994.
57. R. Lee and J. Waltz, "Consider Continuous Sterilization of Bioprocess Wastes", CEP, Dec., pp 44-48, 1990.
58. M. Freemantle: Can we exploit hydrogenases? C&EN, July 22, 2002 pp 35-36.
59. I. Kim, The Promising World of Biooxidation, CEP, Jan. 2004, p 8-11.
60. M. Freemantle, Cover Story, Chemistry for Water, CHEMRAWN Conf., Paris, C & EN., July 19, pp 25-30, 2004.

Chapter

12

CONTROL OF UNDESIRABLE MICROORGANISMS IN BIOSYSTEMS

12.1 INTRODUCTION

In daily life activities human has always tried to control undesirable microorganisms of nature. In sophistication of human life style undesirable microorganisms must be controlled. Also, in producing chemicals/materials, useful for living being, by the useful microorganisms, spoilage of processing material by undesirable microorganism need to be prevented. For keeping living being fit its major essential requirements e.g. water, food/feed, cloths and shelter must be free from undesirable microorganisms. In meeting such requirements human has developed through ages the methods to control the harmful action of undesirable microorganisms either by preventing normal metabolic activity using chemicals or by killing them with various agents.

12.2 METHODS OF CONTROLLING UNDESIRABLE MICROORGANISMS

12.2.1 Preventing Normal Metabolic Activity [1-5]

For controlling the harmful action of biocells like microorganisms they are prevented of normal harmful metabolic activity by treating with agents. The actions of these agents have been defined giving different terminologies as below.

a. *Germicidal*: Any agent that destroys disease organisms, but modern definition is, any agent that destroys microbes but not spores, irrespective of whether they are capable of producing disease.

b. *Bacteriocidal and Bacteriostatic*: Any agent that destroys bacteria but not spores. They are agents which do not kill bacteria but prevents them from multiplication.

c. *Antiseptic:* Any agent that prevents or arrests the growth or action of organisms either by inhibiting their activity or by destroying them.

d. *Disinfection:* Agents which destroy disease bacteria and other harmful microorganisms but not spores.

e. *Viricidal:* Agents which destroy or inactivate filterable viruses.

f. *Sterilization:* Agents that perform complete killing of all organisms including spores.

In process biotechnology and medical biotechnology operations of disinfection and sterilization have been widely practiced.

12.2.2 Control by Disinfection Method

The agents that cause disinfection are called disinfectants. So, disinfectants are the detergents which inactivate the organisms by blocking the normal enzymatic-metabolism so that the ultimate harmful product of metabolism of organisms do not appear. Thus, this process of inactivation of organisms with the help of disinfectant is called disinfection. Among various process biotechnologies the uses of disinfectants in the following are prominent.

- Disinfection of water
- Cleaning gadzets and accessories of process biotechnology
- Keeping the process steps sterile
- Preservation of cosmetics
- Pharmaceutical preparations
- Food preservation

For disinfection most widely used disinfecting agents include the following:

Distilled water	Surface active agents
Acids	O_3, SO_2, Cl_2 and hypochlorite
Alkalies	Quats (Benzal cromium chloride cetrimide)
Salts	Anions, Alkyl sulfonates
Alcohols and ether	Poly phosphates
Soaps	Ethylene oxide
Dyes	H_2O_2, formaldehyde
Salfonamides	Antibiotics

Index of disinfection extent is called phenol coefficient. Phenol coefficient is defined as the killing power of a germicide towards a test organism as compared to that of phenol under similar conditions. For example, considering there was no growth with 2.0% phenol, but growth with 1.8%, the mean is 1.9. Simlarly, suppose there was no growth with 0.457% test disinfectant, but growth with 0.411% of the disinfectant, the mean is 0.434. Thus, phenol coefficient of the test disinfectant $= \frac{1.9}{0.434} = 4.4$.

12.2.3 Mechanism of Disinfection

Disinfection process involves inactivation of enzymes by two ways:

a. Using chemicals which penetrate through cell wall and dislodging the enzyme from getting into the process.
b. Chemicals inhibit the excretion of enzyme out of the protoplasm through the cell wall.

Factors on which disinfection process depends:

1. Nature of organism to be killed and its condition.
2. Nature and condition of disinfectant employed in terms of products that it releases when it is placed in material to be disinfected.
3. The nature of material (water) to be disinfected.
4. Temperature of the material to be disinfected.
5. Time of contact of disinfectant with water material.

Under ideal conditions rate of disinfection depends on the following:

a. Time of contact of disinfectant with water material.
b. Concentration of disinfectant.
c. Number of organisms present.
d. Temperature of water.

12.2.4 The Dynamics of Disinfection [6]

Many investigators working independently showed that the reaction velocity of disinfection to approximate that of a unimolecular reaction. The formula for unimolecular reaction rate constant is

$$k = \frac{1}{t} \log \frac{a}{a - x}$$

Where, k = Constant,
t = Time
a = Amount of substance at the beginning of the reaction and
x = Amount decomposed in time t.

Since plot of t against log (a – x) is a straight line, it is often known as the logarithimic law.

1. Time of contact

When applied to disinfection Chick stated the above law as follows.

"The concentration of population after destruction is a direct function with the cell which are destroyed". Mathematically,

$$\frac{dy}{dx} \propto (N_0 - y)$$

Or
$$\frac{dy}{dx} = k\,(N_0 - y) \qquad (12.1)$$

Where, k = Proportionality constant having unit of $time^{-1}$ or velocity constant at a specific concentration.

y = Number of organisms destroyed/min. Which is proportional to the number of organisms remaining, i.e. N.

N_0 = Initial number of organism

When, y = 0,

t = 0

y = y,

t = t

Integrating equation (12.1)

$$\int_0^y \frac{dy}{N_0 - y} = \int k \cdot dt = k \int_0^t dt$$

or
$$\text{In}\frac{N_0 - y}{N_0} = \ln\frac{N}{N_0} = -kt \qquad [\therefore N_0 - y = N]$$

or
$$\frac{N}{N_0} = e^{-kt}$$

or
$$\log\frac{N}{N_0} = -kt \log_{10}e$$

or
$$k = t \log\frac{N_0}{N} \qquad (12.2)$$

This equation (12.2) shows that plot of t against log N/N_0 is a straight line having a slope of $-k \log_{10}e = -k'$ and intercept – 1 (100%) at t = 0, rate of survival or mean lethal dose = 0.368.

N. B. When conditions are not ideal rate of killing may increase or decrease with time. The increase of killing may be explained in two ways:

(i) As combination of slow diffusion of chemical disinfectants through cell wall and rate of killing dependent upon the material inside the cell.

(ii) On the assumption that the lethal number of centers in cells must be reached by disinfectant.

A linear relationship was developed by plotting log N/N_0 against t^m ($m > 1$) or log N/N_0 against t.

Decrease of Killing May be Explained as Follows: Decrease may be due to variation in resistance of different cells within the same centre of organism. Other factors responsible for decrease may be due to decline of concentration of disinfectant with time. This is very common with O_3.

2. Effect of concentration of disinfectant

The relationship between the concentration and the time taken to kill the organism is exponential i.e. doubling the concentration considerably more than half the rate and the concentration coefficient is greater than 1. If one considers

C = Concentration
n = A constant for the disinfectant, = concentration coefficient and
t = Time required to effect a constant % of inactivation.

Then,

$$C^n t = \text{a constant}$$

or
$$C_1^n t_1 = C_2^n t_2 = \ldots\ldots\ldots = \text{Constant} \tag{12.3}$$

This may be written as

$$n \log C + \log t = \text{a constant} \tag{12.4}$$

This is the equation of a straight line i.e. plotting log c against log t gives a straight line or in other words, the logarithm of the concentration is proportional to the logarithm of the time.

In the equation $C^n t$ = constant may be combined with that for the velocity for disinfection, k = 1/t log N/N_0

i.e.
$$k_t = \log N/N_0 \tag{12.5}$$

Combining, C^n 1/K log N_0/N = constant or C^n/K = constant (12.6)

(for same percent volume) where K = true velocity constant, independent of concentration and therefore different from k.

By inserting K_1 & C_1 & K_2 & C_2 in equation (12.6)

$$n = \frac{\log K_2/K_1}{\log C_2/C_1} \tag{12.7}$$

In order to determine n for any disinfectant it is therefore necessary to obtain velocity constants at two different concentrations at the same temperature.

n for $HgCl_2$ = 1
n for Phenol = 6

Doubling the concentration of $HgCl_2$ half the time of disinfection ($C^n = 2^1 = 2$).

But doubling the concentration of phenol reduces the time of disinfection to 1/64 ($C^n = 2^6 = 64$). A high value for *n*, the concentration coefficient is not necessarily an advantage.

3. Effect of temperature on rate of disinfection

The time-temperature relationship of disinfectant is given by Arrhenius-Vant hoff relationship as

$$\log \frac{t_1}{t_2} = \frac{E\,(T_2 - T_1)}{2.303\, RT_1\, T_2}$$

$$= \frac{E\,(T_2 - T_1)}{4.575\, T_1\, T_2} \tag{12.8}$$

where t_1 & t_2 = times of equal % of kill to be effected at temperature T_1 and $T_2°$ in absolute scale.
E = Activation energy at constant temperature and constant characteristic property of the system.
R = Gas constant = 1.99 cals.
When $T_2 - T_1$ = 10°C ratio of t_1/t_2, called Q_{10}, the temp. coefficient of reaction velocity, is approximately related to E in the vicinity of 20°C as follows :

$$\log Q_{10} = \log t_1/t_2 = E / 39000 \tag{12.9}$$

This means that t_1 and t_2 periods are required for equal % kill at T_1 and T_2 which are 10° apart. Q_{10} is also dependent on the pH of the disinfectant and types of disinfectant as below.

Type of Cl_2	pH	E.Cals.	Q_{10}
Aqueous Cl_2	7.0	82,00	1.65
	8.5	6400	1.42
	9.5	12000	2.13
	10.7	15000	2.50

Q_{10} is also defined by the equation

$$Q_{10} = \frac{K_T + 10}{K_T}$$

$$\approx \frac{5\,\mu}{e^{\{T - (T + 10)\}}} \tag{12.10}$$

Value of Q_{10} increases with the value of μ and decreases with increase in temperature. In a chemical reaction the value of Q_{10} at 20°C = 2 to 4. This corresponds to a value of μ ≈ 12000 to 24000 cals/mol. At 30°C, Q_{10} = 1.2.
In a protein reaction (i.e. denaturation of protein or protein coagulation)

μ = 40,000 to 80,000 cals/mol.

Q_{10} at 20°C = 10 to 100

Equation (12.10) can also be written as

$$\log K_T = A - \frac{\mu}{2.303\, RT} \tag{12.11}$$

Where,

K_T = rate constant at T°A.
μ = Activation energy (cals/mol)
A = Arrhenius constant.

The temperature effect on disinfection also accords with the formula

$$Q_{10} = Q_{T_2 - T_1} = K_2/K_1 \tag{12.12}$$

Where,

Q = Temperature coeficient
K_2 = Velocity constant at T_2°A.
K_1 = Velocity constant at T_1°A.

Interpretation of equation (12.12)

As the temperature rises in A.P. (arithmatic progression) the rate of disinfection increases in G. P.

Q_{10} may be obtained by determining the reaction velocities at two different temperatures.

$$Q_{10} = t_1/t_2 = \frac{1/K_1 \log N/N_0}{1/K_2 \log N/N_0} = \frac{K_2}{K_1}$$

4. Effect of number of organisms

No significant effect has been observed in high or low concentration of disinfectant in killing the organism. Minimum requirement of concentration of disinfectant is

$$C^P/N_r = \text{constant} \tag{12.13}$$

Where, N_r = Concentration of microorganism reduced by given % in a given time.

C = Concentration of disinfectant

P = Exponent of concentration, a direct function of disinfectant.

This equation is valid only if difference is observed in very high cell concentration of microorganisms involved.

Details of standard bacteriological techniques for testing disinfectants :

Test Organism	Rideal–Walker (R.W.) test *B. typhosum* Lister strain NCTC 781	Chick-Martin test *B. typhosum* 'S'strain NCTC 3390	F.D.A *B. typhosum* Hopkins Insecticide strain
Culture medium	2% n-peptone No-1 2% lab. lemco. 1% salt pH 7.4	2% n-peptone No-1 2% lab. lemco. 0.5% salt pH 7.6	1% Armors peptons 0.5% lemco 0.5% salt pH 6.8
Amount of inoculum	0.2 ml	0.1 ml broth culture upto 2.5% with 5% yeast	0.5 ml
Volume of disinfectant	5 ml	2.5 ml	5 ml
Organic matter	Nil	2.4% (by weight)	Nil
Method of determining end point	Dilution showing life in 5 min and no life there after	Mean of dilution which kill and fail to kill in 30 min	dilution showing life in 5 min and none in 10 min.

R.W. test depends on a comparison between the inhibitory effect of phenol and that of agent on the growth of a selected microorganism, under closely controlled conditions. Phenol is quoted as unity and the other is given a R.W. coefficient.

Chick Martin test is now a standard procedure.

Factors influencing germicidal action

1. Test organism
2. H^+ ion concentration
3. Presence of organic matter
4. Surface tension

Evaluation of disinfectants

The following methods are used for the evaluation of germicides.

1. End point of extinction method
2. Counting methods
3. Other methods

12.3 DISINFECTANT DECAY AND BACTERIAL INACTIVATION KINETICS[7-9]

In drinking water disinfection by chlorine it has been demonstrated that the growth of heterotroph plate count of bacteria followed first order kinetics in the water phase of pipe system containing bacterial nutrients. This is valid for a limited stretch of pipe, where the concentration, on the other hand, has been demonstrated to follow a modified Chick's law, in which the concentration of the germicidal agent is incorporated in the first or n-th order. This is valid during the disinfection process, and does not take initial and final effects into consideration. In a study, the effects of growth assumed first order kinetics with respect to the bacterial number, while inactivation assumed first order kinetics with respect to both bacterial number and concentration of the disinfectant. These may be combined in one expression :

$$\frac{dN}{dt} = \mu N - \lambda NC \tag{12.14}$$

where N is the bacterial density in the water l^{-1}; t is time, h; μ is the growth rate constant of the bacterial units in the water h^{-1}, λ is the inactivation rate constant, $lg^{-1}\ h^{-1}$; C is the concentration of disinfectant in the water, gl^{-1}.

12.3.1 Disinfectant Decay Kinetics

Contrary to most inactivation studies where the concentration of disinfectant, C, is assumed to be constant during a relatively short period of time, one study included the decay of disinfectants, which inevitably took place in the water supply systems. The decay was assumed to be first order with respect to the concentration of the disinfectant C, and first order with respect to the sum concentration of disinfectant consuming substances S.

$$-\frac{dC}{dt} = kSC \tag{12.15}$$

Here k is the first order rate constant for decay of the disinfectant, $lg^{-1}h^{-1}$; S is the sum concentration of the disinfectant consuming substances expressed in *g* disinfectant-equivalent/liter.

In order to predict the changes in the concentration of the disinfectant C, implicit information is required about the initial concentration of the disinfectant consuming substances, S. In the chlorination process, S represents the sum of all chlorine consuming compounds in the water, measured in terms of consumed chlorine per unit volume, that is, a parameter comparable to the chlorine demand. The advantage of this transformation lies in the assumption that the change in the concentration of the compounds may be expressed as a change in the concentration of the disinfectant, thus one may express.

$$-\frac{dS}{dt} = -\frac{dC}{dt} \tag{12.16}$$

or

$$S = C - (C_o - S_o) \tag{12.17}$$

By substitution :

$$\frac{dC}{dt} - K\,(C_o - S_o)\,C = -\,kC^{-2} \tag{12.18}$$

This Bernoulli's equation, in situations where C_0 differes from S_0 has the solution :

$$C = \frac{C_o - S_o}{1 - \dfrac{S_o}{C_o}\, e^{-k(C_o - S_o)\,t}} \tag{12.19}$$

12.3.2 Disinfection Kinetics

With C given as a function of t in equation 12.19, equation 12.14 may be solved by substitution of C :

$$\frac{dN}{N} = \left\{ \mu - \frac{\lambda\,(C_o - S_o)}{1 - \dfrac{S_o}{C_o}\, e^{-k(C_o - S_o)\,t}} \right\} dt \tag{12.20}$$

This equation has the solution :

$$N = N_o \left\{ \frac{C_o - S_o}{C_o - S_o\, e^{-k\,(C_o - S_o)\,t}} \right\}^{\frac{\lambda}{k}} e^{[\mu - \lambda\,(C_o - S_o)]t} \tag{12.21}$$

It must be noted that equation (12.19) and (12.21) are not applicable under conditions where C_0 is equal to S_0 that is, where the initial chlorine concentration is equal to the demand. In such cases the differential equation (12.18) is reduced and resolved as follows:

$$-\frac{dC}{dt} = kC^{-2} \tag{12.22}$$

$$C = \frac{C_o}{1 + k\,C_o^t} \tag{12.23}$$

$$\frac{dN}{N} = \left\{ \mu - \frac{\lambda\, C_o}{1 + k\, C_o^t} \right\} dt \tag{12.24}$$

or

$$N = N_o \left(1 + k\, C_o^t\right)^{\frac{\lambda}{k} e^{\mu t}} \qquad (12.25)$$

Contrary to most established kinetic models of growth with inactivation, equations 12.12 and 12.25 are able to simulate the menancing water supply phenomena, of upstream disinfection, decay of chlorine, and downstream regrowth, once the concentration of chlorine is below a certain level.

Control of Microbe by Antimicrobial Drug/Agent:

More recently an avenue to control bacteria through drug - bacteria interaction (DBI) has been presented as scope to process biotechnology.

12.4 REFERENCES

1. R. Cruickshank, *Medical Microobiology*, pp 891, 7th edn. ELBS, 1968.
2. A. J. Salle, *Fundamental Principles of Bacteriology*, 5th edn, McGraw Hill Book Co. Inc., New York and Kogakusha Co. Ltd., Tokyo, 1961.
3. H. Chick, *Investigation on the Laws of Disinfection*, Vol 8, (J. Hygiene), pp 92, 1908.
4. G. Tchobangolous, *Wasterwater Engineering: Treatment, Disposal and Reuse*, 2nd edn., TMH Pub. Co. Ltd., New Delhi, 1972.
5. J.T. O'Connor and S.K. Banerji, "Biologically Mediated Corrosion and Water Quality Deterioration in Distribution Systems", Cincinnatic OH: US EPA, 1984.
6. K. V. Ellis, "Water Disinfection: A Review with Some Consideration of the Requirements of the Third World", Critical Reviews—Environmental Control, 20 (5), pp 341-407, 1991.
7. E. Dahi and J. Thorgensen, *World J. of Microbiology and Biotechnol*ogy, pp 12, 543-547, 1996.
8. J. Thorgensen and E. Dahi, *Ibid*, pp 12, 549-556, 1996.
9. T.C. Hazen and G.A. Toranzos, "Tropical Source Water", *Drinking Water Microbiology*, pp 52-53, (G.A. Mc Feters ed.), Springer-Verlag, New York, 1990.
10. S. Sharma, P. Sen, S.N. Mukhopadhyay and S.K. Guha, colloids and Surfaces B: Biointerfaces (Elsevier Sci), 32, 43-50, 2005.
11. Shivani Sharma, Ph.D. Thesis, I.I.T. Delhi, 2004.

Chapter

13

CELLULOSE PROCESSING RELEVANCE TO PROCESS BIOTECHNOLOGY

13.1 INTRODUCTION

Progress in science and technology of cellulose processing in relevance to process biotechnology has been described in many reviews.[1-6] It is well known that cellulose, the major structural polysaccharides of plants cells (eukaryotic), has high tensile strength. Also, it is recalcitrant to degradation, properties useful to plant cells but not necessarily so to the process biotechnologist for its bioprocessing. The interparticipation between cellulosics, *Trichoderma* sp. and its enzmes (extracellular) cellulases may be depicted as in Fig. 13.1. In this participation cellulosic resource can be of eukaryotic (plant) or prokaryotic (bacterial) origin. The comparative facts of naturally acquired design engineering (NADE) of cellulose biosynthesis in eukaryotic and prokaryotic cells as given[7-9] in Table 13.1 have led to reveal certain chemical and biological complexities of cellulosics as given in Table 13.2.

13.2 CELLULASES : THE COMPLEX RESOURCE CONVERSION AGENT

Awareness of these complexities are associated with many queries, presumptions and some evidence/supports. These are listed in Table 13.3. It is evident that enzymes are essential in cellulose biosynthesis. Few enzymes involved in cellulose biosynthesis and degradation/ conversion are given[7] in Table 13.4. It necessitated to look at the reported cell pathway of the enzyme system action on cellulosics (Figs. 13.2 and 13.3) and regulatory steps involved in cellulase

Cellulosics —→ Contributing significantly to S andT projects of supranation. Its processing/bioprocessing gives important products and by products. Some of which have hightech applications.

Trichoderma —→ Extensively used strain in large scale production of cellulases. Oxygen response/participation in growth is important.

Cellulases —→ Multiple biocatalytic forms and agents of conversion of cellulosics.

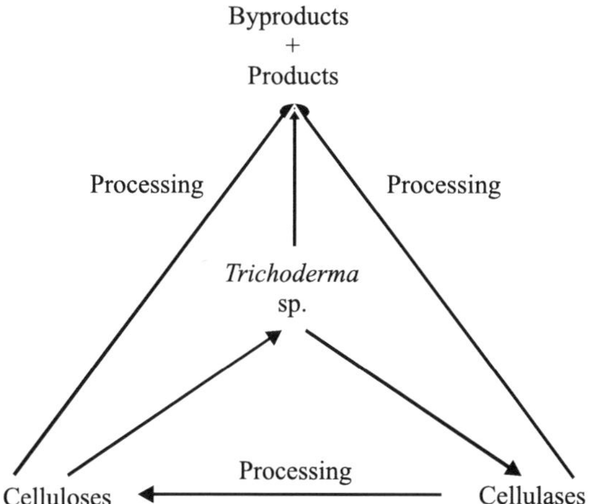

Fig. 13.1 Interparticipation between cellulosic material, *Trichoderma* sp. and cellulases

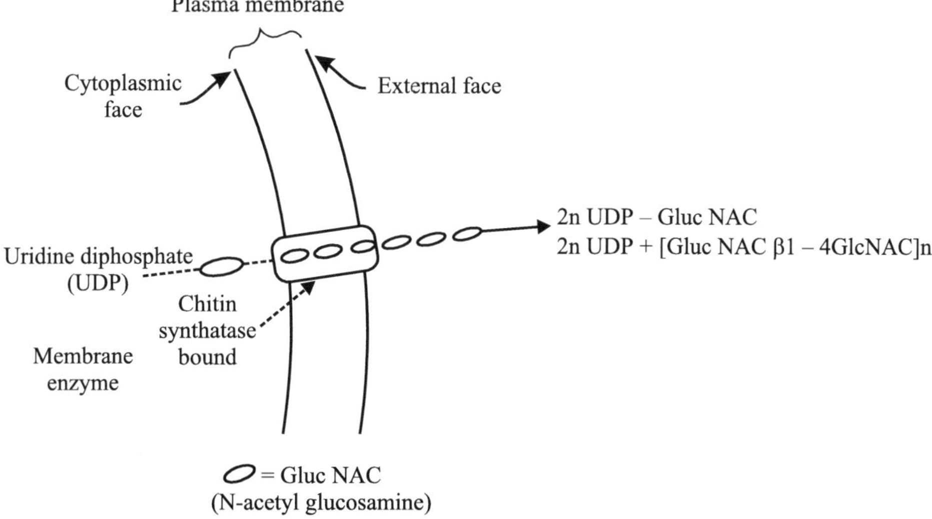

Fig. 13.2 Scheme of vectoral synthesis of chitin through plasma membrane

production (Fig. 13.4). Natural cellulose composition (Table 13.5) shows its complex nature. Besides cellulosics and its related component (hemicellulose), natural cellulose also contains lignin in appreciable quantity. The composition of rice straw, a typical example of a natural

Table 13.1 Comparative facts of cellulose biosynthesis

Facts	*Biosynthetic Sources*	
	Eukaryotic	*Prokaryotic*
• Structural	Basic foundation of the cell wall of almost all plants	Not elucidated clearly
• Synthesis	Synthesized as a primary structural material	Synthesized as a secondary metabolite
• Genetics and • Biochemistry	Complex	Simpler
• Production	Abundant production in nature through photobioreactor investigation	cell cultivation Production in industrial scale-under
• Type of catalytic production	Auto catalytic	Inductive
• Catalysis nature	Hypercyclic	Self replication
• Cellulose nature	Fibrous	Fibriller-called cellulon
• Compositional	Contains lignin, so called ligno-cellulose	Does not contain lignin, so powder cellulose.

Table 13.2 Chemical and biological complexities of celluloses

Chemical	*Biological*
• Linear crystalline polyglycan	Exist in microfibriller forms in cell walls of plants and fungi
• $\beta(1 \rightarrow 4)$) linked polymer of glucose present in composite unit	Microfibril synthesis is under direct cellular control
• Need appropriate organizational judgement for *in vitro* synthesis	Synthesis of cell wall cementing organic material lignin.
	Microfibril generation is enzymic or nonenzymic remains as a topic of further reaserch

cellulose indicate, the same. Lignin, being a complex cell binding molecule in natural cellulose, poses difficulty/resistance in cleavage of cellulose by the cellulase enzyme system action and also to use natural cellulose in cellulase production. For enhancing enzymic cleavage action on cellulosics its pretreatment by various methods has been carried out by many investigators.[9-11] Solvent pretreatment, alkali autohydrolytic pretreatments, steam explosion strategy etc are to produce more pure cellulose material. A typical compositional change by pretreatment of raw rice straw and its yield is shown in Table 13.5. However, cellulase production system is associated with many difficulties as listed in Table 13.6. As these difficulties are concerned with the regulatory steps in cellulase production, it implies that control parameters like pH and temperature need proper profiling strategy. For this strategy progress in bioprocessing through the use of pH cycling and temperature profiling alongwith biological technique of cell redesigning using molecular blending by fussion for biological scale up have been discussed earlier. In this progress of cellulase production process biotechnology two major facts played crucial role. They are (i) enzyme forming system is involved in cellulase biosynthesis and (ii) its production is growth associated but dependent on the bioprocessing strategy. Cellulase producer being an integral part of process biotechnology of cellulose conversions the elemental composition analysis of *Trichoderma reesei* QM9414 was determined with a view to assess its empirical molecular formula as it relates to its chemical quotient (CQ) and respiration quotient (RQ). The chemical analysis of *T. reesei* as given in Table 13.7 provided major elemental components of the cell. Presence of other trace elements and metals was also required to make it more close to one hundred percent. On the basis of results on metabolic physiology of growth of a cellulase deficient *T. reesei* QM 1238 strain in a cultivation medium it was possible to distinguish between CQ of the cellular oxidation reaction and respiration quotient, RQ of the cells.

Table 13.3 Queries, presumptions and evidence on cellulose synthesis

Queries	*Presumptions*	*Evidence*
• How amorphous & crystalline cellulose is synthesized ?	Polymerization and the crystallization or Simultaneous polymerization and crystallization.	Microfibrial synthesis is under direct cellular control.
• What is the *in vivo* site for cellulase synthesis ?	*In vivo* plasma membrane is the site for cellulose synthesis.	Organizational progress. synthesis and degradation of chitin.
• Is there any possibility that other membrane can be induced in cellulose synthesis *in vivo*?	Yes, provided they possess the necessary enzymes/biocatalysts.	In NADE process several enzymes are involved
• What is the precursor of cellulose ?	Nucleotide sugars.	UDP-NAc-Gluc is the donor

Table 13.4 Few enzymes involved in cellulose synthesis and degradation

Synthesis	*Degradation*
• Glucokinase	Exo β1, 4 glucanase
• Phosphoglucomutase	Endo β1, 4 glucanase
• UDP-Glucose-pyrophosphorylase	Exo β1, 4 cellobiohydrolase
• Cellulose synthases	Cellobiase or β glucosidase
• Microfibrillase	Collectively these enzymes are called cellulases/cellulosome

13.3 RQ AND CQ IN *T. reesei*

From the proximate and ultimate analysis of *T. reesei* mycelium the ash-free empirical formula of the cell has been expressed[7] as $C_{86} H_{160} O_{45} N_7$. Cell cultivation medium of *T. reesei* contained cellulose and peptone. The RQ pattern in aerobic cultivation of this organism is shown in Fig. 6.24 measuring RQ as below.

$$RQ = \frac{Q_{CO_2}}{Q_{O_2}} = \frac{\text{Specific rate of } CO_2 \text{ produced}}{\text{Specific rate of } O_2 \text{ consumed}} \tag{13.1}$$

In the process of cell mass formation/participation, however, biooxidation in *T. reesei* could be considered as given below.

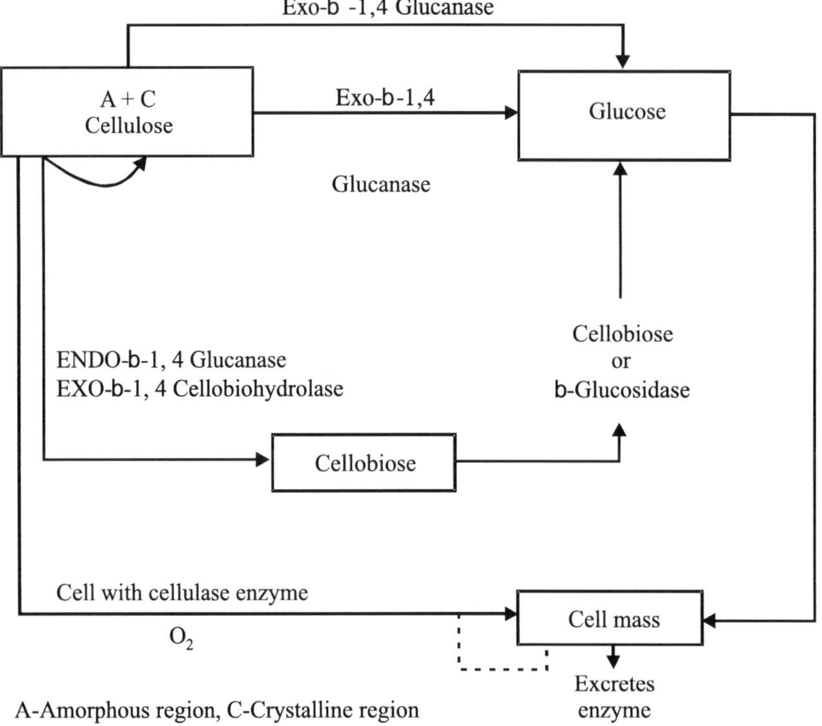

Fig. 13.5 Composition and yield of rice straw before and after treatment

	Raw Rice Straw	*Autohydrolyzed rice straw*	*Solvent degnified rice straw*
Cellulose	35-40%	56%	76%
Hemicellulose/xylan	15-30%	13%	8%
Araban	1.68		
Lignin (Klason)	15%	15%	6%
Ash & others	15%	15.5%	10%
$\text{Yield} = \frac{\text{Wt. of treated straw}}{\text{Wt. of origin straw}}$	1.0	0.70	0.50

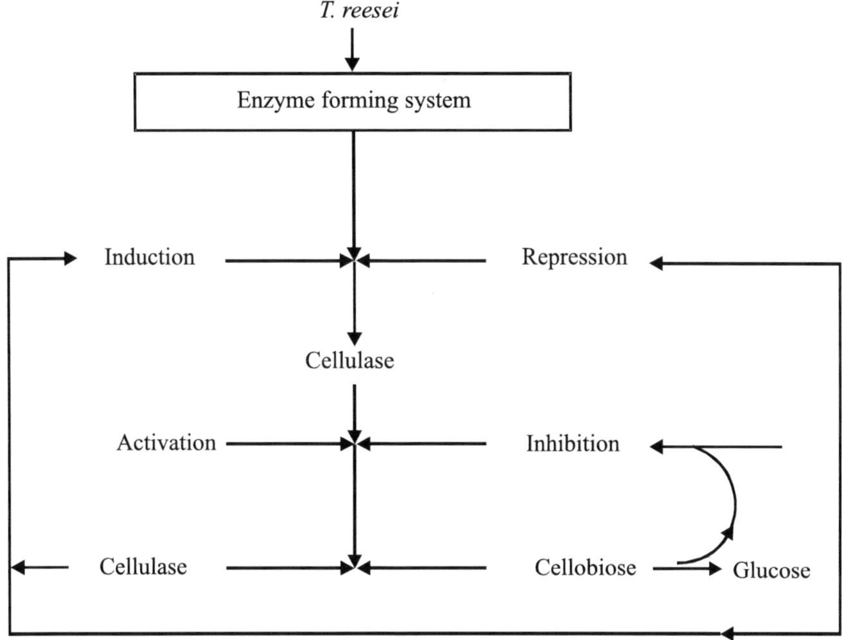

Fig. 13.3 Cell pathway of cellulase action on cellulose

Table 13.6 Difficulties in cellulase production system

- Single organism does not produce all components of cellulases in appropriate pro-proteins.
- Biological scale up of strains by biomoleculer design engineering/protoplast/cell fusion techniques are not well proven.
- Need standardization of bioprocess engineering strategy for enhancement of enzyme productivity.
- Substrate cellulose need be purified in order to enhance substrate uptake by the cellulase producing microorganism.

Table 13.7 Elemental analysis of *T. reesei*

Element	%
Carbon	44.0
Hydrogen	7.2
Oxygen	36.0
Nitrogen	9.5

$$\textit{T. reesei}\text{ cells} \xrightarrow[\text{C-source}]{O_2} \begin{matrix} \nearrow RQ \searrow \\ \searrow CQ \nearrow \end{matrix} CO_2 + H_2O + NH_3 \qquad (13.2)$$

Assuming (endogenous respiration, CQ)

$$C_{nc}\, H_{nH}\, O_{no}\, N_{mn} + a\, O_2 \rightarrow n\, CO_2 + \frac{n_H}{2} + H_2O + \frac{n_H}{3}\, NH_3 \qquad (13.3)$$

gives,
$$CQ = \frac{4n_c}{4n_c + n_H + 2n_o - 3n_N} \tag{13.4}$$

So in cellulose degradative uptake in cell growth/cell fabric the situation in growth phases of the organism may be considered as in Table 13.8. Also, it may entail three possible situations (Table 13.9). In cellulase production enhancement these are important aspects to be considered.

Table 13.8 Situation with C-source and growth conditions of *T. reesei* cultivation

Cultivation Phase	*Status of*		
	Available C-Source	*Cell Mass*	*Carbon Quotient*
Initial growth	Remains in excess	Remains low	Hyper
Nearing growth completion	Relatively limited	Relatively high	Hypo

Table 13.9 Possible CQ situation in *T. reesei*

Situation of CQ	*Possibility*	*Remark (s)*
• > that of cell mass	Overall transformation in C-source → fabric of cells in reduction of catabolism. Excess O_2 is eliminated as CO_2.	C-course having hyper quotient
• = that of cells mass	(a) No reproduction of non cellular organic material. (b) No fixation of organics having hypo-quotient	Cells having hyper quotient only having produced cell
• < that of cell mass	Overall transformation in C-source → fabric of cells is (synthesis or anabolism) oxidation • Oxidative fixation of O_2, no production of non-cellular material having hypoquotient • No fixation of organics having hyper quotient	C-source having hypoquotient (1) Production of growth in cell mass (2) Other carbonaceous products (s) arises.

13.4 APPROACHES OF CELLULOSIC BIOPROCESSING AND CO-PRODUCT UTILITY

When cellulosics are abundantly available and other fermentable sugar containing resources are scanty cellulose cleavage bioprocessing leading to fermentable sugar or hydrolyzate production has been thought to be an alternate route of renewable resource availability through resource engineering approach. Thus cellulose saccharification and utilization gained importance. Also cellulosic cleavage gives fragments of cellulose which have potentials for high tech applications. One of the major approaches of cellulose bioprocessing has been for ethanol production (Fig. 13.5) using various types of cellulosic residues. The reason why this, alternative ethanol production from renewable residual biomass has been given so much importance relates to potential of ethanol in production of various ranges of chemical feed stocks as given in Fig. 13.6. An integrated process biotechnology of lignocellulose bioconversion has been developed.[1,6] Besides ethanol production by this technology it generates, as stated, many coproducts. Utility and value addition scopes of these coproducts are very wide (Fig. 13.7). One of the major high value coproduct is lignin. Industrial value addition scopes with lignin conversion is also very large (Fig. 13.8). After bioconversion of pretreated lignocellulose the residual cellulose, i.e. hemicellulose has been observed to be a very useful coproduct. The property based high tech application of the hemicellulose as given in Table 13.10 indicates its potential.

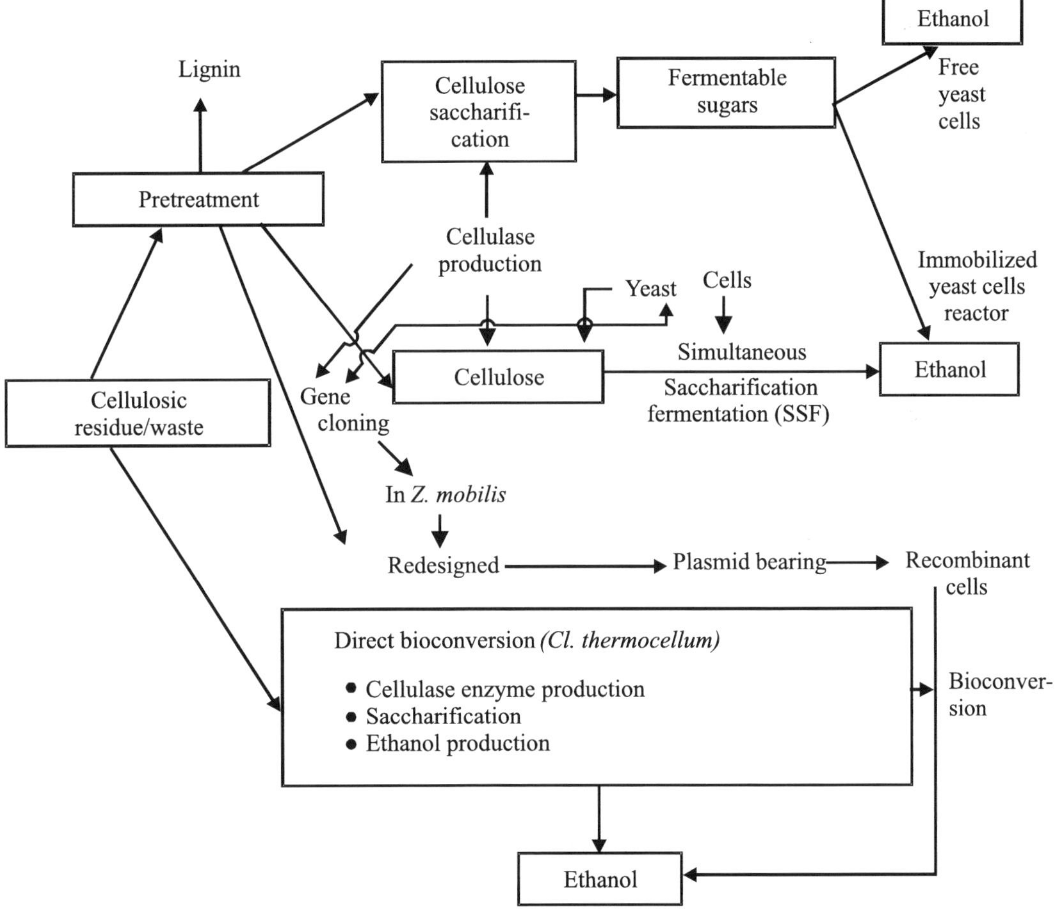

Fig. 13.5 Approach of bioprocessing for ethanol production

Also as shown in Table 13.7 cellulases is an important coproduct of the integrated process biotechnology. The presence of different components in this cellulases as shown in Fig. 13.9 shows that it also has an industrial value addition scope. Although cellulase from various sources have wide application scopes, more rigorous research is in progress towards characterization of cellulolytic complex (cellulosome) produced by prokaryotic cellulases as well as for innovation of further application of the enzyme complex.[14, 15]

13.5 FURTHER SCOPE WITH LIGNOCELLULOSE PROCESSING RESEARCH

From renewable resource engineering point of view lignocellulose is an eukaryotic material of all epochs on the earth. In the deep rain forests many trees may live for thousands of years. However, no individual animal or human is known to live several hundreds of years. It appears, therefore, structurally lignocellulose material, like woodlog may be possessed with physiologically hypercyclic rigid structures in terms of their growth which develops in many cases resin pockets in the log (Fig. 13.10) sections of radiata. These radiata provide an indication of the age of the wood. For providing rigid recalcitrant structure of lignocellulosic woods

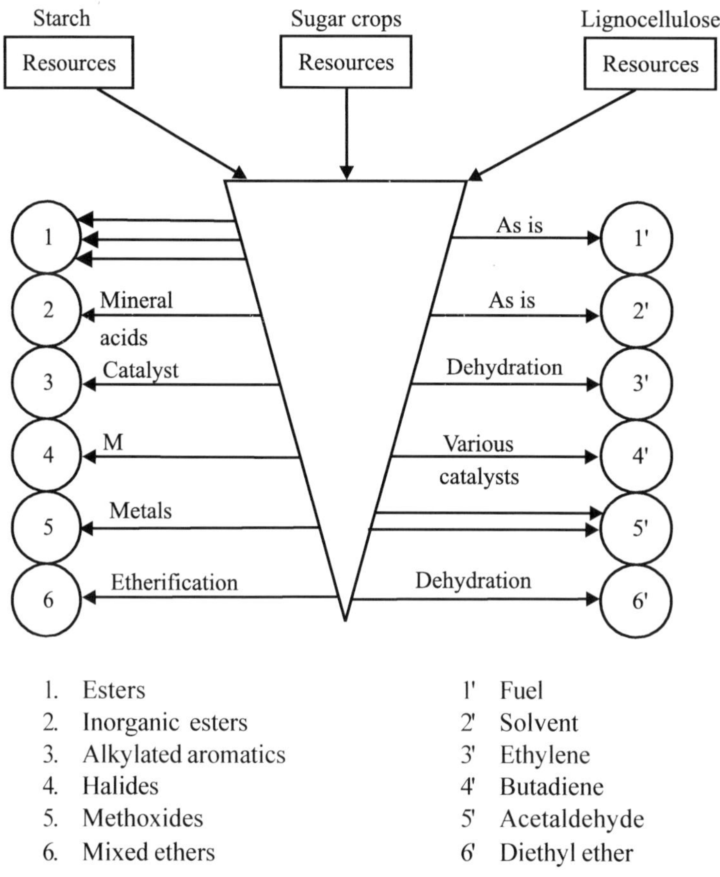

1. Esters
2. Inorganic esters
3. Alkylated aromatics
4. Halides
5. Methoxides
6. Mixed ethers

1' Fuel
2' Solvent
3' Ethylene
4' Butadiene
5' Acetaldehyde
6' Diethyl ether

Fig. 13.6 Potential of ethanol in production of chemical feed stocks

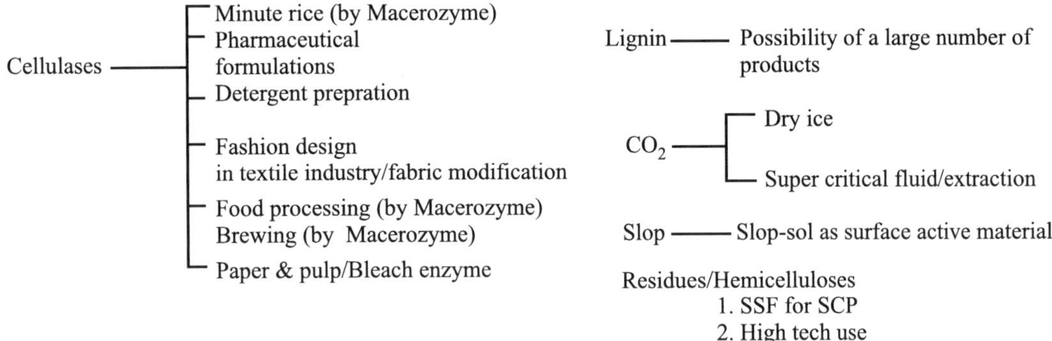

Fig. 13.7 Utility and value addition scopes of coproducts

biological time scales of various magnitude have been proposed considering evolutionary developments (Table 13.11). These biological scales have been involved depending on the system's interaction with cytoskeleton. In lignocellulose since microfibrils is known to be synthesized with a random parallel or crossed parallel orientation with respect to a neighbours participation of these biological time scales is difficult to study by following degradation/cleavage

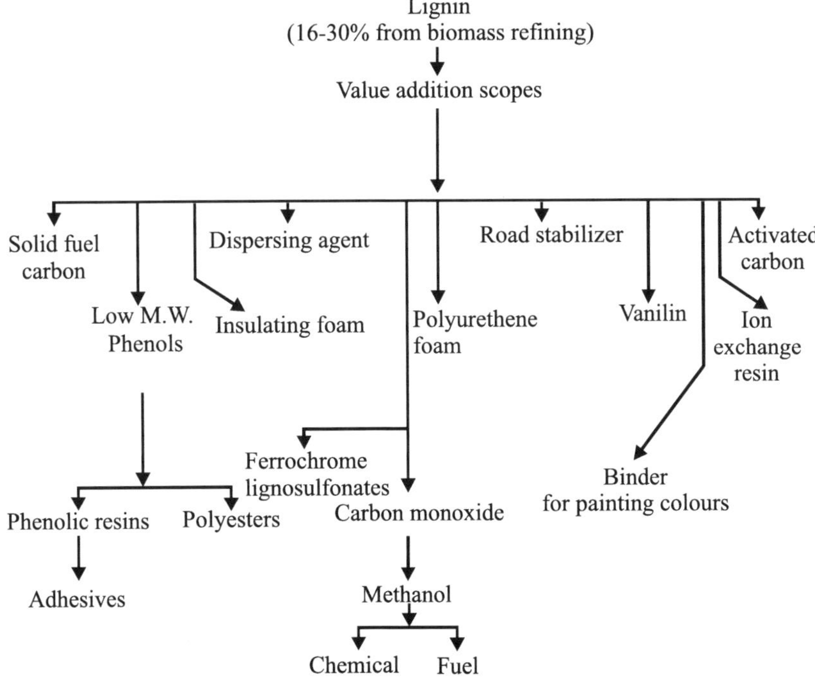

Fig. 13.8 Industrial value addition scopes with lignin conversions (Indian producers: 1. Kalpana chemical, Hyderabad, 2. Hindustan Mcgeobar, Baroda)

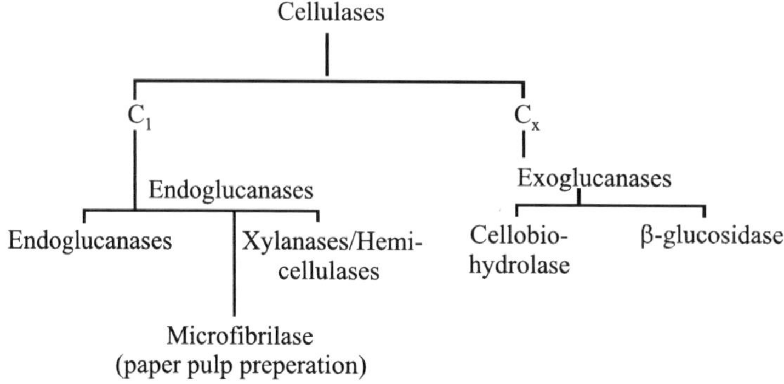

Use of Hemicellulases/Xylanases : (1) In preparation of enzyme bleach for paper and pulp industry
(2) In deinking newspapers for recycling
(3) Component in "Enzone" process technology[13]

Fig. 13.9 Industrial value addition scope of cellulase components

Table 13.10 Property based hightech application of hemicelluloses

Hemicellulose Property	*Product*	*Product/Property*	*Innovative Use*
Under controlled conditions hemicellulose can be convalently linked	Clear cold setting-gels	1. Thermostable, can be heated & sterilized	1. Useful as agent to keep wounds moist, protecting them from infection and speeding up the natural healing processes.
		2. Nontoxic & compatible with animal tissues	2. Useful as a slow release drug delivery system administering a measured dose of antibiotics slowly & steadily to the required site of the body.
		3. Hygroscopic	3. Useful as injectable into the abdomen of diabatic patients to release
		4. Can carry live cells such as Islets of langerhans	precise dose of insulin-over long periods.

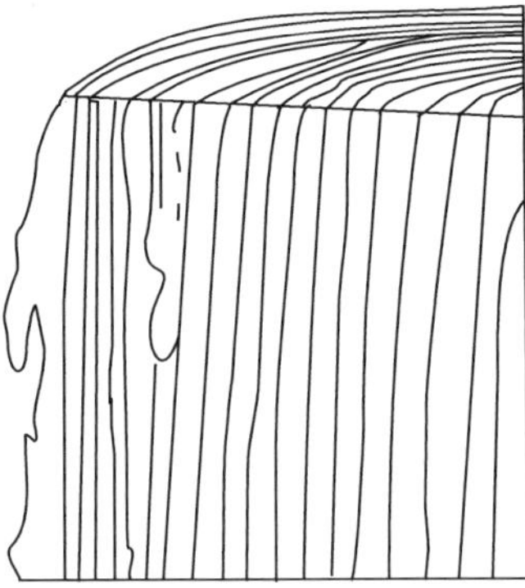

Fig. 13.10 Biomass log section of radiata showing a resin pocket

Table 13.11 Biological time scales of wood log

• The biochemical scale (fraction of a second or less)
• The metabolic scale (in the order of a minute)
• The epigenic time scale (several hours)
• The development scale (days or years)
• The evolutionary scale (thousands to millions of years)

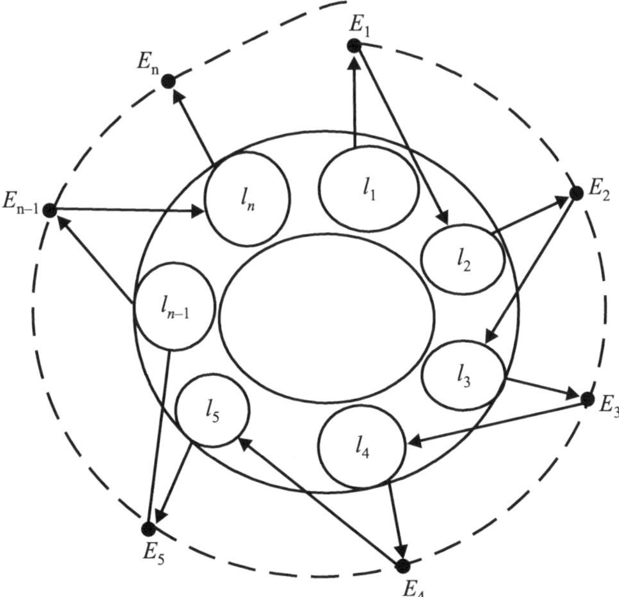

Circles (small — nucleotide quasispecies consisting of two complementary strands interacting as cross catalytic growing kinetics. li-Base pair code for an enzyme E_i, i = 1, 2, 3, . . . n

Fig. 13.11 Conceptual visualization of intracore hypercyclic quasispecies complementary constraint of lignocellulose

of cellulose molecule. This problem becomes more pronounced by the fact that the total number of enzymes involved in the synthesis and degradation of lignocellulose is still unknown. As a result scientists had to depend on the enzymes involved in the terminal stages of cellulose fibril biogenesis which are cell associated. It is not completely understood how the individual glucan molecules polymerize and assemble into the microfibrilar bundles of cellulose. However, the uniformity of micro-fibril size and their orientation in cellular organism at any particular moment in cell development indicate that nucleotidal microfibril synthesis is under cellular control. These features demand to unfold as future scope to explain mechanistically how cellulose microfibrils are formed though simultaneous polymerization and crystallization over-coming hypercyclic quasi species complementation constraints. Its conceptual visualization relates to Fig. 13.11.

13.6 COCKTAIL ENZYME USE IN POLYSACCHARIDE SYSTEMS

Cocktail cellulases in lignocellulose conversion biotechnology are becoming more and more important in recent years. A consortium of enzymes (e.g. endoglucanase, exoglucanase and β-glucosidase (cellobiase)-collectively called cellulases) are needed in cellulose degradation into its constituent glucose monomers.[16-21] According to Proctor and Gamble guar gum—a polysaccharide in the mannase family that is found in many household products—is particularly culpable in stain problems on clothes. Guar gum containing stains that appear to have been washed out are actually still in hiding in the garment, the company says, waiting to stick to dirt that arises during wear or in the wash water and causing the stain to "reappear". Mannase enzymes were developed specifically to address this problem and their introduction in P&G products list helped fuel a 10% rise in third quarter detergent enzyme/cells compared to 1999.

Novozymes predict that mannases may one day be as important to P&G as amylases, cellulases and lipases—all basic cleaning enzymes (including proteases). Total cleanings require "cocktail" of other enzymes as well[22] (Febreze/Cleerbleach).

13.7 REFERENCES

1. Mukhopadhyay, S.N., "Progress in Science and Technology of Cellulose Processing", *Relevance to Process Biotechnology,* Oxford IBH Pub. Co. Pvt. Ltd. (M.J. Mulkey and A. Pandey eds.), *Proc. HLRF-RRL (T) Jt.* Sympo., pp 80-89, 1994.
2. Connon, R. E. and S.M. Anderson, *Critical Reviews in Micobiol.,* 17 (6), pp 435-47, 1991
3. Robinson, D.G. and H. Qnader, *J. Theor. Biol.,* pp 92, 483-95, 1981.
4. Ghose, T.K., "Cellulose Conversion", *Adv. in Food Producing System for Arid and Semi Arid Lands,* pp 225-66, Acad. Press, Inc. 1981.
5. Humphery, A.E., "The Hydrolysis of Cellulosic Material to Useful Products", *Adv. Chem. Series 181,* pp 25-53, Am. Chem. Soc. Washingtion D.C., 1979.
6. Ghose, T.K. "Chemical and Biochemical Reactions: Balance of Energy Inputs and Reaction Times", *CHENRAWN III,* Hauge, 1984.
7. Mukhopadhyay, S.N. and Ajay Shriwastava, *Proc, II ChE. Golden Jubilee Congress,* Vol. I, pp 209-21, (S. Nath ed.), Replica Press, Delhi, 1998.
8. Eveleigh, D.E. Phil. *Trans. Roy. Soc.,* London, A 321, pp 435-47, 1987.
9. Jonas, R and L.F. Farah, *Polymer Degradation and Stability*, pp 59, 101-106, 1998.
10. Cavaco-Paulo, A. and L. Almeida, *Biocatalysis,* pp 353-60, 1994

11. MooYoung, M., D.S. Chahal and D. Valch, *Proc. Bioconv. Sympo.* IIT Delhi, pp 457-465, (T.K. Ghose ed.), 1977.
12. Mandels, M. and J. Weber, *Adv. Chem. Series,* pp 95, 391, 1969.
13. Erikson, K.E. "Enzyme Process Technology", Lecture Delivered at D.B.E.B. IIT Delhi, September 30, 1997.
14. Gal, L. *et al. Appl. Environ. Microbiol.* 63 (3), pp 903-909, 1997.
15. Lamed, R. *et al. Biotechnol, Bioeng. Symp.,* pp 13, 163-81, 1983.
16. Lee, J. J. *Bacteriol*, pp 56, 1-24, 1977.
17. Wheals, A.E. *et al., TIBTECH*, 17 (12), pp 482-487, 1999.
18. Lynd, L.R., *Annu. Rev. Energy & Environ,* pp 21, 403-405, 1996.
19. Tengerdy, R.P., *J. Sci. Ind. Res.*, pp 55, 313-316, 1996.
20. Lee, D, A.H.C., Yu and J.N. Saddler, *Biotechnol & Bioeng.,* pp 55, 547-555, 1995
21. Ingram, L., *Biotechnol & Bioeng.,* pp 58, 204-214, 1998
22. McCoy, M., C & EN, pp 26-31, Jan 15, 2001.
23. C.Vila, G. Garrote, H. Dominguez and J.C. Paroji Hydrolytic Processing of Rice Husks in Aqucous Media: A Kinetic Assessment, Collect, Czech. Commun, 67, 509-530, 2002.

Chapter

14

BIOPROCESSING: USING CELLS UNDER STRESSES

14.1 INTRODUCTION

Tremendous interest has been generated on the stress proteins bioprocessing research and development in recent years because of their technological potential. Exposure of both prokaryotic and eukaryotic cells and/or tissues to a variety of physiological stresses results in the rapid synthesis of a specific class of proteins. This phenomenon is known as stress response, and the newly formed transient proteins have been termed as 'stress proteins' in general.[1-6] These proteins play a significant role in cells and tissues in manifestation of adaptation and may serve as defence mechanism of cells against a variety of stress conditions. However, they may or may not be transient. When these proteins are produced under heat shock (40-60°C) in cells, they are termed heat shock proteins (HSPs) but are inducible by many other stimuli other than heat. The cells that survive after the heat shock exhibit a greater degree of thermotolerance as compared to control cells. Thus, it has been hypothesized that these heat shock-induced proteins play a direct role on both cell stabilization, resistance to injury and disease, and in curative molecule design. Various types or classes of stress proteins of small and large sizes are *de novo* designed in prokaryotes as well as in eukaryotes during different stress conditions. So physiological (prokaryotic or eukaryotic) stress(es) has great biotechnological concern which may be depicted as in Fig. 14.1. There are examples that *de novo* designed small proteins also have some physiological functions.[8-10] In recent years major focus on the role of the stress proteins has been mostly in (a) cell biology in regulatory concerns of protein folding-unfolding and transport, (b) immunobiology on the involvement in the immune response during tissue or cell damage and infectious diseases and (c) pathophysiology and medicine on the effect of stress response in human disease.[1] Although, the mechanism of the stress response in human disease is unclear;

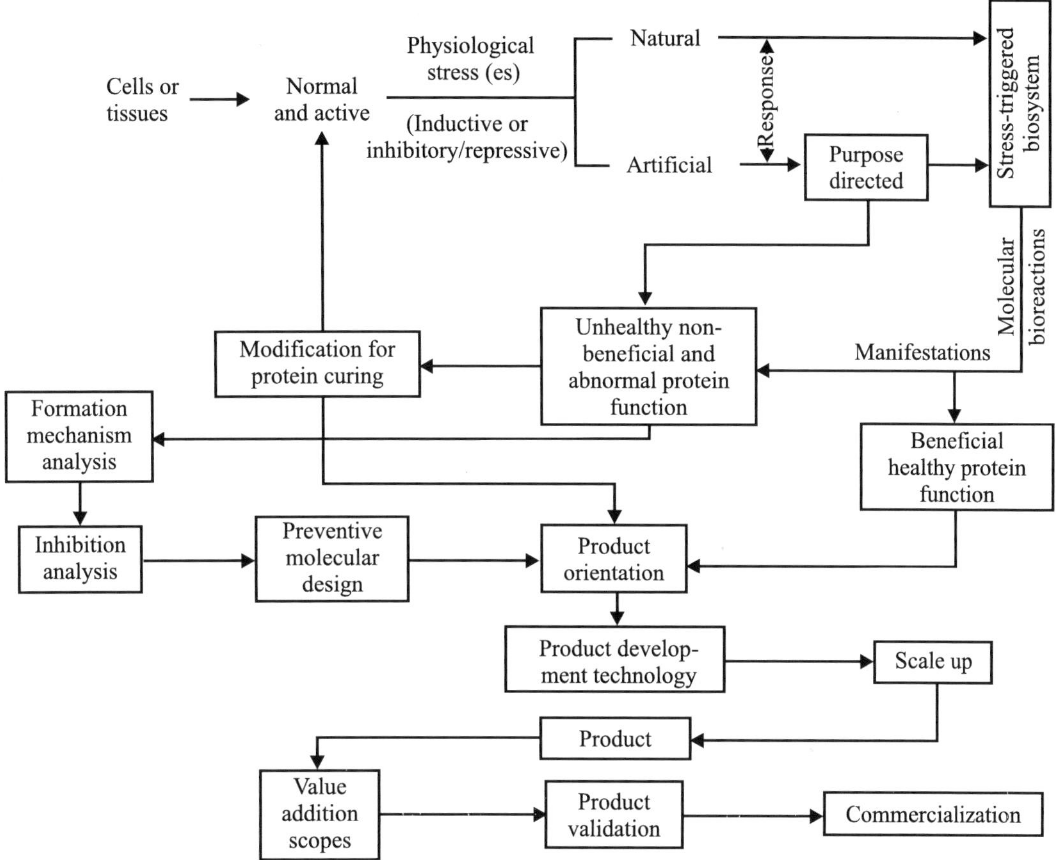

Fig. 14.1 Biotechnological concerns of physiological stressess

but in predictive and diagnostic biotechnology the stress proteins are expected to have high value. When organisms or cells in culture are exposed to adverse conditions that are outside their normal growth range, the response to that change is modulated by many environmental factors. These include parameters such as nutrients (including glucose), oxygen, temperature, and pH of the old and the new milieu, to name more important ones during culture processing. The intrinsic determinant which influences responses to temperature changes is mainly the thermal profile of the organism. Thus, existence of T_{opt}, T_{max}, T_{min} of cell functions is of great significance and relates to value addition scope to cell biotechnology. Value addition scope for commercialization of the biotechnology of the high value low volume stress proteins for different purposes needs, therefore, explorational search. Thus, it seems useful to collate information pertaining to biotechnological concerns of stress proteins.

14.2 STRESS PROTEIN SOURCES AND FAMILY TYPES

Both prokaryotic cells and eukaryotic cells and tissues have been the sources of abnormal stress proteins resulting from the triggering of the activation of stress genes like heat shock gene.[2-5]

These source characters may be shown as in Fig. 14.2. Among the stress proteins, a lot of research has been carried out on heat shock proteins. These investigations enabled classification of the stress proteins into six different classes at present (Fig. 14.3). The source, functional features, and general biotechnological importances of SPs are given in Table 14.1.

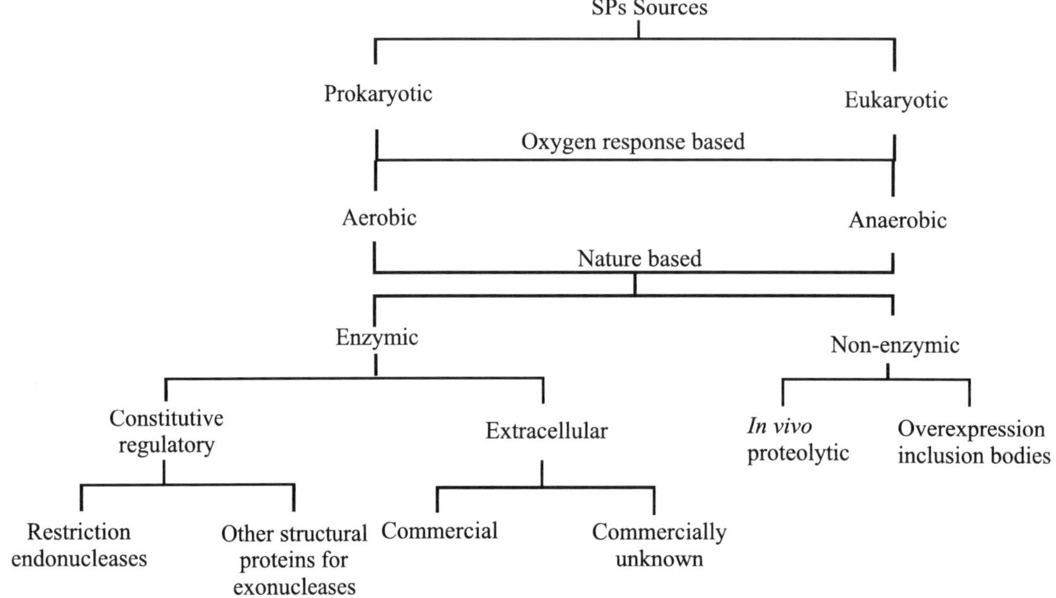

Fig. 14.2 Sources of different super family stress proteins (SPs)

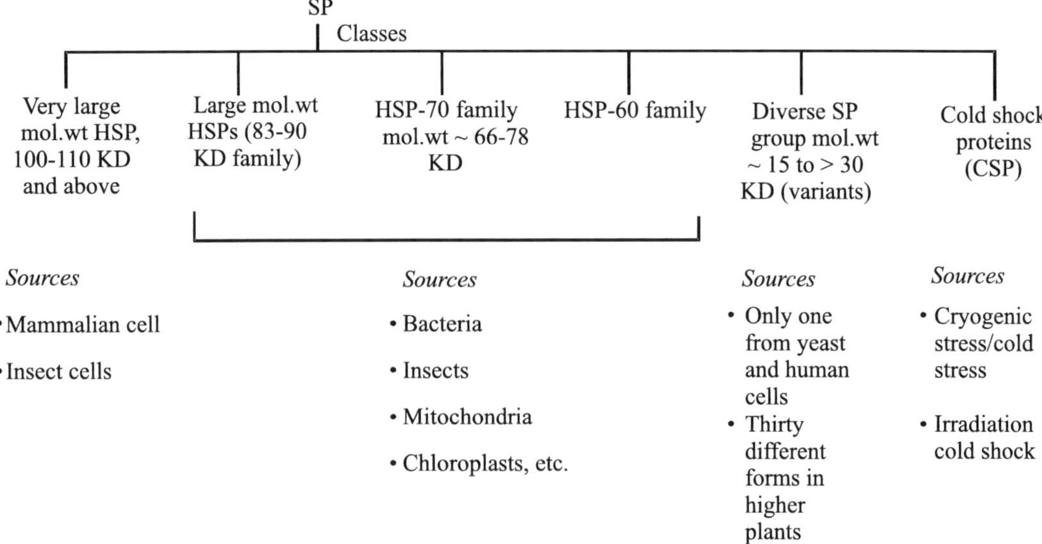

Fig. 14.3 Super family SP classes

Table 14.1 Few stress protein sources, functional features and biotechnological importances

Family/ Major Sources	*Source Designations in Eukaryotes*	*Prokaryotes*	*Remarkable Features*	*Ref.*	*Expected Biotechnological Importance*
HSP 110	Mammalian cells	None	Associated with RAN, Function unknown		
HSP 90, 83, 87	Mammalian cells	HtpG (C 62.5)	Bind to specific polypeptides, and either silence their function (e.g. glucocorticoid receptor), and/or escort them to their proper cellular compartment. Associated with steroid receptors, cellular and viral protein kinases, binds actin and tubulin.	1	Relates to search of enzymes involved in physiological malfunctioning processes like respiratory distress syndrome, rheumatoid arthritis, asthma, etc. for newer preventive drug or medicine design or to produce enzyme inhibitors as potential therapeutic or detector agents in diagnostic and other biotechnology for commercialization of the HSPs.
HSP 70 (Dnak)/ Drosophila (insect)	HSP 68, 72, 73; clathrin uncoating ATP ase; BiP; gap 75, 78, 80; hsc 70; KAR2; SSA 1, 2, 3, 4; SSB 1, 2; SSC 1; SSD 1	Dnak	Dissociate some protien aggregates; maintain some polypetides in unfolded state, thus facilitating their translocation across membranes, and/or accelerating proper folding and oligomerization; bind to specific polypeptides.	1	
HSP 60 (Gro EL)/ *E. coli*	HSP 58; RuBis Co. subunit binding protein; MIF-4	GroEL (MopB)	Maintain some polypeptides in unfolded state, thus facilitating their translocation across membranes, and/or accelerating proper	1	

Family/ Major Sources	*Source Designations in Eukaryotes*	*Prokaryotes*	*Remarkable Features*	*Ref.*	*Expected Biotechnological Importance*
			folding and assembly (by preventing most likely misfolding)		
DnaJ	SEC 63 (NPL) SIS 1	DnaJ	Binds to specific polypeptides, accelerates the release of some of the polypeptides bound to Dnak interacts with DnaK and GrpE.	1	
HSP 27	Mammalian	–	Structurally relates to a-crystaline, function increases.	10	
GrpE	Antigenically related protein is present	GrpE	Interacts with Dnak and DnaJ; accelerates the release of some of the polypeptides bound to Dnak	1	
Small HSPs	HSP 17.5, 22, 23, 26; GENE 3	HtrC	Eukaryotic function is largely unknown; homology to o-crystallin family; HtrC may be necessary for septum formation in prokaryotes.	1, 7	
Ubiquitin	UBI 1, 2, 3, 4	None	Conjugates to and 'tags' unfolded polypeptides destined to be destroyed.	1, 8, 10	

14.3 NOMENCLATURE OF STRESS PROTEINS

There is no universal system of physiologically stress-induced proteins nomenclature so far. However, heat shock-induced genes and proteins are classified with certain nomenclature style. These are identified by three small letters, hsp for the genes and HSP for the corresponding protein with numbers, indicating the relative molecular weights (Mr) of the proteins in kilodalton (KD) on the side. For instance, hsp 70 refers to a gene coding for an HSP of the 70 KD family, HSP 70. Also, the terms hsc/HSC have been used for constitutively expressed members of the eukaryotic HSP families; but their expression in prokaryotes may exist as well. For other stress genes and their corresponding stress proteins other than heat shock proteins, special terms have been used by Nover[7] and other authors[1] in recent books. A list of nomenclatures of a few stress genes and their stress proteins is given in Table 14.2.

Table 14.2 Few commercially important enzymic stress proteins

	Source/Organism	*Enzymes Intracellular*	*Enzymes Extracellular*	*Stress Inducer/ Stress Gene*	*Remark and Application/Potential*
A.	Prokaryotic				
(i)	*E. coli*	–	Protease	Ion gene	–
		MnSOD	–	Only in presence of oxygen	Slow induction
		Lys-tRNA synthatase	–	Lys U-gene	–
(ii)	*Bacillus subtilis*	–	Protease	Ion gene cross-active antibodies	Useful in preparation of protein hydrolysates
(iii)	*B. stearothermophilus* CU 21 (redesigned)	–	Amylases Proteases	Heat shock, hs (55°C)	Rate of induction unknown, used in detergent preparation and other purposes.
(iv)	*B. amyloliquefaciens*	*Bam* H1	–	Heat shock, hs, 37°C oxygen (?)	Rate of induction moderate, used extensively in rDNA technology
(v)	*Clostridium thermocellum* ATCC (anaerobic)	–	Cellulase (ECG)	Heat shock, hs, 50°C colC	Used in digestive tablets, detergents, and other preparations.
B.	Eukaryotic				
(i)	*Saccharomyces cerevisiae* (yeast)	Catalase	–	Heat shock, hs, 37°C	Increase inhibited by CH.
		Ribosomal	–	Glucose deprivation, hs, 37°C	
		Enolase/ Aldolase	–	Corresponds to HSP 48 group	Promoter reveals no heat shock element. Useful in stereoselective enzymic aldol condensation reaction in industry.
(ii)	*T. reesei*	–	Cellulase (CBH 1)	Avicel, sophorose, cbhj	Pharmaceutical and detergent industry.
(iii)	*Neurospora crassa*	Peroxidase	–	hs, 48°C	Confers resistance to 2 mM H_2O_2

14.4 PHYSIOLOGICAL STRESS INDUCERS AND CROSS INTERACTIVE STRESSES

14.4.1 Inducing Agents

In biocells or tissue organs the stress-inducing agents responsible for induction of stress response and abnormal protein formation may be classified[1,6-8] as shown in Fig. 14.4. Chemicals and biochemicals are by far the largest stress conditioning agents, although heat shock is the commonly used one. Microflora indigenous to abyssal depths of the deep oceans are believed to be stress induced by barophilicity and psychrophilicity. So they are uniquely adapted for optimal growth at cold temperatures (<40°C) but at elevated hydrostatic pressures (400-600 atm) by their environment. These microflora may, therefore, be considered unique in stress protein synthesis under baroduric conditions.[9] It is, thus, possible to conceive at *in vivo* stress agents interact and modulate or synergistically effect across functional stress conditioning in *de novo* protein design. Classical examples of synergistic effects of inducers for the induction of hsp mRNAs in Xenopus kidney epithelial cells and in some other systems are reported in a more recent book.[7]

Thermal stress is well known to be an important physical inducer in HSP formation in both prokaryotes and eukaryotes. In biotechnology for biological scale up of cellular capacity in enhancement of commercial proteinous product formation, like enzymes irradiation stressing of cells, has been well practiced for many decades. Irradiation, therefore, is also a well-known, important nonthermal physical 'cold shock' stress protein inducer. The irradiated biological test systems have utilized intact cells or tissue organs. Radiation stress-induced changes in proteins and their *in vivo* refolding or restructuring are concerned primarily with gross DNA/RNA strand breakage, synthesis of new DNA and RNA and re-establishment of perturbed three-dimensional structure of the DNA macromolecule in association with neighboring RNA, proteins, and lipopolysaccharides.[11-15] It has been noticed that the repaired proteinous macromolecule may not function in the same way as before the use of radiation-induced lesions, and misfolding may arise. It may result in formation of wanted and/or unwanted gene products like proteins in their mother or daughter cells. A list of few enzymes that have been produced using stress agents is given in Table 14.2. Several of them have been used commercially.

14.4.2 Concerns of Inducers

At molecular level stress inducers have been stated to cause unfolding and breakage of DNA in cells,[11] and *E. coli* strain was capable of refolding DNA strand breakage (dsb).[12,13] It has also been demonstrated that single strand break (ssb) repair in bacteria was dependent on different repair enzyme and wild strains of *S. typhimurium*, however, are not sensitive to O_2 and grow. It attributes oxygen sensitivity to damage of SOD by heat.

Antibiotics, like novobiocin and many others, at very low dilution may alter stress protein spectrum by acting as an inhibitor of DNA gyrase enzyme in bacteria exposed to irradiation. It appears, therefore, that heat, chemical, and biological agents may induce changes in stress proteins (SPs) by sensitivity response in cells. Irradiation also effects in the variety of conditions with and without oxygen and with and without irradiation dose modifying agents at different stages of the cell cycle.[16-19]

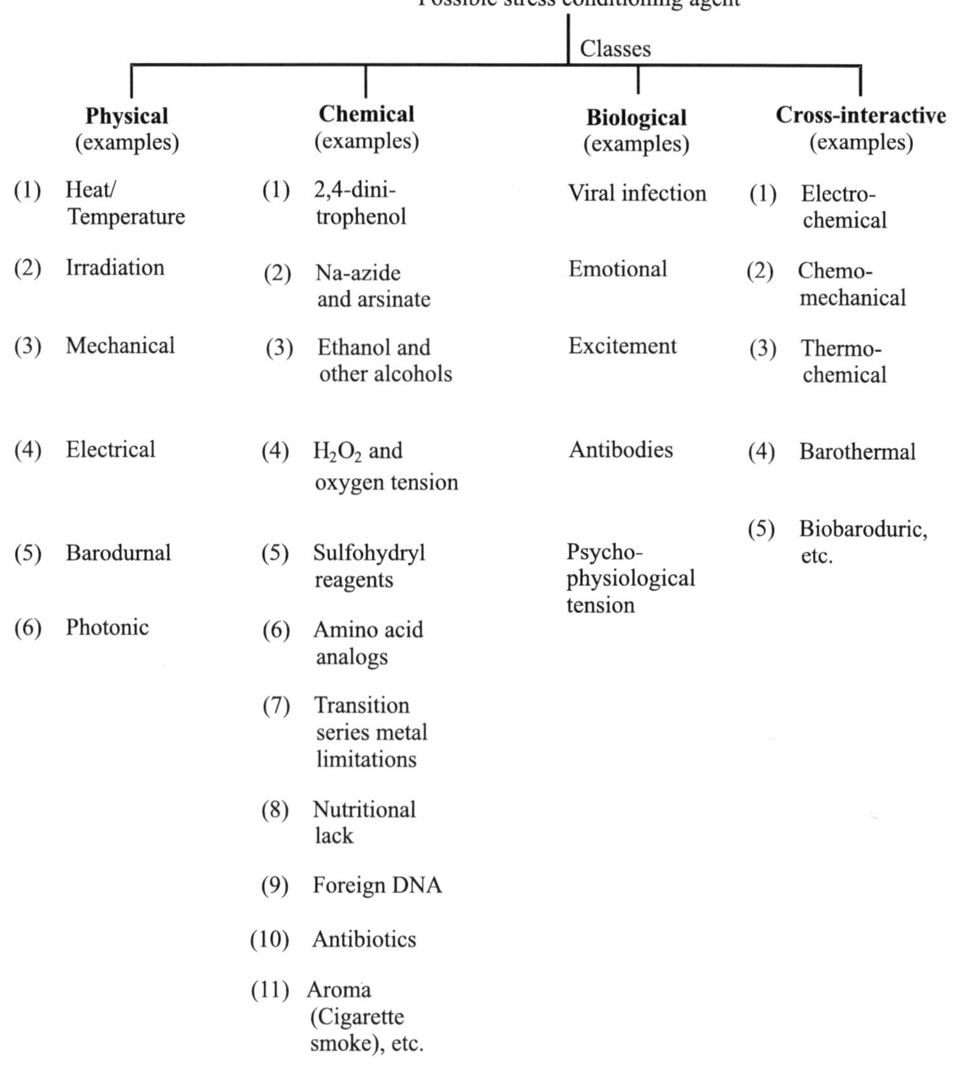

Fig. 14.4 Stress inducers classification

14.5 SPS FUNCTIONAL FEATURES

Different classes of SPs are shown in Fig. 14.4. Much is unknown about the HSPs in the range of 100-110 KD and above. Newer information is gradually accumulating in literatures about their roles in normal cellular processes. Critical insight on the functional features of this class during heat stress and thermotolerence are yet to appear. It is stated that 110 KD HSP is a constitutively expressed protein in eukaryote. Its synthesis increases about five folds after stress conditioning.[20] It is unclear about its involvement in resumption of normal nuclear transcription events during recovery from the heat insult. The synthesis of the protective heat shock proteins produced by eukaryotes in response to high temperature is regulated by the 110 KD heat shock transcription factor (HSTF). Footprinting study results have shown that this protein specially binds to a conserved partially palindromic segment (consensus sequence CNNGAANNTTCNNG) upstream of many known heat shock coding sequences HSTF like sp 1. Also, when bound to its target, sequence stimulates the transcription of the associated gene.[13-16] While protecting some regions of DNA from DNAse 1 digestion, HSTF also renders portions of its bound DNA hypersensitive to this enzyme. The grp 100 KD exhibits considerable sequence homology with HSP 90, a cytosolic protein.[20]

The HSP 90 group is one of the most abundant cytoplasmic proteins present in most types of cells even under nonheat shock conditions. This group may exist in two forms, e.g., HSP 90 α and HSP 90β.[120] The two forms differ slightly in molecular mass and have been identified in mammalian cells. They are encoded by distinct genes which are regulated differently during normal development. Also, they form transient associations with various regulatory and structural proteins including viral oncogene products having tyrosine kinase activity. This associative capacity of HSP 90 indicates them to be regulatory molecules. Their additional accumulation may inhibit inappropriate activation of regulatory cascades during metabolic perturbations caused by hyperthermic and other stresses.[20]

The class of HSP 70 proteins are reported to bind ATP and cause promoter activation. They may have origin from cytoplasm, mitochondria, and endoplasmic reticulum organelles. They are believed to participate in energy-dependent processes such as the disassembly of the clathrin coat of the vesicle, ATP reversible binding of various abnormal proteins, and translocation of proteins across membranes.[20] The HSP70 family of cytoplasmic origin appear to bind directly to nascent polypeptide chains associated with ribosomes during the process of elongation. It is speculated that HSP70 proteins can reversibly interact with internal regions of preexisting proteins that are exposed as the result of thermal denaturation during heat stress and facilitate correct refolding. They may also help reassembly of multiprotein structures damaged by heat. These proteins accumulate in the nucleus primarily in association with the regular region of nucleoli, the location of ribosome assembly. Ribosome assembly, on the other hand, is extremely sensitive to hyperthermia and preaccumulation of some HSP70 in mammalian cells. It is reported to accelerate recovery of nucleolar morphology following heat stress. It is now known that expression of the human HSP 70 gene in the cell cycle regulates and is inducible by both serum and adenovirus Ela protein.[21-22] This regulated expression is predominantly controlled by the CCAAT element at position- 70 relative to the transcriptional initiation site.[23] Its corresponding CCAAT binding factor (CBF) of 999 amino acids cloned recently has been stated to stimulate transcription selectively from the HSP70 promoter in a CCAAT element-dependent manner.[24-25] A more recent publication[24] reports that 192 residues of CBF, when fused to the DNA binding domain of heterogeneous activator GAL-4, are necessary and sufficient to mediate Ela-dependent transcriptional activation. It could show Ela and CBF to exhibit complex formation *in vitro*. It suggested that an *in vivo* interaction between these proteins may be relevant to the well-characterized Ela-induced transcriptional activation of the HSP70 promoter.

The major bacterial HSPs belong to HSP60 class. These are homologous to the *E. coli* groEL gene product. This class is also required in bacteriophage assembly and host DNA replication at normal temperatures. This may be associated transiently with newly synthesized unfolded polypeptides. This class of protein is encoded by a nuclear gene and has site in mitochondria. It is synthesized at elevated levels after shock. During protein import, cytoplasmically synthesized mitochondrial proteins are initially recognized by a mitochondrial form of HSP70 and then passed onto a HSP60 complex upon which final folding and assembly occurs.[20]

The diverse group of small stress proteins have a multiple size range (molecular weight 15 to > 30 KD).[1] In this group charge variants have been stated to exist in lower to higher organisms. In mammalian cells a single small HSP27 has been known to have multiple isoelectric forms. The small HSPs have been reported to associate with mRNA during stress in insect and plant cells. Rapid phosphorylation has been demonstrated in human HSP27 in response to heat shock treatment. It is likely that small HSPs plays a role in both growth signal transduction and thermotolerence. So far little is known about the nature and function of HSP27 as well as other small HSPs.

In many instances functional characteristics of HSPs of prokaryotes are shared by their counterparts in eukaryotes (Table 14.1).

14.6 MOLECULAR BIOLOGY OF CELL PROCESSING UNDER STRESS

14.6.1 Thermal Stress

1. Forewords

A large amount of studies have been carried out in which stress to cells was provided in the form of heat shock, i.e., exposing the cells to elevated temperatures (40-42°C, in some cases up to 60°C as well).[1-15] It is a known fact that prokaryotes possess only a single copy of a heat shock gene. This fact, coupled with the essential function of most heat shock genes, necessitates the constitutive expression under all conditions of most prokaryotes regulatory stress genes.[1] However, in general, eukaryotes possess at least two copies of heat shock genes. Of the two, one is under heat shock regulation and the other is under constitutive control.[1]

2. Stress gene inductive regulation and control mechanism

In prokaryotic cells the heat shock regulon is defined by the rpoH gene.[1] Its product is a 32 KD sigma factor (σ^{32}). For instance, it has been reported that the major heat shock genes of *E. coli* are under the control of the rpoH (htpR) gene which codes for σ^{32} heat shock factor. The σ^{32} factor directs core RNA polymerase enzyme ($E\sigma^{32}$) to recognize the promoters for heat shock genes. The studies on how the cell uses σ^{32} to regulate the heat shock response have provided a great deal of information about the molecular mechanisms involved in mounting a transient, global response to environmental stimuli. The evidence that in *E. coli* RNA polymerase containing σ^{32} ($E\sigma^{32}$) is responsible for nearly all the transcription of the heat shock genes has been shown.[26-32] It indicates that HSPs are required for cell growth at most temperatures. So, the HSPs are involved in thermotolerence and in turn regulation of the heat shock response for the transcription and transition of rpoH mRNA. It also integrates the stability of σ^{32} and is regulated to provide the amount of σ^{32} required for heat shock gene expression in stress protein synthesis. As shown in Table 14.1 the HSPs poses diverse functions at the molecular level ranging from the major

E. coli σ^{32} factor σ^{70} (the rpoD gene product) to a cryptic form of lysyl tRNA synthetase (the lys U gene product). It has been reported that abnormal protein synthesis under adverse conditions, like in sporulation in prokaryotic cells, is accompanied by the appearance of new RNA polymerase specificity factors that read the gene necessary for stress protein formation. It is also stated that the overall structure of RNA polymerase in *B. subtilis* is essentially identical to that in *E. coli* (α_2 β β σ). However, the precise molecular weights of the various subunits differ between gram positive and gram negative bacteria. Vegetatively growing *Bacillus subtilis* has been stated[33-40] to contain multiple σ factors, namely σ^{55}, Q s^{37}, σ^{32} and σ^{28} with molecular weights 55, 37, 32, and 28 KD, respectively. Each of them can bind interchangeably to the core RNA polymerase (σ_2 β β^{1}). This can confer upon it the ability to recognize a different set of promoter sequences. Factors σ^{27} and σ^{32} seem to be involved in switching on genes that are expressed at the very onset of sporulating protein synthesis under stressed environmental condition(s). In exhaustion of nutritional components like carbon, nitrogen, or phosphorous, at least two new sporulation protein specific factors have been stated to be synthesized. One being σ^{29} and the other is probably σ^{37} that dissociates σ^{55} factor from the core RNA polymerase. In this way σ^{29} replaces σ^{55} on core polymerase and permits the transcription of the sporulation protein specific promoter to start functioning. Interestingly, the σ factors determining the expression of specialized sets of genes are appearing as general features of many prokaryotes as diverse as *E. coli*, *Bacillus* and *Streptomyces* species. For example, the expression of heat shock stress genes and nitrogen-regulated genes in *E. coli* is known to be dictated by specific σ factors encoding by genes htpR and ntrA. Also, multiple σ factors are a feature of most complex bacterial viruses such as T4, λ, T7, μ, and *B. subtilis* phage SPO1. More recently, it has been noticed that the rpoH (σ^{32}) gene of *E. coli* can be deleted as long as its culture has been maintained below 20°C. If this culture is, however, shifted to high temperatures, its level of σ^{32} changes in various ways. Firstly, the rpoH mRNA is transiently stabilized; secondly, the rpoh gene transcription is stimulated; and thirdly; the half life of σ^{32} is transiently increased. Because of the very short half life of σ^{32} polypeptide (45 secs), the intracellular level of σ^{32} immediately causes variations in the parameters controlling σ^{32} production and stability. Thus, it is important to know how and which proteins play a role in stress alterations like mutations allowing cell growth at all temperatures to take place. It relates to an organism response at the cellular and molecular level when confronted with sudden changes in environment and molecular adaptation in the ability of the cells to acclimate themselves to the new environment.[41-45]

3. Adaptive expression

Although much information has not been accumulated on this, some light has been thrown on the *E. coli* cell system.[44-45] In this organism three interesting twists in rpoH gene expression have been reported. In the first twist, rpoH is expressed from at least four different promoters. In the second twist, two of the promoters are negatively regulated by the DnaA protein (required for inhibition of *E. coli* DNA replication as well as global regulation). The third promoter is under CAP-CAMP catabolite control, and the fourth is under the control of a more recently known σ^{24} (σ^{E}) factor. The gene coding for σ^{24} has not been identified as yet, it is, however, clear that σ^{24}-promoted transcription is accelerated at high temperature of 50°C range. It indicated that there are at least two heat shock systems in *E. coli.* The conventional one is regulated by σ^{32}, and more currently known under σ^{24} regulation. Heat shock genes at high temperatures like 50°C are transcribed exclusively by either $E\sigma^{32}$ or $E\sigma^{24}$, and $E\sigma^{24}$ levels, are continuously replenished by the σ^{24}-promoted transcription of the rpoH gene. So, it is stated that heat shock gene HtrA (degP) is under the exclusive transcriptional control of $E\sigma^{24}$. Its product is essential for viability of *E. coli* at higher temperatures and remains under heat shock adaptive regulation. It entells that these two heat shock regulons are interconnected. The third twist promises rpoHmRNA translation under negative repression control as well. Signals affecting repressor element activity alters intracellular σ^{32} levels.[46-49]

It appears that adaptive expression of stress has been known for a long time; however, its actual application in biological and physiological systems has been recognized only recently. Adaptive expressions in (a) ischemic stress associated with lethal ischemic injury, (b) pathogenesis in stress-related diseases.[50-51] (c) modifying microenvironment of the lipid bilayer and modulating involved enzyme activities.[52-55] etc., have recently also been known. Participation of stress proteins like HSP70 and HSP68 in cellular adaptive functional expressions has also been shown. Such an adaptation expression process usually takes a long time until the cellular components of living organisms possessing intrinsic molecular mechanism adapt to the stressful situation. The actual molecular adaptive expression, although, is a long term process; many changes can still occur during the initial phase of adaptation. They provide adjustment of cells to the stressful situation and temporarily maintain them in the new environment. However, report are also available regarding short-term adaptive expression in prokaryotic cells to stress conditions. It appears, therefore that adaptive expression depends largely on the source cell as well as the stressor type. For example, the results of a recent study on vascular endothelial cells (VEC) indicated that VEC promptly responded to the stressor if it is in the form of oxidative stress. This prompt response was manifested by synthesizing several oxidative stress proteins including HSP and stimulating antioxidative enzymes. Apparantly, it was to protect the biosystems from the toxic effects of stress allowing them to recover and survive.

14.6.2 Oxidative Stress

1. Forewords

It has been indicated that the constitutive restriction enzyme *Bam* H1 protein biosynthesis in *Bacillus amyloliquefaciens* H1 strain, is greatly influenced by oxygen tension in the cell cultivation liquid.[56-57] The profiles of *Bam* H1 production, as shown in Figs. 14.5-14.7, show that specific growth rate (μ) and specific restriction enzyme protein yield ($Y_{RE/X}$) of this prokaryotic cell varied largely, but $Y_{RE/X}$ to only a little extent under thermal processing stress. The variations of these bioprocess technology state parameters by oxygenation and shear control parameter were seen to be very pronounced. It appeared that formation of Bam H1 involved reactive oxygen species stress gene(s) having functional optimality at specific oxygen tension. In a prokaryotic system, oxidative stress has been found to induce heat shock proteins and

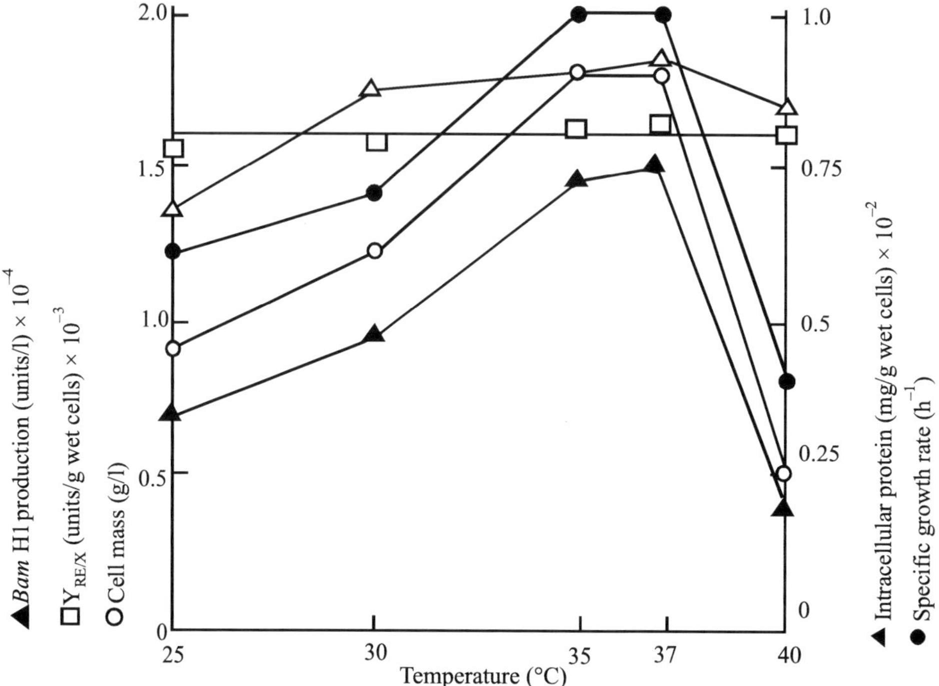

Fig 14.5 Variation of *Bam* H1 production parameters in relation of temperature

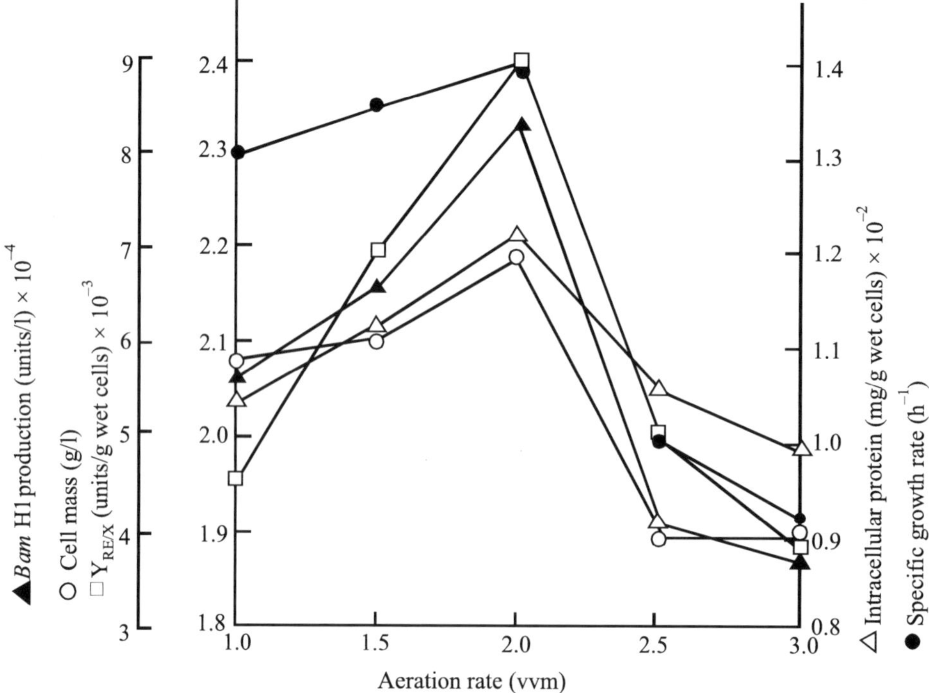

Fig. 14.6 Influence of agitation on parameters on *Bam* H1 production

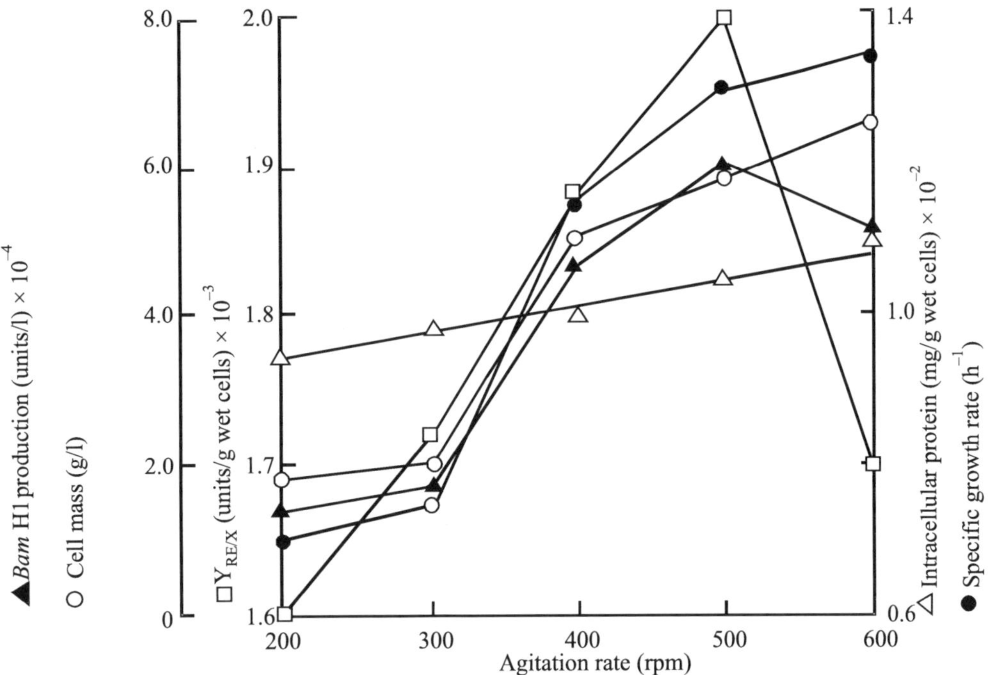

Fig. 14.7 Influence of agitation on parameters of *Bam* H1 production

glucose regulated proteins.[58] This led the scientists to believe that such cellular response in eukaryotic cells may be of great significance, since reactive oxygen species have been shown to play a significant role in a variety of disease processes like heart attack, stroke, arthritis and a few others.[59-62] Reactive oxygen species have also been implicated in ischemic and reperfusion injury to a large variety of mammalian tissues. However, information on the prompt response of eukaryotic cells to the oxidative stress is scanty. Prompt molecular adaptation of vascular endothelial cells to oxidative stress as mentioned earlier is an important piece of information.[63] In *Bam* H1 producing prokaryotic cells, the nature of the oxygen species reactive stress genes and corresponding stress factors in the cell are still not identified. Their identification and involvement in thermotolerence and oxygen stress in *Bam* H1 yield increase (Figs. 14.5 & 14.6) remains as a future reasearch scope in the area of oxidative stress in prokaryotes. It may also be necessary to know in this organism whether the unknown individual HSPs are under the control of constitutive or inducible promoters.

Oxidative stress developed by exposing bacteria (*Salmonella typhimurium*) to low concentration of H_2O_2 induced several new proteins including HSPs and mRNA of catalase.[64] In the process of oxidative stress adaptation, the bacteria becomes resistant to killing by otherwise lethal doses of H_2O_2 and other strong oxidants.[65] Thus, it may appear in mammalian cells that oxidative stress induction creates a defense action against subsequent cellular injury by expressing a distinct group of proteins such as HSP and GRP, etc. This class of special proteins have been collectively termed as 'oxidative stress inducible proteins' (OSIPs). Furthermore, it was shown that among the oxidative stress inducible genes, R_{OXY} gene is a positive regulatory gene for at least 9 different proteins including catalase, hydroperoxide I, glutathione reductase, and alkyl-hydroperoxide reductase.[65] However, many oxidative stress-inducible proteins are not characterized; and their functions are yet unknown.

2. Possible molecular mechanisms

From the influence of dissolved oxygen on constitutive enzyme protein *Bam* H1 formation by *Bacillus amyloliquefaciens* H1 strain as well as prokaryotic systems like *S. typhimurium* and others under oxidative stress, it will be interesting and useful to know about molecular mechanism of the participation of oxygen in such situations. The ambivalent mechanism of oxygen in aerobic organisms is really a paradox. A beneficial effect of oxygen in aerobic organisms up to a certain level has been observed. Above the critical level an adverse effect was observed in many cases including *Bam* H1 production. It tends to suggest that below a certain level ($K_La < 260h^{-1}$) oxygen does not activate the regulon of mRNA of the activator protein to react with its *oxyR* binding site which is responsible for changing the oxidation state. It permits *in vivo Bam* H1 synthesis to continue and increase. On the other hand, above a certain dissolved oxygen level; i.e. for the volumetric oxygen transfer coefficient (K_L a) > $260h^{-1}$, it activates the oxyR binding site of the activator protein. The oxyR protein is, thcrefore, directly activated by metabolic oxygen stimulus, an oxidant becoming a transcriptional inactivatory by generating reactive oxygen species. It is generated from high dissolved oxygen in the medium and interacts with oxyR changing the oxidation state of its binding site. This change perhaps causes conformational change that affects the way in which the proteins interact with their corresponding promoters.

So, the oxyR regulon response to high dissolved oxygen stress is one of the few molecular mechanisms for which the translation of an enviromental stress into transcriptional control has been defined. Some cells were partly resistent to this response to survive harmful metabolic effects of active oxygen species and possibly other oxidants in the medium.

In both eukaryotic and prokaryotic biosystems, molecular oxygen may, therefore, play an ambivalent role. A substantial oxidative stress damage rate to DNA can occur as a part of normal metabolism and of lipid peroxidation in cells.[67] The oxidative DNA damage rate has been measured by thymidine glycol excretion in mammals. In order to cope with oxidative stress, aerobic organisms evolved enzymic and nonenzymic molecular level antioxidant defense mechanisms. These molecular mechanisms within the organisms have been evolved to limit the levels of reactive oxidants and the damage they caused. In cell proliferation the molecular mechanism of oxygen stress dependent pathway has been shown to play a significant role by regulating uridine phosphate mediated ribonucleotide reductase system.[68]

In a most recent study, it was demonstrated that IL-1 can induce SOD activity[69] and also able to express heat shock proteins. [70] IL-1α is also a prominent member of a group of polypeptide mediator called cytokines. IL-1α has recently been found to function as a therapeutic agent when used at low doses. It was also demonstrated recently that IL-1α reduced the myocardial ischemia/reperfusion injury when treated with this cytokine for 48 hours. IL-1α also induces the expression of the mRNA for HSP27 within four hours of treatment.[71]

From various literature informations and the above discussions, the manifestation of molecular mechanisms of oxidative stress possibly may be of the following categories:

a. Inductive oxidative damage and protection (restriction of cell proliferation).
b. Antioxidant protection (by scavenging mechanism).
c. Enzymic control (possibly by gene regulation, e.g., in SPS formation).
d. SOD regulation and control (molecular adaptive mechanism).
e. Metabolic oxygen control coefficient regulation (possibly by induction~repression mechanism of conformational protection, e. g., in restriction endonuclease formation).
f. Therapeutic regulation (possibly delayed molecular adaptation mechanism, e. g., in ischemic heart).

14.6.3 Other Stresses

Cold shock (thermal) and photon stress are shown to be important in transitional stress protein development in phases of some of the plants cell cycle affecting synthetic and organelle activity.[72] These plants growing at subnormal or cold temperatures and under low photonic intensity may have large nucleoli with higher amounts of cellular RNA and increased RNA polymerase activity. Growth of seedlings of *Triptycene aestivum* cv Chinese Spring in darkness between 5°C to 20°C has been cited as an illustrative example.[72,73] The maximum growth rate increased from

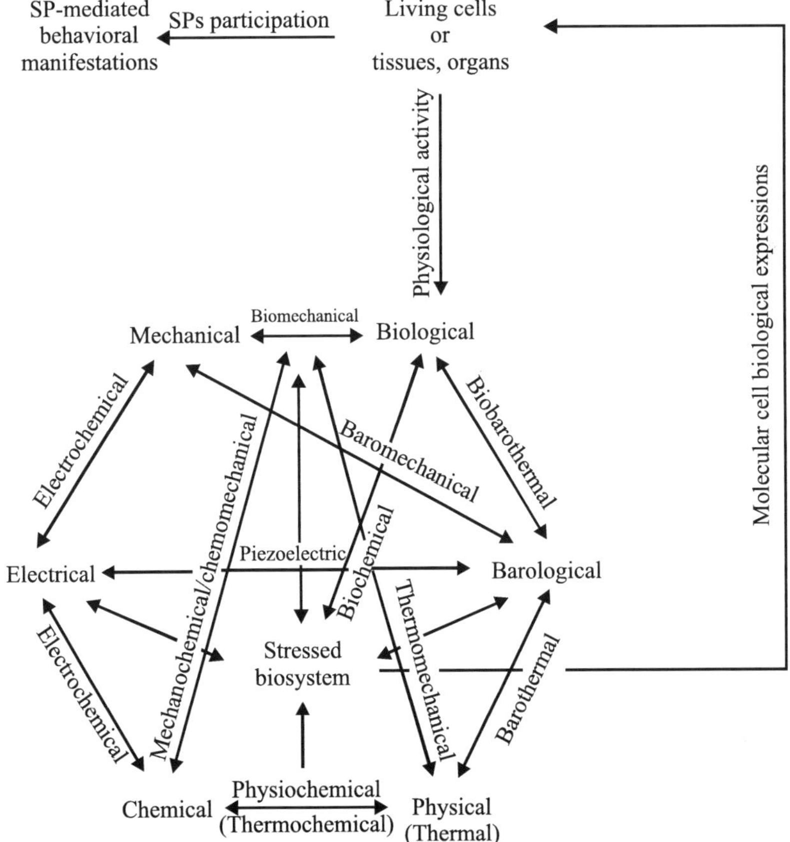

Fig. 14.8 Depiction of possible interactive physiological stress inducing conditions in biosystems

0.6 mgh^{-1} at 5°C to 3.1 mgh^{-1} at 20°C and maintaining this value at 25°C is an indication that the cell cycle would be expected to be longer compared to that at 20° C. So, cells compensate by loosing RNA levels and presumably stress proteins in order to sustain a minimal amount of growth. It is also indicative that cold shock may block the cell cycle and cold shock induced quiescent cells may be different from those of the normal in terms of deficiency of cell cycle related proteins. Generation of stress proteins under cold shock might have prevented the plants from entering into S phase from G1 phase. It may, therefore, appear that in cold perennial plants remain quiescent at temperatures below 5°C accumulating abnormal stress proteins for sustenance until the next favorable climate. A direct usefulness of this may relate to plant biotechnology in having plants remain in quiescent state during long periods of cold and rapidly useful to exploit transient periods of elevated temperatures or rainfall. It will, however, depend on the adaptive expression response of the plant cells. Cold stress proteins, thus, bear important concerns in daily life to infantry in cold regions, marine operations, cryobioepisodes, cold injury, preserved foods, and many others. Until today, however, very little evidence has been shown for induction of transcription of any identifiable gene by cold shock treatment either prolonged or of rapid 'cold shock' type. It, therefore, remains as a big challenge and scope for genetic and metabolic engineers. Possibilities of generations of stress proteins under mechanochemical, electrochemical, and other stresses (Fig. 14.8) do exist in the contraction of skeletal muscle.[74] Two membrane-bound stress proteins, 42 KD and 24 KD, have been reported to be expressed with iron limitation in *Bacteroides gingivalis*[75] at 37°C.

It appears, therefore, that cellular adaptation to a variety of external stresses is essential for the survival of both prokaryotes and eukaryotes. However, unlike HSPs, the majority of cold shock proteins are of relatively low molecular weight. For example in response to cold temperature, *E. coli* rapidly induces several polypeptides including Nus A, Rec A, dihydrolipoamide, acetyl transferase subunit of pyruvate dehydrogenase, polynucleotide phosphorylase, pyruvate dehydrogenase as well as some initiation factors.[76] One of these cold shock proteins, F 10.6 (10KDa), is synthesized only during growth at low temperature. Some of these proteins (viz., Nus A) are likely to be involved in transcription and translation as well as mRNA degradation. Recently a 7.4 KDa protein(CS 7.4) has been found to be induced when *E. coli* culture temperature was shifted from 37°C to 10-15°C.[77] It has been possible to clone the gene for CS 7.4 (csp A) to determine its DNA sequence and to show evidence that CS 7.4 may play a role in protecting cells from cold injury and, thus, may function as an 'anti-freeze protein'. Such anti-freeze proteins (but distinct from CS 7.4) are found at high concentration in the serum of polar-dwelling marine fishes and in the hemolymph of the insects that survive in subfreezing climates.[78] It is known that hypothermia restricts bacterial growth by blocking an early step in protein synthesis.[79] The synthesis of these proteins in response to cold seems to be adaptive in nature.

One of the key questions in the cellular adaptation concerns the molecular mechanisms of differential gene regulation. It is quite possible that cold shock can trigger a cascade of second messengers which can simultaneously induce and inactivate specific sets of genes. The gene encoding cold shock protein has been cloned and characterized.[76] A number of genes induced by cold shock have been identified by a differential hybridization screen of a yeast genomic library.[80] Interestingly, genes for a developmentally regulated membrane protein[81] and for ubiquitin[82] have been shown to be induced in response to both cold shock and heat shock.

Induction of the expression of cold shock proteins has also been demonstrated in eukaryotes. For example, both low and high molecular weight proteins were found to be expressed in the rabbit leg skeletal muscle when the limb was subjected to repeated stress induced by hypothermia (Fig. 14.9). Interestingly, some of these proteins disappeared during subsequent cooling and rewarming (Table14.3).

In a study, the leg of a rabbit was repeatedly cooled by ice, followed by rewarming after each cooling episode. The process was repeated ten times. Such a repeated cooling and rewarming process enabled the leg muscle to withstand the subsequent lethal cold injury significantly better when compared with a normal leg, suggesting that the leg muscle had been adapted to cold by repeated cooling and rewarming.[63] Not only did this process of adaptation make the tissue less susceptible to cold injury, but it was also associated with the reduction of reperfusion injury. It seems reasonable to speculate that the induction of cold shock proteins play a role in the protective mechanism. Recently the major CSP from *Bacillus subtilis* (CSPB) has been overexpressed in recombinant *E. coli* cells.[83] The recombinant cell was developed by using the bacteriophage T7 RNA polymerase/promoter system.

14.7 KINETICS AND DYNAMICS OF STRESS PROTEINS FORMATION

The transient changes of proteins in biosystems is necessary to sustain growth or injury at a stress condition, which, on a kinetic and dynamic basis, would be expected to reduce or increase the concerned rates of reaction. It has been reported that in parallel to generation rate of heat shock proteins there is an increase in the rate of *in vivo* proteolysis as a result of stress.[4] However, the correlation between the stress protein biosynthesis rate and the *in vivo* proteolysis rate appears to be dependent on the specific form of stress imposed.[5] Although this correlation is not clear, it raises the question whether there is any common target of the response, and if so, what its nature is. In order to activate stress genes, living organisms respond at cellular level to unfavorable environmental conditions, e.g., heat shock or other stressful situations of various origins. This is by rapid, vigorous, and transient acceleration in the rate expression of a small system specific genes. Besides the activation of stress genes like heat shock genes, the expression of most other genes is inhibited as a result of stress insult. Thus, stress leads to a perturbation of normal gene expression. Prolongation of the perturbation by stress can have drastic consequences in cellular functions as well. Also these consequences may produce very useful abnormal protein products which are of commercial importance, as indicated in Table 14.1.

Little is known about the identity of stress proteins whose rate of synthesis induced or enhanced by cold shock. However, complements of some commercial enzymes like glutathione reductase, invertase, and ribulose biphosphate carboxylase have been stated to modify during cold shock manifesting newer protein behavior. Both photosynthetic capacity and partitioning to assimilate usually are dynamic parameters during long duration cold shock. It causes the components of the photosynthetic metabolic apparatus and enzymic proteins of carbohydrate metabolism to alter. It is reported that chilling of maize food plant leaves brought about a decrease in photosynthetic capacity, and cold stress induced 31 KD polypeptide was accumulated in the

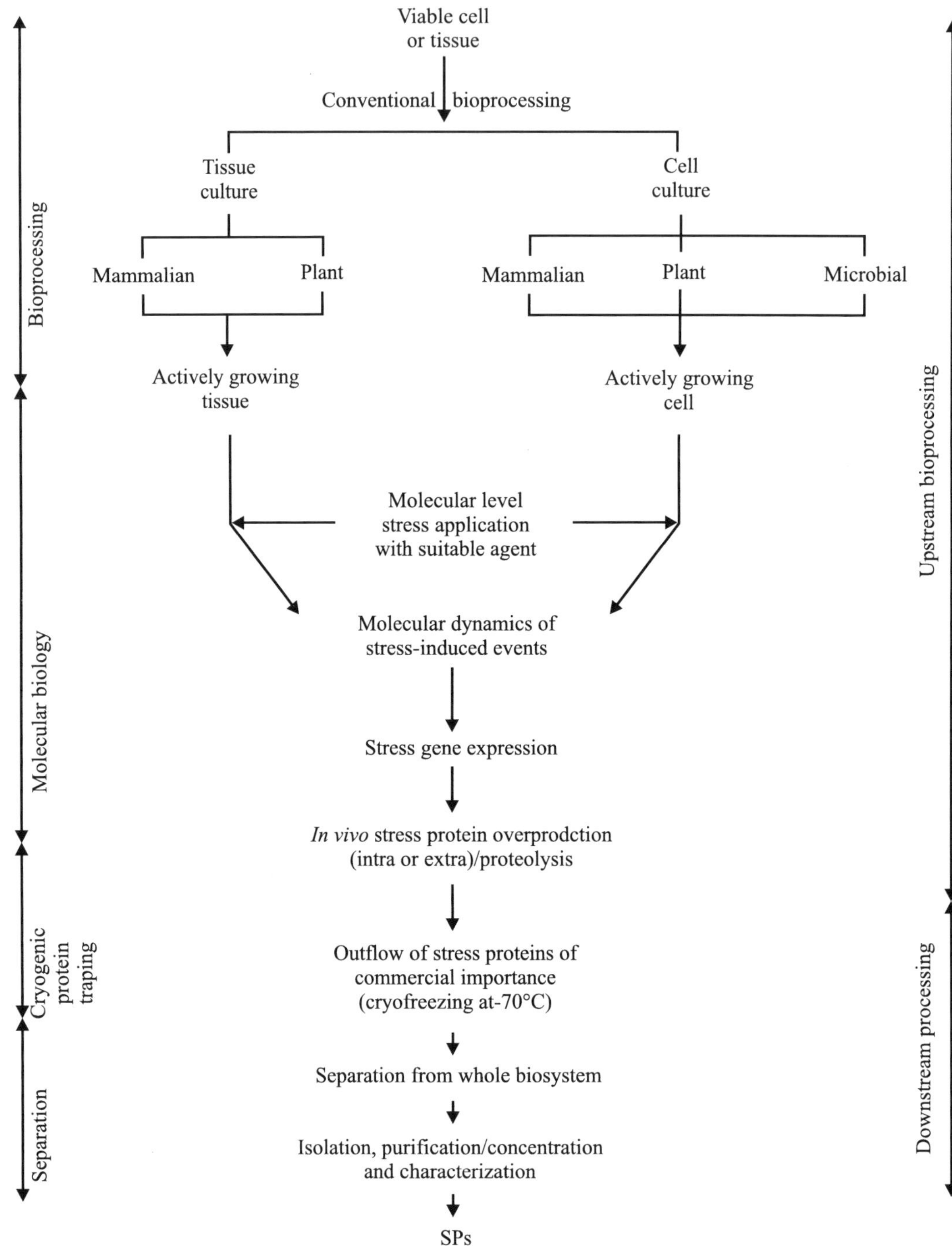

Fig. 14.9 Bioprocessing and biomolecular separation strategy

thylakoids.[72] It has been tentatively identified as a precursor of the smaller chloroplast protein CP29. In producing heat shock proteins (HSP70) by mammalian cells, like CHO cells, by exposing at 45°C for 5-15 mins followed by incubation at 37°C, it was observed that macromolecular synthesis was inhibited following the initial phase of heat exposure; stress protein synthesis resumed in parallel to the development of thermotolerence. The RNA and DNA synthesis rate was slower to recover. The profile of thermotolerence induction could lead to propose that in the dynamics of acquisition of resistance involves two distinct stages: the first being initial signaling (triggering) and the second, processing of the initial step ('development'). A simplistic kinetic model of this cellular thermotolerence in stress protein development has been provided by Hahn and Li.[84]

Table 14.3 Effects of cold adaptation on the antioxidative enzymes in skeletal muscle***

	Cu/Zn-SOD	*Mn-SOD*	*Catalase*	*GSH-Peroxidase*	*GSH-Reductase*
Baseline	35.3+2.2	36.5+6.4	6.6+0.5	67+8.4	6.8+0.9
Cooled & Rewarmed	30.1+3.3	16.9+5.2	5.6+0.6	53+7.0	5.8+0.4
Adapted	40.5+7.5	41.9+2.6	9.7+1.8*	117+7.1*	12.5+0.6*
Adapted & Cooled	31.4+5.6	25.8+8.6	9.9+1.2	92+11.0	11.0+0.7
Adapted, Cooled & Rewarmed	39.2+3.6	18.1+1.8	7.6+0.3**	81.7+4.0**	8.5+0.4**

* $p < 0.05$ compared to baseline; ** $p < 0.05$ compared to unadapted cooled & rewarmed

*** Data supplied by Prof Dipak K. Das

14.8 MOLECULAR AND CELL BIOLOGY (MCB) TECHNIQUES IN STRESS PROTEINS ANALYSIS

14.8.1 Forewords

One of the major reasons for the attraction of recombinant DNA technology relates to gene therapy in prevention of diseases developed under stresses. Among the causes of these diseases in human and other eukaryotes, one has been ascribed to be due to accumulation of abnormal or stress proteins in cells or tissues. These abnormal or stress proteins are formed by over expression of genes in biosystems when the cellular organs or tissues are exposed or given various types of physiological stresses as discussed earlier. However, in prokaryotes imposition of stresses may accumulate abnormal proteins, which may be of importance. Both prokaryotic and eukaryotic stress proteins by proper modulation and molecular redesigning or refolding may prove to be useful in combating diseases and in developing new emerging areas of stress protein biotechnology.[85] Therefore, skillful detection, analysis, and purification of these specific proteins is of prime importance so that upstream bioprocessing and downstream separation can be coherently developed in the form of bioprocess integration. Many precision approaches are gradually being used in developing most modern instrumental and MCB techniques in stress protein biotechnology. A brief description of the techniques that are currently being adapted are discussed below.

14.8.2 Culture Bioprocessing

In order to trap substantial amounts of induced stress proteins during cell growth by stressor, the cell needs to be grown in a culture bioreactor of specific design depending on cell type (microbial, mammalian, or plant) and oxygen response to it. For medically important stress proteins induction in mammalian cells, the suspension culture serum bottle is used in the laboratory. However, large scale production effort of specific stress protein is yet to be reported in a systematic manner.

14.8.3 MCB Techniques in SPs

1. PCR

Since stress proteins are gene-induced products, the study of the structure of individual stress genes in living organisms is very important. Molecular cloning is the technique that permits such study. In microorganisms this technique depends on the replication of DNA of the plasmids and other vectors during cell division. As the amount of DNA is very small and its detection is tedious and difficult, necessity of its amplification procedure is now well known. The procedure is based on an *in vivo* rather than *in vitro* technique. This *in vivo* technique is known as polymerase chain reaction (PCR). For amplifying a specific DNA segment by PCR, the adapted cycle principle has been shown in the literature.[86] It indicates that it is not necessary to know the nucleotide sequence of the target DNA. Heat resistant DNA polymerase has been isolated from *Thermus aquaticus* (*Taq*) and utilized most commonly in PCR technique. In eukaryotic cells the technique of directional cloning cDNA representing mRNA from control and induced cells has been used. The cDNA libraries need to be used to produce ample amounts of DNA and RNA in substractive hybridization for the removal of sequences present in both control and induced cells. The remaining unhybridized sequences are selectively amplified by PCR and cloned to produce the required enriched library. From this library the isolation of cDNA of specific-hsp associated mRNAs needs to be carried out since a family of heat shock genes is activated by various stimuli depending on the type of the cell.[86,87]

2. Northern blotting

In northern blot analysis, the total RNA is extracted from the tissues or cells by various methods.[88,89] Generally, 4-30 mg of total RNA are subjected to agarose- formaldehyde[90] or glyoxylic gel electrophoresis[91] and the RNA separated are transferred to nylon or nitrocellulose membrane. To fix the RNA to the membrane, the dried membrane is either placed between two pieces of 3 MM paper, and it is generally baked for 30 mins to 2 hours at 80°C in a vacuum or conventional oven or the side of the membrane carrying the RNA is exposed to ultraviolet irradiation (254 nm).[92] After fixation, the membrane is prehybridized and then hybridized with the desired^{32P} labeled cDNA probes. The membrane is washed with different concentration of salts (sodium chloride, sodium citrate [SSC] or sodium chloride, sodium dihydrogen phosphate, EDTA [SSPE] at different temperatures (60°C or 55°C) or even at room temperature. Then the autoradiograms are generally obtained after exposing the membrane to x-ray films at 70°C.

RNA is quantitated spectrophotometrically, assuming that 40 μg RNA in 1 ml gives an absorbance of 1.0 at 260 nm. Integrity of RNA preparations and consistent sample loading is verified by ethidium bromide staining of the transferred RNAs.

3. 2-D gel electrophoresis

A very useful analytical technique for the separation of proteins is by two-dimensional polyacrylamide gel electrophoresis. Proteins are separable according to their isoelectric point by isoelectric focusing, in the first dimension; and in second dimension, it separates out according to molecular weight by polyacrylamide gel electrophoresis. 2-D gel electrophoresis is of great merit in mixed protein resolution.

In isoelectric focusing gels are made within glass tubing. Samples (protein) are added on the first dimension isoelectric focusing cylindrical gels. In a typical case, the gels are run at 300 volts for 18 hrs, and then at 800 volts for one hour.[93] If high voltage is applied, the bands become distorted. The sample gels are equilibrated in Farrell's SDS sample buffer for 30 min.[93] The second dimensional gel electrophoresis is the discontinuous SDS gel system.[94] After the preparation of sample gels from one-dimensional gel electrophoresis, they are layered onto second dimensional SDS polyacrylamide slab gels. The gels are generally electrophoresed at 20 mA constant current per gel for 5 hrs until the dye front reaches the bottom of the gel.

If the samples are radio-labeled, the gels, are then dried and exposed to x-ray films, which are processed according to standard procedure.[93] If not, the gels are stained in 0.1% Coomassie blue in 50% methanol, 10% acetic acid for at least one hour and destained by repeated treatment with 7% acetic acid and 10% methanol.

14.9 UPSTREAM BIOPROCESSING AND DOWNSTREAM SEPARATION OF SPs[74]

In forming stress proteins in biosystem processing, the stress induction strategy is usually followed as shown in Fig. 14.9. However, thorough analytical reports of the steps need substantial research extensions.

14.10 FUTURE PROSPECTS OF SPs

The biotechnological importances of SPs in general have been outlined in Table 14.1. Other prospects of SPs may be listed as below:

(i) The development of stable cell lines capable of constitutively expressing individual heat shock proteins is a potentially powerful approach to resolving their function during hyperthermia and thermotolerence development.

(ii) Rat cell lines stably transformed with a human hsp70 gene have also been shown to have increased heat resistance[95] which may have importance in research.

(iii) It is prospective to identify specific heat induced lesions in cell structure or metabolism that are either protected or repaired by individual heat shock proteins. The structural regions of heat shock proteins important for function can then be delineated by conventional site directed mutagenesis. In the case of hsp[27], the importance of protein phosphorylation for thermal protection can be directly ascertained.

(iv) Prospective for selection of transformed cell lines, heat selection was used to isolate stable hamster transformants expressing the human hsp[27] gene. Repeated heat shock could select for cells containing additional mutations affecting survival in addition to expression of the transfected heat shock gene.

(v) Stable transfected cells expressing individual hsps under control of constitutive or inducible promoters should provide important insight into both the mechanism(s) of thermo-resistance and the roles of the individual heat shock proteins.

(vi) For a better understanding of how cells adapt to elevated temperature could lead to more effective use of hyperthermia in clinic.

(vii) The heat shock proteins could also turn out to be targets for new drug design[85] useful to sensitize cells to thermal kill or prevent the development of thermotolerence in tumor cells.

(viii) The stress-induced enzyme cascade has a great prospect to open up avenues in chemistry for bioreaction-like stereoselective stress-induced reaction for aldol condensation for yielding spiro and branched chain reaction.[96]

14.11 CONCLUSIONS

Much more extensive research needs to be carried out in producing, designing, and promoting stress proteins of commercial, beneficial use. The field is emerging for new developments, and some future prospects have been highlighted conceiving novel approaches to the rational design of mechanism-based inactivators for stress proteins like HSPs. Prevention of associated diseases will require more extensive knowledge of the corresponding stress gene(s) active sites of stress proteins of enzymic nature and their kinetics and dynamics. The interactions that are essential for biocatalysis binding substrate analogs and inhibitors need to be documented. Powerful modern instruments and techniques such as NMR, ESR, HPLC, FPLC, PAGE, 2D-gel chromatograph, GCMS, etc., in conjunction with modern techniques of PCR and southern, northern, and western blotting can open up directions in identification of the nature and type of stress and stress protein products, their trapping, isolation and downstream processing for purification; namely, cryogenesis, solid-solid interfacial immobilization (homogenic and heterogenic) like solid phase extraction by either covalent adducting or active site directed agents, etc. These instrumental and MCB analyses in combination with cloning or recombinant DNA overexpression means of protein engineering for active stress proteins, like enzymes of commercial importance, may provide interesting data and value addition scopes to develop this new area of biotechnology rapidly.

14.12 ACKNOWLEDGEMENT

For this part author sincerely thanks Dr. Dipak K. Das, Professor and Director, Cardiovascular Division, for extending an invitation and support as a visiting scientist. Thanks are also due to some of the scientists of Prof. Das group for their kind assistance in preparation of this manuscript. Library facilities of the University of Connecticut Health Center and support received from the Department of Surgery are highly acknowledged. Thanks to members of Dr. Das's group for their cooperation and finally to Laurie Amara for the expert preliminary word processing of this manuscript.

14.13 REFERENCES

1. Morimoto, R.E., A. Tissieres, and G. Georgopoulos, "The Stress Function of the Proteins, and Perspectives I." *Stress Proteins in Biology and Medicine*, pp 1-36, (R. I. Morimoto, A. Tissieres, and C. Georgopoulos, ed.), Cold Spring Harbor Laboratory Press, New York, 1990.
2. Ananthan, J, A.L. Goldberg, and R. Vollemy, "Abnormal Proteins Serve as Eukaryotic Stress Signals and Trigger the Activation of Heat Shock Genes", *Science,* pp 232, 522-24, 1986.
3. Parsell, D.A. and R. T. Sauer, "Induction of a Heat Shock—Line Response by Unfolded Protein", *Escherichia Coli,* "Dependence on Protein Level not Protein Degradation", *Genes Dev.*, 3, pp 1226-32, 1989.
4. Parag, H.A., B. Raboy, and R.G. Kulka, "Effect of Heat Shock on Protein Degradation in Mammalian Cells: Improvement of the Ubiquitin System", *EMBOJ*, 6, pp 55-61, 1987.
5. Westwood, J. T. and R.A. Steinhardt, "Effects of Heat and Other Inducers of the Stress Response on Protein Degradation in Chinese Hamster and Drosophila Cells", *J. Cell. Physiol.*, pp 139, 196-209, 1989.
6. Banerjee, S.S., K. Laing, and R.I. Morimoto, "Erythroid Lineage-Specific Expression and Inducibility of the Major Heat Shock Protein HSP70 During Avian Embryogenesis", *Genes Dev.*, Vol 1, pp 943-53, 1987.
7. Nover, L. Inducers of HSP Synthesis, "Heat Shock and Chemical Stressors", *Heat Shock Response*, CRC Press, Boca Raton, pp 5-40, 1991.
8. Helmke, E. and H. Weyland, "Effect of Hydrostatic Pressure and Temperature on the Activity and Synthesis of Antarctic Ocean Bacteria", *Mar. Biol.*, pp 1-7, 91, 1986.
9. Sasaki, T. and E. T. Kaiser, "Helichrome Synthesis and Enzymie Activity of a Designed Haemoprotein", *J. Am. Chem. Soc.*, pp 111, 380, 81, 1989.
10. Morii, H., K. Ichimura, and H. Udedaira, "Asymmetric Inclusion by De Novo Designed Proteins: Fluorescence Probe Studies on Amphiphilie α-Helix Bundles", *Proteins: Structure, Function and Genetics.*, 11 (2), pp 113-41, 1991.
11. Ahnstrom, G., A.M. George, and W.A. Cramp, "Extensive and Equivalent Repair in Both Radiation Resistant and Radiation Senstitive *E. Coli* Determined by a DNA Unwinding Technique", *lnt. J. Radiat Bioing.*, 34, pp 317-27, 1978.
12. Seeberg, E. and A.L. Steinum, "Repair of X-ray Induced Deoxyribonucleic Acid Single Strand Breaks in Xth Mutants of *Eschenction Coli*", *J. Bacteriol.*, 141, pp 1424-27, 1980.
13. George, A.M. and W.A. Cramp, "The Effects of Ionizing Radiation on Structure and Function of DNA." *Prog. Biophys. Mol. Bioi.*, 50, (3), pp 121-69, 1987.
14. Moore, C. W., "Ligase Deficient Yeast Cells Exhibit Detective DNA Rejoining and Enhanced Gamma Ray Sensitivity", *J. Bacteriol.*, 150, pp 1227-33, 1982.
15. Leaper, S., M.A. Resnik, and R. Holiday, "Repair of Double Strand Breaks and Lethal Damage in DNA of Ustilago Maydis", *Genet. Res. Camb.*, 35, pp 291-307, 1980.
16. Antoku, S., "Chemical Protection Against Radiation Induced DNA Single Strand Breaks in Cultured Mammalian Cells", *Radiat. Res.,* 65, pp 130-38, 1976.
17. Reddy, N.M.S. and B.S. Rao., "Genetic Control of Repair of Radiation Damage Produced Under Oxic and Anoxic Conditions in Diplioid Yeast *Saccharomyces Cerevisiae*", *Radiat. Environ. Biophys.*, 19, pp 187-95, 1981.

18. Budd, M. and R.K. Mortimer, "Repair of Double Strand Breaks in a Temperature Conditional Radiation Sensitive Mutation of *Saccharomyces cerevisiae*", *Mutation Res.*, 103, pp 187-95, 1981.
19. Collins, A. and R. Johns, "Novobiocin: An Inhibitor of the Repair of UV Induced but not X-ray Induced Damage in Mammalian Cells", *Nucleic Acids Res.*, 7, pp 311-20, 1997.
20. Weber, L.A., "Relationship of Heat Shock Proteins and Induced Thermal Resistance", *Cell Prolif* 25 (2), pp 101-13, 1992.
21. Milarski, K. and R. Morilloto, "Expression of Human HSP70 During the Synthetic Phase of the Cell Cycle", *Proc. Natl. Acad. Sci. USA*. 83, pp 9517-21, 1986.
22. Simon, M.C. K. Kitchener, H. T. Kao, E. Hickey, R. "Vollelly, N. Heintz, and J.R. Nevins. Selective Induction of Human Heat Shock Gene Transcription by Adenovirus Ela Gene Products Including 125 Ela Product", *Mol. Cell. Biol.*, 7, pp 2884-90, 1987.
23. Williams, G. T., T.K. McChanahan, and R. Morilloto, "Ela Trans Activation of Human HSP70 is Mediated Through the Basal Transcription Complex", *Mol. Cell. Biol.*, 9, pp 25, 74-87, 1989.
24. Lull, S. Y., S. Hsu, M. Vacwhongs, and B. Wu, "The HSP70 Gene CCAAT Binding Factor Mediates Transcriptional Activation by the Adenovins Ela Protein", *Mol. Cell Biol.*, 12 (6), pp 2599-2605, 1992.
25. Lull, L., L. Sultzman! R. Kaufman, D. Linzer, and B. Wu, "A Cloned Human CCAAT Box Binding Factor Stillutates Transcription from the Human HSP70 Promoter", *Mol. Cell. Biol.* 10, pp 6709-17, 1990.
26. Douglas, B. Y., A. Mehlert, and D.F. Smith, *Stress Proteins in Biology and Medicine*, pp. 131-65, (R.I. Morilloto, A. Tissiers, and C. Georgopoulos eds.), CSHL Press, New York, 1990.
27. Banerjee, S.S., N.G. Theodorakis, and R. Morimoto, "Heat Shock Induced Transitional Control of HSP70 and Globin Synthesis in Chicken Reticulocytes", *Mol. Cell. Biol.*, 4, pp 2437-68, 1984.
28. Neidhart, F.C., R.A. Van Bogelen and V. Vaughn, "The Genetics and Regulation of Heat Shock Proteins", *Annu. Rev. Genet.*, 18, pp 295-329, 1985.
29. Ruger, H.J., "Substrate Dependent Cold Adaptations in Some Deep Sea Sediment Bacteria", *System. Appl. Microbiol.*, 11, pp 90-93, 1988.
30. Arrigo, A.P., J. Suhan, and W.J. Welch. "Dynamic Changes in the Structure and Intracellular Locale of the Mammalian Low Molecular Weight Heat Shock Protein", *Mol. Cell Biol.*, 8, pp 5059-71, 1988.
31. Hershko, A., "Ubiquitin-mediated Protein Degradation", *J. Biol. Chem.*, 263, pp 15237-40, 1988.
32. Lindquist, S. and E.A. Craig, "The Heat Shock Proteins", *Annu. Rev. Genet.*, 22, pp 631-77, 1988.
33. Watson, J.D., N.H. Hopkins, I. W. Roberts, J.A. Steitz, and A.M. Weiner, *Molecular Biology of the Gene*, The Benjamin/Cummings Pub. Co., Inc., Menlo Park, California, 1987.
34. Taylor, W.E. A.D. Straus, Z.F. Grossman, C.A. Burton, and R. Burges, "Transcription from a Heat Inducible Promoter Causes Heat Shock Regulation of the Sigma Subunit of *E. coli* RNA Polymerase", *Cell*, 38, pp 371-81, 1984.
35. Cowing, D. W., J.C.A. Burdwell, E.A. Craig Woolford, R. W. Hendrin, and G. Gross., "Concensus Sequence for *Escherichia Coli* Heat Shock Gene Promotors", *Proc. Natl. Acad. Sci.*, 80, pp 2679, 1985.
36. Yano, R., M. Imai and T. Yura, "The Use of Operon Fusions in Studies of the Heat Shock Response: Effects of Altered Sigma 32 on Heat Shock Promoter Function in *Eschenchia Coli.*", *Mol. Gen. Genet* 207, pp 24, 1987.
37. Grossman, A.D., J. W Erickson and C.A. Gross. "The htpR Gene Product of *E. Coli* is a Sigma Factor for Heat Shock Promoters." *Cell*. 38, pp 383, 1984.
38. Lesley, S., N. Thompson and R. Burgess, "Studies of the Role of the *Escherichia Coli* Heat Shock Regulatory Protein σ^{32} by the Use of Monoclonal Antibodies", *J. Biol. Chem.*, 262, pp 5404, 1987.

39. Straus, D.B., W.A. Walter and C.A. Cross, "The Heat Shock Response of *E. coli* is Regulated by Changes in the Concentration of σ ^{32}" *Nature*, pp 329, 348, 1987.
40. Laudick, R. V., V. Vaughun, E. T. Lau, R.A. Van Bogelin, J. W. Erlckson, and F.C., "Nucleotide Sequence of the Heat Shock Regulatory Gene of *E. Coli* Suggests its Protein Product May be a Transcription Factor", *Cell*, 38, pp 175, 1984.
41. Ostermann, J., A.L. Horwich, W. Neupert, and F.U. Hertl, "Protein Folding in Mitochondria Required Complex Dormation with HSP60 and ATP Hydrolysis", *Nature*, 341, pp 125-130, 1989.
42. Pelham, H.R.B., "Speculations on the Functions of the Major Heat Shock and Glucose Regulated Proteins", *Cell*, 46, pp 959-61, 1986.
43. Pinto, M., M. Morange and O. Bensande, "Denaturation of Proteins During Heat Shock." *In vivo* Recovery of Solubility and Activity of Reporter Enzyme. *J. Biol. Cham.,* 266, pp 13941, 1991.
44. Rotterman, J.E., "Polypeptilde Chain Binding Proteins: Catalysis of Protein Folding and Related Processes in Cells", *Cell*, 59, pp 591, 1989.
45. Morgan, R.W. M.F. Christman, F.S. Jacobson, G. Storz, and B.N. Ames, "Hydrogen Peroxide Inducible Proteins in Salmonella Phimurium Overlap with Heat Shock and Other Stress Proteins", *Proc. Natl. Acad, Sci. USA*, 83, pp 8059, 1986.
46. Lipinska, B., 0. Fayet, L. Baird, L. and C., "Georgopoulos. Identification Characterization and Mapping of the *Eschenichria Coli* htrA Gene whose Product is Essential for Bacterial Growth only at Elevated Temperatures," *J. Bacteriol*., 171, pp 1574-84, 1989.
47. Wada, C., M. Imai and T. Yura, "Host Control of Plasmid Replication: Requirement for the σ Factor σ^{32} in Transcription of Mini-F Replication Initiator Gene", *Proc. Natl. Acad. Dcl.*, 84, pp 8849-53, 1987.
48. Erickson, J. W. and C.A. Gross, "Identificeation of σ E Subunit of *Eschenichia Coil* RNA Polymerase: A Second Alternate σ Factor Involved in High Temperautre Gene Expression", *Gene Dev*., 3, pp 1462, 1989.
49. Georgopoulos, C.P., "The *Eschenichria Coli* DnaA Initiation Protein: A Protein for All Seasons", *Trends Genet*, 5, pp 319-21, 1989.
50 Kubo, T., C.A. Towle, H.J. Maukin and B. V. Treadwell, "Stress Induced Proteins in Chondrocyles from Patients with Osteoarthritis", *Arthritis Rheum*, 28, pp 1140-45, 1985.
51. Melita, H.B., B.K. Popovich, and W.H. Dillman, "Ischemia Induces Changes in the Level of mRNAs Coding for Stress Protein 71 And Creatin Kinase", *M. Cir. Res*., 63, pp 512-17, 1988.
52. Gudon, P. T and L.E. Hightower, "Purification and Initial Characterization of the 71 Kilodalton Rat Heat Shock Protein and its Cognate as Fatty Acid Binding Proteins." *Biochemistry*, 25, pp 3231-39, 1986.
53. Giuidon, P. T. and L.E. Hightower, "The 73 Kilodalton Heat Shock Cognate Protein Purified From Rat Brain Contains Nonesterified Palmitic and Stearic Acids", *J. Cell. Physiol*., 128, pp 239-45, 1986.
54. Guffy, M.M., J.A. Rosenberger I. Simon and C.P. Burns, "Effect of Cellular Fatty Acid Alterations on Hyperthermic Sensitivity in Cultured LI210 Murine Leukemia Cells", *Cancer Res*., 42, pp 3625, 1982.
55. Collier, N.C. and M.J. Schlisinger, "The Dynamic State of Heat Shock Proteins in Chicken Embryo Fibroblasts", *J. Cell. Biol*. 103, pp 1495, 1986.
56. Mukhopadhyay, S.N. "Bioprocessing, Stability and Application of BamH1." *Bioprocess Engineering: The First Generation*, (T.K. Ghose. Ellis Harwood, Chichester eds.) U.K., pp 220-31, 1989.
57. Dubey, A.K. S.N. Mukhopadhyay, V.S. Bisaria, and T.K. Ghose, "Upstream Bioprocessing for Bam H1, Production: Effect of Cell Cultivation Variables", *Ind. Chem. Engr*., 33 (3), pp 16-21, 1991.

58. Welch, W.J., J.I. Garrels, G.P. Thomas, J.J.C. Lin, and J.R. Feramico, "Biochemical Characterization of the Mammalian Stress Proteins and Identification of Two Stress Proteins as Glucose and Ca^{2+} Ionophore Regulated Proteins", *J. Biol. Chem.*, 258, pp 7102-11, 1983.
59. Das. D.K. and R.M. Engelman, "Mechanism of Free Radical Generation in Ischemic and Reperfused Myocardium", *Oxygen Radicals: Systemic Events and Disease Processes*, pp. 97-128, (D.K. Das and W.B. Essmann. Krager, eds.), 1989.
60. McCord, J., "Oxygen Derived Free Radicals in Post Ischemic Tissue Injury", *N. Eng. J. Med.*, 312 (3), pp 159-63, 1985.
61. Pryor, W.A., "Free Radical Reactions and their Importance in Biochemical Systems", *Fed. Proceedings*, 32, pp 1862-69, 1973.
62. Torrielli, M. V. and M.U. Dianzani, "Free Radicals in Inflammatory Disease," *Free Radicals in Molecular Biology, Aging and Disease*, pp 355-79, (D. Armstrong et al. eds.), Raven Press, New York, 1984.
63. Lu, D., N. Maulik, I.I. Moraru, D.L. Kreutzer, and D.K. Das, "Molecular Adaptation of Vascular Endothelial Cells to Oxidative Stress", *Am. J. Physiol.* (*Cell*), In press.
64. Chance, B., H. Sios, and A. Boveris, "Hydroperoxide Metabolism in Mammalian Organs", *Physiol. Rev.*, 59, pp 527-605, 1979.
65. Lowen, P.C., "Requlaticns of Catalse Synthesis in Molecular Biology and Free Radical Scavenging Systerms", *Current Communications in Cell Molecular Biology*, pp. 97-115, (J.G. Scandalios, ed.) CSHL Press, 1992.
66. Meir, E. and E. Yagil., "Regulation of *Eschenchia Coli* Catalases by Anaerobiosis and Catabolic Repression", *Curr. Microbiol.*, 20, pp 139, 1990.
67. Haliwell, B. and O.I. Aruoma, "DNA Damage by Oxygen Derived Species: Its Mechanism and Measurement Using Chromatographic Methods", *Molecular Biology of Free Radical Scavenging Systems*, pp. 47-67, (J.G. Scandalios, ed.), CSHL Press, New York, 1992.
68. Loftler, M.A., "Cytokinetic Approach to Determine the Range of O_2 Dependence of Pyrimidive (deoxy) Nucleotide Biosynthesis Relevant for Cell Proliferation", *Cell Prolif.* 25, pp 169-79, 1992.
69. Ono, M., H. Kahda, T. Kawaguchi, M. Ohkira, C. Seliya, M. Namiki, A. Takeyasu, and N. Taniguchi, "Induction of Mn-Superoxide Dismutase by Tumor Necrosis Factor, Interleukin-1 and Interleukin-6 in Human Hepatoma Cells", *Biochem. Biophys. Res. Commun.*, pp 1100-1107, 1982, 1992.
70. Kaur, P., W.J. Welch, and J. Sakiatvala. "Interleukin-I and Tumor Necrosis Factor Increase Phosphorylation of the Small Heat Shock Protein Effcets", Fibreblasts Hepz and U 937 cells, FEBS Letters, 258 (2), pp 269-73, 1989.
71. Maulik, N., R.M. Engelman D. Lu, J. Wei, and D.K. Das., "Reduction of Mycardial Ischemia Reperfusion Injury by Molecular Adaptation of Heart With Interleukin–1α." Circulation in press.
72. Francis, D. and P. W. Bariow, "Temperature and the Cell Cycle", *Plants and Temperature,* pp. 181-201, (S.P. Long and F.I. Woodword. eds.) *Soc. For Expt. Biol.,* 1988.
73. Dulhunty, A.F., "The Voltage Activation of Contraction in Skeletal Muscle", *Prog. Biophys. Mol. Biol.* 57 (3) pp 181-223, 1992.
74. S.N. Mukhopadhyay, Proc. 3rd *A.P. Biochem. Engg.* pp. 511-513, NUS, Singapore, 1994.
75. Barua, P.K. D. W. Dyer, and M.E. Neiders, "Effect of Iron Limitation on Bacteroids Gingivalis" *Oral Microbiol. Lmmunol.* 5, pp 263, 1990.
76 Jones, P.G., R.A van Bogelen, and F.C. Neidhardt, "Induction of Proteins to Low Temperature in *Eschenichia Coli.,*" *J. Bacteriol.*, 169, pp 2092-95, 1987.
77. Goldstein, J., N.S. Pollitt, and M. Inouye, "Major Cold Shock Protein of *Eschenchia Coli.*", *Proc. Natl. Acad. Sci. USA*, 87, pp 283-87, 1990.

78. Duman, I. and K. Horwath, "The Role of Hemolymph Proteins in the Cold Tolerence of Insects," *Annu. Rev. Physiol.*, 45, pp 261-70, 1983.
79. Broeze, R.J., C.J. Solomon, and D.H. Pope, "Effects of Low Temperature on *in vivo* and *in vitro* Protein Synthesis in *Escherichia Coli* and Pseudomonas Fluorescens", *J. Becteriol.*, 134, pp 861-74, 1978.
80. Kondo, K, and M. Inouti., "TIPI: A Cold Shock Inducible Gene of Saccharomyces Cerevisial", *J. Biol. Chem.*, 266, pp 17537-44, 1991.
81. Mauiak, M. and W. Nollen, "A Developmentally Regulated Membrane Protein Gene in Dictyostelium Discoideum is Also Induced by Heat Shock and Cold Shock", *Mol Cell. Biol.*, 8 (1), pp 153-59, 1988.
82. Taubenberger, A.M., I. Hamann, A. Noegel, and G. Gerisch, "Ubiquitin Gene Expression in *Dictyostelium* is Induced by Heat and Cold Shock, Cad Mum and Inhibitors of Protein Synsthesis", *J. Cell. Sci.*, 90, pp 51-58, 1988.
83. Schindelin, H., M. Herrler, G. Willimsky M.A. Marahid, and U. Heinemann, "Over Production, Crystallization and Preliminary X-ray Diffraction Studies of the Major Cold Shock Problem From *Bacillus subtilis* cspB.", *Proteins: Structure, Function and Genetics*, pp 120-24, 1992.
84. Hahn, G.M. and G.C. Li. *Thermotolerance, Thermoresistance, and Thermosensitization in Stress Proteins in Biology and Medicine*, (R.I. Morimoto, A. Tissieres, and C. Georgopoulos, eds.), CSHL Press, pp 79-100, 1990.
85. Mollenhauer, J. and A. Schulmelster, "The Humoral Immune Response to Heat Shock Proteins", *Experientia,* 48, pp 644, 1992.
86. Amheim, N., "Polymerase Chain Reaction Strategy", *Ann. Rev. Biochem.*, 61, pp 131-36, 1992.
87. Owens, G.P., W.E. Hahn and J.J. Cohen, "Identifications of mRNAs Associated with Programmed Cell Death in Immature Thymocytes", *Mol. & Cell. Biol.*, 11 (8), pp 41, 77, 1991.
88. Chemczynskl, P. and N. Sacchl, "Singel Step Method of RNA Isolation by Acid Quanidinium-Thiocyanate-Phenol-Coloroforrn Extraction", *Anal. Biochem.*, 162, pp 156-59, 1987.
89. Gilisin, V., R. Crkvenjakov, and C. Byus, "Ribonucleic Acid Isolated by Cesim Chioride Centrifugation", *Biochemistry*, 13, pp 2633, 1974.
90. Samlerook, J., E.E. Fritsch, and T. Maniatis. *Molecular Cloning: A LAboratory Manual*, pp. 743-45, CSHL Press, New York, 1983.
91. McMaster, G.K. and G.G. Carmichael, "Analysis of Single and Double-Stranded Nucleic Acids on Polyacrylamide and Agarose Gels by Using Glyonal and Acridine Orange", *Proc. Natl. Acad. Sci.*, 74, pp 4835, 1977.
92. Khandjian, E. W., "Optimized Hybridization of DNA Blotted and Fixed to Nitrocellulose and Nylon Membranes", *Biotechnoiogy*, 5, pp 165, 1987.
93. O'Farrell, P.H., "High Resolution Two-Dimensional Electrophoresis of Protein", *J. Bioi. Chem.*, 250 (10), pp 4007-4021, 1975.
94. Laemmli, U.K., "Cleavage of Structural Proteins During the Assembly of the Head of Bacteriophage", *Nature*, 227, pp 680-85, 1970.
95. L.I. G.C. Li, Y.K. Liu J. Y. Mak, L. Chen, and W.M. Flee, "Thermal Response of Rat Fibroblasts Stably Transformed with Human 70 KDa Heat Shock Protein Encoding Gene." *Proc. Natl. Acad. Sci. USA*. 88, pp 1681, 1991.
96. St. S., "Enzymatic Cascade Yields Novel Saccharides", C&EN, pp 34, 1992.

Chapter

15

BIOPROCESS PLANT DESIGN CALCULATIONS: PENICILLIN PRODUCTION SYSTEM

15.1 INTRODUCTION

In any process technology industry the needs of design engineers and consultants as well as those of students/personnel with adequate background is essential. Process Biotechnology is no exception for the same. This chapter is based upon my experience gained in consultancy at IDPL, Rishikesh. I was actively involved in teaching courses in process biotechnology equipment design at IIT Delhi for a long time. I have supervised research and development of fermenters, and have acted as consultant in the field.

The purpose to include this chapter in the book is to consolidate the basic/fundamental concepts, industrial practices and theoretical relationships useful in the design of fermentation processing equipment. Thus objective in this chapter is to expose the readers/students systematically on the steps involved in upstream design process calculations and downstream processing calculations for separation/recovery of the product.

The computational approaches presented here is with respect to penicillin fermentation case. I wish to express my appreciation to the then IDPL, Rishikesh industry authority who took active interest in industry-academia interaction to foster the growth of process biotechnology in the country.

15.2 DEFINING THE DESIGN PROBLEM

15.2.1 Statement

A plant is to be designed for the manufacture of 10,000 kg annum of Amine penicillin salt from a fermentation broth containing 5000 units/ml whole broth.

15.2.2 Raw Materials

Fermentation broth at 5000 u/ml whole broth commercial H_2SO_4 98% pure by weight. Butyl acetate 99% pure by weight with specific gravity of 0.88 at 20°C in aqueous buffer solution.

15.2.3 Services

Dry saturated steam at 4 atm. absolute. Compressed air at 3 atm. absolute at a temp. of 70°C which can be assumed to have no water content. Cooling water at 18°C. Electricity of 440 V 3-phase 50 Hz and ambient air temp. 15°C

15.2.4 Description of Process[1-15]

Penicillin is manufactured by a fermentation process batchwise at a temperatuere of 25°C in agitated vessels supplied continuously with sterile air. The biochemical engineering design of the process need not be carried out and for this design problem the fermenter broth at a potency of 5000 u/ml whole broth is the starting point of the extraction process.

The broth from the fermenter is passed to a filter which separates the solid (mycelium) from the aqueous liquors. A 5% water wash is used on the filter and added to the broth to improve the efficiency of the process. The solids from the filter are discarded and the aqueous product containing the penicillin in passed forward for concentration and purification by liquid/liquid extraction and then for crystallisation, filtration and drying to produce an amine salt of penicillin which is later recrystallised under sterile conditions to yield a high purity product.

The liquid/liquid extraction is carried out in three steps. The first step is carried out by adjusting the pH of the aqueous phase from the filter with acid betwen 2.4 & 2.5 and extracting the penicillin into butyl acetate to yield a half rich butyl acetate solution. The spent aqueous solution from this first step is passed for recovery of the dissolved butyl acetate.

At step two, the half rich butyl acetate is extracted with buffer at a pH of 6 to yield a penicillin rich buffer solution. The butyl acetate phase from step two is passed for recovery of the butyl acetate.

At step 3 the pH is again adjusted with acid to a low pH and the penicillin reextracted into butyl acetate to yield a solution of potency of 50,000 u\ml. The aqueous phase is fed with the aqueous phase from step one for recovery of the butyl acetate.

For the purpose of this question the design can be considered complete at the rich butyl acetate solution of 50,000 u/ml. Normally amine salt of pencillin is precipitated from this rich butyl acetate solution. The efficiency of this precipitation process can be considered to the 75% giving a penicillin amine salt of potency 1300 u/mg.

The solvent recovery is undertaken using two seperate columns. The first column is a pot still used to recover the solvent resulting from step two of the extraction train together with the solvent recovered from the crystallisation process. The second column is a stripping column used for recovering solvent from aqueous stream resulting from steps one and three of the extraction train. In this second column the feed is passed to the column through a heat exchanger and the aqueous bottom from the column are passed through this exchanger to recover the heat before dumping to drain. The product from this second column is obtained as an azeotrope which is seperated in a decanter to yield a clean solvent product. The bottom phase from decanter is fed back to the column for recovery of the associated solvent.

15.2.5 Data Listing

Input power to fermenter liquor : 1Kw/m^3 of fermenter volume. Airflow : 1m^3 every 5 mins measured at 0°C & 1 atm/m^3 of fermenter vol. Mycelial concentration 20% v/v.

Table 15.1 Effect of pH on half-life of penicillin G at 20°C (time in hours to inactivate 50%)

pH	2.0	3.0	4.0	5.0	5.8	6.0	7.0	7.5	8.0
Time, hr	0.31	1.7	12	92	315	336	281	178	125

Table 15.2 Distribution of penicilin G between equal volumes of butyl acetate and aqueous solution at various pH values (Assume independent of temperature.)

pH of aqueous phase.	1.1	2.1	3.3	4.4	4.8	5.8	6.6
Distribution ratio. $\frac{\text{Concentration in butyl acetate}}{\text{Concentration in aqueous phase}}$	64	25	10.4	1.38	0.595	0.102	0.0204

The buffer solution can be assumed to give the correct pH at step two of the extraction for any volume ratio. It can also be assumed to have a sp. gravity of 1.0. The acid added at steps one and three of the extraction can be assumed to be 2% by volume of the aqueous penicillin stream.

Sp. gravity fermenter broth : 1.03
Sp. heat of fermenter broth : 1.0
Thermal conductivity of fermenter broth : 0.34 Btu ft/ft^2.°F/hr
Viscosity of fermenter broth : 1000 centipoises

The heat evolution of the fermenter broth varies through the cycle but for case of calculation can be taken as constant throughout the fermentation at 3.5 kW/m^3 of broth.

From harvesting a fermenter to rebatching, it takes two weeks which includes 288 hrs actual fermentation.

Fermenter working volume : 20m^3
Fermenter agitator speed : 100 rev/min.
Solubility of butyl acetate in water :
at 15°C 0.8% w/w
at 20°C 1.0% w/w
Solubility of water in butyl acetate :
at 10°C 1.2% w/w

at 15°C	1.28% w/w
at 20°C	1.37% w/w
at 30°C	1.55% w/w

Interfacial tension of butyl acetate-water at 20°C :	14 dynes/cm
Surface tension of butyl acetate at 20°C :	27.6 dynes/cm
Viscosity of butyl acetate at 20°C :	0.7 c.p.
Azeotropic butyl acetate/water is 73.3/26.7 w/w	
Boiling:	90.2°C
Specific heat of butyl acetate :	0.459 cal/g at 20°C
Specific gravity of butyl acetate :	0.88 at 20°C

Table 15.3 Vapour pressure of butyl acetate

Temperature (°C)	– 16	0	10	15	20	40	60	68	100	118	126.5
Vapour pressure (mm Hg)	1	3	5.7	7.5	10.0	30	70	100	340	600	760

15.2.6 Plant Design Scopes

1. Prepare a material balance for the extraction train including the solvent recovery, expressed in kg/m.
2. Prepare a heat balance for the fermentation, extraction and solvent recovery but excluding the crystallization and subsequent stages.
3. Prepare a complete process flow diagram. This diagram must show :
   (a) All item of equipment approximately to scale and as far as possible in correct elevation. Only one fermenter need be shown in this diagram. The type of internal construction of vessels such as plates, packing, heating and cooling coils, etc., should be indicated. All items must be numbered to correspond with the equipment schedule.
   (b) All major pipelines. One specimen pipe size calculation only need be given.
   (c) Detailed instrumentation of the liquid-liquid extraction process and the solvent recovery systems only need be given.
4. Prepare a detailed chemical engineering design of :
   (a) The liquid/liquid extraction stages calculating the flow ratio, at each of the steps. Compare the performance characteristics of pulsed columns, mixer settlers Podbielniak contactors and produce reasoned recommendations for the choice of unit. Write notes on the pilot plant investigations that would be necessary in the development of full scale plant.
   (b) The heat transfer system in the fermenter and calculate the number of fermenters required.
   (c) The butyl acetate stripping column to recover the solvent from steps one & three of the extraction train. Determine the size of the heat exchanger for heat recovery and design the condenser system. Include a sketch of the installation showing the

column; heat exchanger and decanter. In the design of the column special care has to be exercised to the material causing heavy fouling of the surfaces.

5. Make the necessary calculations for the drailed design of one fermenter which is basically a vertical cylindrical tank with a control stirred and internal cooling coil. The shaft and impellers should be designed to give the correct power input assuming the broth is a Newtonian fluid but it is not required to design the gear box and motor drive. Submit detailed dimensional sketch suitable for submission to a drawing office.
6. Prepare an equipment schedule listing all items of equipment giving approximate sizes, capacities, etc.

15.3 FERMENTER DESIGN CALCULATION ITEMS[6-18]

15.3.1 Number of Fermenters

Quantity of amine salt of penicillin required per year 10,000 kgm.
Quantity of penicillin in salt, 1300 u/mg.
Unit of penicillin required per year.

$$= 10{,}000 \times 1300 \times 1000 \times 1000$$

$$= 13 \times 10^{12} \text{ units.}$$

Assuming over all efficiency of 45% and giving ample time for plant cleaning and maintenance, a year has been taken equivalent to 44 working weeks. No. of times a fermenter can be harvested in a year is 22. Qantity of penicillin available from the fermenter per harvesting.

$$= 5000 \times 20 \times 1000 \times 1000 \text{ units}$$

$$= 10 \times 10^{10} \text{ units}$$

$$\text{No. of fermenters required} = \frac{3 \times 10^{12}}{5000 \times 1000 \times 1000 \times 20 \times 22 \times 0.45}$$

$$= 14$$

One fermenter can be harvested daily.

15.3.2 Related Design Aspects

1. Specifications of fermenter

The following specifications have been selected.

Dia.	= 8' – 6" (8 ft 6 in)
Area of cross section	= 56.6 ft^2
Working Height	
Vol. of broth.	= 20 M^3 = 707 ft^3.
Vol. of tubes & accessories	= 30 ft^3.
Total vol.	= 737 ft^3.

Working height $= \dfrac{737}{56.6} = 13$ ft.

Actual height = 18 ft.

Height of fermenter = 18 ft.

Working pressure = 5 psi (G)

2. Power input calculations

Power input was worked out with various sizes of impellers and the following size was found suitable.

The agitator is composed of three flat-six bladded radial flow turbines attached to a shaft rotated at 100 rpm.

D_i = Diameter of impeller = 3'

D_t = Diameter of tank = 3' 6"

H_w = Working height of tank = 13'

W_i = Width of the blade = 7.2"

L_i = Blade length = 9"

$D_t/D_i = 2.833$

$H_w/D_i = 4.333$

$W_i/D_i = 0.2$

$L_i/D_i = 0.25$

Width of baffle = 10"

The bottom impeller is located 40" above the tank bottom and distance between succeeding impeller is 56".

A. Aeration :Aeration rate is $1M^3/M^3$ of broth every 5 mins

at NTP = 20/5 = 4 M^3/min at N.T.P.

$$= \frac{4 \times 298 \times 760}{273 \times 1010} = 3.286 \text{ M}^3\text{/min at } 25°\text{C and } 5 \text{ lb/in}^2$$

Power for agitation :

Modified Reynold's number is given by

$$R_e = \frac{n \cdot D_i^2 \cdot \rho}{\mu}$$

Where n = No. of revolution per hour

= 6000

$$D_i^2 = 9 \text{ ft}^2$$

Density of broth $\rho = 62.4 \times 1.03$

$= 64.4 \text{ lb/ft}^3.$

Viscosity of broth μ = 1000 c.p. = 2420 lb/ft.hr

$$R_e = \frac{6000 \times 64.4 \times 9}{2420} = 1440.$$

Now, reading corresponding to the value of the Power Number from the Fig. 15.1, N_P = Power No. = 5

$$N_P = \frac{P_g}{\rho \cdot n^3 \cdot D_i^5}$$

where P = Power required by impeller.

g = Acceleration due to gravity

N_P = 5

ρ = 64.4 lb/ft3.

$$n = \frac{100}{60} = 1.666 \text{ rev./sec}$$

$$P_g = \frac{N_p \cdot \rho \cdot n^3 \cdot D_i^5}{g} = \frac{5 \times 64.4 \times 1.666^3 \times 3^5}{32.2 \times 550} = 20.4 \text{ H.P.}$$

Since the geometrical ratio in this case deviates from the curve used for power number a correction factor is applied which is approximately expressed as below:

$$\text{Correlation factor } F_c = \sqrt{\frac{(D_t/D_i)*(H_w/D_i)*}{(D_t/D_i)\cdot(H_w/D_i)}}$$

where * are the values for the tank in question.

$$F_c = \left\{\frac{(2.833 \times 4.333)}{2.83 \times 4.3}\right\}^{1/3} = 1.168$$

∴ Corrected H. P. = 20.4 ×1.168 = 23.8 HP.

Based on the observation[13] that from the base upward the three identical impellers take some, 60, 30 and 10 percent of the total shaft power respectively one can then compute the total power (P_g) input

$$P_g = \frac{23.8}{0.6} = 39.6 \text{ H.P.}$$

(ii) Aeration Number : Aeration number can be calculated as follows[6]

$$N_a = \frac{Q}{n \times D_i^3}$$

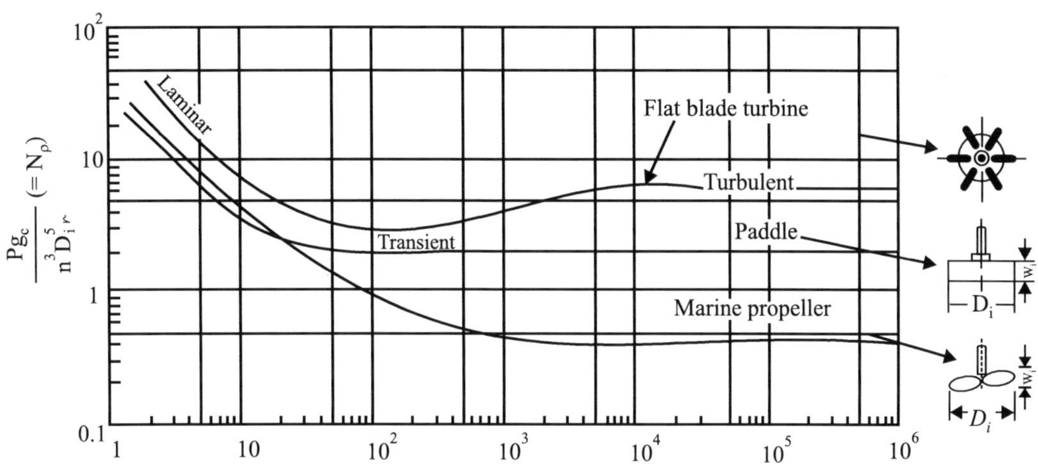

Fig. 15.1

Where Q = Aeration rate, vol/unit time

n = No. of rev./unit time

D_i = Dia. of impeller

N_a = Aeration number

Q = 3.286 M^3/min

= 3.286 × 35.3/4 = 116 ft^3/min

n = 100, D_i = 3 ft.

$$N_a = \frac{116}{100 \times 33} = \frac{1.16}{27} = 4.3 \times 10^{-2}$$

From the Fig. 15.2 using curve A we get.

$P_g/P = 0.69$

P_g = Power input in gassed broth

P = Power input in unaerated broth

Hence

$P_g = P \times 0.68$

$= 39.6 \times 0.68 = 26.95$ H.P.

$= 26.95 \times 0.7457$

$= 20.05$ kW

$= 20$ kW power input by impeller.

Percentage hold up of air can be calculated from Fig. 15.3.

P_g/V = power input/unit vol. of ungassed liquid

$= 39.6.20$ HP/M^3.

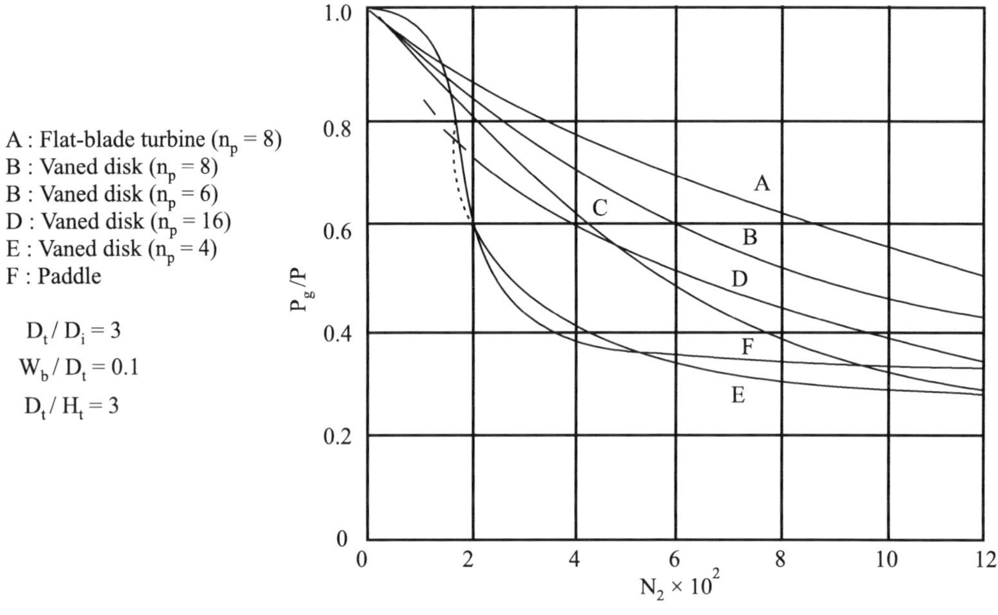

Fig. 15.2

Aeration rate = 116 ft^3/min

V_g = velocity of air on empty vessel basis

$= 116 \times 60/56.6 = 123$ ft/m.

$$(P_g/V)^{0.4} \times V^{0.5} = (39.6/20)^{0.4} \times (123)^{0.6}$$

$= 8.6$

Air hold up, $H_0 = 7.5\%$ from Fig. 15.3

The motor required for driving the impeller shaft should be of 60H.P. variable speed which can be started only at 60 rpm and the speed can be increased to 100 rpm when aeration starts.

Since the rheological property of penicillin fermentation broth by *P. chrysogenum* increases from Newtonian to highly non-Newtonian range (30 cp to > 1000 cp) it required to consider variable speed motor of high rating as a safety factor and that is why 60H.P. has been considered.

3. Heat transfer design of fermenter

(i) Heat Input : (1) By air.

Vol. of air = 20 × 60/5. = 240 tr^3/hr at N.T.P.

Weight of air = 240 × 29/22.4 = 310.8 kg/hr.

Air inlet temp. = 70°C.

Air outlet temp. = 25°C.

Sp. heat. of air at mean temp. = 0.238.

Heat lost by air = 310.8 × 2.203 × 45 × 0.238

= 7300 lb-cal/hr.

(2) Heat of fermentation = 20 × 3.5 = 70 kW.

(3) Heat input due to agitation (assuming that 5 – 10% of the power input is converted into heat)

= 2 kW.

$$\text{Total of (1) + (2) + (3)} = \left(72 \times 3414 \times \frac{1}{1.8}\right) + 7300$$

$$= 140500 + 7300$$

$$= 147800 \text{ lb} - \text{cal/hr}$$

(ii) Heat Output : (i) By evaporation of water

Pw_0 = Vapour pressure of water at 25°C = 24 mm Hg.

P = Air pressure = 1010 mm Hg.

Humidity of saturated air.

$$= \frac{Pw_0}{P - Pw_0} \times \frac{M_w}{M_a} \begin{matrix}\text{(Mol. wt. of water)} \\ \text{(Mol wt. of air)}\end{matrix}$$

$$= \frac{24}{1010 - 24} \times \frac{18}{29} = 0.01511$$

Quantity of dry air = 310.8 kg/hr.

Quantity of water evaporated = 310.8 × 0.01511

= 4.7 kg/hr.

= 10.34 lg/hr.

Latent heat of water at 25°C = 583 cals.

Heat removed by cooling water = 147800 – 6000

= 142000 lb – cal/hr.

Fermenter is insulated from outside and no loss or gain of heat, is assumed, from any other source.

Cooling water (c.w.) temp, = 18°C

If c.w. exit temp. = 22°C.

$$\text{Quantity of cooling water required} = \frac{14\,2000}{22-18} = 35500 \text{ lb/hr}$$

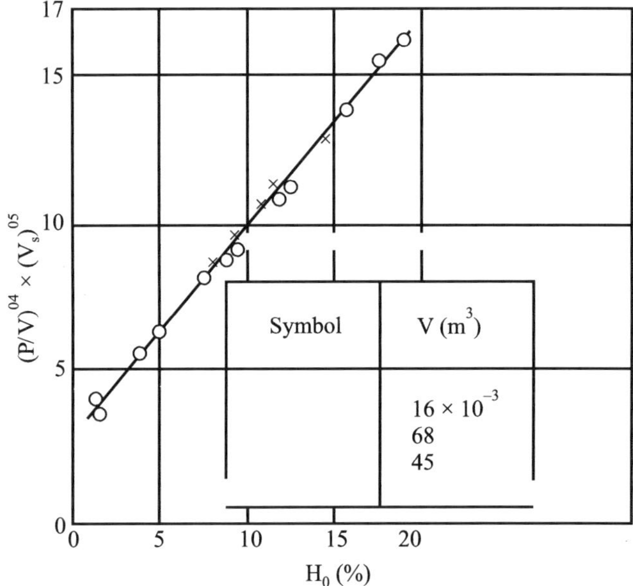

Fig. 15.3 Estimation of hold-up, H_0, with power input per unit volume of ungassed liquid, P/V, and nominal linear velocity of V_s of air

Sp. gravity of water at 20°C = 0.997

$$\text{Vol. of water required} = \frac{35500}{3600 \times 0997 \times 62.4}$$

$$= 0.136 \text{ ft}^3/\text{sec}.$$

If water velocity = 3 ft/sec.

Area of cross section required for flow

$$= \frac{0.136 \times 144}{3} = 6.5 \text{ in}^2.$$

Area of flow of a 2" N.B. Pipe.

$$= 3.35 \text{ in}^2.$$

Area of flow of two pipes

$$= 3.35 \times 2 = 6.7 \text{ in}^2.$$

Two pipes in parallel of 2" N.B. will serve the purpose.

(iii) Heat Transfer Coefficient [14] : Assuming an over all heat transfer coefficient of 80 lb-cal/hr-ft^2. °C The following pipe size is selected. Normal pipe size IPS shedule no. 40 (Table II from Kern)[14].

O.D. = 2.38"

I.D. = 0.067"

Flow area = 3.35 in^2.

Outside surface = 0.622 ft^2/ft

Weight = 3.66 lb/ft.

$$\text{L.M.T.D.} = \frac{(25-18)-(25-22)}{\ln 7/3} = 4.7°\text{C}.$$

A. Calculation of coil inside film coefficients

The inside film coefficient is given by the relation[19]

$$h_i = k/d\left(1+3.5\frac{d}{dc}\right) \times 0.023\,(u\,\rho d/\mu)^{0.8}\,(C_p\,\mu/k)^{0.4}$$

Where h_i = Inside film heat transfer coefficient.

d = Internal diameter of the tube = 2/12 ft.

k = Thermal conductivity of water

= 0.35 lb-cal/hr ft^2 °C/ft. [from Kern]

d_c = Dia. of coil = 6 ft = 72".

u = Vel. of water = 3 f.p.s.

ρ = Density of water = 62.4 lb/ft^3.

μ = Viscosity of water = 2.40 lg/ft-hr.

C_p = Sp. heat of water = 1.

$$h_i = \frac{0.35\times 12}{2}\left(1+3.5\frac{2}{72}\right)\times 0.023\left(\frac{3\times 3600\times 62.4\times 2}{12\times 2.40}\right)^{0.8}\times\frac{(1\times 2.4)^{0.4}}{0.35}$$

$$= 2.1 \times 1.0928 \times 0.023 \times (49790)^{0.8} \times (6.857)^{0.4}$$

$$= 2.33 \times 0.023 \times 5448 \times 2.16$$

$$= 632 \text{ lb - cal/hr ft}^2\ °\text{C}.$$

B. Calculation of coil outside film coefficient

Chilton, Drew & Jebens gave the following relation for heat transfer to fluid in agitated vessels, heated or cooed by submerged coil or jackets.[15]

$$\frac{\lambda \cdot D_i}{k} = a \cdot \left(\frac{L^2 \cdot N\rho}{\mu}\right)^{0.66} \times \left(\frac{C \cdot \mu}{\rho_k}\right)^{0.6} \times \left(\frac{\mu_b}{\mu_s}\right)^{0.14}$$

Ackley (Chem. Engg. 67, 133 (1960)) has shown that this type of equation can be used to estimate film coefficients for both inner wall of the vessel and the outer wall of tubular surface contained within the vessel.

Average value of coefficient ‘a’ for turbine agitator and coil surface has been given as 1.50.

$$\frac{L^2 \cdot N\rho}{\mu} = \text{Reynolds No. for agitated liquid}$$

$$\frac{\mu_b}{\mu_s} = \frac{\text{Viscosity in bulk}}{\text{Viscosity in wall}}$$

D_j = I .D. of vessel = 8' 6".

K = Thermal conductivity of broth

= 0.34 lb - cal/hr/t^2 °C/ft.

a = 1.5.

Re No. = 1440. Calculated earlier.

c = Sp. heat of broth = 1.0.

μ = Viscosity of broth = 1000 c.p. = 2420 lb/ft.hr.

μ_s = Since the temp. difference is small and the viscosity index is not known the ratio $\frac{\mu_b}{\mu_s}$ is assumed to be equal to 1.

h_0 = Outside film coefficient of coil.

$$h_0 \times \frac{17}{2 \times 0.34} = 1.5\ (1440)^{2/3} \times \left(\frac{1 \times 2420}{0.34}\right)^{1/3} \times 1$$

or
$$h_0 = \frac{1.5 \times 127.619.23 \times 2 \times 0.34}{17}$$

$$= 147 \text{ lb-cals/hr. ft}^2\text{. °C}$$

C. Heat transfer in two phase flow[16]

Kudrika *et al.*[16] have presented rates in terms at h_{TP} / h_L [the ratio of two phase to single phase heat transfer coefficients] which illustrates effectively the increase in heat transfer rates caused by the addition of gas phase to liquid flow.

The experiment was done with water-air and ethylene glycerol-air system. with L /D = 14.

If gas holdup is an indication of the term u_g/u_L (ratio of gas/liquid flow) the ratio in fermenter is 0.07 and the curve of Re. No. 1700 in Fig. 15.4 will give a ratio h_{TP} / h_L = 1.3.

Viscosity of broth = 1000 c.p. which can be due to solid mycelia.

Another contribution to turbulence by air is high pressure drop, and subsequent high velocity while entering the liquid phase.

The air has not cooled before coming to fermenter because at high temperature the kinetic energy will be more and 70°C is not an unsafe temperature especially when it rapidly drops of broth temperature. Moreover cooling of air to broth temperature before it enters the fermenter will be uneconomical.

So aeration will increase the true outside film heat transfer coefficient and as a conservative estimate a value of

$$h_{TP} / h_L = 1.2 \text{ is assumed.}$$

$$h_0 = 147 \times 1.2 = 176 \text{ lb-cal/hr-ft}^2 \text{ °C.}$$

Overall heat transfer coeffi. based on outside area of the coil is given by

$$\frac{1}{u_0} = \frac{1}{h_0} + \frac{x_w\, d_0}{k_w\, d_w} + \frac{d_0}{k_i d_i} + R_0 + \frac{R_i\, d_0}{d}$$

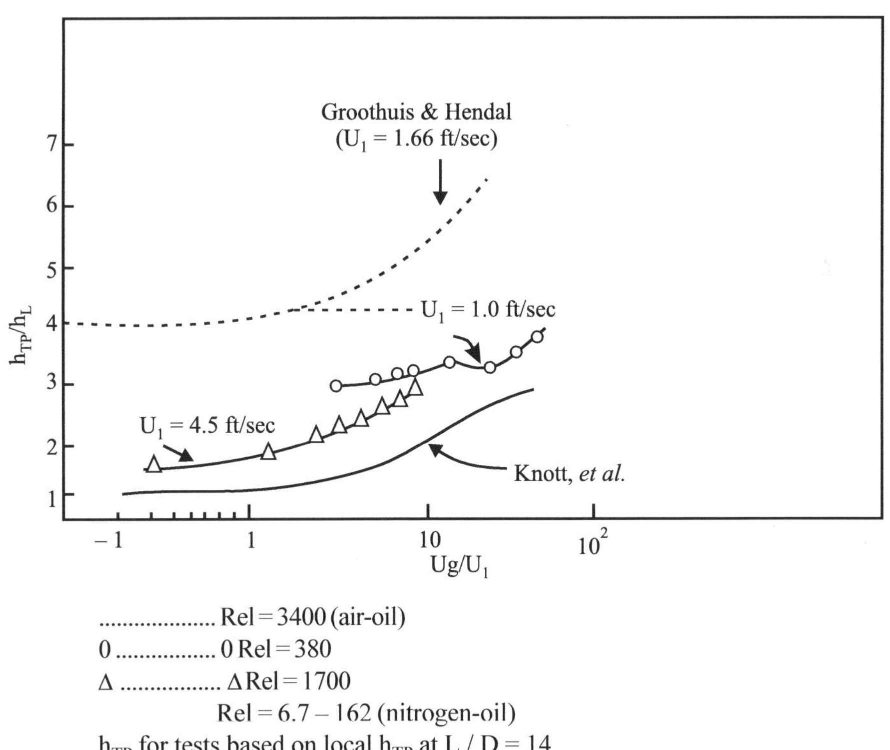

.... Rel = 3400 (air-oil)

0 .... 0 Rel = 380

Δ .... Δ Rel = 1700

Rel = 6.7 – 162 (nitrogen-oil)

h_{TP} for tests based on local h_{TP} at L / D = 14

Fig/ 15.4 Comparison of air-ethylene glycerol results

Where K_w = Thermal conductivity of tube wall

x_w = Thickness

h_0 = 176 lb-cal/hr ft^2 °C

$$x_w = \frac{0.19}{12}\text{ ft}$$

d_w = 2.19", d_0 = 2.38". d = 2".

h_i = 632 lb-cal/hr ft^2 °C

R_0 = 0.003 assumed

R_i = 0.001

k_w = 96. lb-cal/hr ft^2 °C (from kern)

$$\frac{1}{u_0} = \frac{1}{176} + \frac{0.19 \times 2.38}{12 \times 26 \times 2.19} + \frac{2.38}{2 \times 632} + 0.003 + \frac{0.001 \times 2.38}{2}$$

$$= 0.0056 + 0.000633 + 0.00188 + 0.003 + 0.0019$$

$$= 0.01238$$

u_0 = 80 lb-cal/hr ft^2 °C

Q = u . A . ΔT

Q = 142000 lb-cal/hr.

u = 80 lb-cal/hr. ft ± 2°C

ΔT = 4.7°C

$$A = \frac{142000}{80 \times 4.7} = 378 \text{ ft}^2.$$

Surface area of tubes = 0.622 ft^2/ft^2

Length of pipe required = $\frac{378}{0.622}$ = 607 ft.

Length of one tube = 18.75 ft.

No. of tubes = $\frac{607}{18.75}$ = 32.4 = 32 tubes (say)

Two sets of coils with 16 turns each is used

Coil dia. = 6′

If height to be covered is = 12′

Pitch of turns = $\frac{12 \times 12}{32}$ = 4.5″.

Clearance between turn = 4.5 – 2.38 = 2.12″.

which is a satisfactory arrangement.

4. Chemical engineering design of fermenter[15]

Pr. Drop Across Coils

$u = 3$ ft/sec. $= 3 \times 3600$ ft/hr

$\mu = 2.42$ lb/ft hr.

$\rho = 62.4$ lb/ft^3.

$$\text{Re no.} = \left(\frac{u \cdot \rho \cdot d}{\mu}\right) = \frac{3 \times 3600 \times 62.4 \times 2}{12 \times 2.42}$$

$$= 46400.$$

$$\frac{d_c}{d} = \frac{\text{diameter of coil}}{\text{diameter of tube}} = \frac{72}{2} = 36. \text{ It lies between } 15 - 860.$$

$$N_{Re} \text{ crit} = 20000 \times \left(\frac{d}{d_c}\right)^{0.32}$$

$$= 6353$$

Re no. is $> N_{Re}$ crit.

$$N_{Re}\left(\frac{d}{d_c}\right)^2 = \frac{46400}{(36)^2} = \frac{46400}{1296} = 35.8$$

Since it lies between 0.034 to 300, the following equation applies:

f_c = Friction factor.

$$f_c\left(\frac{D_c}{D}\right)^{1/2} = 0.0073 + 0.076\left[N_{Re}\left(\frac{D}{D_c}\right)^2\right]^{-\frac{1}{4}}$$

$$f_c\,(36)^{1/2} = 0.0073 + 0.076\,(35.8)^{-1/4}$$

$$= 0.0064$$

$$F = \left(\frac{4 \cdot f_c \cdot l}{D}\right) \cdot \frac{v^2}{2g}$$

F = Loss in ft lb force/ft. of fluid flowing

l = Length of pipe = 303 ft.

v = Fluid velocity.

D = Temperature dia.

g = Acceleration due to gravity

$$F = \frac{4 \times 0.0064 \times 303 \times 12}{2} \times \frac{9}{32.2}$$

$$= 13.9 \text{ ft.}$$

$$\Delta p = F \times \rho = 13.9 \times \frac{62.4}{144}$$

$$= 6 \text{ lb/in}^2 \text{ (satisfactory)}$$

Heat balance over fermenter in terms of *k*-cal/hr. Datum temp. (0°C).

Heat in				*Heat out*			
	Qty. kg/hr	Temp. °C	Heat k-cal		Qty. kg/tr.	Temp. °C	Heat k-cal.
Air	310.8	70	4680	Air	310.8	25	1670
Fermentation & agitation			63700	Evaporation			2710
Cooling water	16100	18	290000	Cooling water	16100	22	354000
	Total		358380		Total		358380

This completes the heat transfer design of fermenter.

5. Mechanical design of fermenter

Fermenter is a vertical pressure vessel made of stainless carbon steel[17]. Its operating pressurre is 5 lbs/in^{2}g but during sterilization, heating is done to above 15 bl/in^2 steam psig.

It is equipped with cooling coils, baffle plates, a turbine type agitator and a sparger for introduction of air/steam.

I. Dimensions

a. Dia = 8′ 6″

b. Height = 18′

Height between tangent to tangent = 19′

c. Agitator.

Shaft of S.S. O. D. = 4″ & I.D. = 3″.

Fitted with three sets of turbine type impellers. The bottom impeller is located at 11″ from the bottom of vessel and distance between succeeding impeller is 56″.

Dia. of impeller = 3′
Width of impeller blades = 7.2″.
Length of blades = 9″.

Diameter of central disc = 2′ 3″
No. of blades = 6

d. Baffles

4 No. of baffles 10" wide equally spaced. Clearence between wall & baffles = 2"
Thickness of plates = ¼″
Height of plates = 12′.

e. Sparger

1 ft. diameter of 2" N.B. tube in which 170 holes of 1/8" diameter are drilled in two rows.

f. Cooling water coils:

Two sets of coils of 2" N.B. tube. No. of turns in each set = 16
Coil dia. = 6 ft
Both the coils are connected in parallel with inlet & outlet pipe of 3" N.B.

II. Operating pressure and Design pressure
Static pressure at fermenter base = 5.8 lb/in^2.
Maximum operating pressure = 15 lb/in^2.
Total = 20.8 lb/in^2.
Design temperature = 125°C.

III. Material of construction

(1) Shaft & turbines – Stainless steel.
(2) Fermenter body – Carbon steel.
(3) Others – Mild steel (M.S.)

IV. Skirt height = 6 ft

V. Accessories :

Motor to be secured at the top of the fermenter. One cagged ladder to fermenter top.
H.P. of motor = 60 H.P.
Motor should have variable speed arrangement so that it can be started only at 60 rpm. Speed can be increased to 100 rpm when aeration starts.
Design of shaft for impellers18–20

The design of impellers has already been given in the Chem. Engg. Design of fermenter. Now the shaft is designed.

Stainless steel, hollow shaft closed at bottom is selected.

O.D. = 4″ = D

I. D. = 3″ = d

f_s = Permissible shear stress. = 64000 lb/in^2.

N = rpm = 100

H = H.P. to be transmitted.

If J is the moment of inertia

$$\frac{J}{R} = \frac{198000 \times H}{\pi N \cdot f_s}$$

$$\frac{\pi (D^4 - d^4)}{32 \times D/2} = \frac{198000 \times H}{\pi N \cdot f_s}$$

or
$$H = 87$$

If angle of twist in a length of 20" dia. is not to exceed 1 degree (As is the general requirement)

$$J = \frac{198000 \times H \cdot l}{\pi \cdot N \cdot C \cdot \theta}$$

where

$$C = \frac{\text{Shear stress}}{\text{Shear strain}} = 12 \times 10^6$$

$$\theta = \text{Angle of twist} = 1° = \frac{1}{57.3} \text{ Radian.}$$

$$l = \text{Length of shaft} = 20 \text{ ft say.}$$

$$H = \frac{\pi (D^4 - d^4)}{32} \times \frac{\pi \cdot 100 \cdot 12\, 10^6 \cdot 1}{57.3 \times 198000 \times 20 \times 4} = 70.$$

So, the shaft can take a load of 70 H.P. with 1° angle of twist in 20" diameter.
The shaft proposed is satisfactory.

Design of sparger

Height of liquid = 13 ft.

$$\text{Pressure due to liquid head} = \frac{13 \times 64.4}{144} = 5.8 \text{ lb/in}^2.$$

Pressure in ressel = 5 lb/in^2.

Total pressure at the bottom of vessel = 10.8 lb/in^2.

Air pressure P_1 = 14.7 × 3 = 44.1 lb/in^2 Abs.

Pressure at bottom P_2 = 10.8 + 14.7 = 25.5 lb/in^2 Abs.

The velocity of flow[19]

$$u_2^2 = \frac{2P_1}{v-1} \; v_1 \, . \, v_1 \left\{1 - \left(\frac{P_2}{P_1}\right)^{\frac{v-1}{v}}\right\}$$

where, u_2 = Vel. of flow at pressure P_2.

$$v = \frac{C_p}{w} = 1.4,\; v_1 = \text{Sp. volume at } P_1.$$

$$\therefore \qquad u_2^2 = \frac{2 \times 1.4}{1.4 - 1} \times 44.1 \times 144 \times 3.29 \left\{1 - \left(\frac{25.5}{44.1}\right)^{\frac{1.4-1}{1.4}}\right\}$$

u_2 = 14.6 ft/see.

Area required for this flow

$$A_2 = \frac{G \times v_2}{u_2} \cdot \text{ Where } v_2 \text{ is mass flow rate of air}$$

$$= \frac{685}{3600} \times \frac{5.7}{14.6} \times 144 = 1.7 \text{ in}^2.$$

Taking into consideration the pressure losses in pipe and orifice. $A_2 = 2.1$ in^2.

Area of 1/8″ hole = 0.0123 in^2.

$$\text{No. of 1/8″ holes} = \frac{2.1}{0.0123} = 170$$

Holes to be drilled in a sparger of 1′ dia. (coil) made of 2″ N. B. tube, two rows of holes at a pitch of 0.4″.

Welding Joints : It is recommended that double welded buff joints to be made where ever possible. Longitudinal welds to be radio graphed. Stress relieving is not necessary.

Over all joints efficiency factor

Gross joint efficiency = J_i = 0.95

Weldability discount factor = J_w = 0.

Stress reliance factor = Js = 0.04

Radiograph factor = J_r = 0.03

Minimum mechanical test & inspection factor = J_t = 0.13.

Therefore $\quad J = J_i - (J_2 + J_s + J_r + J_t)$

$= 0.95 - (0 + 0.04 + 0.03 + 0.13)$

$= 0.80$

Vessel Thickness : Thickness of shell is calculated from equation 3 class 62 of B.S.S., 1500 code equation for this shell.

$$t = \frac{pD}{2f(j-p)} + c$$

. Symbols have same significance as given in B.S. 1500 code.

$$= \frac{50 \times 102}{2 \times 19600 \times 0.8 - 50}$$

$$= 0.288 \text{ in.}$$

Nelson[21] states (Petroleum Refinery Engg.) that the thickness of a taken shell is estimated from consideration of corrosion resistance rather than working pressure. Shell thickness is 1/2″ for a column greater than 5ft diameter Hence a shell thickness of 1/2″ is recommended.

Thickness of Domed End : Domed end shape I is reommended for bottom of the vessel in which the crown radius is to be equal to the vessel diameter & knuckle radius is 10% of the vessel diameter

$$\frac{R_i}{D_i} = 1, \ \frac{r_i}{D_i} = 0.1$$

Thickness of domed end is given by the equation.

$$t = \frac{p \cdot D_0 \, k_1 k_2}{2 \, f \cdot J \, k_3}$$

$$k_1 = 2, k_2 = 1.15, k_3 = 0.95$$

$$t = \frac{50 \times 103 \times 2 \times 1.15}{2 \times 19600 \times 0.8 \times 0.95} = 0.395 \text{ in}$$

This is without corrosion allowance. The thickness of domed end recommended is 1/2" which is same as shell plate thickness.

Top : The top is to be flanged and standard disked[11]

The various dimensions are

t = Thickness = 0.5"

S_f = Standard flange = $2\frac{3''}{4}$.

r = Inside crown radius = 1.5".

I.D. = 102".

O.D. = 103".

Thickness of Flanges : Top flange of shell matching with flanged and standard T of the flange is calculated from the equation.

$$T = \sqrt{\frac{2p\,D_0\,L}{k_f}}$$

$$D_0 = 103$$

$$2\,L = 2\,[0.5\,(D_b - D_0)] \text{ where } D_b = \text{p.c.d.} = 107''.$$

$$= 4''$$

$$k = 1.44 \text{ (BSS 1500).}$$

$$T = \sqrt{\frac{50 \times 103 \times 4}{1.44 \times 19600}} = \sqrt{7.3} = 2.75''.$$

Bolt Pitch Circle

d = Bolt dia = 1"

B = Inside diameter of vessel at flange.

$j = \text{Filled weld leg} = \frac{11''}{16}$ in

$$c = B + 2\,(t + j + d) + \frac{1}{4}$$

$$= 102 + 2\left(\frac{1}{2} + \frac{11}{16} + 1\right) \approx 107''$$

Pitch of bolt

$$p = \frac{7d + T}{2} = \frac{7 \times 1 + 2.75}{2} = 4.37''$$

No. of bolts required

$$= \frac{\pi \cdot 107}{4.37} = 46 \text{ Bolts}$$

Inspection Manway : A 18" diameter circular Manhole is recommended at the top disked end. The centre of Manway being at a distance of 30" from center of vessel.

According to BSS 1500, single openings of 3" and below do not require compensation.

The Manway must be compensated. Area of compensation required

$$= d \times tr = 18 \times 0.5 = 9 \text{ in}^2.$$

Dimensions of Manway :

I.D. = 18".

O. D. of flange = 25"

Flange thickness = $1\frac{9''}{16}$.

Wall thickness = 0.5".

Height of bolts = 6" is recommended.
A sight glass is also to be fitted in top disked end. Other nozzle required at top are :
Feed inlet, air inlet to sparger, air outlet, topping of P.I. thermowell, light for sight glass, Antifoam agent inlet.
From side-sample point. At bottom-cooling water in and out, fermented broth exit.
This concludes the mechanical design calculation of fermenter.

Diameter of Pipes : (1) Vapour line from top of solvent recovery part I.

$$\text{Temperature} = 96°\text{C}$$

$$\text{Vapour rate} = 8.4 \text{ kg moles/hr}$$

$$= 8.4 \times 2.203 \text{ lb moles/hr}$$

$$= 8.4 \times 2.203 \times 359 \times \frac{369}{273}$$

$$= 9000 \text{ ft}^3\text{/hr}$$

Vapour velocity = 50 ft/sec [Perry 3rd edition].

$$= 180{,}000 \text{ ft/hr.}$$

$$\text{Area of cross section required} = \frac{9000 \times 144}{180{,}000} = 7.2 \text{ in}^2.$$

$$\text{Diameter of pipe} = \left[\frac{7.2}{0.7854}\right]^{1/2} = 3.03 \text{ in. Use } 3\frac{1''}{2} \text{ diameter pipe.}$$

(2) Vapour line from S.R. No. II top. temp. = 90°C.

$$\text{Vapour rate} = 20 \text{ kg mol/hr.}$$

$$= 20 \times 2.203 \times 359 \times \frac{363}{273}$$

$$= 21000 \text{ ft}^3\text{/hr}$$

$$\text{Vapour velocity} = 50 \text{ ft/sec.}$$

$$= 180{,}000 \text{ ft/hr.}$$

$$\text{Area of cross section required} = \frac{21000 \times 144}{180{,}000} = 16.8 \text{ in}^2.$$

$$\text{Diameter of Pipe} = \left[\frac{16.8}{0.7854}\right]^{1/2} = 4.6''. \text{ Use } 5'' \text{ diameter pipe.}$$

15.4 DOWNSTREAM PROCESS FOR RECOVERY BY FILTRATION [6,7,20,22,23]

15.4.1 Filter Design Calculations

A continuous rotary vaccum filter will be used.

Vol. of whole broth = $20M^3$.

Vol. of Mycelia = 20% = $4M^3$

Let the voidage of filter cake = 0.25

Vol. of beer left in cake after filtration = $\dfrac{4 \times 25}{75}$ = 1.33 m^3.

Quantity (Qty) of penicillin left in filter cake = 8333×10^6 units.

Vol. of beer = 16 m^3.

5% water wash = 1 m^3.

The efficiency of wash = 50%

Qty. of penicillin lost with cake = 4166×10^6 units.

Vol. of beer as filtrate = 14.667 M^3. Pen.

Vol. of beer as after wash = 15.667 m^3.

Qty. of penicillin in beer after wash = $(91667 + 4166) \times 10^6 = 95884 \times 10^6$ units.

$$\text{Percentage loss of penicillin} = \frac{4166 \times 100}{100{,}000} = 4.166\%.$$

(Total quantity of penicillin in one fermenter = 100 × 109 units). This beer is collected in a storage tank, after passing through a heat exchanger which cools the beer to 20°C.

Capacity of tank = 20 M^3.

Flow rate = 653 kg/hr

Penicillin = 6.115×10^6 units/liter.

For continuous operation of filtration and recovery section, or to meet process hazard or any abnormality it assumed that a quantity of $10M^3$ of beer is kept in beer tank. Since the data for various properties of penicillin is available at 20°C, only the extraction process will be carried out at this temp.

However, if the beer is chilled and kept at a low temperature the decay rate will be less and consequent losses will be small. But refrigeration will add to the cost of the process.

Penicillin loss due to decay in storage tank

Residence in storage = $\dfrac{10 \times 24}{15.677}$ = 15.3 hrs. or say, the total time taken after leaving the fermenter to the inlet of extraction train = 17 hrs. Penicillin is kept at pH6 in the tank. Half life period of penicillin at pH6 = 366 hrs.

If P_i = initial number of units of penicillin and P = No. of units at time t.

Decay unit time is given by $= -\dfrac{dp}{dt} = lp$

where λ = Decay constant or proportionality const. Integrating we get.

$$-\int_{P_1}^{P} \frac{dp}{p} = \lambda \int_0^t dt$$

$$\text{In}\ \frac{P_1}{P} = \lambda^t \text{ or } P = P_1\ e^{-\lambda t1/2}$$

To relate half life period with decay constant.

Setting $$P = P_{1/2} \text{ and } t = t_{1/2}$$

$$P_{1/2} = P_1\ e^{-\lambda\, t1/2}.$$

or $$\lambda\ .\ t_{1/2} = \text{In}\ 2 = 0.693$$

$$t^1\!/_2 = \frac{0.693}{\lambda}$$

In above case, $$\lambda = \frac{0.693}{336}$$

$$t = 17 \text{ hrs.}$$

$$P = P_1 e^{-\lambda t}$$

$$= P_1\ .\ e^{-\left(\frac{0.693}{336}\right)\times 17} = P_1\ (2.718)^{-\frac{0.693}{14.7}}$$

$$= P_1 \times \frac{1}{1.635} = P_1 \times 0.964$$

or 3.6% of penicillin will decay.

$$\text{Loss} = \frac{6115 \times 3.6}{100} = 215 \times 10^3 \text{ units/liter}$$

Total quantity of penicillin lost per fermenter.

$$= 215 \times 10^3 \times 653 \times 24 = 3.369 \times 10^9 \text{ units}$$

$$\text{Loss in filtration} = 4.166 \times 10^9 \text{ units}$$

$$\text{Total loss} = 7.535 \times 10^9 \text{ units}$$

Beer will be fed to extraction train or 653 litres/hr with penicillin quantity of 5900 u/ml.

The losses have been assumed high which can considerably be reduced in smooth operation of rotary vaccum filter. It is assumed that filtration time for broth from one fermenter = 10 hrs.

Vol. of broth = 20,000 liters

Rate of filtration = 2000 litres/hr.

Mycelia 20% = 400 liter/hr. = 14.14 ft^3/hr.

If rotation speed of drum = 1 Rev./6 min

$$\text{Mycelia to be removed} = \frac{14.14 \times 6}{60} = 1.414\ ft^3/\text{Rev.}$$

Assuming that 1/2" layer of mycelia thickness is built on surface.

$$\text{Drum surface covered} = 1.44 \times 24 = 34\ ft^2.$$

If 20% of surface is submerged in broth[15]

$$\text{Drum surface} = \frac{34}{0.2} = 170\ ft^2$$

A rotary vaccum filter of following specification is suitable, length = 10 ft.

Dia. of 6 ft.

Surface = 181 ft^2

Material of construction = Stainless steel.

15.5 DOWNSTREAM PROCESSING FOR EXTRACTION[7,22]

Podbielniak (Pod) extractors have been selected for use in extraction.

Performance tests have shown that Pod units have the equivalent of 3 to 6 theoretical stages [Ref. Chem. Engg. Prog. May 1957]. But a more reliable account about the performance of such equipment has been given in CEP May 1953. It was found that while extracting from water into alcohol [in another system] with a ratio of light liquid to heavy liquid of 0.33 to 0.66 gave the number of theoretical (Th) stages from 1.23 to 1.65.

No. of sample calculations have been made as shown below.

x_f = Concentration of penicillin in feed = 5900 u/ml.

x_n = Concentration in Raffinate

y_s = Concentration in solvent = 0

y_1 = Concentration in extract = ?

A = Heavey liquid rate = 100 liter/hr (say).

B = Light – liquid rate (B.A.) = 30, 40, 50. 60,

n = No. of Th. stags = 1.3, 1.4, 1.5, 1.6 (say)

m = Distribution rate at pH 2.1 = 25

$$\Sigma = \frac{m \times B}{A}$$

In case I

$$\frac{x_f - x_n}{x_f - y_s/m} = \frac{\Sigma^{n+1} - \Sigma}{\Sigma^{n+1} - 1}$$

or

$$\frac{5900 - x_n}{5900 - 0} = \frac{7.5^{2.3} - 7.5}{7.5^{2.3} - 1}$$

$x_n = 5900 - 5520 = 380$ u/ml. [Loss in Raffinate].

$$y_1 = \frac{5570}{0.3} + y_s$$

$= 18400$ u/ml

Case No.	$x_n = u/ml.$	$y_l = u/ml$
1	380	18400
2	210	14225
3	120	11560
4	60	9733

In case No. 4 the loss of penicillin in Raffi. is low but the concentration in extract is also less. The duty of machine will be more due to high flow rate.

[as will be shown later that a Pod. machine of different capacity will have to be selected].

Without actual pilot plant data, it is difficult to estimate the performance which changes with different conditions and systems.

However, as a conservative estimate, the light liquid to heavey liquid rate of 0.4 has been selected and no. of these stages assumed at 1.5.

Note : A 10% concentration solution strength of H_2SO_4 is added instead of concentration acid, as otherwise there will be heavey decay of penicillin by the line acid mixer with beer.

The quantity of acid calculated at 2% v/v for 10% strength. This is a preliminary estimate of extraction duty. Later, the acid thus changed to 20% at less liquid flow. A lead lined tank will be required for dil. H_2SO_4.

PVC pipes to be used for carrying to booster pump inlet where it mixes with beer.

A non-return valve on beer line to be provided. Temperature of mixture (Acid-Base) asumed at 20°C.

Beer flow rate = 653 litres./hr.

$$\text{Vol. of acid added at 2\% v/y} = \frac{653 \times 2}{100} = 13.06 \text{ liter.}$$

Sp . gravity of acid = 1.84 (Perry)

Wt. of acid = 24 kg.

Wt. of 98% acid = 245 kg.

Sp. gravity of 10% acid = 1.066.

Vol. of 10% acid = 243.5 liter.

Vol. of Beer + Acid = 653 +243.5 = 896.5 liters.

Flow of heavy liquid = 896.5 liter/hr

Flow light/heavy liquid = 388.6 liter/hr

Total flow rate = 1285.1 liter/hr = 5.656 liter/min

[Ref. Perry. Page 21 – 35].

A Pod. Extraction of Series 9600 will have to be used for this duty. The minimum hold up is 7 gals which means a residence time of 1.24 min.

At a pH. 2.1 the half life period of panicillin is 0.35 hrs. The % decay will be = 4%

If the total flow rate is reduced to 4 gals/min, it will be possible to use extractor of series 6000 with a hold up of 1–2 gallons, and consequently the % decay will be above 1% and other advantages will be less costlier equipment and power consumption.

Wt. of 20% acid added = 122.5 kg.

Sp. gravity of 20% acid = 1.14 (Perry)

Vol. of acid = 107.5 liters/hr.

Total vol. flow rate of 20% acid + Beer = 653 + 107.5 = 760.5 liter/hr.

Vol. flow rate of Butylacetate required = 304.2 liters/hr.

Total flow rate = 760.5 + 304.2 = 1064.7 liter/hr = 4.688 gals/min

Extraction of series 6000 is selected with following specification

Diameter = 25"

Width = 2"

Vol. hold up = 1 – 2 galls.

Flow capacity = 1 – 5 gpm.

Power = 1 – 2 H.P.

Light liquid in press = 80 – 165 lb/in^2

Heavy liquid in press = 20 – 125 lb/in^2

Let rpm = 5000

rps = 5000/60 = 83.33

If w = Angular velocity.

g = Acceleration due to gravity.

r = Effective radius of rotor

ρ_{hL} = Density of heavy liquid

$\rho_{L.L}$ = Density of light liquid

Pressure exerted at periphery of rotor due to heavy liquid.

$$= \frac{w^2r^2}{2g} \times \rho_{hL}$$

Pressure due to light liquid $= \dfrac{w^2r^2}{2g} \cdot \rho_{L.L.}$

Additional pressure required for light liquid to enter periphery of rotor.

$$= \frac{w^2r^2}{2g} (\rho_{hL} - \rho_{LL})$$

w = 2π rps., $g = 980.6$ dyne/sec^2

r = 30 cms (assumed)

ρ_{hL} = 1.01 gm/c.c, $\rho_{LL} = 0.88$ gm/c.c.

$$\rho_L \text{ in} = \frac{4\pi^2 (83.33)^2 \times 30^2 (1.01 - 0.88) \times 14.2}{2 \times 98.6 \times 1000}$$

$$= 232.8 \text{ lb/in}^2$$

which is in excess of the pressure limit of the equipment. A lower R.P.M. is selected.

R.P.M. = 4000.

R.P.S. = 66.66

$$\rho_L \text{ in} = \frac{4\pi^2 (66.66)^2 \times 30^2 \times 0.13 \times 14.2}{2 \times 980.6 \times 1000}$$

$$= 137.8 \text{ lb/in}^2.$$

Hence an RPM 4000 is selected. Heavey liquid exit is opened to atmospheric pressure. Light liquid exit pressure is controlled and regulated according to process condition assumed at 80 lb/in^2.

Note : All pressure units are in lb/in^2 guage.

(1) Heavy liquid in press = 80 lb/in^2 G.

(2) Light liquid in press = 138 lb/in^2 G.

Pump requirement for (2) 320 liter/hrs cap. 140 lb/m. G. cap — Light liquid

Pump for (1) 760 liter/hrs. cap. 140 lb/m. G. cap — Heavy liquid

$$\text{Maximum residence time} = \frac{2}{4.7} + \frac{1}{6} \text{ [minutes after mixing with acid up to extract unit]}$$

$$= 35 \text{ secs} = 0.6 \text{ min.}$$

$$= 0.01 \text{ hr.}$$

Half life period of penicillin at pH 2.1 = 0.35 hrs.

$$\text{Decay constant } \lambda = \frac{0.693}{0.35}$$

$$P = P_1 \; e^{-\left(\frac{0.693}{0.35}\right)\times 0.01}$$

$$= P_1 \, . \, e^{-0.693.35} = P_1/1.020.$$

$$= P_1 \times 0.9804$$

∴ Decay = 1.96%.

This is an estimate based on higher side of residence time. Actually after about half of the residence time, most of penicillin will be in butyl acetate.

Qty. of penicillin at heavy liquid inlet after adjusting for decay

$$= \frac{5900 \times 0.9804 \times 653}{760.5} = 4967 \text{ units/ml}$$

Extraction Step I

x_f = Concentration of penicillin in feed = 4967 u/ml

x_m = Concentration of penicillin in feed = 4967 Raffinate = ?

y_s = Concentration of penicillin in feed = 4967 so heat = 0

y_1 = Concentration of penicillin in feed = 4967 Extract.

A = Heavy liquid rate in feed = 4967 = 760.5 liter/hr

B = Light liquid rate in feed = 4967 = 304.2" liter/hr

η = No of the stages = 1.5 (assumed)

m = Distribution ratio at pH 2.1 = 25.

Assuming :

(1) Distribution ratio to be constant in the range of concentration encountered.

(2) Solubility of aqueous solution and organic solvent as negligible.

(3) Vol. changes on penicillin transfer are negligible.

$$\text{Extraction factor } \Sigma = \frac{mB}{A} = \frac{25 \times 304.2}{760.5} = 10$$

as $S \neq 1$.

$$\frac{x_f - x_n}{x_f - y_s/m} = \frac{\Sigma^{n+1} - \Sigma}{\Sigma^{n+1} - 1}$$

Substituting the values, we get

$$\frac{4967 - x_n}{4967 - 0/25} = \frac{10^{2.5} - 10}{10^{2.5} - 1}$$

or $$x_n = 4967 - 4825 = 142 \text{ u/ml.}$$

Further $$A/B = \frac{y_1 - y_s}{x_f - x_n} = \frac{y_1 - 0}{4967 - 142} = \frac{y_1}{4825}$$

$\therefore$ $$y_1 = \frac{4825 \times 760.5}{304.2} = 12062 \text{ u/ml.}$$

Liquid in :

Aq. phase = 760.5 Lit. hr, ρ = 1.02 gm/c.c.

Wt. = 775.5 kg/hr.

Butyl acetate = 304.2 lit/hr. ρ = 0.88 gm/c.c.

Wt. = 267.7 kg/hr

Solubility of B.A. in water at 25°C (Assumed) = 1.2% W/w.

[There will be some rise due to wash out.]

$$\text{Qty. of B.A. dissolved in water} = \frac{775.5 \times 1.2}{100} = 9.22 \text{ kg/hr} = 10.48 \text{ liter/hr.}$$

Liquid out :

Aq. phase = 784.72 kg/hr = 770.98 liter/hr

Butyl acetate = 258.48 kg/hr. = 93.72 liters/hr.

B.A. used has been obtained from decanter of distillation column and hence is already saturated with water. So it can not dissolve more quantity of water.

Recalculating on the basis of above flowrate and taking into consideration the solubility of B.A. in water we get.

$$y_1 = 12640 \text{ u/ml.}$$

Concentration of penicillin in extract phase at liquid out pressure will be about 80 lb/in^2 G. It is fed to the section of booster pump for Extraction Step II.

Extraction Step II

The above reference says that while extracting from organic aqueous phase the number of Th. Stages is considerably more. While extracting from alcohol to water (in another system) from a light liquid to heavy liquid with flow ratio of 1 to 3.25, the number of stages obtained was 2.79 to 1.74.

A light to heavy liquid ratio of 3 is kept in step II of extraction and number of stages assumed at 4.

x_f = 12640 u/ml

x_n = ?

y_s = 6000 u/ml (estimated)

y_1 = ?

A = 293.72 Lit/hr (B.A.)

B = 97.9 (Buffer)

n = 4.

$$m = \frac{15.15 \times 979}{293.72} = 5.051 = S \neq 1.$$

The solution obtained as mother liquor after crystal separation is treated with buffer to extract penicillin.

Extract obtained from mother liquor joins the buffer solution at the inlet of booster pump for heavy liquid. The penicillin content of buffer has been estimated at 6000 u/ml. So by substituting the various values in

$$\frac{x_f - x_n}{x_f - y_s/m} = \frac{\Sigma^{n+1} - \Sigma}{\Sigma^{n+1} - 1}$$

we get, $$x_n = 12640 - 12230 = 40 \text{ u/ml.}$$

$$y_1 = \frac{12230 \times 293.72}{27.9} + 6000$$

$$= 42690 \text{ u/ml}$$

The butyle acetate (spent) is sent to solvent recovery part II.

The extract in buffer is collected in tank of $3m^3$ capacity for use in Step III extraction.

Qty. of buffer from mother liquor - extraction = 60 lb liter/hr, assumed $\rho = 1$.

This buffer is saturated with B.A. quantity remaining buffer to be saturated with B.A. = 37.9 kg/hr.

$$\text{Wt. of B.A. dissolved} = \frac{37.9 \times 1.2}{100} = 0.455 \text{ kg/hr} = 0.52 \text{ liter/hr}$$

Liquid in

Buffer = 97.9 lit/hr. = 97.9 kg/hr
B.A. = 293.72 lit/hr = 258.48 kg/hr

Liquid out

Buffer = 98.42 lit/hr = 98.9 kg/hr

B.A. = 293.2 lit/hr = 257.98 kg/hr.

Penicillin in buffer out = 42460 u/ml in 98.42 lit/hr. of Extract.

At extractor of same series is selected at Extraction Step I.

Extraction Step III

The volumes are selected so as to make the use of Pod. Extract of series 6000 possible, with a minimum low rate of 1gpm.

Vol. at buffer from Step II = 98.42 lit/hr.

Vol. of acid (a) 2% v/v = 1.97 lit./hr, ρ = 1.8 gm/c.c.

Wt. of acid = 3.546 kg.

Wt. of 98% acid = 3.62 kg.

Vol. of 6% acid = 58.2 liters.

Total vol. = 9842 + 58.2 = 156.62 liter/hr.

Decay of penicillin at 1 min. residence in acid phase = 3% approx.

Penicillin in buffer = 42460 u/ml.

Decay = 42460 × 0.03 = 1274 u/ml

Penicillin left = 41186 u/ml.

$$\text{Penicillin in liquid inlet to extractor} = \frac{41186 \times 98.42}{156.62} = 25900 \text{ u/ml}$$

Vol. of B.A. used = 78 liter/hr.

x_f = 25900 u/ml

A = 156.62 lit/hr.

B = 78 lit/hr

m = 25, pH = 2.1, n = 15 (assumed)

$$\Sigma = \text{Extraction factor} = \frac{25 \times 78}{156.62} = 12.48$$

$$\frac{x_f - x_n}{x_f - y_s/m} = \frac{\Sigma^{n+1} - \Sigma}{\Sigma^{n+1} - 1}$$

or
$$\frac{25900 - x_n}{25900 - 0} = \frac{12.48^{2.5} - 12.48}{12.48 - 1} = \frac{537.5}{549}$$

$\therefore$
$$x_n = 25900 - 25900 \times \frac{537.5}{549} = 550 \text{ u/ml}$$

$$y_1 = \frac{25350 \times 156.62}{78} = 50800 \text{ u/ml}$$

Concentration of penicillin in extract. from Step III = 50800 u/ml.

Liquid in	*lit/hr*	*kg/hr*
Buffer	98.42	98.4
Acid 6%	58.2	60.33
B.A.	78	68.70
Buffer 157.42	159.43	
B.A	77.20	68.00

1.2% w/w of B.A. dissolved in dil. acid soln.
In all of above extract. stages the wt. of penicillin has not been accounted for.
The weight is estimated at 1.4 kg./hr. [Ref. Chem. Engg. Practice]
If efficiency of precipitation process = 75%
Quantity of penicillin left in mother liquor = 12600 u/ml.
Some B.A. is lost in crystal separation, the remaining mother liquor is extracted for penicillin with buffer.
The quantity of penicillin in buffer phase is estimated as 10,000 u/ml after taking into consideration all losses including decay.
Penicillin in 97.9 liter/hr or buffer at Extraction Step II

$$= \frac{60 \times 10{,}000}{97.6} = 6120 \text{ u/ml}$$

Hence earlier estimate of 6000 u/ml is correct.

Total quantity of penicillin recovered in 24 hr per fermenter

$$= 50800 \times 77.2 \times 24 \times 10^3 \times 0.75$$
$$= 70 \times 10^9 \text{ units/day.}$$

Quantity of penicillin in one fermenter = 100×10^9 u
$\therefore$ Percentage of recovery = 70%
If penicillin is not recovered from mother liquor and extracted at Step II.
Percentage recovery = 56%.

Qantity of buffer/beer going to spent tank, Kg/hr

	Step I	Step. III	Total
Buffer/Beer	751.00	153.89	904.89
B.A. (dissolved)	9.22	1.92	11.14
78% Acid	24.50	3.69	28.12
Total	784.72	159.43	944.15

Material balance over extraction train, Kg/hr

Extraction	In	Out
Step I		
Beer.	653.00	653.00
98% Acid	24.50	24.50
Water	98.00	98.00
Butylacetate	267.70	258.40
B.A. dissolved in aqueous phase	—	9.22
Total	1043.20	1043.20
Step II		
B.A.	258.48	257.98
Fresh buffer.	37.48	97.18
Buffer pressure	59.28	
Mother liquot		
B.A. dissolved	0.72	1.22
Total	356.38	356.38
Step III		
Aq-buffer	97.18	97.18
Dissolved B.A.	1.22	1.92
98% Acid	3.62	3.62
Water	56.71	56.71
Butyl acetate	68.70	68.70
Total	227.43	227.43

Butyle acetate has all along been assumed saturated with water.

Neutralization of spent Beer/Buffer (B.B.) is carried out by 10% solution of $Na_2\ CO_3$. Flow of carbonate solution is controlled by a pH meter installed at inlet of solution vessel.

Mol. Wt. of $H_2SO_4 = 98$

$Na_2CO_3 = 106.$

Qty. of Na_2CO_3 required to neutralise 98% acid.

$$= 28.12 \times \frac{106}{98} \times 0.98 = 29.8 \text{ kg.}$$

Quantity of 10% carbonate solution used = 298 kg/hr.

Total quantity of solution for recovery of B.A.

= 944.15 + 298 = 1242 kg/hr including 11.14 kg of B.A.

Wt. % of B.A. = 0.90% approx.

Water from decanter of Step II solvent recovery

= 143 kg/hr. (assumed) containing 1% of B.A.

Total quantity of solution = 1242 + 143 = 1385 kg/hr.

Quantity of B.A. in solution = 0.1082 kg mol,

Water = 76.244 l

This quantity of solution is sent to solvent recovery Part I from recovery of dissolved butyl acetate.

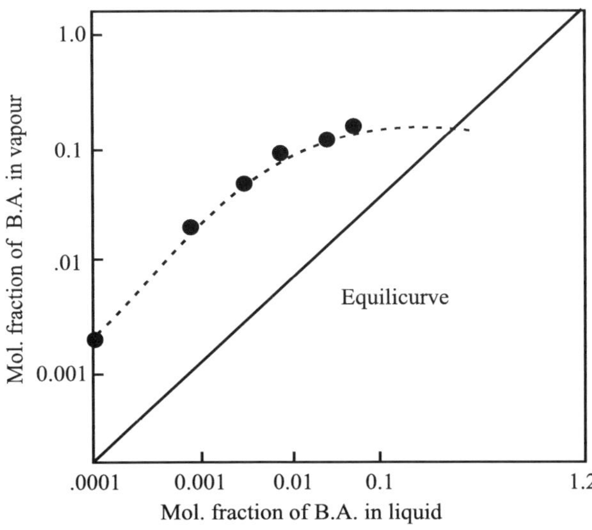

Fig. 15.5 Vapour liquid equilibrium curve. B.A. water system on log-log scale

Vapour Liquid Equilibrium

System : B.A. – water

No published data was available for this system. Even the solubilities at high temperature were not available.

Van Laar method has been used to evaluate the vapour-liquid equilibrium.[24] (Fig. 15.5) Azeotropic composition at 90.2°C.

	Wt.	*Mol. Wt.*	*Mols*	*Mol. Fraction*	*Vap. Press.*
B.A.	73.3	116	0.630	0.296	033
water	26.7	18	1.486	0.704	523

γ = Activity coeff.

p = Partial pressure.

x = Mol. fraction in liquid phase

y = Mol. fraction in vapour phase.

π = Total pressure

Subscripts 1 & 2 stand for B.A. & water respectively

$$v_1 = \pi\, y_1 / P_1 x_1$$
$$\gamma_2 = \pi\, y_2 / P_2 x_2$$

at Azeotropic composition

$$y_1 = x_1 \,.\, \&\, y_2 = x_2$$

Hence $$\gamma_1 = \frac{\pi}{P_1} = \frac{760}{233} = 3.265$$

$$\gamma_2 = \frac{\pi}{P_2} = \frac{760}{525} = 1.455$$

The reference substance graph for vapour pressure of B.A. and water has been drawn on a log-log paper and attached Fig. 15.6. A variation of ± 3 mm Hg (press.) has been neglected.

$$\log 3.265 = 0.5139$$
$$\log 1.445 = 0.1628$$

Van Laar constants C_1 & C_2

$$C_1 = \log \gamma_1 \,[1 + x_2 + \log \gamma_2 / x_1 \log \gamma_1]^2$$

$$= 0.5139 \left[a + \frac{0.7012 \times 0.1628}{0.2988 \times 0.5139} \right]$$

$$= 0.5319 \times 1.743^2 = 1.562.$$

Similarly[24]

$$C_2 = \log \gamma_2 [1 + x_1 + \log \gamma_1 / x_2 \log \gamma_2]^2 = 0.896.$$

The table 15.4 shows the range of immiscibility in symmetrical system. By the help of this table we can roughly find out the range of immiscibility at azeotropic one, (A_z) composition, the activity coefficient of which has already been evaluated from A_z data.

By Van Laar const. $c_1 = 1.562$, the range of immiscibility of B.A. in water has been estimated at 0.40 – 0.96 mol. fraction.

The corresponding value of γ_1 at $x = 0$ should be betweeen 27 and 59, preferably 35 for the above range of immiscibility.

A study of above table shows that immiscibility of B.A. in water is very low at Azeotropic state.

Solubilitry data at high temperature is not available and from solubilities at 15°C & 20°C, no reliable estimate can be made.

On the same page a method is mentioned to evaluate constants of Redlist - Kister equn. but the procedure neglects effect of temperature on ratio of activity coefficients.

However, the activity coefficient at different temperature and composition have been evaluated and $x - y$ curve has been drawn, covering the solubility range of B.A in water. The log-log graph on which the curve is drawn has been attached. (Fig. 15.6.).

Vapour pressure of pure substances were estimated from reference substance graph as (Fig. 15.6) recommended by Othmer.[2]

The results are tabulated as below (Table 15.4) corresponding to the step by step method used.

$$C_1 = 1.562$$

$$C_2 = 0.896$$

$$\log v_1 = C_1 / \left[1 + \frac{c_1 x_1}{c_2 x_2}\right]^2$$

$$\log v_2 = C_2 / \left[1 + \frac{c_2 x_2}{c_1 x_1}\right]^2$$

Size of Pumps

No. 8 : Pumping beer from filter to beer tank.

Flow rate = 200 lits/hr. = 4406 lits/hr.

Total Head = 30 ft. (say)

$$\text{Work done} = \frac{4406 \times 30}{33000 \times 60} = 0.064 \text{ H.P.}$$

Power of pump required assuming 60% efficiency.

$$= \frac{0.064}{0.6} = 0.107 \text{ H.P., Say } 0.5 \text{ H.P.}$$

No. 10 : Pumping beer + Acid to extractor I.

Flow rate = 775.5 kg/Hr. = 1710 lb/hr

$$\text{Volume (in terms of water)} = \frac{1710}{62.4} = 26.8 \text{ ft}^3/\text{hr}.$$

Pressure against which pumping is required = 80 lb/in^2 + 5 lb/in^2 (other losses)

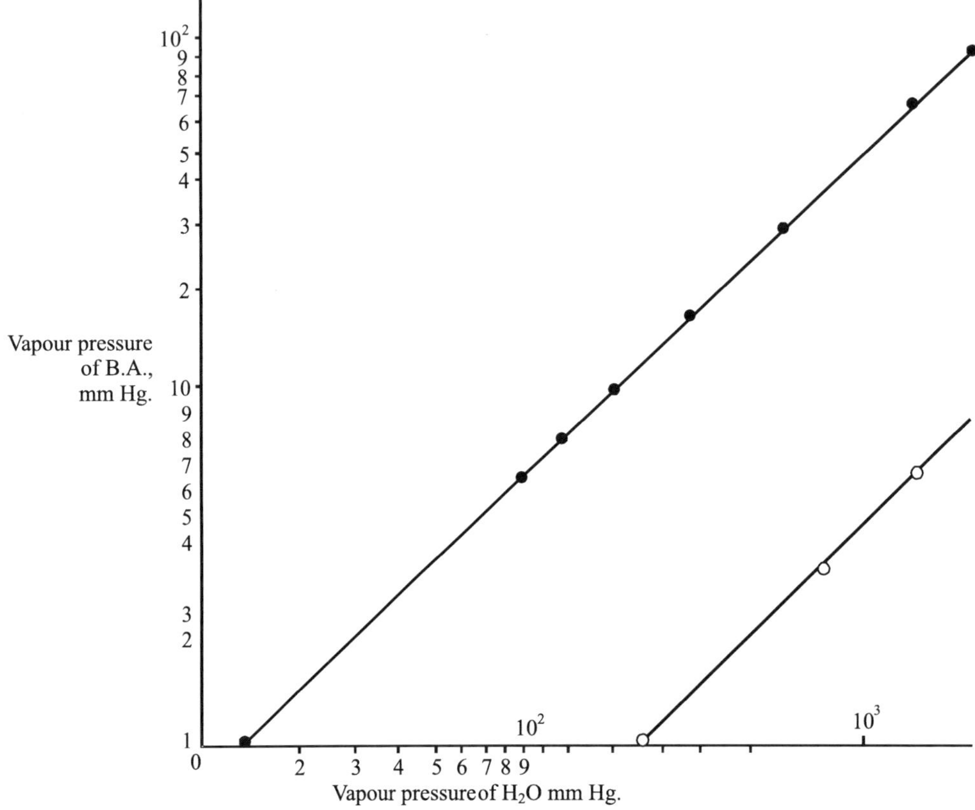

Fig. 15.6 Reference substance plot for vapour pressure of B.A.

Table 15.4

$$\log v_1 = c_1 / \left[a + \frac{c_1 x_1}{c_2 x_2}\right]^2 \qquad \log v_2 = c_2 / \left[a + \frac{c_2 x_2}{c_1 x_1}\right]^2$$

x_1	x_2	$c_1 x_1$	$c_2 x_2$	$\left[a + \frac{c_1 x_1}{c_2 x_2}\right]^2$	$\left[a + \frac{c_2 x_2}{c_1 x_1}\right]^2$	$\log \gamma_1$	$\log \gamma_1$	γ_1	γ_2
0	1	0	196	1α	α	1.562	0	36.48	1
1	0	1.562	0	α	1	0	.896	1	7.9
.001	.999	.00156	.895	1.0003	33000	1.561	.000006	36.39	1
.01	.99	.0156	.886	1.004	3400	1.555	.00024	35.89	1.0004
.02	.98	.0312	.878	1.071	840	1.456	.001	28.18	1.002
.02	97	.0468	.869	1.111	380	1.410	.00236	25.70	1.006
.04	.96	.0624	.860	1.15	218	1.360	.0041	22.91	1.009

Temp. (°C)	99.55	96.5	94.3	92.5	91.8
x_1	.001	.01	.02	.03	.04
x_2	.999	.99	.93	.97	.96
v_1	36.39	34.09	28.18	25.70	22.91
v_2	1	1.0004	1.002	1.006	1.009
P_1 mm Hg	325	290	272	256	249
P_2 mm Hg	749	675	617	577	569
$P_1 x_1 v_1$	.0364	.341	.563	.770	.917
$P_2 x_2 v_2$	748	663	605	563	534
π	760	762	759	760	762
y_1	0.016	0.13	0.225	0.26	0.276

From reference substance graph (Fig. 15.6) $P_1x_1v_1$, $P_2x_2v_2$ were evaluated. If the sum of both is 760 ± .3, the temperature assumed is correct, else,the procedure was revised.

$$y_1 = \frac{P_1\ x_1 v_1}{\pi}$$

At value of $x_1 = 0.04$, $y_1 = 0.295$ i.e. nearly Azeotrop. composition in vapour and at $x = 0$, $v_1 = 36.48$ which means that immiscibility predicted above is correct.

The above forms x – y curve of B.A. & water for low mol fraction of B.A. in water.

$$\text{Work done} = \frac{85 \times 144 \times 26.8}{33000 \times 60} = 0.1657 \text{ H.P.}$$

Power of pump required at 60% efficiency

$$= \frac{0.1657}{0.6} = 0.276 \text{ H.P., say } 0.5 \text{ H.P.}$$

No. 9 Pumping Butylacetate to Extractor I.

Flow rate = 267.7 kg.hr. = 590 lb/hr = 9.45 ft^3 [in terms of water].

Work done in pumping against 140 lb/in^2 pressure.

$$= \frac{9.45 \times 140 \times 144}{33000 \times 60} = 0.11 \text{ H.P.}$$

Power of pump required = say 0.5 H.P.

Rise of Temperature in Extractor

Assuming work done on liquid in Extractor I = 1 H.P.

Total work done by pump & Extractor.

$$1 + 0.166 + 0.111 = 1.276 \text{ H.P.}$$

If whole of it converts into heat corresponding head = 1.276 × 2545.

= 3250 BTU

= 2340 lb - cal. = 1060 k – cal/hr.

Total flow = 1043 kg/hr.

Temp. rise = 1°C.

There is no need of coolers after extractors. Power requirement of other pumps was also calculated as above and included in equipment schedule. No pump has been provided for broth from fermenter to filter. The flow can be achieved by applying air pressure in the fermenter.

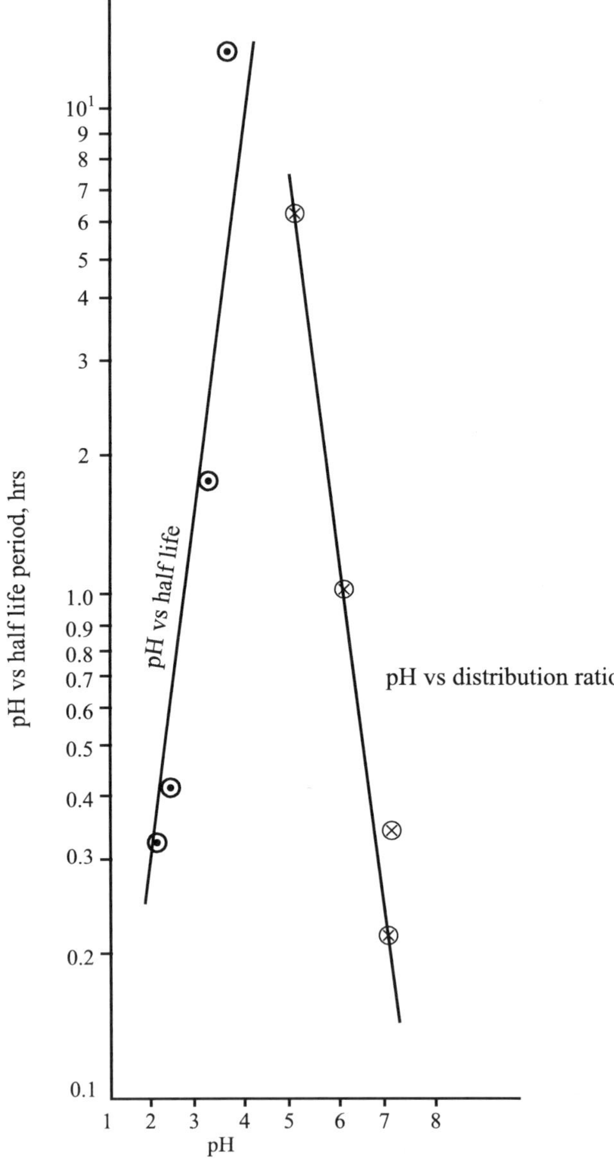

Fig. 15.7

Optimum Value of pH to be Maintained

A plot of pH vs. log-half life period of penicillin (Fig. 15.7) was drawn on a semi-log paper and found to be a straight line. The various values of half life period were noted between pH 1.8 to 2.6 (Fig. 15.8).

The plot of pH vs. log distribution ratio on a semilog paper was a straight line for high pH value (Fig. 15.7)

The curve of log pH vs. log distribution coefficient between pH of 1 to 3 was a straight line. The various values of distribution coefficient at different pH values were noted.

An analysis was made about the yield of penicillin at different pH values taking the following values of constants.

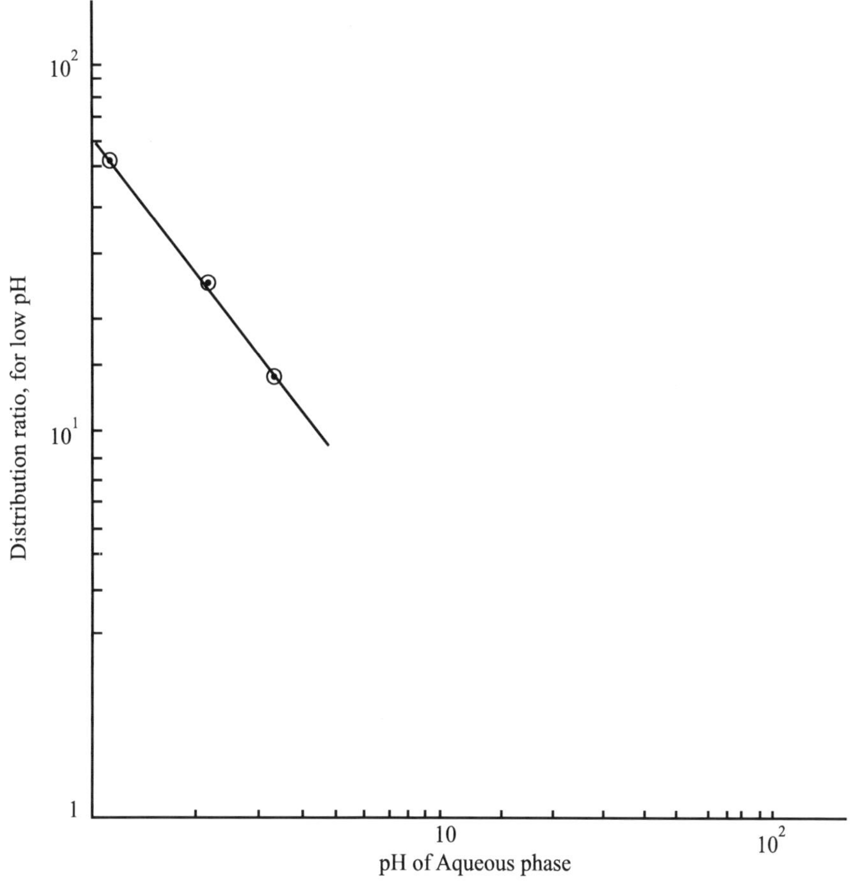

Fig. 15.8 (Ref. Table 15.2)

(1) Residence time = 0.01 hr.

(2) No. of Th. stages = 1.5

(3) Ratio between flow rate of B.A and beer = B/A = 0.4.

Case No.	1	2	3	4	5	6
pH	1.8	2	2.1	2.2	2.4	2.6
Distribution ratio, m.	31.5	27	25	223.7	21	19
Half life period, hr	0.21	0.31	0.35	0.41	0.6	0.84
Decay constant λ.	3.3	2.236	1.98	1.69	1.55	0.825
$e^{-\lambda(.01)}$	0.966	0.977	0.980	0.984	0.988	0.992

Let the quantity of penicillin originally present = 1000 u/ml.

Case (1) Penicillin left after decay = 966 u/ml

$$m.B/A = 31.5/4 = 12.6.$$

$$\frac{x_f - x_n}{x_f} = \frac{12.5^{2.5} - 12.6}{12.6^{2.5} - 1} = 547.5/559$$

$$x_n = 966 - \frac{966 \times 547.5}{559} = 966 - 940$$

$$y_1 = \frac{940}{0.4} = 2350 \text{ u/ml.}$$

e_f = Concentration of penicillin in feed.
x_n = Concentration of penicillin in Raffinate
y_1 = Concentration of penicillin in extract.

Case No.	*pH*	*Yield in u/ml (Conc. of Penicillin in Extract)*
1	1.8	2350
2	2.0	2382.5
3	2.1	2392.5
4	2.2	2388
5	2.4	2385
6	2.6	2375

It is quite clear from above that keeping either values constant, the yield of penicillin is maximum at a pH value of 2.1

Hence this value is recommended while extracting penicillin from beer/buffer to solvent B.A. in acid medium.

Downstream Processing for Solvent Recovery: Part I

Spent beer/buffer, after being neutralized with 10% solution of Na-Carbonate is sent to this section. In it is also mixed the water layer from Step II of recovery section.

The feed temperature has been assumed at 20°C. Feed is first heated in condenser of distillation column & then heated to almost its boiling point in heat exchanger for residue exit.

The design of column and accessories follows step by step.

		Feed.	
	kg./hr.	*kg. mol/hr.*	*mol Fraction*
B.A.	12.57	0.1082	0.00142
water	1372.43	76.2444	0.99858
Total	1385.00	76.3526	

Material Balance

Basis : 100 mols/hr

F = Feed, D = Distillate, W = Residue.

d_c, d_x, x_w are molecular fractions of B.A. in feed, distillate & residue. y is molecular fraction in vapour phase.

Since heavy fouling is expected, the column should have large number of plates. A value of $x_w = 0.0001$ will give a large number of plates in stripping section.

So $x_w = 0.0001$ has been selected.

Many calculations were made with different values of x_d and diff. reflux ratios.

The following arrangements of composition was found satisfactory.

$x_f = 0.00142$

$x_d = 0.131$

$x_w = 0.0001$

By material balance

$F = D + W$

$\therefore D = 100 - W$

$F.\ x_f = D.\ x_d + W.\ x_w$

$\therefore 100 \times 0.00142 = (100 - W) \times 0.131 + 0.0001\ W$

From which we have

$W = 98.99$

$D = 1.01$

Minimum reflux ratio was found from the following equation[26].

$$R_{min} = \frac{x_d - y_f}{y_f - x_f} = \frac{0.131 - 0.021}{0.021 - 0.00142} = 5.6$$

On economic ground Gilliland has recommended a reflux ratio of 1.3 to 2 times the minimum reflux. By trial & error to find the required product composition, a reflux ratio of 9.9 has been selected.

Reflux ratio, R = 9.9

Equation of Operating Lines

With the usual assumption of constant molar heat of vapourisation (B.A. = 8850 & W = 9700 cals/hr) no heat losses, no heat of mixing, the following equations worked satisfactory.

While taking into consideration the feed composition, reaction between H_2SO_4 & $Na_2\ CO_3$ has been neglected and it is assumed that feed consists of only B.A. & water. Since the feed has been assumed nearly at its B.P. q-line will be vertical. & q = 1.

Stripping Section

Below feed plate, liquor on m-plate

$$L_m = RD + F.$$
$$= 9.9 \times 1.01 + 100 = 110 \text{ moler/hr}$$
$$V_m = D\ (R + 1)$$
$$= 1.01\ (9.9 + 1) = 11.009 \text{ mole/hr}$$

$$y_m = \frac{L_m}{V_m} \cdot x_{m+1} - \frac{W}{V_m} \cdot x_w$$

$$= \frac{110}{11.009} \cdot x_{m+1} - \frac{98.99}{11.009} \times .0001$$

or $$x_{m+1} = \frac{y_m + .0009}{99.92}$$

Plate to Plate Analysis

Plate no.	x_m	y_m	x_{m+1}
Still	0.0001	0.0016	0.00025
2	0.00025	0.004	0.00049
3	0.00085	0.0133	0.00142
4	0.00142		Feed plate

Rectifying Columns

Eqn. of operating lines for rectifying column is

$$y_n = \frac{L_n}{V_n} \cdot x_{n+1} + \frac{D}{V_n} \cdot x_d$$

$$= \frac{R}{R+1} x_{n+1} + \frac{x_d}{R+1}$$

$$= \frac{9.9}{9.9+1} x_{n+1} + \frac{0.131}{9.9+1}$$

or $$x_{n+1} = \frac{y_n - 0.01202}{0.908}$$

Plate to Plate Analysis

Plate No.	x_n	y_n	x_{n+1}
4	0.00142	0.0215	0.0102
5	0.0102	0.134	Vapours to condenser

Since the material can cause heavy fouling,if a reboiler is used there will be heavy fouling on outside of its tubes.

It is recommended to use open steam. For steam stripping, approx. one plate will be required more. Hence all 6 theoretical plates are required, the feed plate will be 5th from bottom.

The product quality was checked with other values of reflux and found as under.

Assumed value. of x_d	Reflux Ratio	Calculated x_d	No. of plates
0.13	9	0.20	7
0.13	9.9	0.142	6

Since feed temperature is slightly lower than its B.P. the pitch zone will be in the bottom portion of the columns.

Material balance on solvent recovery I.

Feed = 76.3526 kg. moles

L_m = 110 × 0.763526 = 83.990 kg - moles.

V_m = 11.009 × 0.763526 = 8.407 kg - moles.

D = 1.01 × 0.763526 = 0.772 kg - moles.

W = 98.99 × 0.763526 = 75.58 kg - moles.

The mean properties were calculated on the basis of water in stripping columns & 50% B.A. in rectifying columns. B.P. of liquid in stripper has been assumed at 104°C due to solution of Na-sulphate. Other properties have been assumed same as that for water.

$$\text{Vapour density at top} = \frac{18 \times 0.87 \times 273}{359 \times 369} + \frac{116 \times 0.13 \times 273}{359 \times 369} = 0.0634 \text{ lb/ft}^3.$$

$$\text{Vapour density at bottom} = \frac{18 \times 1 \times 273}{359 \times 373} = 0.0367 \text{ lb/ft}^3.$$

Maximum vapour,

Top = 8.407 kg moles.

$$= 8.407\ (0.83 \times 18 \times 0.13 \times 111)\ \text{kg}$$

$$= 573\ \text{lbs/hr}$$

$$\text{Bottom} = 8.407 \times 18 \times 2.203 = 334\ \text{lb/hr.}$$

Maximum vapour rate

$$\text{Top} = \frac{573}{0.0634 \times 3600} = 2.52\ \text{ft}^3/\text{sec.}$$

$$\text{Bottom} = \frac{334}{0.0367 \times 3600} = 2.53\ \text{ft}^3/\text{sec}$$

Maximum liquid rate

Top 1.035 gals/min (gpm)

Bottom 5.850 gpm.

The data has been tabulated as below :

Data	*Top*	*Bottom*
Pressure psi (A)	15	20
Temperature °C	96	104
σ = Surface tension dynes/cm	30	50
ρ_L = Liquid density, lb/ft^3	53	59.5
ρ_V = Vapour density, lb/ft^3	0.0634	0.0367
Internal reflux, L/v	9.9	–
Maximum vapour rate, lb/hr	0.573	334
Maximum liquid rate, lb/hr	597	3340
Maximum vapour rate, ft^3/see	0.00276	0.0156
Maximum liquid rate, gpm	1.035	5.850
Tray spacing	10 in	10 in

Design of Perforated Tray

Where the calculation appears on the same line, left hand side is for top trays & right hand side is for bottom (stripping columns) trays.

Foaming has been assumed in the system.

Top *Bottom*

Flow parameter

$$P_F = \frac{L}{V}\left[\frac{\rho_v}{\rho_L}\right]^{0.5}$$

$$= \frac{597}{573}\left[\frac{0.0634}{53}\right]^{0.5} \qquad = \frac{3340}{334}\left[\frac{0.0367}{59.5}\right]^{0.5}$$

$$= 0.0314 \qquad = 0.253$$

Plate spacing = 10″

From Fig. 13 – 21 (VW)[25]

$$\text{Vap. velocity } U_{VM} = \left(\frac{\rho_v}{P_L - \rho_V}\right)^{0.5}$$

Capacity factor

$P_c = 0.19$ $\qquad$ $P_v = 0.15$

I. Surface Tension Correction

Top $\qquad$ Bottom

P_c (corres.) for 6 $\qquad$ P_c (corres.) for 6

$$= 0.19\left[\frac{30}{20}\right]^{0.2} \qquad = 0.15\left[\frac{50}{20}\right]^{0.2}$$

$$= 0.206 \qquad = 0.18$$

For 100% of flood

$$U_{VM} = P_c\text{ (corres.)}\left(\frac{\rho_L - \rho_V}{\rho_v}\right)^{0.5}$$

$$= 0.206\left[\frac{53 - 0.0634}{0.0634}\right]^{0.5} \qquad = 0.18\left[\frac{59.5 - 0.0367}{0.0367}\right]^{0.5}$$

$$= 0.18 \times 40.2 = 7.24 \text{ f.p.s.}$$

For 70% of flood. (Table – 15.2 VW)[25]

Net vapour flow area between plates.

$$= A - Ad - A_N = \frac{Q.V}{U_{VM} \times 0.7}$$

$$= \frac{2.52}{5.93 \times 0.7} \qquad = \frac{2.53}{7.24 \times 0.7}$$

$$= 0.608 \text{ ft}^2 \qquad = 0.497 \text{ ft}^2$$

Area of down commer = A_d = 0.1A (assumed)

Area of column $= A = A_N + 2A_d$

$A = 0.608 + 0.2A$ | $A = 0.497 + 0.2A$

$0.8A = 0.608$ | $0.8A = 0.497$

$A = 0.76\ ft^2$ | $A = 0.62\ ft^2$

Tower diameter

$D = \left(\frac{0.76}{0.7854}\right)^{0.5}$ | $D = \left(\frac{0.62}{0.7854}\right)^{0.5}$

$= 0.984$ ft | $= 0.89$ ft

Tower diameter selected = 1 ft

Percent flood | Percent flood

$= \frac{2.52 \times 100}{0.6283 \times 5.92} = 68\%$ | $= \frac{2.53 \times 100}{0.6283 \times 7.24} = 56\%$

Area of column $= A = 0.7854\ ft^2$.
Area of downcomer $= A_d = 0.0785\ ft^2$
Active area for bubbling $= A_A = 0.7854 - 2 \times 0.0785 = 0.6783\ ft^2$
Plate thickness $= t_P = 0.125$ in
Hole diameter $= d_h = 0.75$ in
Hole area/hole = ah. = 308 in^2.
Pitch of holes $= p = 3 \times 0.75 = 2.25$ in
[Equilateral triangular pitch]
Weir height $= h_w = 1.5$ in
Weir length $= l_v - 10.39$ in [Table 14 – 10 V.W. for. H/D = 0.25, L/D = 0.866 or L_w = 0.866 ft.]

II. Entrainment

From Fig. 13 – 26 van winkle (v.w.)
$P_F = 0.0315$ flow parameter $P_F = 0.253$
$\psi = 0.06$ mols/mol of down flow. Entrainment $\psi = 0.004$.
Which is a satisfactory arrangement.

III. Pressure Drop

Height of crest over weir $= h_{ow}$

Top : | Bottm

$$h_{ow} = 0.48\ F_w \left(\frac{Q_L}{L_w}\right)^{0.67}$$

Liquid Load gpm./ (weir length ft)$^{2.5}$

$Q_L/(L_w)^{0.5}$

$= \dfrac{0.035}{(1.866)^{2.5}}$ $\qquad$ $= \dfrac{5.85}{(1.866)^{2.5}}$

$= 1.49$ $\qquad$ $= 8.4.$

F_w = weir construction correction factor from fig. 13-7 V.W. for $\dfrac{D_w}{D} = 0.866$

$F_w = 0.01$ $\qquad$ $F_w = 1.03$

$h_{ow} = 0.48 \times 1.01 \times \left[\dfrac{1.035}{10.4}\right]^{0.64}$ $\qquad$ $h_{ow} = 0.48 \times 1.03 \times \left(\dfrac{5.85}{10.4}\right)^{0.64}$

$= 0.111$ in $\qquad$ $= 0.3355$ in

Top $\qquad$ $h_w = 1.5$ in $\qquad$ Bottom

h_G = Equivalent surface tension head lost.

$$= \frac{0.04 \times 6}{\rho_L \times d_L} \quad \text{[Eq. 13 – ww V.W]}$$

$= \dfrac{0.04 \times 30}{53 \times 0.75}$ $\qquad$ $= \dfrac{0.04 \times 50}{59.5 \times 0.75}$

$= 0.0302$ in $\qquad$ $= 0.045$ in

h_0 = Equiv. head lost through holes.

$$= 0.186 \, \frac{\rho_v}{\rho_L} \left(\frac{u_h}{C_0}\right)^2 \quad \text{[Eq. 13 – 16 V.W]}$$

$t_p = 0.125$ in $d_h = 0.75$ in $t_p / d_h = 0.167$

Let. $A_h / A_A = 0.1$ [A_h is total hole area]

From Fig. 13 – 18 V.W.

Discharge coefficient. $C_0 = 0.69$

$A_h = 0.1 \times 0.6283 = 0.0628$ ft^2.

U_h = Velocity of vapour through holes.

$U_h = \dfrac{2.52}{0.0628}$ $\qquad$ $U_h = \dfrac{2.52}{0.0628}$

$= 40.2$ f.p.s. $\qquad$ $= 40.3$ f.p.s.

Vapour rate

$= 2.52$ ft^3/hr $\qquad$ $= 2.53$ ft^3/hr

$h_0 = 0.186 \left(\dfrac{0.0634}{53}\right)\left(\dfrac{40.2}{0.69}\right)^2$ $\qquad$ $h_0 = 0.186 \left(\dfrac{0.0367}{59.5}\right)\left(\dfrac{40.3}{0.69}\right)^2$

$= 0.755$ in $\qquad$ $= 0.382$ in

From fig 13-16 (V.W.).

Aeration factor

$\beta = 0.72$ $\qquad$ $\beta = 0.8$

Total pressure drop = $\Delta H_T = b(h_w - h_{0w}) + h_0 + h_a$

$= 0.72\ (1.5 + 0.111) + 0.755 + 0.0302$	$= 0.8\ (1.5 + 0.335) + 0.382 + 0.045$
$= 0.72 \times 1.611 + 0.7852$	$= 0.8 \times 1.835 + 0.427$
$= 1.945$ in	$= 1.895$ in

IV. Check for Weak Point

$A_h/A_A = 0.1$

$h_w + h_{0w} = 1.945$ in		$h_w + h_{0w} = 1.835$
	from Fig. 13 – 22 V.W.	
$h_0 + h_G = 0.45$ in		$h_0 + h_G = 0.50$in
	Calculated values.	
$h_0 + h_G = 0.7852$ in		$h_0 + h_G = 0.427$

Only top section operation above weak point to rectify the defective area for vapur flow in bottom trays is reduced as under.

$$A_h = 0.08 \times 0.6283 = 0.050264 \text{ in}^2$$
$$U_h = 50.5 \text{ f.p.s.}$$
$$h_0 = 0.598 \text{ in}^2$$

Hence $h_0 + h_G = 0.598 + 0.045 = 0.643$ in

Total head lost $= \Delta H_T = 1.468 + 0.643$

In bottom trays $= 2.111$ in botton

V. Liquid Backup in Downcommer

Top Bottom

$$H_D = \left[\Delta H_T + \beta\,(h_w + h_{0w}) + \beta\frac{\Delta}{2} + h_d\right]\frac{1}{\phi d}$$

Liquid gradient is negligible for small diameter perforated trough [Ref. V.W.] and has been accounted for. Assume 1.5" clearence under aprox.

A_{AP} = Area for liquid flow under aprox.

$$= \frac{1.5 \times 0.866}{144} = 0.903$$

$$H_D = 0.03\left(\frac{Q_L}{100 \times A_{AP}}\right)^2$$

$= 0.03\left(\dfrac{1.035}{100 \times 0.0903}\right)^2$	$= 0.03\left(\dfrac{5.850}{100 \times 0.0903}\right)^2$
$= 0.01011$ in	$= 0.02215$ in

H_D for top

$$= [\Delta H_T + \beta\ (h_w + h_{0w} + \Delta/2) + h_d]\frac{1}{\phi d}$$

$$\Delta H_T = \beta\ (h_w + h_{0w}) + h_0 + h_G.$$

Neglecting Δ and substitution values of ΔH_T in above equation

$$H_D = [2.\ \beta(h_w + h_{0w}) + h_0 + h_6 + h_d]\frac{1}{\phi d}$$

$$\phi_D = \text{Broth density in downcomer for clear liquid}$$

Top :

$$H_D = [2 \times 0.8\,(1.5 + 0.111) + 0.753 + 0.0302 + 0.01011]$$
$$= 2 \times 0.72 \times 1.611 + 0.7953 = 3.1153$$

Bottom :

$$H_D = [2 \times 0.8\,(1.5 + 0.335) + 0.382 + 0.045 + 0.0241]$$
$$= 1.6 \times 1.835 + 0.451 = 3.39 \text{ in}$$

Assuming $\phi\ d = 0.5$

Height of foam back up a downcommer.

Top = 1.23 in

Bottom = 6.78 in

VI. Liquid Gradient

$$\Delta = \frac{f \cdot v_f^2 \cdot 2L}{12 \cdot g \cdot R_L}$$

It is negligible & has not been calculated/accounted.

VII. Liquid Residence Time in Downcomer

$$A_d = 0.0785 \text{ ft}^2$$

$H_D = 3.1153$ in $\qquad H_D = 3.39$ in

Liquid Load in downcommer.

$\Theta'_{Ld} = 0.00276$ ft³/sec $\qquad \Theta'_{Ld} = 0.0156$ ft³/sec

$$\text{Residence time} = \frac{\text{Volume of downcomer}}{\text{Flow rate}}$$

$$= \frac{(0.0785)\,(3.115/12)}{0.00276} = 7.39 \text{ secs.} \qquad = \frac{(0.0785)\left(\frac{3.39}{12}\right)}{0.0156} = 1.42 \text{ secs.}$$

Residence time in stripping section is below the recommended line for vapour disengagement. One way to increase it is by decreasing the apron clearance. Since the fouling is expected to be heavy it is not advisable to decrease apron clearence. Sloping of apron can also increase residence.

A slope of $7\frac{1}{2}^{\circ}$ with vertical plane is recommended.

Summary

Tower dia. = 1ft

Tray spacing = 10 in

Active area = 0.6283 ft².

Area of holes top → 0.0628 ft², bottom → 0.05003 ft².

Area of downcomer = 0.0785 ft².

A_h/A = Top → 0.08 Bottom → 0.06
$A_{d/d}$ = Top → 0.1 Bottom → 0.1
A_h/A_A = Top → 0.1 Bottom → 0.1
d_h = 0.75 in
l_w = 10.39 in.
h_w = 1.5 in
Downcommer clearance = 1.5 in
Sloping apron for stripping section t_p = 0.125 in

Cross Flow Design

Holes clearance
Hole-tower well - 1.5 in.
Hole-weir – 2 in.
Hole-apron – 2 in.
This completes the design of perforated trays.

Tray efficiency

(1) *By Drickamer Bredford Method*

$E = 0.17 - 0.616 \log \mu'_{av}$
μ' for water at 95°C = 0.27
μ' for B. A. at 95°C = 0.25
μ'_{av} = 0.26 c.p.
∴ E = 0.17 – 0.616 log 0.26 = 0.53
∴ Efficiency = 53%

(2) *From O. Cornell*

$$\frac{mM_L\mu'}{\rho_w} = \frac{16 \times 18 \times 0.26}{58} = 1.29$$

From graph E = 40% [The graph is for Bubble cap (Ref. Traybal–Mass Transfer Operation[23]), tray absorber]

(3) *English & Van Winkle Method* [25]

Van Winkle has given an equation (no. 13–80) which is applicable to the following type
Column type – Bubble cap, perforated trays.
Column diameter – 1 to 24 inches
% free area – 2.7 to 18.5
Plate spacing – 2 to 36 in
Hole diameter – $\frac{1}{16}$ to $\frac{7}{8}$ in
Weir height – $\frac{1}{2}$ to 6 in
G = 100 to 1000 lb/hr ft^2

L = 100 to 1000 ”

L/V = 0.6 to 1.0

Nomenclature is same as given by Van Winkle

Efficiency

$$E = 10.84(FFA)^{-0.28} \times \left(\frac{L}{V}\right)^{0.024} \times h_w^{0.241} \times G^{-0.013} \times \left(\frac{\sigma}{\mu' LU'_v}\right)^{0.044} \times \left(\frac{\mu' L}{\rho'_L D'_L}\right)^{0.137} \times \alpha^{-0.028}$$

FFA = Fractional Free Area.

α = Relative Volatility.

In solving this equation liquid – liquid diffusivity of B.A. and water is required.

Traybal “Mass trans. op.” has given a method of Winkle & a graph correlating diffusivity to dil. solution of non-electrolyte.

$$\frac{T}{D_{AB} - \mu_B} = F \text{ [eqn. 2.38]}$$

T = Abs. temp. °k

M. Wt. of B.A. = 116

Molar Vol. of B.A. = $\frac{116 \times 1}{0.88}$ = 132 c.c/gm.mol

For water as solvent ϕ = 1.0.

From Fig. 2.4, F = 3.8×10^{-7}

$$D = \frac{373}{0.26 \times 3.8 \times 10^{-7}} = 37.8 \times 10^{-5} \text{ cm}^2 \text{ sec}^{-1}$$

The various properties and data for top & bottom of column are given as under

	Top	*Bottom*
D'L	= 37.8×10^{-5} cm²/sec	= 37.8×10^{-5} cm²/sec
$^L/_V$	= 0.92	= $\frac{3840}{334}$ = 10
h_w	= 1.5 in	= 1.5 in
G	= 573 lb/hr ft2	= 570 lb/hr. ft2
μ'L	= 0.25 c.p.	= 0.27 cp.
σ	= 30 dynes/cm	= 50 dynes/cm
ρ'L	= 0.9 gm/cc	= 0.96 gm/c.c.
α	= 16	

$$FFA = \frac{A_h}{A} = \frac{\text{Total hole area}}{\text{Cross section area of column}} = 0.08$$

Top:

Solving for above eqn. we get

$$(FFA)^{-0.28} = (0.08)^{-0.28} = 2.028$$

$$(^L/_V)^{0.024} = \left(\frac{527}{573}\right)^{0.024} = 0.9977$$

$$h_w^{0.241} = (1.5)^{0.241} = 1.103$$

$$G^{-0.013} = (573)^{-0.013} = 0.927$$

$$\left(\frac{\sigma}{\mu'_L\, D'_v}\right)^{0.044} = \left[\frac{30}{34 \times 0.25}\right]^{0.044} = 1.057$$

$$\left(\frac{\mu'_L}{\rho'_L\, D'_L}\right) = \left[\frac{0.25}{37.8 \times 10^{-5} \times 0.9}\right]^{0.137} = 2.358$$

$$\alpha^{-0.028} = 16^{-0.028} = 0.926$$

$\therefore$ E = 10.84 × 2.028 × 0.9977 × 1.103 × 0.927 × 1.057 × 2.358 × 0.926 = 51.5%

[If α is taken as 10 (Rectifying column) E = 52.5%]

Since bottom portion does not satisfy $\frac{L}{V}$ parameter, the tray efficiency has not been calculated by this method. Drickamen & Bredford method and English and Van Winkle equation give nearly similar results.

Hence for rectifying section, a plate efficiency of 50% is selected.

For stripping section an efficiency of 40% is selected.

$$\text{No. of plates in stripping column} = \frac{4}{0.4} + 1 = 11$$

$$\text{Rectifying plates in stripping column} = \frac{1.5}{0.5} = 3$$

Feed plate is number 11 from bottom.

This completes the steam stripping column design. Design of condenser & preheater follows.

Steam Requirement:

Max. vapour rate = 8.407 kg moles

Assuming constant molar vapour flow

Steam used = 8.407 kg. moles/hr

W = 75.580

$$\text{Water for steam} = \frac{8.407}{83.987} \text{ kg moles/hr}$$

Actually about 10% more steam is consumed.

Design of Column Condenser

The heat exchanger which is to be used as the condenser is required to condense 8.4 kg moles/hr. of B.A. & water vapours.

B.A. in distillate = 0.772 × 0.131 × 116 = 11.75 kg/hr

Water in distillate = 0.772 × 0.869 × 18 = 12.01 kg/hr.

Qty. of B.A. in condensing vapour = 8.4 × 0.131 × 116 = 127.7 kg/hr = 281.5 lb/hr

Qty. of water in condensing vapour = 8.4 × 0.869 × 18 = 131.7 kg/hr = 290.0 lb/hr

Latent heat of B.A. = 75 cal/gm at 96.7°C

Latent heat of water = 546 cal/gm

Heat load on condenser

For B.A. = 281.5 × 75 = 171122 lb cals./hr

For water = 290 × 546 = 128340 lb cals/hr

It is proposed to use the feed to distillation column as a cooling medium in this condenser. Before sending distillate to decanter, it is cooled to 20°C. The cooling medium is water.

Heat Load in Cooler

$$\text{For B.A} = \frac{281.5}{10.9}\,[96 - 20] \times 0.459 = 900$$

$$\text{For water} = \frac{290}{10.9}\,[96 - 20] \times 1 \quad = 2000$$

Total 2900 lb cals/hr

Condenser

Heat load = 178200 lb-cal/hr

Qty. of feed (cooling medium) = 3060 lb/hr.

$$\text{Temp. rise of feed} = \frac{178200}{3060} = 57.5°\text{C}$$

The properties of spent beer/buffer has been assumed same as that of water.

Feed inlet temp. = 20°C

Feed exit temp. = 77.5°C

The overhead vapour is a mixture of single compound and steam and so the condensation occurs isothermally (Kern. P – 338)

If a condenser tube of 3/4 in N. B. is used the various dimensions of the tube are as followes:

O.D. = 1.05". I.D. = 0.824 in $A = 0.534\ \text{in}^2$

Kern[14] has given an equation for outside heat transfer co-efficient condensing organic compounds with steam.

$$h = 61\left[\frac{\text{wt.\% } A/\lambda A + \text{wt.\% } B/\lambda B}{\text{wt.\% } A \times D_0}\right]^{1/4}$$

$$= 61\left[\frac{\frac{49.2}{75} + 50.8/546}{49.2 \times 0.0875}\right] = 655\ \text{lb-cals/hr ft}^2\ °\text{C}$$

Assuming an over all heat transfer coefficient for condenser

$U_D = 150\ \text{lb-cals/hr. ft}^2\ °\text{C}$

Temps

	In	*Out*
Hot medium	96	96
Cold medium	20	77.5
Difference	76	18.5

L.M.T.D = 38.6°C. (Log Mean Temp. Difference)

Area required for heat transfer

$$= \frac{178200}{38.6 \times 150} = 30.8 \text{ ft}^2$$

$$\text{Feed rate} = \frac{3060}{62.4} = 49 \text{ ft}^2/\text{hr}$$

Assuming a vel. = 2 ft/sec.

Tube of 3/4 in O.D of B.W.G. – 10 is selected

$$\text{I.D.} = 0.482 \text{ in}$$

Flow area = 0.182 in^2

Surface per linear foot = 0.1963 ft^2/ft

$$\text{No. of tubes} = \frac{49 \times 144}{0.18821 \times 3600 \times 2}$$

$$\text{Tube length required} = \frac{30.8}{5 \times 0.1963} \text{ in}$$

Use of 4 passes 8 ft. length of tube.

Total number of tubes = 5 × 4 = 20

Tube sheet lay out:

Shell I.D. = 8 in.

No. of passes = 4.

Tubes in each pass = 5

Tubes to be arranged on 1 in sq. pitch.

Baffle spacing = 8 in.

Segment of baffles = 25% cut

Shell Side Heat Transfer Coefficient

The cross flow area (from Kern)

$$= \frac{\text{I.D.} \times e'B}{p_T \times 144} = \frac{8 \times 0.25 \times 8}{144 \times 1} = 0.111 \text{ ft}^2$$

Mass vel. $= G_s = \dfrac{3060}{0.111} = 27550$ lb/hr ft^2

$h_{iD} = 395$ [see for tube side coefficient]

$h_0 = 600$ [estimated]

$$\text{Tube wall temperature} = \frac{600}{995}[96-49]+49 = 77°C$$

Properties of condesing vapours at 77°C
Mean properties

$$\text{Thermal conductivity } K = \frac{0.09+0.385}{2} \text{ [Kern]}^{14} = 0.0237. \text{ lb cal/hr. ft}^2/°C$$

$$\text{Viscosity} = \frac{0.32+0.37}{2} = 0.35 \text{ c.p [Conlson Richardson (C.R.) vol – 1]}$$

$$\text{specific heat} = \frac{0.85+0.97}{2} = 0.91 \text{ [Perry]}$$

Kern[14] states that use of LMTD is justifiable for a mixutre of immiscible liquid

$$G'' = \frac{W}{L.N.t^2/3} \text{ [Eqn. 12 – 63 from Kern]}$$

$$= \frac{3060}{8\times 7.36} = 52 \text{ lb/hr. linear ft.}$$

From Fig. 12.9 of Kern
h = 700 lb cal/hr ft^2 °C

Tube Side Heat Transfer Coefficient

$$\text{Flow rate per pass} = \frac{5\times 0.182}{144} = 0.00632 \text{ ft}^2$$

$$G_T = \frac{3060\times 144}{5\times 0.182} = 485000 \text{ lb/hr. ft}^2$$

$$\text{Re. No.} = \frac{485000\times 0.482}{12\times 0.76\times 2.42} = 1.06\times 10^4$$

From Fig. 24. of Kern
$J_N = 40$

$$\text{Pr no } 1/3 = \left(\frac{C_p\cdot\mu}{k}\right)^{1/3} = \left(\frac{1\times 0.75\times 2.42}{0.482}\right)^{1/3} = 1.71$$

$$h_i = \frac{J_N k}{D}(P_r)^{1/2} = \frac{40\times 0.36\times 1.71\times 12}{0.482} = 615 \text{ lb. cal./hr. ft}^2\ °C$$

$$h_{i0} = \frac{615 \times 0.482}{0.75} = 395 \text{ lb. cal/hr. ft}^2\ °\text{C}$$

Assuming a dirt factor $R_D = 0.003$, over all heat transfer coeffi.

$$\frac{1}{U_0} = \frac{1}{700} + \frac{1}{395} + 0.003$$

$$\therefore \quad U_0 = 145 \text{ lb. cal/hr. ft}^2\ °\text{C}$$

The heat exchanger proposed above is satisfactory from heat transfer point of view.

(a) Pressure Drop in Shell

Temperature of vapour = 96°C
Mean viscosity = 0.0152 c.p.
= 0.0152 × 2.42 lb/ft. hr.
= 0.0368 "

Equivalent diameter (from Kern.) = 0.95 in = 0.08 ft

$$\text{Re. No.} = \frac{0.08 \times 27550}{0.0368} = 6000$$

f = 0.00175 (from Kern)

$$\text{No. of crosses} = \frac{8 \times 12}{\rho} = 12$$

Mol wt. of vapours. 62

$$\rho_r = \frac{62}{357} \times \frac{373}{469} = 0.137 \text{ lb/ft}^3$$

$$\text{I.D. of shell} = \frac{2}{3} \text{ ft}$$

$$\Delta p = \frac{\frac{1}{2} + G^2 D_S (N+1)}{522 \times 10^{10} \times D_0 \times S}$$

$$= \frac{1}{2} \times \frac{0.00175 \times 7.6 \times 10^8}{5.72 \times 10^{10} \times 0.08} \times \frac{2}{3} \times \frac{12 \times 63.2}{0.137}$$

$$= 0.515 \text{ lb/in}^2$$

(b) *Pressure Drop in Tubes*

$$\text{Re. No.} = 1.06 \times 10^4$$

f = 0.00027 (from Kern)[14]

$$\Delta P_T = \frac{f \cdot G_R^2 \cdot L \cdot N_t}{5.22 \times 10^{10} \times D \times S \times \phi}$$

$$= \frac{0.00027 \times 4.85^2 \times 10^{10} \times 8 \times 4}{5.22 \times 10^{10} \times 0.04 \times 1 \times 1}$$

$$= 0.975 \text{ lb/in}^2$$

ΔP accross 4 return bends

$$= \frac{4 \cdot n \cdot v^2}{5.2g} \text{ p.s.i [Kern Eq. 7-24]}^{14}$$

$$= \frac{4 \times 4 \times 2^2}{1 \times 2 \times 32.2} = 0.995 \text{ lb/hr}^2$$

$$\text{Total pressure drop} = 1.97 \text{ lb/in}^2$$

Both the pressure drops are low.

Distillate After Cooler

Cooler duty = 2700 lb-cal/hr
Distillate = 23.85 kg/hr = 52.7 lbs/hr
Distillate is to be cooled from 96°C to 20°C

$$\text{Cooling water required} = \frac{2700}{25 - 18} = 386 \text{ lb/hr}$$

	In	*Out*
Hot flux temp.	96	20
Cold flux temp.	out 25	in 28
Difference	71	2
LMTD = 19.3°C		

This is designed on same principles as feed heated outside tube = $1\frac{1}{2}$ in N.B. IPS. Schedule no. 40.

Inside tube of O.D. = 3/4 in
Tube of length = 8 ft.
Double tube heat exchanger
Overall heat transfer coefficient = 80 lb-cal/hr. ft^2 °C.

Design of Feed Heat Exchanger

The feed before entering distillation column is passed through the annulus of this heat exchanger. Hot residue from distillation column is passed through the inner tube.

A double pipe heat exchanger is proposed for it. The temperature of residue from distillation column has been assumed at 104°C

Qty. of residue = 75.580 + 9.4 kg mole of steam
= 85 ”
= 3380 lb/hr

The feed temperature is required to be raised to 98°C. This unit has been purposely designed for less heat load and feed pre-heated in condenser, so as to keep the unit small.

Hot fluid	Cold fluid	Temperature difference
104 Higher temperature	98	6
80.5 lower temperature	77.5	8
18.5 Differences	20.5	2
$T_1 - T_2$	$t_2 - t_1$	$\Delta t_2 - \Delta t_1$

L.M.T.D = 19.5°C

Heat load = 3060 × 20.5 = 52800 lb-cal/hr. Since heat load is low, a double pipe heat exchanger will be designed on the same principles as given by Kern,[14]. The nomenclature used by him is followed here.

A check on both the streams shows that neither is viscous than the cold terminal and the temperature range and differences are moderate. The heat transfer coefficient will be evaluated at arithmatic mean temperature and value of $(\mu\ /\mu_s)^{0.14} = 1$.

LMTD = 19.5°C

T_{av} hot = 94.75°C

T_{av} cold = 87.75°C

Since precaution against scaling is to be taken, and tubes are easy to clean from inside, the outgoing residue will pass through tubes and feed through the annulus.

Assume velocity of residue = 2 ft/sec.

$$\text{Vol. flow rate} = \frac{3380}{62.2} = 54.3\ \text{ft}^3/\text{hr}$$

Area of cross section required for flow = 1.09 in^2

A hair pin of outside pipe 2 in IPS and inside pipe of $1\frac{1}{4}$ in IPS is selected.

Tube N.B. $1\frac{1}{4}$ in O.D = 1.66 D,

2 in I.D. = 2.06 D^2

$a_a = 1.77\ m^2$ (area of annulus × section)

Cold fluid annulus

3060 lb/hr

Flow area 1.17 in^2

= 0.00812 ft^2

Equiv. diameter = D_e

= $D_2^2 - D_1^2/D_e$

= 0.075 ft

Mass velocity

Hot fluid inner pipe

3380 lb/hr

Flow area = 0.0104 ft^2

Mass velocity $Gp = \frac{w}{a_a}$

$$G_p = \frac{w}{a_a}$$

$$= \frac{3060}{0.00182} = 340500 \text{ lb/ft. hr}$$

At. 87.75°C

$\mu = 0.31$ c.p.

$= 0.75$ lb/ft. hr

$$\text{Re. no.} = \frac{340500 \times 0.075}{0.31 \times 2.42}$$

$$= 34100$$

$J_m = 105$

At 87.75°C, k = 0.4

Sp. heat = 0.93

$$p_r^{1/3} = \frac{C_p \, \mu^{1/3}}{k} = \left(\frac{0.937}{0} \frac{0.75}{1}\right)^{1/3}$$

$$= 1.2$$

$$h_0 = Jm \frac{k}{D_c} \times p_r^{1/3} \times \left(\frac{\mu}{\mu_s}\right)^{0.14}$$

$$= \frac{105 \times 0.4}{0.075} \times 1.2 \times 1$$

$$= 623 \text{ lb cal/hr ft}^2 \text{ °C}$$

$$= \frac{3380}{0.0104}$$

$$= 32500 \text{ lb/hr. ft}^2$$

At. 94.75°C

$\mu = 0.28$ c.p.

$= 0.68$ lb/ft – hr.

$$\text{Re. no.} = \frac{325000 \times 0.115}{0.28 \times 2.42}$$

$$= 57200$$

$J_m = 160$

k = 0.41

Sp. heat = 0.92

$$p_r^{1/3} = \left(\frac{0.68 \times 0.92}{0.41}\right)^{1/3}$$

$$= 1.15$$

$$h_i = J_M \times \frac{k}{D} \times p_r^{1/3} \left(\frac{\mu}{\mu_s}\right)^{0.14}$$

$$= \frac{160 \times 0.41 \times 1.15 \times 1}{0.0140} = 724$$

$$h_{i_0} = \frac{72451.38}{1.66} = 600 \text{ lb cal/hr ft}^2 \text{ °C}$$

Clean over all coefficient.

$$= \frac{h_{i_0} \times h_0}{h_{i_0} + h_0} = \frac{623 \times 600}{1223} = 305$$

Assuming a dirt factor $R_d = 0.005$

Design over all coefficient,

$$\frac{1}{U_D} = \frac{1}{U_C} + 0.005$$

$$U_D = 118 \text{ lb-cal/hr. ft}^2 \text{ °C}$$

Summary

623 h outside 600

$$U_c = 305$$

$$U_D = 118$$

Surface area required = $A = \dfrac{Q}{D_D \times \Delta T} = \dfrac{62800}{118 \times 19.5} = 27.3\ ft^2$

From table 11 of Kern. $1\dfrac{1}{11}$ in IPS pipe surface area

$= 0.435\ ft^2/ft$ of pipe length

Required length of tube = $\dfrac{27.3}{0.435} = 63$ ft

Fin tubes (double) of 12 ft. lenght will be O.K. Actual design coefficient

$$= \frac{67800}{60 \times 0.435} = 123 \text{ lb-cal/hr. ft}^2{}^\circ C$$

Pressure Drop

Annulus

D'_e for pr. drop = $D_L - D_1$

= 0.0345 ft.

$$Re. = \frac{0.0345\ 5\ 340500}{0.75}$$

= 15700

f = 0.00807. (Kern)

S = 0.93 sp. ht.

$\rho = 62.5 \times 0.08 = 61.7$ ft/ft3.

$\Delta f_a = 4f\, G^2L/2g\rho\ ^2 .\ D'_e$

$$= \frac{4 \times 0.0081 \times 340500^2 \times 60}{2 \times 4.18 \times 10^8 \times 612^2 \times 0.0345}$$

= 18.4 ft

Inner pipe

Re. = 57200

$$f = 0.0035 + \frac{0.764}{(D_e\ \mu)^{0.42}} \text{ (Eqn. 3 – 476 Kern)}$$

$\therefore$ F = 0.0061

S = 0.92

$\rho = 62.5 \times 0.97 = 60.6$ lb/ft3

$$\Delta f_a = \frac{4f\, G_\rho^2 \cdot L}{2 \cdot g \cdot \rho^2 \cdot D}$$

$$= \frac{4 \times 0.0061 \times 325000^2 \times 60}{2 \times 4.18 \times 10^8 \times 60.6^2 \times 0.115}$$

= 4.5 ft

$$\Delta P = \frac{4.5 \times 60.3}{144}$$

$= 1.875\ lb/in^2$

$$V = \frac{G}{3600\,\rho} = \frac{340500}{3600 \times 61.2} = 1.55 \text{ fps}$$

$$F = 5\left(\frac{V^2}{2g}\right)$$

$$= 5 \times \frac{(1.55)^2}{2 \times 32.2} = 0.186 \text{ ft}$$

$$\text{APG} = \frac{(18.4 + 0.2) \times 61.2}{144} = 7.92 \approx 8 \text{ lb/in}^2$$

To be cared while designing pump.

Length of hair pin has been kept low for ease of cleaning. The unit is a small one and if plugging of tubes take place earlier than the cleaning required for distillation column it will be economical to have a double tube heat exchanger of above duty as a stand by.

Decanter

The decanter proposed is a cylindrical vessel of type C in Fig. 21–27 mentioned by Perry.[15]

A decanter of 200 liters capacity will give about $3\frac{1}{2}$ hr for liquid layers of B.A. & water to separate.

Quantity of distillate to be handled = 52.7 lb/hr = 1 ft^3/hr

Dimensions of decanter

Diameter = 1'6 in
Height = 4'3 in
Distance of heavy liquid outlet from bottom = 47 in
Distance of light liquid outlet from bottom = 50.6 in

Material Balance Over Solvent

Recovery Part I

Material balance in kg/hr

	In	*Out*	
		Distillate	*Residue*
Butylacetate	12.57	11.73	0.84
Water	1372.43	12.10	1360.33
Steam	159.00	–	159.00 (Condensate)
Total	1544.00	23.83	1520.17

The water layer from decanater is sent for recovery of B.A. along with spent beer/buffer. It is a very small quantity (0.16 kg/hr.) and is ultimately recommended (Not cited in material balance separately). B.A. is sent to B.A. holding tank.

Quantity of steam consumed and heat balance

Unit of heat = k – Cals.

Datum temp. = 0°C

Heat Input

(1) By column feed = 27700 kcal/hr.

(2) By steam = Q × 654

Heat Output

(1) By distillation = 360 k-cal/hr.

(2) Bottom residue = (1361.5 + 159) × 85.5 = 130000 kcal/hr.

(3) By after cooler = 12.20

Q × 656 + 27700 = 130000 + 1220 + 360

Qty. of steam used = Q = 159 kg/hr

Heat Balance in k-cal/hr Datum temp. 0°C.

	In				*Out*		
	Wt.(kg)	*Temp. °C*		*Heat (kcal)*	*Wt (kg)*	*Temp. °C*	*Heat kcals*
Feed	1385	20	27700	Distillate	23.8	360	
Steam	159	–	103900	Residence	1520.0	85.5	130000
Cooling Water	175	18	3100	Cooling Water	175	25	4340
	Total		134700				134700
			k-cal/hr				k-cal/hr

Solvent Recovery Part II

B.A. from step II of extraction process together with mother liquor from crystallisation section will be returned in a pot still.

If B.A. is to be recovered in anhydrous state using one column only it will be in bottom product, but then the impurities in it will remain in the product. Another way is to mix it with water and use two columns, one for water and the other for B.A. But this will be a costly affair. If water is present in B.A. corresponding to its solubility limit at 20°C i.e. 1.37% w/w, it will not effect the extraction process. So, we can do without anhydrous B.A.

If water is mixed in B.A. and a continuous process is used for recovery, the number of stages and reboiler load will be very high.

Batch distillation is proposed for it. The B.A. will be mixed with water & distilled in a still of 15 M^3 capacity which can take the load of 24 hrs. of one batch of fermenter.

The liquid left as residue when contains 0.0005 mol. fraction of B.A. will be drained.

However, there is great flexibility in its operation and if the local by-laws do not allow the effluent containing more than 0.0001 mol fraction or less, it can be achieved at the cost of more reflux/steam.

Distillation is [24,25] carried out at atmospheric pressure.

During operation, the temperature at top will be the least guiding factor.

B.A. from Step II

Of Extraction	=	257.98 kg/hr
B.A. from M.L	=	65.02 kg/hr
Total	=	323.00 kg/hr

$$\text{Quantity of dissolved water} = \frac{223 \times 1.33}{100} = 4.4 \text{ kg}$$

Anhydrous B.A. = 378.6 kg.

Weight of water mixed = 210.0 kg.

Feed

	Wt. in kg/hr	Mol. wt.	kg Mol.	Mol. fraction
B.A.	318.6	116	2.745	0.187
Water	214.4	18	11.910	0.813
Total			11.655	

Feed/day = 14.605 × 24 = 351.72 kg mols/day. The distillation is carried out in three steps. *Step I* : Simple distillation till residue contains 0.04 mol fraction of B.A. Distillate will contain 0.226 mol fraction of B.A.

Step II : Starting of reflux and increasing reflux ratio to 3.

During this operation, distillate will be of purtiy 0.296 mol fraction of B.A. Top temperature will be kept steady at 20.2°C. At the end residue will be left with 0.005 mol fraction of B.A.

Step III : Keeping the reflux ratio constant at 3 and collecting second cut of distillate, the operation will be continued till the bottom product is left with 0.0005 mol fraction of B.A.

Step I : Feed to still per batch = 351.72 kg mol.

$x_f = 0.18$

Since the composition of distillate remains constant due to Azeotrope formation, the quantity of distillate & residue can be calculated by simple material balance.

If f = Mols. of feed

x_f = Mol. fraction

D & W = Mols. of distillate & residue respectively, x_d & x_w = Mol. fraction of B.A. in distillate & residue.

If F = 100 mols.

F = D = w, D = 100 – w

$F\,x_f = D\,x_d + W\,.\,x_w$, $x_f = 0.18$ $x_d = 0.276$

$\therefore\ 100 \times 0.18 = (100 - w) \times 0.296 + w \times 0.06\ x_w - 0.04$

W = 42.56

D = 57.44

Qty. of B.A. in distillate = 57.44 × 3.5172 × 0.296 × 116
= 6952 kg/day

Qty. of water in distillate = 57.44 × 3.5772 × 0.704 × 18
= 2560 kg/day

Heat Duty

(1) Heat required to raise the feed temperature from 20° to 96°C (Av)
For B.A. = 318.6 × 24 × 76 × 0.454 = 254000 kcals
For water = 214.4 × 24 × 76 × 1 = 376000 kcals.

(2) Heat supplied by boiler for evaporation duty
For B.A. = 6952 × 73.8 = 513000 kcals
For water = 2560 × 545 = 1395000 kcals

(3) Heat removed in condenser same as no. (2).

(4) Heat removed after cooler.
From. B.A. = 6952 × 70 × 0.454 = 221000 kcals
From water = 2560 × 70 = 179200 kcal

Total heat load (k cals)

Boiler	*Condenser*	*After cooler*
254000	513000	221000
376000	1395000	179200
513000		
1395000	1908000	400200
2538000		

Step II : Const. product, Variable reflux
[Ref: Coulson & Richardson, Chem. Eng., vol. II Eq. 18-126]

D_b = Amt. of product obtained

S_1 = No. of moles originally present in still

S_2 = Moles. of risidue

x_{s_1} = Mol. fraction of B.A. in start up

x_{s_2} = Mol. fraction of B.A. after each fraction

x_d = Mol. fraction of B.A. in distillate

ϕ = Intercept on Y-axis

$$R = \text{Reflux ratio}$$

$$D_b = S_1 \left[\frac{x_{s_1} - x_{s_2}}{x_d - x_{s_2}}\right], \text{ Assume } S_1 = 100 \text{ mols}$$

$$\text{For } R = 1, \phi = \frac{x_d}{R+1} = \frac{0.296}{2} = 0.148$$

$$D_b = 100 \left[\frac{0.04 - 0.012}{0.296 - 0.012}\right] = 9.87$$

The various values at different flux ratio were evaluated and tabulated as under.

R	ϕ	x_s	D_b
0.0	0.296	0.04	0.0
0.5	0.197	0.017	8.25
1.0	0.148	0.012	9.87
2.0	0.095	0.007	11.40
3.0	0.074	0.005	12.00

Qty. of distillate = 12 × 1.4972 = 17.97 kg mol

Qty. of distillate in residue = 131.75

Wt. of B.A. in distillate = 17.97 × 0.296 × M. wt. of B.A.

= 617.2 kg. wt. of B.A.

Wt. of water in distillate = 1797 × 0.704 × 18

= 227.8 kg

Reflux:

For 100 mole feed

$$\int_{R=0}^{R=3} R_1 \, D_b = 6$$

Reflux = 6 × 1.4972 = 8.77

Heat Duty

Heat duties of Reboiler & Condenser are same.

(1) *For Reflux*, quantity of heat supplied by boiler

From B.A. = 8.77 × 0.296 × 116 × 73.8 = 22230 kcals

From water = 8.77 × 0.704 × 18 × 545 = 60570 kcals

(2) For distillate heat supplied

From B.A. = 6.17 × 2 × 73.8 = 45550 kcal

From water = 227.8 × 545 = 124220 kcal

Total heat load. k-cal

Boiler	*Condenser*	*After Cooler*
45550	252570	19650
124220		15950
22230		35600
60570		
252570		

Step III : Const. Reflux Variable Distillate

In step III the distillation is carried out with a constant reflux ratio of 3 till the bottom product left is 0.0005 mol fraction, of B.A. (Refer to Coulson & Richardson vol II).

$$\ln \frac{S_1}{S_2} = \int_{x_{s2}}^{x_{s1}} \frac{dx_2}{x_d - x_s}$$

Material Balance for Part II Solvent Recovery

Feed = 351.72 kg mol/day

B.A. = 0.18 mol fraction

Qty. of B.A. = 7646.4 kg/day

	Distillate				*Residue*	
	Distillate kg-mols	*Mol fr. B.A.*	*B.A. kg*	*Water kg*	*Residue kg-mol*	*Mol fr. B.A*
I Step	202	0.296	6952.0	2560	149.72	0.04
II Step	17.9	0.296	617.2	227.8	131.72	0.005
III Step	4.55	0.130	69.1	79.2	127.2	0.0005
		Total =	7638.3	2867.0		

kg/day	*Present in feed*	*Present in distillate*	*Qty. left*
B.A.	7646.4	7638.3	8.1
Water	5145.6	2867.0	2278.6

Analysis of Residue

$$\text{Qty. of B.A.} = 0.0005 \times 127.2 \times 116 = 7.4 \text{ kg}$$

$$\text{Water} = 0.4995 \times 127.2 \times 18 = 2285$$

The difference is due to slide rule error or graphical integration. The quantity of B.A. removed is taken as

$$= 7638.3 + (8.1 - 7.4) = 7639 \text{ kg/day}$$

Total heat load in kcal/day

Step	1 Heat input	2 Heat removed	3 Heat removed	4 Heat left in
I	2538000	1908000	400200	
II	252570	252570	35600	
III	192800	192800	7800	19640
Total =	2983370	2353370	443600	

Equipment for solvent recovery part II

(1) Still volume = 10 m^3
Heat load = 2500,000 kcals/hr
The design should be able to meet the above requirement.
It is well evident from these calculations that as number of stages increases beyond 3, no significant benefit occurs.
The nomenclature used by Coulson & Richardson has been used here.

Nature of x_d, x_s, $x_d - x_s$, $\frac{1}{x_d - x_s}$ are tabulated as below.

These data were used for graphical integration and various values.

x_s	x_d	$x_d - x_s$	$\frac{1}{x_d - x_s}$
0.003	0.296	0.291	3.44
0.0027	0.16	0.1573	6.35
0.0022	0.13	0.1278	7.83
0.0017	0.1	0.0983	10.17
0.00085	0.05	0.04915	20.35
0.0005	0.02	0.0195	51.20

$$\ln \frac{s_1}{s_2} = \int_{0.0005}^{0.005} \frac{dx_s}{x_d - x_s} = 0.0355$$

$$\frac{s_1}{s_2} = 1.036, \; s1 = 131.75; \; s2 = 127.20$$

Distillate = 4.55 kg mole
Mole of B.A. in distillate

$$= x_1 s_1 - s_2 x_2$$
$$= 0.005 \times 131.75 - 0.0005 \times 127.20$$

$$= 0.6588 - 0.0636 = 0.5952$$

Average composition of distillate

$$= \frac{0.5952}{4.55} = 0.130$$

Wt. of B.A. in distillate $= 0.5952 \times 116 = 69.1$ kg

Wt. of water in distillate $= 3.9548 \times 18 = 79.2$ kg

(2) Heat Duties

Heat required to provide reflux and evaporation of distillate

$$= (3 + 1)(69.1 + 73.8)\ 337.29$$

$$= 4 \times 48200 = 192800 \text{ k. cals/day}$$

Heat removed in after cooler

$$= 69.1 \times 70 \times 0.454 + 79.2 \times 70 \text{ cals/day}$$

No. of theoretical stages required = 3

No. of theoretical plates required = 2

If plate efficiency = 4%

No. of plates required = 5

Max. vapour rate = 615 m^3/hr = 6 ft^3 sec. A column of 2 ft dia. filled with 5 perforated plates having ¼" holes on 0.75" pitch should be enough. Plate spacing = 1.5 ft.

(3) Condensers

Heat duty requirement of condenser = 19100 k cal hr, the cooling water (C.W) used will first pass through cooler and then through this condenser C.W entry temp will be 25°C and quantity of C.W used = 40000 kg/hr.

(4) After cooler heat duty = 4000 k cal/hr

(5) Decanter used will be same type as provided in S.R. part I

Liquid in condenser is not to be cooled below 90°C and a part of distillate will be used as reflux if and when needed.

Time requirement for solvent recovery part II

If vapour boil up rate = 20 kg. mols/hr approx., time requirement for batch distillation operation will be

(1)	Heat up	—	2 hrs
(2)	Step I	—	10 hrs
(3)	Step II	—	1.5 hrs
(4)	Step III	—	1.0 hrs
	Total	=	14.5 hrs

The chemical requirement in design of still and accessories have not been asked for and so they have not been designed in detail. However, the design will be on the same basis as done for S.R. Part I.

Material balance over solvent recovery (S.R. Part II)

Kg/day	*Anhydrous B.A.*		
	In	*Out*	
		Distillate	*Residue*
B.A.	7646.4	7639	7.4
Water	5145.6	2867	2278.6
Total	12792.0	10506	2286

Heat balance over S.R. Part II kcal/day (datum temp. = 8°C)
Over all material balance in terms of hydrated butyl acetate (B.A.)

(1) Qty. of B.A. recovered from part II of solvent recovery (S.R.)

$$7639 + \frac{7639 \times 1.37}{100} = 7744.5 \text{ kg/day.}$$

(2) Qty. of B.A. sent to S.R. Part I. (B.A. dissolved in water layer in decanter of S.R.

$$\text{Part II} = \frac{2286 \times 1}{100} = 22.86 \text{ kg/day.}$$

(3) Qty. of B.A. sent to storage from S.R. Part II.
$= 7744.5 - 22.86 = 7721.64$ kg/day

(4) Qty. of B.A. lost in residue in S.R. Part II

$$= 7.4 + \frac{7.4 \times 1.37}{100} = 7.5 \text{ kg/day.}$$

(5) Qty. of B. A. sent to S.R. II was assumed at $1.43 \times 24 = 34.32$ kg/day
Hence yield is S.R. I will be less by $34.32 - 22.86 = 11.46$ kg/day.

(6) Correct quantity of B.A. recovered from S.R. Part I.
$= 281.52 - 11.46 = 270.06$ kg/day

(7) Total quantity of B.A. sent to storage
$= 7721.64 + 270.06 = 2991.7$ kg/day

Qty. of B.A. lost

(a) In S.R. I	=	20.16	kg/day
(b) In S.R. II	=	7.50	kg/day
(c) Crystal section	=	54.24	kg/day
Total		81.90	kg/day loss

Qty. of B.A. drawn from storage

(a) Extraction Step I.	=	267.70	kg/hr
(b) Step III	=	68.70	kg/hr
Total		336.40	kg/hr

Total B.A.	=	(7744.5 – 7.5) + 336.4
	=	8073.40 kg/day
Qty. of B.A sent back	=	7991.70
Qty. of B.A. lost	=	81.70 kg/day

15.6 REFERENCES

1. Steel, R., *Biochemical Engineering.,* London, Heywood & Co. Ltd., 1958.
2. Kirk, T.K. and D.F., Othmer., *Encyclopedia of Chemical Technology* 2, 3rd edn., John Wiley & Sons, New York, 1978.
3. Benedic, R.G. W.H., Schmidth and R.D. Coghill. *J. Bact.* pp 3, 51, 1946.
4. Flynn, E.H. and C.W. Godzerki, "Penicillins and Calplolosporis." *Antibiotics,* Vol 1, (D. Gottlieb and P.D. Show eds.), Springer Verlag, New York Inc., pp 1-39, 1967.
5. Presoctt, S.C. and C.G. Dunn, *Industrial Microbiology* 3rd edn., (Intern. student eds.), McGraw Hill Book Co. Inc, New York, 1959.
6. Aiba S., A.E. Humphrey and N.F. Millis, *Biochemical Engineering* 2nd edn., Univ. Tokyo Press, 1973.
7. Blakebrough, N. (ed), *Biochemical and Biological Engineering Science*, Vol. 1, Acad. Press., 1969.
8. Bailey, J.E. and D.F. Ollis, *Biochemical Engineering Fundamental*, 2nd edn, McGraw Hill Book Co., New York, 1986.
9. Atkinson, B. and F. Mavituna, *Biochemical Engineering & Biotechnology Hand Book*., 2nd edn., M. Stocktor Press, Hamp Shire, England, 1991.
10. Van't Riet, K. and J. Tramper, *"Basic Bioreactor Design*, Marcel Dekkar, Inc. New York, 1991.
11. Brownell, L.E. and E.H. Young, *Process Equipment Design, Vessel Design*; John willey & Sons Inc., New York, pp 76 -97, 1959.
12. Walas, S.M. *Chemical Reaction Engineering Hand Book of Solved Problems*, Gordon and Beach Pubs., Australia, pp 798-814, 1995.
13. Chain, E.B., *World Health Org. Bult.,* pp 673, 1952
14. Kern, D.Q., *Process Heat transfer*, MacGraw Hill., New York, 1950.
15. Perry, R.H. and C.H. Chilton, *Chemical Engineers' Hand book* 4th edn., pp 10-25, 1963.
16. Kudrika A.A., R.J. Grosh and P.W. McFadden, "Heat Transfer in Two-Phase Flow of Gas-Liquid Mixtures", *Ind. Eng. Chem.* 4(3), pp 339-344, 1965.
17. Solomons, G.L., *Materials and Methods in Fermentation,* Acad. Press., London and New York, 1969.
18. Timoshenko, S. and G.H. MacCullough, *Elements of Strength of Materials* 3rd ed., D. Von Nostrand Princeton, New Jersey, 1949.
19. Coulson, J.M., and Richardson. *J.F. Chem. Engg*., Vol. I, Pergamon Press, 1962.
20. McCabe W.L., J.C. Smith and P. Harriot, *Unit Operations of Chemical Engineering*, McGraw Hill, New York, 1985.
21. Nelson, W.L. *Petroleum Refinery Engineering*, 4th edn., pp 25-58, 1985.
22. Liddell, J.M., "Solvent Extraction Processes for Biological Products", *Engineering Processes for Bioseparations*, pp 166-201, (Weatherly, L.R. ed.), 1994.

23. Treybal, R.E. *Mass Transfer Operations*, McGraw Hill, New York, 1980.
24. Hougen, J.A. K.M. Watson *Chem. Process Principles*, Part II Asia Pub. House Bombay, pp 954, 1962.
25. Van Winkle, *Distillation*, McGraw Hill Book Co., N. Y.
26. Gillil, E.R. *et al., Ind. Eng. Chem.*, pp 32, 1220, 1940.

Chapter

16

BIOPROCESSING PRACTICE TUTORIALS

16.1 INTRODUCTION

The process biotechnology for productions of materials has been recognized based on high scientific excellence. Biotechnological processes and research have witnessed enormous progress over the last few decades. The engineering sciences of biotechnology have grown significantly. Computation processes for the same are also not lagging behind and no longer limited to descriptive sciences. In this new era of Biochemical engineering and Biotechnology encompasing areas like engineering biology, upstream bioprocessing, fermentation technology, downstream processing, biocatalytic processing, bioseparation, bioprocess monitoring sensors and devices, bioprocess scale up, simulation and control, bioprocess design and calculations etc have advanced significantly. In these research based subjects teaching, it is essential to set elucidatory numerical problems on various concerns and provide large number of multichoice questions to introduce students of various levels and researchers to parametric computational approaches. The necessity of such provision in the book appears frequently in the mind of biotechnologists with bioscience background for reasons concerned with arguments based on efficiency, examination of process models and strong quantitative inference. If a text book is contained with rich sources of problems and questions it is well suited for setting examination papers at various levels. Readers particularly students, must therefore get acquainted with the techniques for solving problems and answering questions. To this end the numerical problems and multichoice questions (MCQ) provided in this chapter have been prepared mostly based on the long research and teaching experiences at UG, PG and pre Ph.D levels and available informations from research papers published in peer reviewed journals, books as cited in the bibliography. These will aid in provoking thoughts in the minds of the readers of this book.

16.2. MICROBIAL PURE CULTURE BIOPROCESSING

16.2.1 Engineering Biology in Bacterial Biotechnology

Prob. 1 In host cells of *E. coli* the recombinant plasmid PBR 322 T leu which contained β iso-propyl malate dehydrogenase gene of *T. thermusthermophilus* HB27 was cloned. For assessment of stability of the plasmid in host cells the following scheme was proposed by Imanaka and Aiba in a medium substrate S $mgml^{-1}$ and inoculum contained number concentrations of plasmid carrying cells, P cells ml^{-1}, and cells without plasmid had number of concentrations N cells ml^{-1}.

$$aS + P \rightarrow (2 - P)\,P + N;\ (N = pP) \tag{16.1}$$

$$bS + N \rightarrow 2N \tag{16.2}$$

The terms a and b in the above reaction scheme are coefficients having units of cells $(mg\ subtrate)^{-1}$ in terms of process biotechnology and p is the probability of deprivation of plasmid.

a. What assumptions are needed to formulate the above scheme and why?

b. From the above scheme express the following

(i) Number of concentration of plasmid carrying cells.

(ii) Number of concentration of cells without plasmid in relation to plasmid carrying cells.

c. Fraction of cells carrying plasmid in total population.

Prob. 2. In the problem 1 arrive at expressions for part c in a

(i) batch culture for nth generations of cells

(ii) chemostat

Prob. 3. The restriction enzyme *Bam* HI cut the recognition sequences as in its standard cleavage figure below.

5' — G — G — A — T — C — C — 3'

3' — C — C — T — A — G — G — 5'

Bam H1

a. After cut indicate the 5' and 3' ends of the fragments of DNA molecules.

b. Is it possible to modify the cut molecules? If so, how would the ends be modified if one would have indicated the cut molecules with DNA polymerase in presence of all four dNTPS?

c. It is further necessary to redesign the molecule by joining. Is it still possible to join the *Bam* H1 ends together?

d. Does this redesigning of the part c will regenerate *Bam* H1 site?

Prob. 4. What are restriction fragments? A microorganism's plasmid carries gene that confers resistance to several antibiotic markers. The restriction digests of the plasmid and its restriction enzyme fragment's electrophoretic mobilities on agarose gels indicated the size of the fragments as in the Table 16.1.

From the above informations construct the restriction map of the plasmid.

Table 16.1

Participating Restriction Enzyme	*Fragment Size (kb)*
*E. co*R1	5.4
Hind III	2.1, 1.9, 1.4
Sal I	5.4
*E. co*R1 + *Hind* III	2.1, 1.4, 1.3, 0.6
*E. co*R1 + *Sal* I	3.2, 2.2
Hind III + Sal I	1.9, 1.4, 1.2, 0.9

Prob. 5 What do you mean by replication fork in chromosomal replication? Compute the minimum and maximum number of replication forks in a contiguous chromosome of an *E. coli* that is dividing every (a) 25 minutes, (b) 80 minutes

Prob. 6. In an experiment it was found that at 37°C a culture of *E. coli* gave 0.67 mutations per 10^8 cells per hour. Assuming there is only one gene to mutate per bacterium, calculate the half life of the genes in years.

Prob. 7. Define 'Morgan' unit of gene separation. A study in cell biology revealed 0.15% separation and recombination of two genes in a bacteriophage.
a. Assuming that 10^{-5} Morgan is 30Å calculate the separation between the genes.
b. Another pair showed a 15% figure. Assuming those to lie at opposite ends of the linkage group calculate the length of the genetic line required.
c. The phage has a head of diameter 750Å and a tail of the same length. Comment on the molecular nature of the "gene string".

Prob. 8. In a cell growth study with *E. coli* two identical *E. coli* cultures were incubated at 37°C. One of them was infected with phage T_{4_o} and the other with phage T_{4_r} II 73. The multiplicity of infection was found to be 1 ml suspension (containing 2×10^{10} cells/ml) per 1000 ml (4×10^8 cells per ml). While the T_{4_r} II 73 infected culture was found to be lysed and decreased but the cell density to T_{4_o} infected culture did not decrease. After chloroform addition and centrifugation the phage titre in the crude lysate was found to be 1.2×10^{11}/ml $T4_0$ and 0.3×10^{11}/ml T_{4_r} II 73. What inference can you draw from these data? Also, calculate; (a) multiplicity factor of infection, (b) growth rate constant, (c) number of generations, generation time.

16.2.2 Catabolic Repression

Prob. 9. From the relation of specific invertase activity vs dilution rate (Fig. 16.1) in a chemostat cultivation of *S. carlsbergensis* on a glucose medium dual control of induction and repression on two sities of the operator genes for invertase biosynthesis has been proposed, Fig. 16.2. Assuming synthesis of invertase was initiated only when functions of both O_1 and O_2 genes worked conveniently on a chromosome the chemical equilibrium of the reactions shown in Fig. 16.3 were given by :

$$Q_1 = \frac{[O_1]}{[O_2]_t} = \frac{1 + K_1\, s_1^m}{1 + k_1\,[R_1]_t + k_1 s^m} \tag{16.3}$$

and

$$Q_2 = \frac{[O_2]}{[O_2]_t} = \frac{1 + K_1\, S_1^n}{1 + (1 + k_2\,[R_2]_t + k_2 s_2{}^n} \tag{16.4}$$

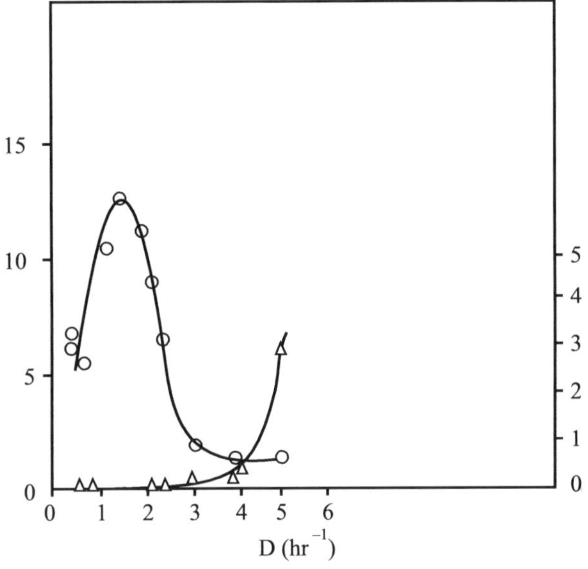

Fig. 16.1 Invertase specific activity vs. the dilution rate (*S. carlsbergensis*)

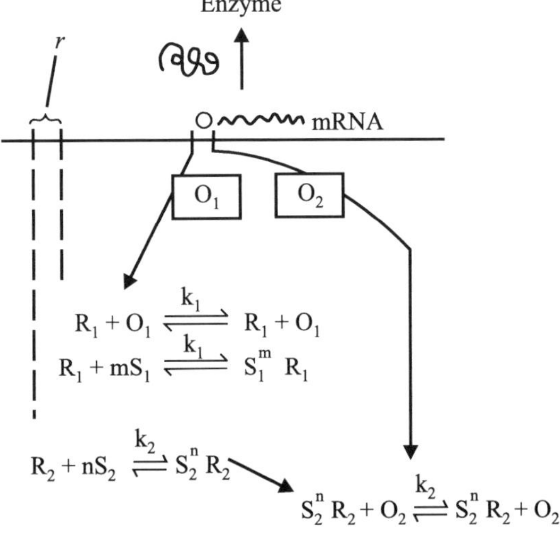

Fig. 16.2 Schematic representation of the dual control mechanism

where Q_1 and Q_2 are ratios, $[O_1]$ is number of induced gene, $[O_2]$ number of non-repressed gene and $[O_1]_t$ and $[O_2]_t$ are total number of each operator gene considering fraction of invertase specific activity (Q) is the ratio of actual (E / X) value to theoretical maximum value with full induction and no repression being equivalent to product of Q_1 and Q_2. Estimate at lower dilution rates values of m, n, K_1, K_2, k_1 and k_2 which are the constants for the stoichiometry and adsorption equillibrium in the binding process among the molecules R_1, R_2, S_1, S_2, O_1, O_2 and $S_2^n R_2$ (assuming the value of S_1 same as glucose).

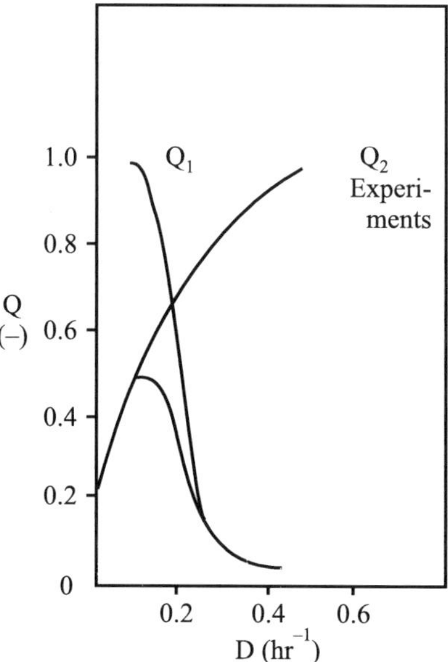

Fig. 16.3 The extent of induction (Q_1) and repression (Q_2) estimated hypothetically from the experimental results shown in ig. 16.1

16.2.3 Homogenic Cell-Cell Interactions

Prob 10. In the production of cellulase in a batch laboratory stirred tank bioreactor (CeCa) by *Trichoderma reesei* QM9414 the organism formed pellets by cell-cell multiinteractions. The pellet diameter varied with cultivation time. The bioreactor diameter was 15 cms and impeller operated at 300 rpm had a diameter 5 cms. The multiinteractions caused pellet formation to be started from first day of cultivation when liquid density was 1.1 gl^{-1}. Average weight of a wet pellet was 0.03 g. The average weight of a pellet on 9th day of cultivation was 0.09 g and the density of the liquid increased to 1.30 gl^{-1}. Considering the ratio of consistency index to liquid viscosity as of Newtonian nature calculate the value of homogenization efficiency index and pellet diameter of *T. reesei* QM 9414 on the nineth day of cell cultivation, [Assure the ratio, $\alpha = 0.7$ and liquid height in fermenter = diameter of the fermenter].

Prob 11. The dynamics of two species/component multiinteracting biosystem near a steady state could be given by the following system equation.[2]

$$\frac{d\lambda_1}{dt} = a_{11}\lambda_1 + a_{12}\lambda_2$$
$$\frac{d\lambda_2}{dt} = a_{21}\lambda_1 + a_{22}\lambda_2 \qquad (16.5)$$

(a) Deduce to show that this equation system has the following solution system

$$\lambda_1(t) = \frac{c_1 a_{12}}{\sigma_1 - a_{11}} e^{\sigma 1(1-t0)} + c_2 e^{\sigma 2(1-t0)}$$
$$\lambda_2(t) = c_1 e^{\sigma 1(1-t0)} + \frac{c_2 a_{21}}{\sigma_2 - a_{22}} e^{\sigma 2(1-t0)} \qquad (16.6)$$

(b) Under what condition the equation system (16.6) will show linearity ?

16.2.4 Miscellaneous Aspects

1. Scale up

Prob. 12 A gluconic acid fermentation yielded optimum conditions in a 5 *l* bioreactor (internal diameter D_t = 7.5 cm) where aeration rate at 2.5 *l*-air/min and agitation at 500 rpm was used. This is to be scaled up to a bioreactor of 40,000 *l* (D_t = 112 cms) of similar geometry. If the power input per unit volume is to remain constant and if the aeration rate in the large bioreactor is to be 10,000 *l*/min because of flooding conditions what will be the recommendation of the agitator speed for large scale bioreactor on the basis of the following criterea of scale up, maintaining

(a) Constant K_La ?
(b) Constant impeller tip speed ?
(c) Constant mixing quality ?

Prob. 13 A 10 *l* (H/D = 1.4), 500 rpm, 1 vvm, bioreactor is to be scaled up to 10,000 *l* on similar geometry equal aeration rate basis. Compute the speed of agitation in the scale up vessel.

2. Energetics

Prob. 14 Assuming the biosynthetic ability in *E. coli* cell as given in the table 16.2, ideal energy coupling growth be proceeding estimate how much cells is possible to be synthesised when 1g mole ATP is utilized.

Prob. 15 In an anaerobic biocell the bioconversion of glucose to lactate/lactic acid is coupled to formation of 2 moles of ATP per mole of glucose. Assuming standard free energy of conversions as below

Glucose → Lactic acid ($\Delta G°$ = – 52000 cals/mole)
ATP → ADP + Pi ($\Delta G°$ = – 7,300 cals/mole)
Glucose → CO_2 + H_2O ($\Delta G°$ = – 686,000 cals/mole)

Calculate

(a) $\Delta G°$ of the overall reaction

(b) the efficiency of energy conservation.

(c) how many moles of ATP per mole of glucose can be obtained in an aerobic organism at 40% efficiency of energy conservation ?

Table 16.2 Biosynthetic ability of *E. coli*

Chemical Composition	*Content %*	*Av. M. Wt*	*Molecule Numbers*	*Rate of Synthesis (Molecule Per sec.)*	*Rate of ATP Required (Molecule Per sec.)*	*Fraction of ATP Required (%)*
DNA	5	2×10^9	4	3.3×10^{-3}	6×10^4	2.5
RNA	10	1×10^6	1.5×10^7	12.5	7.5×10^4	3.1
Protein	70	6×10^4	$1.7\ 10^6$	1.4×10^3	2.12×10^6	8.8
Fat	10	1×10^3	1.5×10^7	1.25×10^4	8.75×10^4	3.7
Polysaccharides	5	2×10^5	3.9×10^4	32.5	6.5×10^4	2.7

The data given are as below.

Water content in *E. coli* = 75%

Cell size = 1 × 1 × 3 microns

Cell weight = 2.5×10^{-13} g/cell

Doubling time = 20 mins.

3. *Phase-plane analysis*

Prob. 16 In a prey (x_1)–predator (x_2) interacting system the rate of population variation may be expressed by Lotka-Voltera equation as below.

$$\frac{dx_1}{dt} = \alpha\, x_{1e}\,(x_2' - x_{2e})$$
$$\frac{dx_2}{dt} = f\alpha\, x_{2e}\,(x_2 - x_{1e}) \qquad (16.7)$$

where α is a positive proportionality constant, f is the fraction of cells of predator that hatch, x_1 and x_2 are numbers of prey and predator at time t = 0, where as x_{1e} and x_{2e} represent their values at equilibrium state. Simplify equations (16.7) by displacing x_1 and x_2 from equilibrium state to a value of p and q so that

$$p = x_1 - x_{1e}$$
$$q = x_2 - x_{2e}$$

and show that phase-plane representation of x_2 vs x_1 follows an elliptical path whose centre is at the origin in *pq* plane.

Prob. 17 Starting from a transient chemostat behaviour as given below Humphrey and Koga

$$\frac{dx}{dt} = x\left[\frac{\mu_m s}{K_s + s} - D\right] \qquad (16.8)$$

$$\frac{ds}{dt} = D\,[S_R - S) - \frac{X}{Y}\,\mu_m \left[\frac{S}{k_S + S}\right] \tag{16.9}$$

obtained its phase plane (X – S) diagram as shown in Fig. 16.4 in which α, β indicate, steady state values.

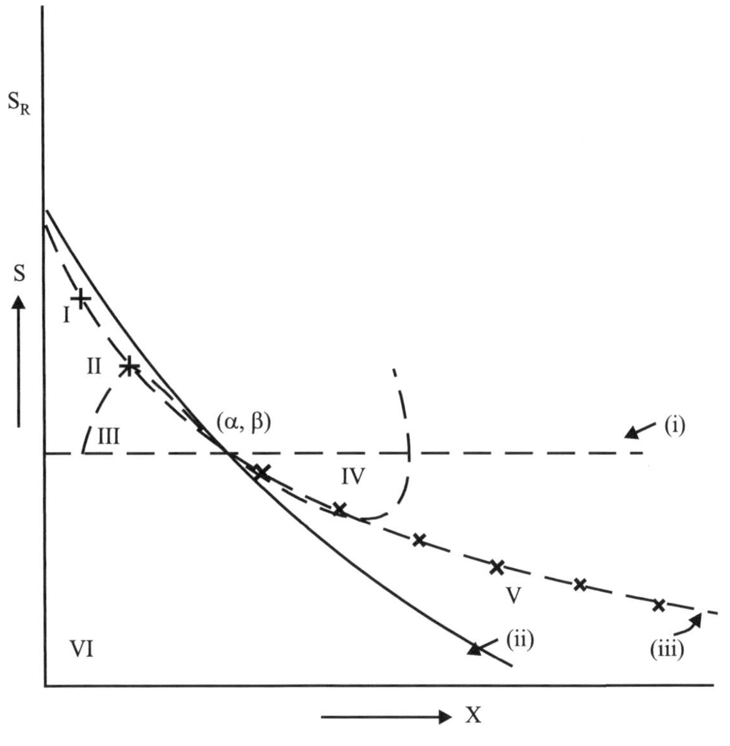

Fig. 16.4

From the above equations, considering steady state in the chemostat, and stability by singular point find out the match equations, giving steps, of the profiles (i), (ii) and (iii) in the figure (in the equations X is the cell populations, S is substrate concentration, S_R is the inlet substrate concentration, D is the dilution rate, μ is specific growth rate, Y is yield coefficient and K_s is a constant).

4. Computer simulation

Prob. 18 Fermentative bioconversion of glucose to gluconic acid by *Pseudomonas ovalis* B1486 was as given in the Table 16.3. Based on these experimental results the kinetic behavior of the fermentative bioconversion could be expressed by the following equations.

$$\frac{dc_s}{dt} = -\frac{1}{Y_s}\left(\frac{dc_x}{dt}\right) \tag{16.10}$$

$$\frac{dc_x}{dt} = \frac{\mu_m c_s}{k_s + c_s} . c_x \quad (16.11)$$

$$-\frac{dc_G}{dt} = \frac{k_m (t) c_G}{k_1 + c_G} . c_x \quad (16.12)$$

$$\frac{dc_P}{dt} = a' c_{GL} \quad (16.13)$$

Table 16.3 Batch fermentation data of gluconic acid production by *Ps. ovalis* in HRF.

Fermentation Time (hrs)	*Cell Concentration (UOD ml^{-1})*	*Ammonium acetate concentration (mg ml^{-1})*	*Glucose concentration (mg ml^{-1})*	*Gluconic acid concentration (mg ml^{-1})*	*Gluconolactone concentration (mg ml^{-1})*
t	c_x	c_s	c_G	c_P	c_{GL}
0	0.10	1.0	51.0	–	–
1.0	0.11	0.995	49.61	0.12	0.20
1.5	0.133	0.979	49.15	0.24	0.45
2.0	0.168	0.986	48.80	0.60	0.58
2.5	0.190	–	–	0.82	0.79
3.0	0.217	0.936	47.58	1.10	1.00
3.5	0.280	–	–	1.50	1.28
4.0	0.317	0.872	45.81	1.90	1.55
4.5	0.400	–	–	2.55	2.15
5.0	0.479	0.784	43.18	3.28	2.50
5.5	0.652	0.700	–	4.48	3.48
6.0	0.875	0.648	39.15	5.88	4.22
6.5	1.090	0.550	36.62	7.59	5.00
7.0	1.2400	0.448	34.15	9.63	6.58
7.5	1.491	0.330	30.72	12.82	–
8.0	1.732	0.280	26.71	15.08	9.25
8.5	2.00	0.123	22.08	19.02	10.35
9.0	2.200	0.094	17.20	22.02	11.50
9.5	2.200	–	–	–	–
10.0	2.200	–	10.00	30.86	1060
10.5	–	–	–	34.20	9.50
11.0	–	–	6.25	37.05	8.52
11.5	–	–	–	39.68	7.20
12.0	–	–	3.33	42.11	5.90
12.5	–	–	–	44.00	5.08
13.0	–	–	1.00	45.30	3.24
13.5	–	–	–	46.20	2.65
14.0	–	–	–	46.82	2.85

$$\frac{dc_{GL}}{dt} = \alpha' \frac{dc_G}{dt} - b.\ c_{GL} \tag{16.14}$$

In these equation c_S in the limiting nutrient concentration, Y_s is the yield coefficient, c_x is the cell concentration, c_G is the glucose concentration, c_p is the product (gluconic acid) concentration, c_{GL} is intermediate (gluconolactone) concentration, k_m (t) is the Michaelis-Menten coefficient as a function of time; a', and b are stoichiometric coefficients and α' is a proportionality constant.

Develop a computer programme giving the detailed flow chart for computer simulation of the above fermentative bioconversion kinetics and check the appropriateness of the kinetic models. Also, examine the extent of accuracy for a chosen time interval of 0.01 sec in computational iteration.

5. Bioconversions

(i) *Cellular*

Prob. 19 Bioconversion of glucose to gluconic acid by *Pseudomonas ovalis* B1486 is a consecutive reaction where the intermediate product accumulates to some extent before the product is formed and is represented by the following scheme

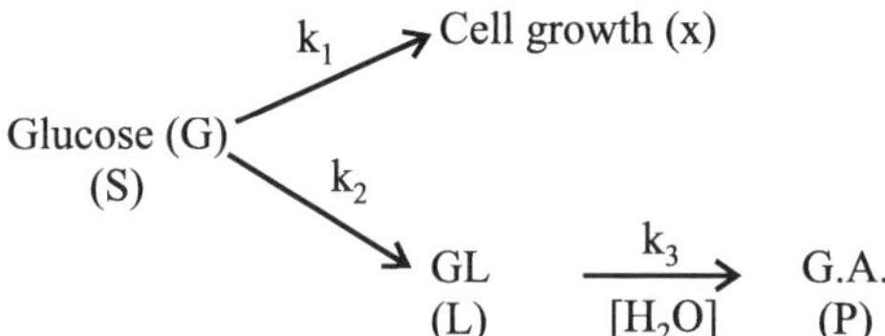

Where k_1, k_2 and k_3 are rate constants for cell yield, lactone formation and product yield respectively. If the rate equation is given by

$$-\frac{ds}{dt} = f_1 \left[\frac{k_1 s}{k_s + s}\right] + f_2 \left[\frac{k_2 s}{k_m + s}\right] \tag{16.15}$$

show that

$$\frac{dP}{dt} = f_3\, k_3\, .\, L \tag{16.16}$$

where f_1, f_2, and f_3 are stoichiometric constants.

Prob. 20 In a bioconversion reaction the total change of the substrate was expressed by the following relationship

$$V_c \frac{ds_i}{dt} = J_{in} \left(\frac{s}{k_1 + s}\right) V_c - J_{out} \left(\frac{s}{k_2 + s_i}\right) V_c - J \left(\frac{s_i}{k_3 + s_i}\right) V_c \tag{16.17}$$

In this relation V_c is the unit cell volume (m^3), J_{in}, J_{out} are fluxes of substrate uptake and discharge respectively, ($g/m^3/h$); J is maximum reaction rate of substrate metabolism, ($g/m^3/h$); s is the substrate concentration in the system (M); s_i is the substrate concentration in the cell (M); k_1, k_2 and k_3 are constants. Assuming that $k_2 \doteqdot k_3$, $S \ll k_1$; $s_i \ll k_2$ and

$$\mu = k\,J\left(\frac{s_i}{k_3 + s_i}\right) = J'\left(\frac{s_i}{k_3 + s_i}\right) \qquad (16.18)$$

in which k is a constant and J' = kJ, show that the relationship between μ (specific growth rate) and s can be expressed as a first order lag.

Prob. 21 In a hydrocarbon bioconversion by *Candida tropicalis* the following data were recorded
(*i*) Maximum oxygen uptake rate (OUR) = 12 m mole O_2/hr. g cell.
(ii) Cell concentration at the time of maximum OUR = 10 g/*l* (for 1% hydrocarbon source)
(iii) Critical O_2 concentration for this organism is 0.032 m mole O_2/*l*.
(iv) Saturation O_2 concentration in the broth is 0.544 m mole/*l*.
From these data determine the value of the minimum volumetric oxygen transfer coefficient (K_La) required to supply sufficient dissolved oxygen.

Prob. 22 In the bioconversion of glucose to gluconic acid by *Pseudomonas ovalis* B 14 86 in a horizontal rotary fermenter (HRF) the change of dissolved oxygen concentration and percentage oxygen in HRF exit gas measured by DO probe and paramagnetic oxygen analyser (DCL Servomex) as a function of rotation speed of HRF is given in Table 16.4 below. Determine, using (Table 16.4) oxygen balance method of Mukhopadhyay and Ghose,[8] values of K_La, rX and C* values at each rotation speed of the HRF and comment on the observed data given in the table and results obtained.

Table 16.4

Fermentation Time (hrs)	*Rotation Speed of HRF, rpm*					
	50		*100*		*120*	
	C_L-ppm	*% O_2 in exit*	*C_L ppm*	*% O_2 in exit*	*C_L ppm*	*% O_2 in exit*
0	5.9	21.0	5.9	21.0	5.9	21.0
2	5.5	20.9	5.7	20.9	5.8	20.9
4	4.9	20.8	5.2	20.8	5.4	20.7
6	4.0	20.5	4.3	20.4	4.4	20.4
8	2.5	20.1	2.5	19.8	2.8	19.5
9	1.4	19.8	1.7	19.2	2.0	19.0
12	2.4	20.2	2.0	19.5	2.1	19.3

Prob. 23 Growing *Aspergillus oryzae* cells on different substrates the reactions occured and products formed is shown below.

Substrate	*Bioreaction*	*Products*
Glucose	$C_6H_{12}O_6 + 6O_2$	$6CO_2 + 6H_2O$
Formic acid	$HCOOH + 1/2\ O_2$	$CO_2 + H_2O$
Ethanol	$C_2H_5O_6 + 3O_2$	$2CO_2 + 3H_2O$
Leucine	$C_6H_{13}O_2N + 7.5\ O_2$	$6CO_2 + 5H_2O + NH_3$

considering general cell reaction to be

$$C_{nc}\,H_{nH}\,O_{no}\,N_{nN} + aO_2 \rightarrow\; n\,CO_2 + \frac{nN}{2}H_2 + \frac{nH}{3}NH_3$$

empirical cell formula as $C_{409}\,H_{717}\,O_{233}\,N_{46}$ and empirical cell weight 9997. (i) Determine list values of Chemical Quotient (CQ) and Respiration Quotient (RQ) of the cellular reactions. Assume definition of

$$CQ = \frac{n_c}{a} = \frac{4n_c}{4n_c + n_H - 2n_0 - 3n_N} \text{ and } RQ = \frac{Q_{CO_2}}{Q_{O_2}}$$

(ii) Determine specific rate of CO_2 produced/Sp. rate of O_2 consumed. What conclusion one can draw from the results?

(ii) Enzymic/iwc

Prob. 24 The bioconversion of sucrose by the enzyme sucrase at room temperature resulted in the batch reaction data given in the table 16.5 below.

Table 16.5

C_s, $\frac{\text{m moles}}{l}$	1.0	0.84	0.68	0.53	0.38	0.27	0.16	0.09	0.04	0.018	0.006	0.0025
t, hr	0	1	2	3	4	5	6	7	8	9	10	11

The initial enzyme concentration used was 0.01 m. moles/*l*. Determine whether these data can reasonably fit the Michaelis-Menten kinetics

$$-r_A = \frac{k_3\,C_3\,C_E}{C_S + k_m} \tag{16.19}$$

where k_m is Michaelis-Menten constant. If the fit is reasonable determine the constants k_3 and k_m.

Prob. 25 Considering the following bioconversion by an immobilized enzyme

$$E + S \underset{k_2}{\overset{k_1}{\rightleftharpoons}} E\,S \xrightarrow{k_3} E + P \tag{16.20}$$

Derive an expression representing the ratio of the amount of immobilized enzyme required in CSTBR and PFBR.

Prob. 26 A sequential isomerization bioreaction has been represented as below and has

$$A \xrightarrow{k_1} B \xrightarrow{k_2} C \tag{16.21}$$

been carried out in two stage CSTBR as per diagram given on page 529.

If both the reactors are operated at the same temperature what is the composition of the effluent from

a. The first CSTBR?

b. The final effluent composition?

Prob. 27 During performance of two bioreaction systems in immobilized whole cell (IWC) bioreactors, various types of data were collected as given in the table 16.6. Examine whether film resistance has any significant role for the following IWC systems. If not, check what resistance is controlling during bioreaction.

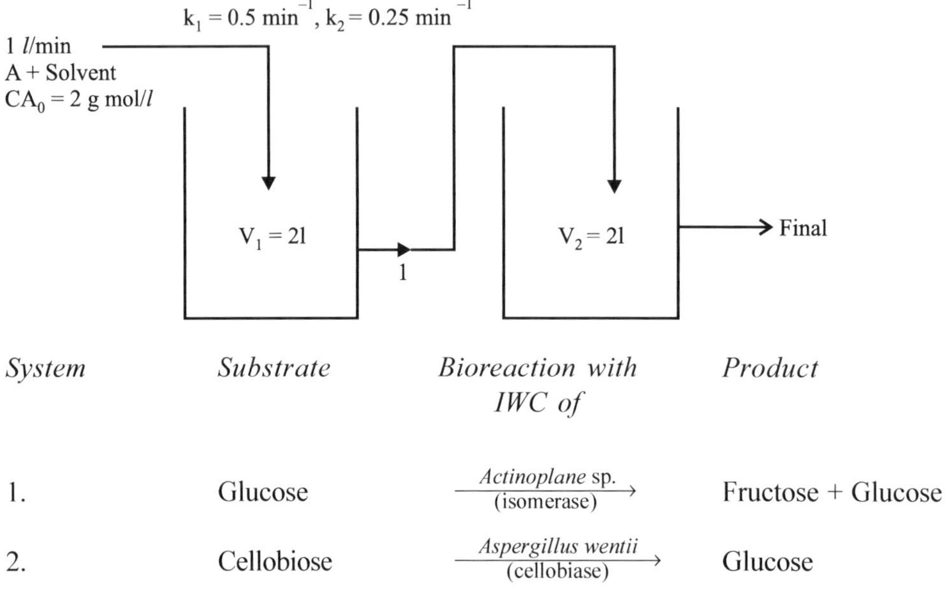

System	*Substrate*	*Bioreaction with IWC of*	*Product*
1.	Glucose	*Actinoplane* sp. (isomerase) →	Fructose + Glucose
2.	Cellobiose	*Aspergillus wentii* (cellobiase) →	Glucose

Table 16.6 Available data on IWC bioreaction

Sl. no.	*Item*	*System 1*	*System 2*
1.	Bed height	22.5 cms	3 cms
2.	Feed rate	42 ml/hr	20 ml/hr
3.	Conversion efficiency	43%	50%
4.	Feed concentration	36% glucose (w/v)	0.01 M cellobiose
5.	Feed viscosity	0.94 c.p.	0.8 c.p.
6.	Feed density	1.2036 gm/ml	1.0083 gm/ml
7.	Diffusivity	1.18×10^{-5} cm^2/sec	2.5×10^{-5} cm^2/sec
8.	Particle diameter	1.48 cm	0.009 cm
9.	Void fraction	0.44	0.45
10.	Reaction order	First	First
11.	Effective diffusivity	1.11×10^{-5} cm^2/sec	0.79×10^{-5} cm^2/sec
12.	Area/vol	4.05 cm^2/c.c	333 cm^2/c.c.
13.	Column diameter	5 cms	1 cm
14.	Bulk concentration	2 M	0.01 M
15.	Surface concentration at biocatalyst surface	1 M	—
16.	Equilibrium Constant	1.04	—
17.	Intrinsic reaction rate	95.5 μm/min/gm	108.9 μm/min/gm
18.	Product concentration	15.5% fructose	0.18% glucose
19.	Thiele Modulus	<2.8	*K* 2.0

16.3 MIXED MICROBIAL CELL CULTURES

16.3.1 Heterogenic Cell-Cell Interactions

Prob. 28 In a prey [*Colpodium stenii* (protozoa)] x_1- predator (*E. coli*) x_2 heterogenic biosystemic multi-interactions, the Lotka-Voltera equation could be expressed by the following rate equations.

$$\left.\begin{aligned} \frac{dx_1}{dt} &= -\alpha x_1 x_2 \\ \frac{dx_2}{dt} &= x_2(-\delta + f\alpha\, x_2) \end{aligned}\right\} \qquad (16.22)$$

Discuss the problems of this interacting system by finding dx_1/dx_2 and sketching the trajectories in the x_1 x_2 phase plane for the following cases when

(a) the birth rate = death rate of x_1

(b) none of the parasitic infection hatch. Comment on the trajectories.

16.3.2 Treatment Biotechnology of Industrial Waste Water and Water

Prob. 29 An industrial plant discharges a waste water with a flow of 1.3 mG (million gallons) day and an average BOD of 785 mg/*l*. Regulatory discharge criteria have estabilished an average effluent BOD of 30 mg/*l* and a maximum BOD of 60 mg/*l*. Design an activated sludge treatment plant to meet average effluent quality and specify equalization requirements to maintain the effluent BOD below the maximum allowable level. Given information :

So (av) = 785 mg/*l*

Prob. 30 A waste water is to be treated in an activated sludge process. The waste flow rate in the plant is 200 *l*/day and it has a strength of 10,000 mg BOD per liter. The process loading factor and detention time have values of 0.40 lb BOD//lb MLVSS and 1 day respectively. Calculate from these data the following design parameters.

a. Concentration of the MLVSS.

b. Total oxygen requirement in the process.

c. Total power input when O_2 requirement is thrice the value obtained in (b)

d. Volumetric process loading rate in lbs/1000 ft^3/day

Assume the following in calculations.

(i) Yield coefficient = 0.55 g cells synthesised per g BOD removed

(ii) Actual O_2 consumption in energy requiring synthesis reaction is 35% of the theoretical O_2 requirement.

Prob. 31 Ozone is to be used in disinfection treatment to obtain 99.9% kill of bacteria in water with a residual of 0.5 mg/*l*. Under these conditions the reaction rate constant (k) is 2.5×10^{-2} sec^{-1}. Determine the contact time of this treatment process.

Prob. 32 It is required to treat 500000 g.p.d (gals/day) of water with 0.3 mg/*l* of chlorine disinfection. The chlorine disinfectant is in the form of bleach that contains 33.33% of available chlorine. Estimate how many pounds of the bleach are needed to treat the daily flow of water.

Prob.33 In drinking water treatment by chlorine (in winter) its concentration has been correlated with contact time in batch systems at constant levels of survival, temperature and pH as given by equation 16.23. For small water supplies the adequate disinfection is given by this dose contact time relation for complete kill of coxsacie virus A-2. Values of constant k are as in the table 16.7 below. A chlorine constant operates at 20 g pm witha free chlorine residual 1.0 mg/*l* and meeting bacteriological standards for drinking water, what changes in operation may be required if the capacity of the system is scaled up to 60 gpm ?

Table 16.7

Max pH	*Values of k*	
	0 – 5°C	*10°C*
7 - 7.5	12	8
7.5 - 8.0	20	15
8.0-8.5	30	20
8.5-9.0	35	22

Prob. 34 In drinking water supplies *E. coli* bacteria is a common contaminant. In chlorination treatment of water these organisms are inactivatd. The chlorine inactivation of *E. coli* has been observed as given in the table 16.8 below.

Table 16.8

Cl (mg/l)	*Time of contact, min*				
	0.5	*2*	*5*	*10*	*20*
0.14	52	11	0.7	–	–
0.07	80	56	30.0	0.5	0
0.05	25	85	65.0	21	0.31

From the above data examine which of the following deactivation rate equation is valid for the chlorine.

(a) $$-\frac{dN}{dt} = kN + k^1 N (N_0 - N) \qquad (16.23)$$

(b) $$-\frac{dN}{dt} = k_t N \qquad (16.24)$$

(c) $$-\frac{dN}{dt} = \left(\frac{k}{1+\alpha t}\right) N \qquad (16.25)$$

Prob 35 An activated sludge process with 3000 mg/*l* MLVSS treats a waste with an ultimate BOD of 1000 mg/*l* and 350 mg/*l* VSS which are 90% biodegradable. The plant effluent contains 30 mg/*l* ultimate BOD and 20 mg/*l* VSS. Determine the daily VSS accumulation and oxygen requirement for a flow of 0.1 m^3/sec if the synthesis constant is 0.55 and the endogenous respiration constant is 0.15.

Prob. 36 An organic waste water is being treated by an activated sludge process. It has a flow of waste water 8,600 m^3, concentration 850 mg BOD/*l* and an effluent concentration 30 mg BOD/*l*. Activated sludge concentration in aeration tank is 3000 mg MLSS/*l*. The experimental data collected is shown in the table 16.9. Estimate the aeration tank volume from these data.

Table 16.9

S_0 *mg BOD/l*	*S* *mg BOD per l*	*X* *mg MLSS per l*	*O* *(hr)*	*SVI* *ml g MLSS*	r_x *mg O2 l.day*	*Excess x return rate mg MLSS day*
800	100	1200	10	250	1320	960
750	50	1500	15	175	975	600
750	50	1000	40	80	440	200
750	50	1000	50	110	350	150

16.4 MAMMALIAN CELL CULTURE SYSTEM

16.4.1 Kinetics

Prob. 37 Assuming the adsorption of vaccinia virus on the cytodex 1 microcarrier culture of vero 76 cells as per following Table 16.10 [at 37°C for 1.5 hrs] examine what adsorption isotherm fits these data.

Table 16.10

Virus conc. (mg/*l*)	0.01	0.02	0.03	0.06	0.10
Adsorption on vero cells anchored on cytodex (mg/cm^3)	5.28	7.26	8.49	11.08	13.68

Prob. 38 Adsorption of vaccinia virus on Vero 76 cells at different cellular activity parameter (P) provided results as given in the following Table 16.11.

Table 16.11

$P\left[\left(=\dfrac{\mu_t}{\mu_{max}}\times 10\right)\right]$	0.1	0.2	0.5	1.0	2	4	6	8	10
% virus adsorbed	20	30	38	40	46	46	44	45	44

What is the significance of P in this relation? Is there any linkage of P in terms of the data in Problem 37? Comment also on the profile (μ indicates specific growth rate).

16.4.2 Mammalian vs Microbial Cell Function

Prob. 39. Assuming metabolism to be proprotional to amount of surface area, compare the rate of metabolism in man, whose surface area is abot 260 sq. cm per kg. of body weight, with that of a cylindrical shape bacteria whose size is 1μ × 2 μ. Assume its specific gravity as 1.0. Comment on the result.

16.5 PLANT CELL CULTURE

Prob. 40 By exposing a *Cantharanthus roseus* cell cultivation mash (100 gl^{-1} wet weight) to a constant shear rate of 290 sec^{-1} using a Contravas Rheomal 115 viscometer the variation of apparent viscosity of the suspension was as shown in the figure 16.5. Examine the behavior of this cell cultivation mash, put down the conclusion and estimate corresponding shear stresses.

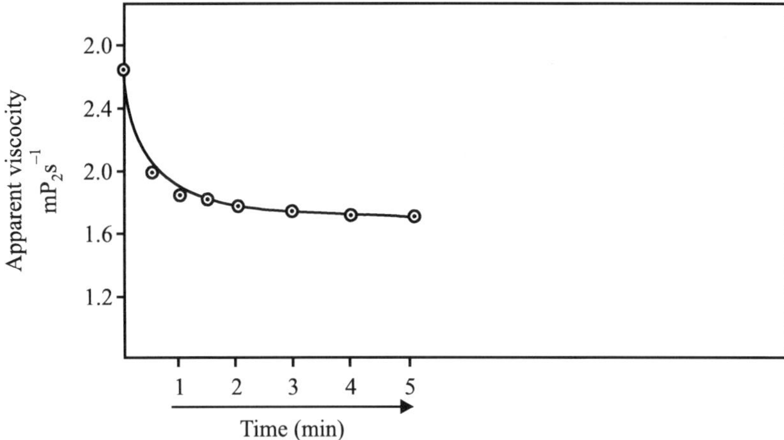

Fig. 16.5

16.6 BIOPRODUCT RECOVERY

Prob. 41 The ultrafiltration rate for purification of pepsin using HF 200 membrane could be represented by the following expression

$$\frac{dV}{dt} = \frac{A\,\Delta P}{R_m + k_1 V} \tag{16.26}$$

where V is the volume of filtrate, t is the time, A is the membrane area, ΔP is pressure drop across the membrane, R_m is the resistance of the membrane and k_1V is equal to the fouling resistance (R_e) of the deposited material on the membrane, k_1 being a constant, a characteristic for a given material deposited. Filtration performance using a membrane area of 33.30 cm^2 and a pressure drop 100 psi at 25°C provided data as given in the Table 16.12 below.

Table 16.12

Filtration time, (hr)	*Filtrate vol. (ml)*	*Filtration rate (ml min^{-1})*
0	–	–
0.5	3.0	6.00
1.0	4.4	4.40
1.5	6.0	4.00
2.0	7.6	3.80
3.0	9.0	3.00
4.0	11.6	2.90
5.0	14.0	2.80
6.0	16.8	2.78
6.5	18.0	2.77

From these data determine R_m, k_1 and R_e at 4.5 th hour of filtration.

Prob. 42 A fermentation liquid is to be recovered by clarification using a leaf filter. A leaf filter with 20 ft^2 of filtering area produced following results during constant filtration at 50 psi (Table 16.13).

Table 16.13

Time (min)	*Filtrate volume (ft^3)*
10	100
30	163
45	213
60	258
90	235

The fermentation slurry before filtration was found to contain 5 lb of solids per 100 lb of liquid. The densities of the solid and the liquid were 78.5 lb/ft^3 and 62.4 lb/ft^3 respectively. The viscosity of the slurry was 2 c.p. The cake of filtration was found to be incompressible. Determine the specific resistance, *r* of the cake and the equivalent length of the filter cloth. [Hint. use Carman's correlation].

Prob. 43 In the above problem the specific resistance was found to vary with pressure and following results were observed (Table 16.14).

Table 16.14

Pressure *(psi)*	*Specific resistance* *(sec^2/gm)*
251.2	7.943×10^9
316.2	9.550×10
398.1	1.222×10
501.2	1.380×10
631.0	1.585×10
794.3	1.905×10

Using Carman's equation $r = r' P_s$ determine the coefficient of compressibility and the constant of variation (r').

16.7 ADDITIONAL PRACTICE TUTORIALS

Prob. 44 In absence of temperature control mode an assesment of the temperature profile in batch aerobic cultivations of genetically recombinant strain of *E. coli* was made. With reasonable assumptions the following differential equations could represent the cultivation dynamics.

$$\rho_b C_D \, dT_b/dt = (-\Delta H^*) \, dx/dt - UA \, (T_b - T_r)/V - a \, (N_h + \lambda_H N_K) \quad (1)$$

$$dx/dt = \mu x = \mu_{max} \, xs/K_s + s \quad (2)$$

$$- ds/dt = 1/ \, Y_{x/s} \, . \, dx/dt \quad (3)$$

in which

$$aN_h = GK_Ga \, / \, G + K_GA \, (G_H T_b - C_g T_r) \quad (4)$$

$$aN_K = GK_Ga/ \, G + K_Ga. \, H_s \quad (5)$$

$$H_s = M_v/M_G \, P_s/ \, P - P_s \quad (6)$$

Use initial conditions as

S_0 = Initial glucose concentration = 10 kgm^{-3}

X_0 = Inoculum size = 0.01 kgm^{-3}

Solving equation 1 to 3 develop suitable algorithm/computer programming and trace the temperature profiles of the cultivation liquid with time interval of 0.001 hr.

[Assume the following values in computation

ρ_b = 1×10^1 kg broth m^{-3},

C_b = C_C = 1 kcal., kg of liquid^{-1}°C^{-1},

ΔH^* = Fermentation heat,

kcal Kg drycell^{-1} = $- \Delta H_g . \, Y_{x/s}^{-1} - \Delta H_a$,

$-\Delta H_g$ = 3.74×10^3 kcal kg glucose$^{-1.19}$,

$-\Delta H_a$ = 5.3×10^3 kcal kg drycells$^{-1./18}$,

C_g = 0.24 kcal kg dry air^{-1}, °$C^{-1.17}$,

G = 77.41 kg dry air^{-1} h^{-1} (vvm)

K_Ga = 2 kg water vap. $m^{-1}h^{-1}$. ΔH^{-1}
M_g = 28.9 kg. kmol of air^{-1}
M_v = 18 kg. kmole of water vap.$^{-1}$
K_s = 0.1 kg glucose m^{-3}
$Y_{x/s}$ = 0.45 kg dry cell. kg glucose^{-1}
P = 760 mm, Hg = Total pressure
T_r = 25°C, T_b = Temperature of broth,
P_s = Saturation vapour pressure of water, mmHg
μ_{max} *E. coli* = W. T_b exp $\{a_1 + a_2 / (T_b + 273.15)\}$
1; $T_b < (a_1 - 1)/a_4]$

16.7.1 Problem on Control of Undesirable Microorganisms

Prob. 45 In a disinfection process with chlorocresol using *Staphylococcus aureus* as the test organism the following data were obtained. (Table 16.15)

Table 16.15

Strength of Solution	*Temp. T. (°C)*	*Initial No. of Organism, N_0*	*No. of Surviving Organism, N*
0.04%	20°	3,350,000	2,165,000
0.08%	20°	3,350,000	12,600
0.04%	30°	3,350,000	1,440,000

t = 5 mins = time of contact.
Evaluate from the data
(i) Concentration coefficient, n,
(ii) Temperature coefficient, Q_{10}

16.7.2 Problems on Air Sterilization

Prob. 46. An air filter is to be designed for a given fermentation, which runs for 100 hrs and used 1.6 cubic meter air per min. The intake air is expected to have a microbial load of 10,000 microorganisms per cubic meter. Assuming a reasonably safe operation that is low probability of a single organism for every 1000 passing the filter and that filter packing material of choice has L_{90} value of 4.3. How thick should the air filter be?

Prob. 47. For a 20000 gal fermenter (batch) working for 96 hrs with intake of air 1 vvm with an incoming microbial load of 3000 cells/ft^3 of air and a probability that a single organism for every 10^3 held back penetrates. Compute the value of sterilization required to attain this degree of sterilization. What should be the length of the filter bed?

Prob. 48. It is required to supply sterile air at the rate 500 CFM (ft^3/min) for a fermentation, the duration of which is 100 hrs. Assume that the air entering the filter has a bacterial count of 30 per ft^3. Calculate the required bed for the sterilization, pressure drop across this bed and diameter of the tube used.

Data available :

(a) Chance of infection of organism is 1 in 1000.
(b) Air velocity for maximum K is 1.2 to 1.8 ft per second over which range value of K is 0.61.
(c) Pressure drop across 10 in filter at 1.5 ft/sec = m15 in W. G and pressure drop across 8 in filter at 1.5 ft/sec = 12" W.G. (water guage)

Calculate the following :

(a) Single fibre collection efficiency
(b) Overall collection efficiency
(c) Pressure drop across the bed.

Prob. 49. In a laboratory air filtration experiment was carried out with glass wool and the following observations were made :

Length of the filter tube	=	50 cm
Length of the filter bed	=	35 cm
I.D. of the tube	=	3.5 cm
Void volume of the bed	=	140 c.c.
Particle diameter, d_p	=	1 μ
Fibre diameter, d_f	=	20 μ
No. of particles in intake air	=	100/m^3
Allowable penetration	=	1 in 1000
Air velocity at the time of expt.	=	6 cm/sec
Assuming air viscosity at the time of expt.	=	1.8×10^{-4} cm/g.sec and
Air density	=	1.20×10^{-3} gm/c.c

Determine :

(a) Single fibre collection efficiency
(b) Overall collection efficiency
(c) Pressure drop across the bed.

Prob. 50. A filter is to be designed to sterilize 250 cu.ft air/min. Assume that the incoming air contains a maximum of 500 phage particles/cu.ft. The efficiency demanded of the filter is not that organism will be allowed to pass in 75 hrs. Instead, the design is based on 7500 hrs, so that the chance that a virus will pass the filter during the first 75 hrs is only 1 in 100. A linear air velocity of 2 ft/sec is assumed fixing the bed diameter at about 20 inches. The glass fibres employed have an arithmetic mean diameter of 9.0 microns and the fraction fibre in the mat is 0.04. Compute the filter bed depth required fulfilling above condition.

Prob. 51. In an experiment of transport phenomenon of sterilization (20°C) of air by fibrous filtration following data are obtained.

Size of the particles to be removed	1.25 microns
Particle density	2.5 g/c.c
Air velocity	2.5 cm/sec
Air density	0.017 c.p
Fibre diameter	20μ
Void fraction of fibre	0.03
Filter depth	2.54 cm

Variation of drag coefficient as a function of Reynolds number in the filter was as shown in Fig.16.6.

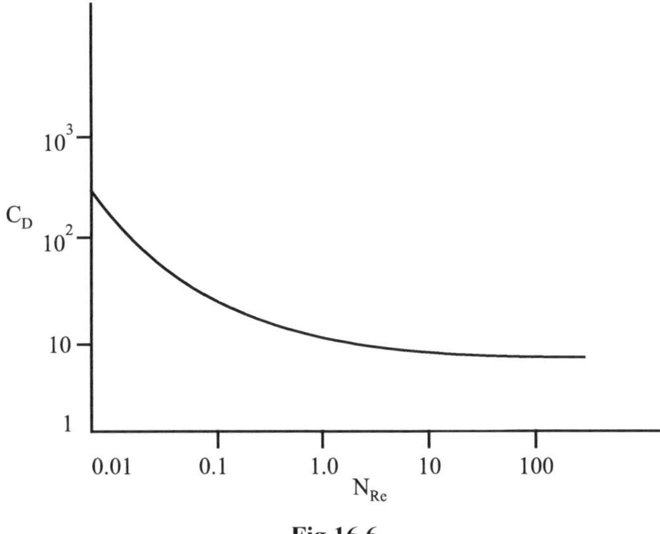

Fig.16.6

From these data determine the overall efficiency of the air filtration, pressure drop across the filter bed and value of coefficient of diffusion for the particles of 0.5 micron in diameter suspended in air at atmospheric pressure (Assume R = 8.314 × 10 atmospheric, N = 6.02×10^{23} molecules/gm. Mole. and mean free path λ = 0.1 micron).

Prob. 52. It is required to determine the depth of a fibrous filter necessary to remove 99% of the particles from an aerosol. Experiment was performed (at 20°C) with

(i) Particle density d_f is 1 gm/c.c.

(ii) Fibre diameter, d_f, is 2μ and fraction solids 5% and

(iii) Air velocity, v_o, is 10 cm/sec.

From these data determine the filter bed depth for the diameter of the particles in aerosol 0.1m.

In the calculation assume, air viscosity at 20°C = 1.808×10^{-4} gm/cm.sec, air density = 1.2×10^{-3} gm/c.c., and the value of Cunnigham's Correlation factor, C = 2.6.

Prob. 53. A 10,000 gal working capacity fermentor will be used to carry out a fermentation lasting 4 days. It has been decided a volumetric air flow rate equivalent to 0.1 vvm be used. The incoming air contains on an average 150 microorganisms per cuft at an average bacteria diameter of 1 μ. Fibrous filter material having average fibre diameter of 19 μ and a void fraction fo 0.95 is available for the construction of an air filter. An allowable risk of 0.001 had been designated in terms of bacterium penetration. Estimate the length of filter required.

16.7.3 Problems on Media Sterilization

Prob. 54. It has been proposed that the 14l. New Brunswick fermenter be operated continuously to produce SCP. To maximize the productivity, the fermenter will be operated at a dilution rate D = 1.0 hr^{-1} with a medium volume of 10 liters. To sterilize the medium continuously, the pilot plant fermenter will be used as a continuous sterilizer. Steam in great excess will be available to the fermenter jacket at 135°C. The overall heat transfer coefficient for the jacket was found to be 1/3 kcal per m^2 per litre per°C. The maximum heat transfer area for the sterilizer is 1.4 m^2.

Medium is changed to the pilot plant fermenter at 25°C. Assume the density and specific heat of the medium are respectively 1.0 gm/ml and 1.0 Cal/gm°C and does not change significantly with temperature. Calculate the minimum volume of medium required in the sterilizer in order to achieve the following microbial destruction.

Inlet contamination = 150 organisms/liter

Desired outlet contamination = 0.01 organism/liter. See attached (Fig. 16.7) thermal inactivation curve. Please state all reasonable assumptions.

Prob. 55. In the sterilization of a fermentation medium in a given fermenter heating and cooling rates are as follows:

Heat up from 100°C to 121°C is 25 min.
Cooling from 121°C to 100°C is 15 min.
The characteristic value of K and ∇ at different temperatures are provided in the table (16.16). If the total ∇ value required for the whole sterilization process is 45.0, how long the medium should be held at 121°C?

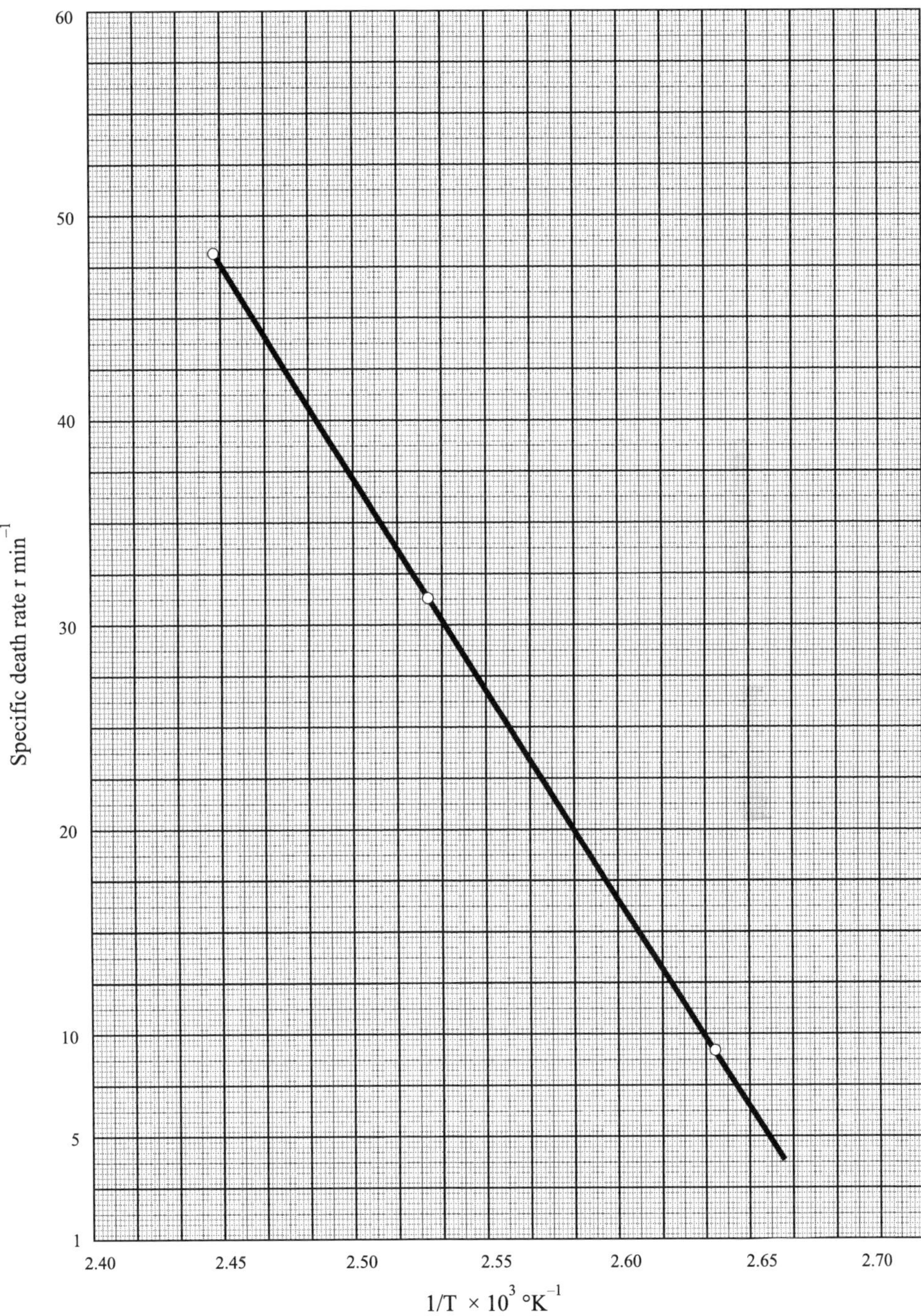
60
50
40
30
20
10
5
1
Specific death rate r min^{-1}
2.40
2.45
2.50
2.55
2.60
2.65
2.70
1/T × 10^3 °K^{-1}

Fig.16.7

Table 16.16

$T°C$	$Kmin^{-1}$	∇	$T°C$	$Kmin^{-1}$	∇
100	0.019	–	101	0.025	0.044
102	0.032	0.076	103	0.040	0.116
104	0.051	0.168	105	0.065	0.233
106	0.083	0.316	107	0.105	0.420
108	0.133	0.553	109	0.168	0.420
110	0.212	0.932	111	0.267	1.199
112	0.366	1.535	113	0.423	1.957
114	0.531	2.488	115	0.666	3.154
116	0.835	3.983	117	1.045	5.034
118	1.307	6.341	119	1.633	7.973
120	2.037	10.0	121	2.538	12.5
122	3.160	19.6	123	3.929	24.5
124	4.881	30.5	125	6.056	38.0
126	7.506	47.5	127	9.293	58.8
128	11.494	73.0	129	14.200	90.0
130	17.524	–			

Prob. 56. A fermentation mash was to be sterilized in batches of 50,000 *l*. Three separate examples of unutilized mash, which were made using different batches of raw materials gave total bacterial count of 5×10^6, 1×10^7 and 2×10^5 per ml. Supposing that 1 in 10^4 of a single organism out of those present in batch of mash surviving the heat treatment. Calculate the degree of sterilization of the process.

16.7.4 Problems on Aeration

Prob. 57. *Dynamic differential gassing out* : The following data (Table 16.17) of DO concentration, measured by a DO probe, was obtained in a yeast fermentation. Using dynamic differential gassing out technique determine

(a) K_La in the broth
(b) rC_x value and
(c) C*.

Table 16.17 D.O. Trace.

	Air off										Air on						
Time (secs.)	0	10	20	30	40	50	60	70	80	90	100	110	120	130	140	150	160
C_L (ppm)	5.2	5.2	5.2	5.2	4.7	4.2	3.7	3.1	2.6	2.0	1.5	0.9	2.8	3.8	4.2	4.4	4.5

Prob. 58. *Dynamic Integral Gassing Out*: The time of course of change DO concentration (by DO probe) during a small interruption of a batch fermentation using *Aerobacter aerogenes* at 30°C was recorded by Fujio and his associates (1973)[20] as given in Table 16.18.

Table 16.18 DO Concentration as a function of time

Air off		*Air on*	
Time (secs.)	*DO cove (ppm)*	*Time (secs.)*	*DO cove (ppm)*
10	3.7	50	0.15
15	3.7	55	1.7
20	3.7	60	2.41
25	3.7	65	2.9
30	3.7	70	3.2
35	3.2	75	3.3
40	1.8	80	3.41
45	0.8	85	3.52
		90	3.59
		95	3.61
		100	–

From these data determine the following by dynamic integral gassing out technique.

(a) K_La,

(b) rC_x

(c) C*.

Prob. 59. *Oxygen Balance Method*: Mukhopadhyay and Ghose (1976) conducted gluconic acid frementation in a 4 in diameter HRF using *Ps. ovalis* B1486 as fermenting organism. Fermentation conditions were as follows:

Working Vol.	0.91
Air flow rate	0.5 vvm
Fermentation temperature	29 ± 1°C
Fermenter rotation speed	120 rpm

Data recorded during fermentation is given in Table16.19. From these data evaluate K_La, rC_x and C* values by oxygen balance technique of Mukhopadhyay and Ghose. Assume air density at 29 ± 1°C = 1.2×10^{-3} g/c.c.

Table 16.19 Relation of C_L with $(f_i - f_o)$

C_L (ppm)	$(f_i - f_o)$
6.48	0.2×10^{-2}
5.76	0.6×10^{-2}
5.20	1.0×10^{-2}
2.40	2.20×10^{-2}
0.60	4.2×10^{-2}

Prob. 60. *Probe Response Method :* Oxygen at 20°C was passed through a solution of 0.25 Kg mol/m^3. Sodium sulfite in an agitated fermenter (agitator speed 4.17 rev. sec^{-1}) at the rate of 2.8×10^{-4} m^3 sec^{-1}. Inorder to determine K_La by Linek (1972) modified technique of Heineken Theory the following data was collected using a dissolved oxygen probe (having different membrane thickness) in the liquid. Compute K_La from the data given in the table 16.20.

Table 16.20 Membrane thickness in relation to parametric values.

Membrane/types and thickness (microns)	*K*	*Time of gassing (secs.) t*	*L values*
Teflon, 50m	0.05	148	0.625
Polypropylene, 25m (pp)	0.149	57.1	0.306
ppp, 15m	0.314	69.5	0.409

Prob. 61. (a) Using the constructed Zimm's plot as given in figure below for vaccinia virus show by calculation the values of Mr (relative molar mass), M_W (weight av. molar mass) and hydrodynamic diameter of the organism.

(b) What is the significance of scattering vector in Zimm's plot relation?

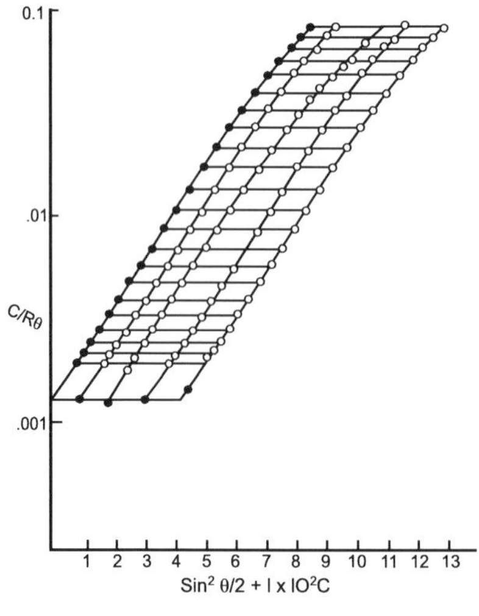

Fig. Log Zimm plot of vaccinia virus for concentration ranges from c = 0.88 – 4.4μg/ml. (– O –) Experimental points, (– • –) extrapolated. Reproduced, by permission of the publisher, from Ref. (35)

Prob. 62. (a) In examining the polydispersed phase of a starch characteristics DMSO solutions by DLS Zimm's plot could be constructed as shown below. Using the figure compute the values of Mr, M_W, Rg and hydrodynamic diameter of the particles in solution. Consider Debye equation and its parameters

$$\frac{KC}{R_q} = \frac{1}{M_W}\left(1+\frac{1}{3}q^2\left(R_q\right)_2+.....\right)+2A_2C+3A_3C^2.....$$

where $$K = \frac{4\pi^2 n_0^2\left(\frac{dn}{dc}\right)^2}{N_A\lambda_o^4}$$

and $$R_q = \frac{r^2 i_\theta}{I_o}$$

Here parameters have their usual significances. Also evaluate the value of the second virial coefficient A_2 making suitable assumption.

(b) What is the difference between Zimm's and Berry's plots?

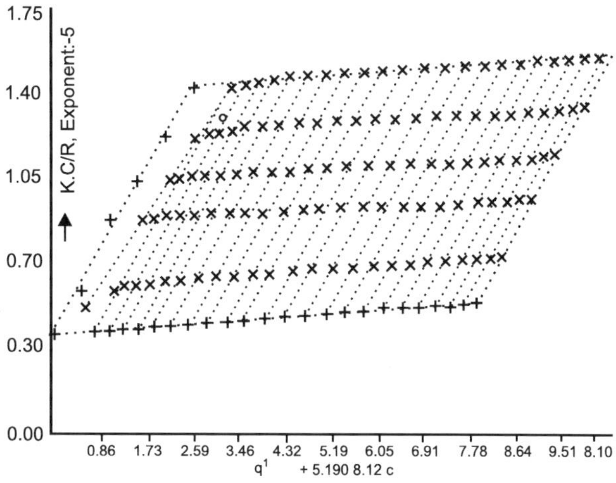

Fig. Zimm plot for A-S1 in DMSO at 25°C

Prob. 63. Anaerobic digestion of MSW at 35°C in a 28*l* CSTR having HRT 15 days produced biogas containing CH_4, CO_2 and H_2. Stripping of biogas components was followed assuming that generated rising gas bubbles have similar composition. The mass of gaseous component i transferred from the liquid to the gas phase $\left(\rho_{l_i}\right)$ could be expressed by the following relation.

$$\rho_{l_i} = K_L a_i (C_L - C_{L_i})$$

where $$C_{L_i} = \rho_i\left(\frac{MGi}{H_i RT}\right)$$

In these relations C_L is the bulk dissolved gas conc., C_{L_i} is dissolved gas concentration at the boundary layer interface, P_i is gas density, H_i is the Henry's constant between 30°C to 60°C, R is gas constant (8.314×10^{-5} bar m^3 gas mol^{-1}K^{-1}) and T is absolute temperature. Considering the given relations and data determine the following.

1. $K_L a_{CO_2}$, $K_L a_{CH_4}$, $K_L a_{H_2}$
2. Total volume specific dry biogas flow q_{tot}(m^3 gas. m_{CSTR}^{-3} d^{-1})
3. Computed values at thermophilic temp. (55°C)

Given Relations:

$$K_La = \left(\frac{D}{dl}\right)a, \; K_La_i = K_La_{CO_2}\left(\frac{Di}{D_{CO_2}}\right)$$

$$D_i \simeq D_{i35} \exp\,[0.03(T-35)]$$

$$q_{tot}, 1\text{ bar} = q_{tot} \cdot \sum pi$$

$$q_{tot} = K_p\left[\sum P_i - \left(p_{tot} - p_{H_2O}\right)\right]$$

$$pH_2O = 0.08\, e^{-0.05T}$$

$$K_p > 100\, q_{tot}.$$

Given Data:

$$D_{CO_2,35} = 2.3 \times 10^{-4} \quad m^2d^{-1}$$

$$D_{CH_4,35} = 1.8 \times 10^{-4} \quad m^2d^{-1}$$

$$D_{H_2,35} = 6.8 \times 10^{-4} \quad m^2d^{-1}$$

Prob. 64. In an aerobic cultivation of *Aerobacter aerogenes* in minimal medium with different substrates the results obtained are given in the table below. Comment on the results.

Table 16.21 Growth yields of *A. aerogenes*

Substrate (S)	*Molecular Formula of (S)*	*g cell / mole S* $(Y_{X/S})$	*g cell / mole* O_2 $(Y_{X/O})$	ΔS *(momole/l)*	ΔX *(mg cell/l)*
Maltose	$C_{12}H_{24}O_{12}$	149.2	48.2	Glucose:	
D-Manitol	$C_6H_{14}O_6$	95.5	38.0	2	97
D-Glucose	$C_6H_{12}O_6$	72.7	35.4	4	150
D-Fructose	$C_6H_{12}O_6$	76.1	46.8	6	210
D-Ribose	$C_5H_{10}O_4$	53.2	31.2	8	280
Succinate	$C_4H_6O_4$	29.2	20.2	Glycerine:	
Glycerine	$C_3H_6O_3$	41.8	31.0	4	100
DL-Lactate		16.6	11.8	8	165
				12	250
Pyruvate	$C_3H_4O_3$	17.9	15.2	16	310
Acetate	$C_2H_4O_2$	10.5	10.0	Lactate:	
				8	70
				16	110
				24	200
				32	225

Estimate from the given data the following:

1. Available electrons
2. Enthalpy changes

for each substrate to undergo cellular biochemical reaction.
[Ref. L.P. Hadjipetrou *et al*; J. Gen. Microbiol. 36, 139, 1964]

16.8 MISCELLANEOUS MULTICHOICE QUESTIONS

1. Morphologically cell envelopes of bacteria (both gram-positive and gram-negative) are composed of macromolecules of complex nature. Which of the statements given below describes both gram-positive and gram-negative cell envelopes?
   (a) They contain significant amount of teichoic acid.
   (b) Their antigen specificity is determined by the polysaccharide O antigen
   (c) They act as a barrier to the extraction of crystal violet iodine by alcohol.
   (d) They are a diffusion barrier to large charged molecules.
2. Plasmids are small extrachromosomal genetic elements that contain all the factors except
   (a) Resistance factors
   (b) Colicin factors
   (c) Transfer factors
   (d) Sex factors
3. What many be a reason for the relative success of bacterial forms?
   (a) Rapid multiplication in number
   (b) High surface area to volume
   (c) Rapid metabolic rates
   (d) All of them
4. After incubation of a bacterial culture for 132 minutes, the number of bacteria present is 20,000. What is the generation time?
   (a) 2 minutes
   (b) 10 minutes
   (c) 30 minutes
   (d) Greater than 30 minutes.
5. A microbial cell requires glucose (G) as carbon source and $(NH_4)_2\ SO_4$ (N) as nitrogen source for its nutrition. How much glucose and $(NH_4)_2\ SO_4$ would be required to produce 20 gram of the cell having its cellular composition 50% carbon and 40% protein and assuming 50% of the substrate carbon converted into cell material?
   (a) 45 g. 3.33 g
   (b) 50 g 6.03 g
   (c) 25 g 8.00 g
   (d) 59 g 12.00 g
6. In addition to cytoplasm and genome which compound is present in the core of a bacterial spore that confers its resistance to adverse environment.
   (a) Adipic acid
   (b) Muramic acid
   (c) Calcium di-picolinate
   (d) Nucleotide
7. What are the roles of ATP in a cell?
   (a) Driving all of the energy requiring reactions of cellular metabolism.
   (b) Activation of a compound prior to its entry into a particular reaction.
   (c) Cycling energy rich phosphate groups.
   (d) All above
8. How the number of molecules of a substrate terms formed to a product by one molecule of an enzyme per second is defined?
   (a) A formation number
   (b) Biot number
   (c) Turn over number
   (d) Ping Pong number
9. If a metabolic reaction of a cell requires 5000 calories of energy in order to occur, will the hydrolysis of

terminal phosphate bond of ATP supply enough energy to drive the reaction?
(a) No
(b) Yes, just sufficient
(c) Yes, in excess
(d) None of the above

10. How many ATPs are derived from the oxidation of one molecule of pyruvate via krebs cycle and the electron transprot system?
(a) 12
(b) 14
(c) 15
(d) 20

11. What is the heat of formation of 100 gram of yeast if the chemical formula of the cells is given by $C_{3.92}H_{6.5}O_{1.94}$ and the heat of combustion of carbon = 394.133 KJ mol^{-1} Hydrogen = 285.767 KJ mol^{-1}?
(a) 1010 kJ
(b) 1308 kJ
(c) 1403 kJ
(d) 1501 kJ

12. How is the cooperative interaction of two microbial systems producing the total effect greater than the sum of the two effects taken independently defined?
(a) Symbiosis
(b) Commensalism
(c) Synergism
(d) Ammensalism

13. By what mechanism detol exerts its control of microorganisms?
(a) Pasteurization
(b) Disinfection
(c) Sterilization
(d) Inactivation

14. Proposed reaction model of microbial cell growth given by the following equation $\frac{dx}{dt} = \mu_m \frac{(s/x)}{\left(k_s + \frac{s}{x}\right)} \cdot x$ is called.
(a) Monod model
(b) Teissler model
(c) Moser model
(d) Contois model

15. Why is electron balance identical to oxygen balance under acrobic conditionas of cell cultivation?
(a) Oxidation does not depend on oxygen as terminal electron acceptor
(b) Oxidation depends on oxygen as a terminal electron acceptor.
(c) Redox balance is dependent only on the redox state
(d) None of the above

16. Maximum specific growth rate in Monod growth equation depends on
(a) Microbial strain
(b) Microbial species
(c) Culture conditions
(d) All of the above

17. For compairing batch and continuous cell cultivation the useful index is
(a) Cell quota
(b) Maximum specific growth rate
(c) Gain factor
(d) Respiration quotient

18. In cell growth on C_2 substrate operation of the essential cycle linked with the TCA cycle is called
(a) Calvin cycle
(b) Glyoxalate cycle
(c) Amphibolic cycle
(d) All of the above

19. The genetic properties of microbial cells are preserved
(a) In mRNA
(b) In tRNA

(c) In DNA
(d) In all above

20. Viruses require a specific host cell for their multiplication often killing the host cell in the process so they are
(a) Obligate conjugate
(b) Obligate parasite
(c) Obligate transfection agent
(d) None above

21. A mutant bacterial strain which requires a supplement of nutrients not required by the original cell type is known as
(a) Phototroph
(b) Chemotroph
(c) Auxotroph
(d) Heterotroph

22. What is transferred from the Hfr bacterium to F bacterium during a bacterial conjugation?
(a) The F factor
(b) Portions of the Hfr chromosome
(c) The F factor and portions of the Hfr chromosome
(d) None of the above

23. What is the optimum pH for growth in most bacteria?
(a) 2.5 – 3.5
(b) 3.5 – 4.5
(c) 4.5 – 6.5
(d) 6.5 – 7.5

24. In assessing random distribution of spontaneous mutations of cell population the best numerical distribution is given by
(a) Malthusian distribution
(b) Gaussian distribution
(c) Poisson distribution
(d) All of the above

25. In microbial production of chemicals by fermentation based on the nature of fermentation reaction type they are classified as
(a) Simple reaction
(b) Simultaneous reaction
(c) Consecutive reaction
(d) Stepwise reaction

26. In a fermentation by *Candida tropicalis* the data recorded were as below (at steady state): Maximum oxygen uptake rate = 12 m mole O_2/hr $(OTR)_m$; cell concentration at $(OTR)_m$ = 10 grams/liter
Critical oxygen concentration for this organism = 0.032 m mole O_2/ liter
Saturation oxygen concentration in the broth = 0.544 m mole O_2 per liter.
What is the value of volumetric oxygen transfer coefficient (K_La) in the system in hour^{-1}?
(a) 155
(b) 215
(c) 235
(d) None of above

27. Most important factors that affect the value of K_La in a continuous stirred tank bioreactor operating at a controlled temperature and pH are
(a) Air flow rate
(b) Agitator speed and type
(c) Cell nature
(d) All above

28. In a CSTBR (continuous stirred tank bioreactor) the inactivation of immobilized catalase enzyme by H_2O_2 followed the equation

$$-\frac{dE}{dt} = k_d E$$

in which E = percent activity of catalase, k_d = its specific inactivation rate constant and t is the time. Assumig k_d to be 6.8×10^{-3} sec^{-1}. What will be the time required for the activity to fall by 10%?

(a) 2.22 mins
(b) 3.6 mins
(c) 5.6 mins
(d) None above

29. In a CSTBR what will be the value of dilution rate (D) at wash out condition if $\mu_m = 1\ h^{-1}$, $k_s = 0.2\ gl^{-1}$ $Y = 0.5$ and $S_0 = 10\ gl^{-1}$, μ_m is maximum specific growth rate constant, k_s is substrate affinity constant, Y is yield coefficient and S_0 is initial substrate concentration.
(a) $0.23\ h^{-1}$
(b) $0.45\ h^{-1}$
(c) $0.72\ h^{-1}$
(d) $0.98\ h^{-1}$

30. In controlling *Anthrax* spore by deactivation with phenol (5%) it followed the following equation

$$-\frac{dN}{dt} = \frac{kN}{1+at}$$

where k is decay constant, t is the time of contact, N is the number of cellspores, α is a constant. Considering its validity for *E. coli* sterilization the data obtained is as below.

t (mins)	0.5	2	5.8
% variable cells	80	56	30

What is the value of k in min^{-1}?
(a) 0.11
(b) 0.25
(c) 0.37
(d) 0.48

31. A 10 *l* fermenter with 500 rpm agitation speed and 1 vvm aeration rate is to be scaled up to 10,000 *l* on similar geometry basis. What is the speed of agitation in the scale up fermenter?
(a) 59 rpm
(b) 109 rpm
(c) 185 rpm
(d) 209 rpm

32. Enzymes catalysing the joining together of two molecules coupled with the hydrolysis of pyrophosphate bond in ATP or similar phosphates are called
(a) Tranferases
(b) Mutases
(c) Ligases
(d) Epimerases

33. The enzymes which catalyse geometric or structural changes within one molecule are called
(a) Hydrolases
(b) Isomerases
(c) Enolases
(c) Catalases

34. In the design of a continuous fermentation medium sterilization system the crucial requirement is to employ
(a) Temperature time profile
(b) Residence time distribution
(c) Peclet number constancy
(d) All of the above

35. The distance corresponding to unit probability of separation of two genes has been termed by the unit
(a) Morgan
(b) Angstrom
(c) Nanometer
(d) None of above

36. It was found that at 37°C a culture of *E. coli* gave 0.67 mutations per 10^8 bacteria per hour. If there is only one gene to mutate per bacterium what is the half life of the gene in years?
(a) 100
(b) 1000
(c) 10000

(d) 11807

37. What will be the frequency of cut of a restriction endonuclease (RE) recognizing 6 base pair (bp) sequence?
    (a) 1056 bp
    (b) 2096 bp
    (c) 3016 bp
    (d) 4096 bp

38. Plasmids carrying the genetic determinants for their own intra-cellular transfer through conjugation belong to the type of
    (a) Relaxed
    (b) Transmissible
    (c) Non transmissible
    (d) None of above

39. During sterilization of medium in a fermenter, the heat up from 100°C to 121°C took 25 mins, while cool-down period from 121°C to 100°C took is 15 mins. The characteristic values of rate constant (k) and the degree of sterilization in the temperature range $\left(\Delta^{100-121°C}_{1°C/min}\right)$ = 12.549 respectively. If the total value of ∇ required for the whole sterilization process is 45 the holding period at 121°C would be
    (a) 3.3 mins
    (b) 5.6 mins
    (c) 8.3 mins
    (d) 9.5 mins

40. For mass transfer into a suspension of neutrally buoyant particles in a culture medium the Froude number has been defined by the dimensionless group (N_i – impeller speed, D_i – impeller diameter, L – fermenter height, D – bubble diameter, μ_{rms} – root mean square fluid velocity)
    (a) $\frac{N_i^2 D_i^2}{gL}$
    (b) $\frac{\mu_{rms}^2}{gD}$
    (c) $\frac{N_i^2 D_i^2}{g}$
    (d) None above

41. In bioprocess engineering the use of momentum factor as scale up criteria was first proposed by
    (a) Norman Blakebrough and K. Sambamurthy
    (b) Suichi Aiba
    (c) T. K. Ghose
    (d) Arther E. Humphrey

42. Continuous separation of enzymic saccharification products via ultrafiltration membrane was first proposed by
    (a) T. K. Ghose
    (b) D.I.C Wang
    (c) S. Sourirajan
    (d) E. L. Gaden. Jr.

43. The operon model of genes regulation was first proposed by
    (a) Jacob and Monod
    (b) Eigen
    (c) H. Martinez
    (d) L. Wolpert

44. 'Mixing Rate Number.' as a scale up criteria was first introduced by
    (a) J. Oldshue
    (b) O. Levenspiel and S. Khang
    (c) H. Taguchi
    (d) A. Fiechter

45. Use of a radio flow follower in characterization of mixing in fermenters was first proposed by
    (a) A. B. Metzner

(b) P. Sykes
(c) J. Bryant
(d) V. W. Uhl

46. In a fully aerated-agitated fermenter the liquid phase oxygen mass transfer coefficient (K_L) computed from Dankwerts surface renewal theory is larger to that computed from Higbie's penetration theory by
(a) 1.13 times
(b) 1.24 times
(c) 1.33 times
(d) 1.51 times

47. In a highly aerated and agitated fermenter the rate of transfer of oxygen from gas phase to liquid phase is proportional to
(a) Available bubble surface area
(b) Partial pressure of oxygen
(c) $1/K_L$
(d) All above

48. Shear stress vs shear rate behavior of Newtonian and non-Newtonian fermentation liquids has been modeled by Power Law containing n as power law index whose value may be above, equal to or below unity. When the value of n is less than unity the fermentation fluid is called shear stress vs shear rate relation passing through origin.
(a) Newtonian
(b) Dilatant
(c) Pseudoplastic
(d) None above

49. The scheme of technologically redesigning living microorganisms was given by
(a) Stanley Cohen
(b) George Wald
(c) David Baltimore
(d) James Watson

50. Joining of DNA molecules by DNA ligase can be achieved by
(a) Covalently annealing the cohesive ends
(b) Catalysing the formation of phosphodiester bonds between blunt ended fragments
(c) Utilizing the enzyme terminal deoxynucleotidyl transfer
(d) All above

51. A genetic unit consisting of adjacent genes that function coordinately under the joint control of an operator and a repressor has been termed.
(a) Codon
(b) Regulon
(c) Operon
(d) Neuron

52. An unicellular organism lacking membrane-bound nucleus is called
(a) Autotroph
(b) Eukaryote
(c) Heterotroph
(d) Prokaryote

53. Extra chromosomal, autonomous, self replicating, circular segments of DNA, as well as some viruses used as 'vectors' for cloning DNA in bacterial host cells are called
(a) Cosmids
(b) Phasemids
(c) Plasmids
(d) None above

54. A technique used for transferring DNA, RNA or protein from gels to a suitable binding materix is known as
(a) Cloning
(b) Blotting
(c) Annealing
(d) Transfecting

55. A bioreactor in which steady state growth of microorganisms/cells is maintained over prolonged periods of time under sterile conditions by providing the cells with a constant input of nutrients and continously removing effluents with cells as output is called
    (a) Bistat
    (b) Turbidostat
    (c) Chemostat
    (d) Oxystat
56. Combined process of cell differentiation, growth and morphogenesis is called
    (a) Ontogenesis
    (b) Phylogenesis
    (c) Biosynthesis
    (d) None above
57. In computer aided design of a bioprocess computer and control functions define
    (a) Analog-Digital (A/D) converter, multiplexer, D/A converter
    (b) Hardware, software
    (c) Process sensor, monitor, controller, final control element
    (d) All above
58. The phase of metabolism that encompasses the synthesis of low molecular weight precursors and from that the synthesis of macromolecular cell component is called
    (a) Syntrophism
    (b) Catabolism
    (c) Anabolism
    (d) Synergism
59. A disinfection by ozone following Chick's law showed 99.9% kill of bacteria in water with a residual concentration of 0.5 mg/*l*. Assuming disinfection reaction rate constant to be 2.5×10^{-2}/sec. What will be the contact time for disinfection?
    (a) 1 min
    (b) 1.5 mins
    (c) 2 mins
    (d) 2.5 mins
60. A carbohydrate composed of a straight chain of glucose units has been called
    (a) Xylose
    (b) Amylose
    (c) Trehalose
    (d) None above
61. Lactase hydrolyzes lactose to form
    (a) Glucose
    (b) Glucose and fructose
    (c) Glucose and Galactose
    (d) Galactose and fructose
62. *Idli* is a
    (a) Natural food
    (b) Nonvegeterian food
    (c) Fermented food
    (d) Baked food
63. Milk sol is transformed fermentatively into milk gel and the product is called
    (a) Curd
    (b) Cheese
    (d) Panir
    (d) Kefir
64. In thermal processing of a food by Ball's method the data collected are; f_h = 12.9, j = 1.51 IT = 160°F, RT = 250°F, F_0 = 2.78, log g = 0.75. From these data computed process time of the food is
    (a) 12.15 mins
    (b) 13.25 mins
    (c) 16.25 mins
    (d) 18.15 mins
65. Specific nutrients traverse the cytoplasmic membrane of bacteria by

(a) Active transport
(b) Facilitated diffusion
(c) Group translocation
(d) All of the above

66. Bacteria that ferment substrates to single end product are called
(a) Oxidative fermenters
(b) Homofermenters
(c) Obligately anaerobic fermenters
(d) None of the above

67. Which species of RNA may be processed in prokaryotes?
(a) mRNA
(b) rRNA
(c) tRNA
(d) All above except (a)

68. Given that the average gene is coded for a polypeptide whose chain length is 300 amino acids long and that 4000 such genes exist in a (hypothetical) bacterial chromosome, what would be the probability that a forward mutation would occur in a given gene?
(a) 1/300
(b) 1/3000
(c) 1/400
(d) 1/4000

69. Restriction enzymes are found only in
(a) Gram positive bacteria
(b) Gram negative bacteria
(c) In both (a) and (b)
(d) In none of the above

70. The part of the bacterial growth curve that reflects an adjustment to the medium and a replenishment of the pools of metabolic intermediates is the
(a) Lag phase
(b) Exponential phase
(c) Stationary phase
(d) Death phase

71. A gene that codes for an enzyme is called
(a) Jumping gene
(b) Structural gene
(c) Regulatory gene
(d) None of the above

72. A pathway that converts two carbon compounds to carbon dioxide transferring electrons to NAD^+ and other carriers has been called
(a) Krebs cycle
(b) Amphibolic cycle
(c) HMP pathway
(d) None of the above

73. A trickling filter involves a method of
(a) Primary waste water treatment
(b) Secondary waste water treatment
(c) Combined waste water treatment
(d) All above

74. The characteristic property that distinguishes cream style corn from waxy corn is the property of
(a) Saccharification
(b) Gelling
(c) Cross linking
(d) None above

75. Vinegar is a
(a) Nutrient
(b) Condiment
(c) Supplement
(d) Adjunct

76. For a turbine impeller mixer the mixing rate number, $\left(\frac{N}{K}\right)\left(\frac{D_i}{D_t}\right)^{0.23}$ is related to power number by the value (N–impeller speed, K–amplitude decay rate constant, D_i–impeller diameter, D_t–tank diameter)

(a) $\dfrac{Pg_c}{\rho N^3 D_i^5}$

(b) $0.1\left(\dfrac{Pg_c}{\rho N^3 D_i^5}\right)$

(c) $1.5\left(\dfrac{Pg_c}{\rho N^3 D_i^5}\right)$

(d) None of the above

77. The capsid of a virus weighing 3.5 × 107 daltons has 2150 protein molecules. If one amino acid weighs 125 daltons, how many amino acids will be there per protein molecule in the capsid?
    (a) 100
    (b) 112
    (c) 128
    (d) 150
78. A fully turbulent laboratory fermenter having following design dimensions was used in cellulase production. How much power in horse power (h.p.) is required in mixing? D_i = 6.2 cms, D_t = 13 cms, n_b = number of blades = 6, V = liquid volume = 1 liter viscosity of fluid = 2 c.p., density of fluid = 1.1 g/c.c. and impeller rotation speed = 700 rpm (revolutions per minute)
    (a) 1.1 h.p.
    (b) 0.51 h.p.
    (c) 0.144 h.p.
    (d) 0.052 h.p.
79. Straight dough method is used in
    (a) Deep fat frying
    (b) Bread making
    (c) Idli making
    (d) Freeze drying
80. Synthesis of protein using mRNA as template is termed
    (a) Translation
    (b) Transcription
    (c) Transfection
    (d) Translocation
81. A class of microorganisms which can be subdivided into methanogenic, halophilic and thermoacidophilic groups characterized by special constituents like ether-bound phytane containing lipids and special coenzymes is called
    (a) Eubacteria
    (b) Archaebacteria
    (c) Sulfate reducing bacteria
    (d) Purple sulfur bacteria
82. Macerozyme is a food enzyme used in processing of
    (a) Meat
    (b) Fish
    (c) Minute rice
    (d) Cauliflower
83. Penicillinase enzyme from an organism inactivates 6-amino penicillinic acid by breaking the following numbered bonds shown below

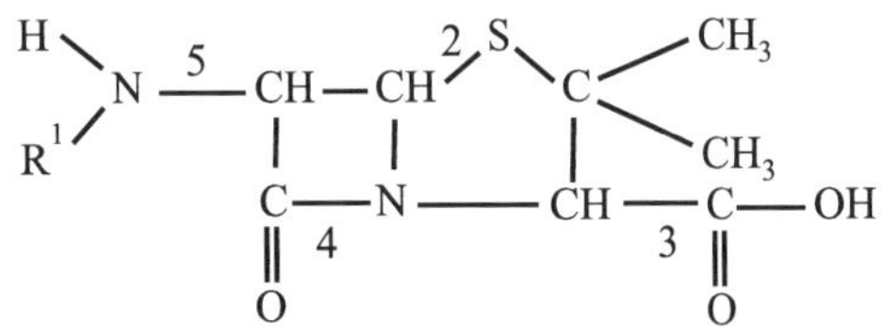

H, R^1 — N —5— CH — CH —2— S — C(CH_3)(CH_3); CH — C(=O) —4— N — CH —3— C(=O) — OH

    (a) 1
    (b) 2
    (c) 3
    (4) 4
84. A first wash of an aliquot of *Escherichia coli* with EDTA on analysis showed to contain alkaline phosphatase, DNA and penicillinase. The physiological area of the cell affected by the EDTA is

(a) Periplasmic space
(b) Mesosomal space
(c) Chromosome
(d) Plasma membrane

85. The value of a haemocytometer constant is
(a) 100
(b) 1000
(c) 2.5×10^{-7}
(d) 1.6×10^{-4}

86. In water pollution control BOD test is used to measure
(a) The total dissolved solids
(b) Sludge volume index
(c) Strength of pollution
(d) Suspended solids

87. A portion of 5 ml sample of a waste water was diluted to 300 ml in a BOD bottle. The dissolved oxygen content of the mixture was 8 mg/*l*. If after 5 days of incubation at 20°C the dissolved oxygen content of the mixture is 3 mg/*l*, what will be the value of BOD $_{5(20°C)}$ of the waste water?
(a) 50 mg/*l*
(b) 100 mg/*l*
(c) 200 mg/*l*
(d) 300 mg/*l*

88. An organism following Monod kinetic equation and having $\mu_m = 0.5\ h^{-1}$ and $K_s = 2\ gl^{-1}$ in a continuous perfectly mixed bioreactor at steady state showed no cell death. At what dilution rate it will produce maximum total rate of cell population? (Consider $S_0 = 50\ gl^{-1}$)
(a) $0.1\ h^{-1}$
(b) $0.3\ h^{-1}$
(c) $0.4\ h^{-1}$
(d) $0.62\ h^{-1}$

89. It has been estimated that in a multistage fermenter concentration of microbial cells in the second fermenter can not be greater than that in the first fermenter by a factor of
(a) 1.21 times
(b) 1.348 times
(c) 1.718 times
(d) 1.818 times

90. Citranellol is a food flavour obtained by distilling
(a) Mustard oil
(b) Orange peel oil
(c) Lard oil
(d) Lemon grass oil

91. Psychophysical law is used in testing
(a) Food flavour
(b) Food texture
(c) Food maturity
(d) Food acidity

92. Diacetyl is the flavouring component in
(a) Milk
(b) Curd
(c) Butter
(d) Cheese

93. If a can of food is spoiled by increased acidity by microorganisms without gas production and the can looks normal in outward appearence the spoilage is said to be due to
(a) Stack burning
(b) Pin holing
(c) Flat sour
(d) None of the above

94. The microorganism which is used in industrial fermentative production of terramycin is
(a) *Penicillium chrysogenum*
(b) *Streptomyces griseus*
(c) *Streptomyces rimosus*
(d) None of the above

95. Mustard oil is adulterated by
 (a) Til oil
 (b) Sesame oil
 (c) Argemone oil
 (d) Orange peel oil
96. The colour of tomato is due to the presence of the pigment
 (a) Anthocyanin
 (b) Carotin
 (c) Lycopin
 (d) Xanthin
97. Methyl propionate is the flavouring compound of the fruit
 (a) Mango
 (b) Cherry
 (c) Pineapple
 (d) Guava
98. In sucrose, glucose and fructose are bound in 1 : 1 linkage leaving no free reducing group. So sucrose is
 (a) Reducing sugar
 (b) Nonreducing sugar
 (c) Amino sugar
 (d) None of the above
99. The protein present in wheat is called
 (a) Albumin
 (b) Gluten
 (c) Casein
 (d) Kerratin
100. The time in minutes at a specific design temperature (250°F) needed to kill a population of cells or spores in food processing is termed as
 (a) Z-value
 (b) F-value
 (c) Q_{10}-value
 (d) None of the above
101. Cytological dimension of nuclear material to bacterial cell volume is about.
 (a) $\frac{1}{3}$
 (b) $\frac{1}{2}$
 (c) $\frac{1}{4}$
 (d) None of the above.
102. The fermentation pattern of three microbial strains of gram negative cocci is given below. Only strain C grows on plain nutrient agar. The data indicate that the strain A is

Strain	Acid produced from		
	Maltose	Dextrose	Sucrose
A	+	+	—
B	—	+	—
C	—	—	—

 (a) *Branhamella catarrhails*
 (b) *Neisseria flavesceus*
 (c) *N. meningitis*
 (d) *N. sicca*
103. *Staphylococcus aureus* can produce a severe food poisoning that results from the injestion of
 (a) Enterotoxin
 (b) Coagulase
 (c) Penicillinase
 (d) Hemolysin
104. Which of the tests would best provide specification for a manitol positive, slide coagulase negative *Staphylococcus*?
 (a) Lactose fermentation
 (b) Lipase activity
 (c) Phage typing
 (d) Thermostable endonuclease
105. Botulism food poisoning symptoms include double vision, inability to speak, and respiratory paralysis which are consistent with

(a) Secretion of an enterotoxin
(b) Endotoxin shock
(c) Ingestion of a neurotoxin
(d) None of the above.

106. The biochemical responsible for heat resistance of a bacterial spore is
(a) Pantothenate
(b) Calcium dipicolinate
(c) Ascorbate
(d) None of the above.

107. Bacterial spore component which is responsible for its chemical resistance is
(a) Coat
(b) Core
(c) Exosporium
(d) None above.

108. The difference between prokaryotic and eukaryotic cells lies in that the former lacks
(a) A plasma membrane
(b) Ribosome
(c) Endoplasmic reticulum
(d) A cell wall

109. Molecular weight of ribosomes is
(a) 8.5×10^2 Da
(b) 6.1×10^4 Da
(c) 2.8×10^6 Da
(d) None above

110. The birth time of a bacterial cell is given by
(a) The reciprocal of its specific growth rate
(b) Its doubling time
(c) Its maximum specific growth rate
(d) None above.

111. Under special case where all of the substrate collected is laid down and retained as cell material the "cell quota" in growth is
(a) Equal to specific substrate uptake rate (maximum)
(b) Equal to reciprocal of true growth yield
(c) Equal to specific cell yield
(d) None above

112. Appearance of stationary phase in the growth cycle of a microbial cell may be due to
(a) Lack of nutrients
(b) Lack of biological space
(c) Accumulation of toxic metabolites
(d) All above

113. In a microbial fuel cell the reaction

$$C_6H_{12}O_6 + O_2 \xrightarrow{\text{Cells}} 6CO_2 + 6H_2O$$

has been used to produce electrical energy. This reaction produces 673 kilo calories per mole glucose. Considering 1K cal = 1.16 Watt hour the amout of electrical energy produced by this fuel cell is
(a) 1.5 wh
(b) 2.0 wh
(b) 3.0 wh
(c) 6.0 wh

114. An aerobic organism is incubated in the presence of acetic acid, which is used as a carbon and energy source. Analysis of the metabolic pathway intermediates reveals, among other substances, succinic acid, acetyl CoA, but no pyruvate. The series of biochemical reaction responsible for such a pattern of metabolites is called
(a) Krebs cycle
(b) TCA cycle
(c) Glyoxalate cycle
(d) Succinate cycle

115. During gram stainning of *Staphylococcus* by mistake the iodine fixation step was missed. The most likely result is that the bacteria would appear
    (a) Pink
    (b) Colourless
    (c) Blue
    (d) None above.
116. A biotechnologist after disinfecting a culture of *Mycobacterium tuberculosis* by chloroform treated it by acid-fast stain and counter-stained by methylene blue. He/she could see
    (a) Blue organisms against a red background
    (b) Blue organisms against a blue background
    (c) Red organisms against a blue background
    (d) Colourless organisms
117. Variable volume cell cultivation by submerged process has been termed
    (a) Batch cultivation
    (c) Continuous cultivation
    (d) Fed batch cultivation
    (e) Bistat cultivation
118. A hemispherical colony of a cell culture without magnification showed 0.2 mm diameter. Assuming that cells in the colony are cylindrical with 1 micron length and 0.5 micron diameter one can compute to show that maximum number of cells in the colony is
    (a) 10^4
    (b) 10^3
    (c) 10^7
    (d) 10^{12}
119. In an aerobic treatment of waste water with high organic content it was observed that first stage BOD removal was independent of organic substrate concentration. For this BOD removal kinetics is
    (a) Mixed order
    (b) First order
    (c) Second order
    (d) Zero order
120. In an activated sludge process of waste water treatment the ratio of pound BOD applied per day to pound mixed liquor volatile suspended solids in aeration tank has been called
    (a) BOD loading rate
    (b) Process loading rate
    (c) Hydraulic loading rate
    (d) None above
121. The amount of oxygen that can be dissolved per unit power expenditure to the aerated culture liquid is called
    (a) Oxygenation capacity
    (b) Aeration economy
    (c) Aeration number
    (d) None above
122. Considering cell growth follows geometric progression for increase of biomass in cell, the ratio of nuclear volume to the difference between cell volume and nuclear volume has been called
    (a) Sludge density index (SDI)
    (b) Nucleoplasmic index (NPI)
    (c) Sludge volume index (SVI)
    (d) Cell compaction index (CCI)
123. Exposing spores of a bacteria at a given temperature and considering that most probable life span distribution of spore is logarithmic than denaturation rate constant of spores will be
    (a) Proportional of mean life span
    (b) Reciprocal of mean life span
    (c) Having no correlation
    (d) None above

124. The concentration of a non-competitive inhibitor, having $K_i = 4 \times 10^{-6}$ M, that will be required to yield 65% inhibition of an enzyme catalysed reaction is
   (a) 1.25×10^{-5} M
   (b) 2×10^{-7} M
   (c) 7.45×10^{-6} M
   (d) None above
125. In fabrication of stream sterilizable dissolved oxygen probe the used membrane thickness is one mil which is equal to
   (a) One inch
   (b) Half of an inch
   (c) 0.00254 inch
   (d) 1×10^{-3} inch
126. In Polymerase Chain Reaction (PCR) formula given by SDNA = 2n –2 where SDNA stands for short fragment DNA and n for number of cycles, state in which cycle the number of SDNA molecules will equal the number of the other two types DNA in total DNA molecules.
   (a) 1st cycle
   (b) 2nd cycle
   (c) 3rd cycle
   (d) 4rth cycle
127. The concept of metabolic engineering in fermentation process biotechnology was proposed by
   (a) James E. Bailey
   (b) R.K. Finn
   (c) A.E. Fiechter
   (d) None above
128. In biosynthetic pathways utilizing precursors that are not true intermediates are called
   (a) Anabolic pathway
   (b) Amphibolic pathway
   (c) Salvage pathway
   (d) Catabolic pathway
129. Lamberts-Beer law was held good in measuring optical density of a suspension containing 200 mg dry weight per liter of microbial cells having optical density (OD). One in 1 cm cuvette at 450 nm. So for a cell suspension having 30% transmission in a 3 cm cuvette its OD will be (Assume OD $\propto$ cell dry weight)
   (a) 15.5
   (b) 25.4
   (c) 17.4
   (d) 8.5
130. One of the ways of overcoming the problem of catabolite repression in alcohol fermentation is by
   (a) pH cycling
   (b) Vaccum cycling
   (c) Cell recycling
   (d) None above
131. In hydrocarbon fermentation scale up the most suitable criteria of maintaining similar oil drop sauter mean diameter was proposed by
   (a) R.K. Bajpai
   (b) D Ramakrishna
   (c) A. Prokop
   (d) All above
132. the concept of transfectional fermentation process biotechnology has been proposed in more recent years by
   (a) S.N. Mukhopadhyay
   (b) G. Goma
   (c) A. Moser
   (d) S.K. Majumdar
133. Bubble column bioreactor is not suitable for animal cell cultivation due to shear force exerted by
   (a) Liquid circulation
   (b) Bubble coalescence
   (c) Cell fragility
   (d) All above

134. The number of regimes considered in nonlinear modelling and control of gluconic acid fermentation by *Pseudomonas ovalis* is
    (a) 2
    (b) 3
    (c) 4
    (d) 5
135. For ecological safety it is required to treat 500000 gals per day of water with 0.3 mg per liter of chlorine. If the disinfectant is in form of bleach that contains 33.33% of available chlorine the amount of bleach in pounds needed to treat the daily flow of water is
    (a) 2.25
    (b) 1.75
    (c) 3.75
    (d) 4.18
136. In phase-plane analysis of a continuous culture bioprocessing the dynamics of cell growth always manifests stability by singular point
    (a) Yes
    (b) No
    (c) Sometimes
    (d) None above
137. The formula given below is the structure of the antibiotic

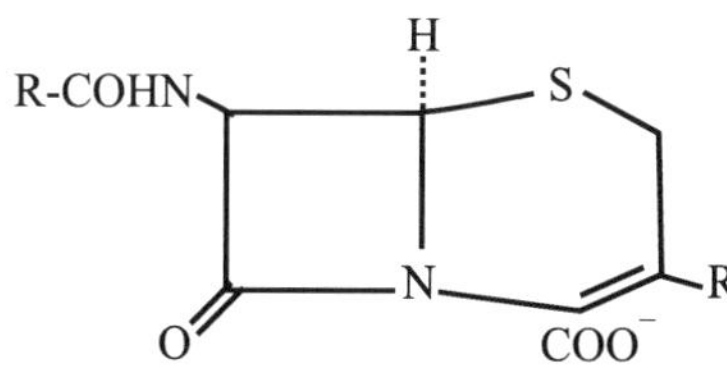

    (a) Erythrocin
    (b) Rifamycin
    (c) Cephalosporine
    (d) Tetracyclin
138. The microorganism used in fermentative production of Rifamycin is
    (a) *Steptomyces fradae*
    (b) *Steptomyces mediterranei*
    (c) *Streptomyces griseus*
    (d) None above
139. Erythromycin is a

Erythromycin
Produced by
Streptomyces erythreus

    (a) Macrolide antibiotic
    (b) Broad spectrum antibiotic
    (c) Fungal antibiotic
    (d) None above
140. Expression of an eukaryotic gene in prokaryotes requires
    (a) A SD sequence in mRNA
    (b) Absence of introns
    (c) Regulatory elements upstream of the gene
    (d) All above
141. Oxygen vector pathway for enhanced oxygen mass transfer in biosprocessing liquid has been proposed by
    (a) G. Goma
    (b) A. Moser
    (c) S. N. Mukhopadhyay
    (d) Bo Mattiason
142. In batch ethanol fermentation of cellulose by *Clostridium thermocellum* for overcoming the problem of product inhibition vaccum cycling strategy has been proposed by

(a) S. Kundu
(b) S. N. Mukhopadhyay
(c) T. K. Ghose
(d) All above

143. Surface renewal theory of oxygen mass transfer in liquid from air bubbles was proposed by
(a) W. G. Whitman
(b) R. Higbie
(c) P. V. Danckwerts
(d) M. M. Sharma

144. In mixed sugar fermentation by yeast the principle of microbial rejection has been proposed by
(a) B. S. M. Rao
(b) R. K. Bajpai
(c) T. K. Ghose
(d) All above

145. Dynamic differential gassing out method of determination of volumetric oxygen transfer coefficient was developed by
(a) B. Bandyopadhyay
(b) A. E. Humphrey
(c) H. Taguchi
(d) All above

146. Based on fluid regime consideration in mixing in a stirred tank baffled bioreactor where a vortex is formed the value of power factor θ is obtained from the value of

(a) $\dfrac{Pg_c}{PN^3\,D_i5}$

(b) $\dfrac{Pg_c}{PN^3\,D_i5}\left(\dfrac{D_i\,N^2}{g}\right)^{-q}$

(c) $\dfrac{K}{g_c}\,\rho\;N^3D_i^5$

(d) None above

147. For demostration that plants are living being Sir J.C. Bose designed the instrument called
(a) Fairnograph
(b) Sismograph
(c) Crescograph
(d) Demograph

148. Which of the following is not part of cells' complete life cycle?
(a) Mitosis
(b) G_1 phase
(c) S phase
(d) P phase

149. The genetic code of a cell is
(a) Commaless
(b) Degenerate
(c) Non-overlapping
(d) All of the above

150. A bacterium contains 3690 amino acids. Given the information that 4 is the average number of amino acids per polynucleotide for this bacterium, what is the good estimate for the total number of genes of this organism?
(a) 160
(b) 330
(c) 990
(d) 1320

151. The genes which serve as a binding site for RNA polymerase are called
(a) Operator genes
(b) Structural genes
(c) Promoter genes
(d) Regulatory genes

152. By infecting mice with smooth and rough strains of *Pnemococcus* in 1928 Griffith demonstrated the phenomenon of
(a) Transfection
(b) Translation
(c) Transformation
(d) Translocation

153. Intercellular protoplasmic channels in plant cells are known as
    (a) Cellulosome
    (b) Gap junctions
    (c) Plasmodesmata
    (d) Desmosomes
154. The number of molecules of a substrate transformed to a product by one molecule of an enzyme per second is called enzyme's
    (a) Biot number
    (b) Trunover number
    (c) Access number
    (d) None above
155. In the process of wine making the fact that yeast is
    (a) An aerobe
    (b) A facultative anaerobe
    (c) An obligate anaerobe
    (d) None above
156. In solid state fermentation an example of a fruiting body is a mushroom. Once it is formed, does it detach completely from the non-reproductive part?
    (a) Yes
    (b) No
    (c) Sometimes
    (d) None above
157. In conversion of glucose to gluconic acid by *Ps. ovalis* where the intermediate gluconolactone accumulates to some extent befor the product is formed by the following scheme

$$\text{Glucose} \xrightarrow[\text{[O]}]{k_1 \cdot k_2} \text{Gluconolactone}$$

$$\xrightarrow[\text{[H}_2\text{O]}]{k_3} \text{Gluconic acid (P)}$$

in which k_1, k_2 & k_3 are rate constants for cell yield, intermediate formation and product yield respectively. If its substrate uptake rate equation is given

$$\text{by} - \frac{ds}{dt} = f_1\left[\frac{k_1 s}{k_s + s}\right] + f_2\left[\frac{k_2 s}{k_m + s}\right]$$

in which f_1, f_2 and f_3 are stoichiometric constants and k_m is Michaelis-Menten constant state wheather its rate of product formation is proportional to
    (a) Gluconolactone concentration
    (b) Substrate uptake rate
    (c) Oxygen uptake rate
    (d) Product concentration
158. Pizza is a
    (a) Fermented food
    (b) Non fermented food
    (c) Cooked food
    (d) None above
159. The enzymes that catalyze the covalent linking together of two molecules, coupled with the breaking of a pyrophosphate bond as in ATP are
    (a) Lyases
    (b) Glucanases
    (c) Ligases
    (d) None of the above
160. The equation to estimate critical concentration of fission promoting metabolite in cell for minimizing the length of lag time for a good cell cultivation process design was proposed by
    (a) E.L. Oginsky
    (b) W.W Umbreit
    (c) J.E. Bailey and D.F. Ollis
    (d) A.C.R. Dean and C. Hinselwood
161. If in the cultivation of a bacteria in a medium having ammonium sulfate as sole nitrogen the harvested cells show nitrogen content 8% by weight and amount of growth is 10 kg per meter cube then neglecting buffering action

of the medium and initial concentration of hydrogen ion (10^{-7} M) the value of pH of the broth will be
(a) 2.12
(b) 1.00
(c) 1.24
(d) 3.28

162. In recombinant DNA technology the frequency of recombination serves as an index for
(a) Mapping sites
(b) Map distance
(c) Map function
(d) All above

163. Discoverer of the first enzyme was
(a) J.B.S. Halden
(b) Planche
(c) E. Duclank
(d) None above

164. In computer aided fermentation sensor signals from the fermenter are amplified and displayed on digital panel meters using computer
(a) Limit switch
(b) Binary coded decimal signal in digital form
(c) Data acquisition system
(d) None above

165. In comparing batch and continuous cell cultivation system the ratio of the maximum rate of production in continuous run over batch has been called
(a) Growth modulus
(b) Gain factor
(c) Yield factor
(d) None above

166. The specific rate at which cells respire increases with increase in the dissolved oxygen concentration upto a point which has been termed
(a) Bulk dissolved oxygen concentration
(b) Apparent dissolved oxygen concentration
(c) Critical dissolved oxygen concentration
(d) Saturation dissolved oxygen concentration

167. Hagen-Poiseuelle law is applicable in handling flow through a circular tube in biosystems. Few assumptions that are implied in the development of this law include
(a) The flow is laminar
(b) The density of fluid is constant
(c) The flow is independent of time
(d) All above

168. Using recombinant DNA technology besides chromosome fractions plasmids may be introduced into living bacteria by
(a) Transformation
(b) Transduction
(c) Transfection
(d) None above

169. In eukaryotic organisms, it is possible to cross strains with different genetic properties and look among the progeny of the cross for those which have acquired, by recombination during DNA replication, the desirable properties from
(a) The donor strain
(b) The acceptor strain
(c) Both parents
(d) None of them

170. A potentially self perpetuating open system of linked organic reactions, catalysed step-wise and almost isothermally by complex and specific organic catalysts which are

themselves produced by the system may be defined as

(a) Bioorganic catalyst
(b) Life
(c) Gene
(d) Nucleus

171. The logarithmic rate of death of cells in medium sterilization is directly proportional to the number of viable cells if the morphological form of the cells in the medium be

(a) Vegetative
(b) Spores
(c) Septate mycelia
(d) None above

172. In a bubble column bioreactor the air-water experiments reveal that the air bubbles rising through the liquid will coalesce into slugs if the gas volume fraction exceeds a critical value of

(a) one
(b) 0.5
(c) 0.3
(d) 0.1

173. Flow injection technique has been used in optimization of bioprocessing system by

(a) Off line analysis
(b) On line analysis
(c) Transient analysis
(d) All above

174. The trend in entropy generation in microbial cell growth is to reach

(a) An equillibrium state
(b) A transient state
(c) A pseudo steady state
(d) None above

175. Case hardening is not observed in foods preserved by

(a) Solar drying
(b) Freeze drying
(c) Tray drying
(d) All above

176. Liquid membranes are useful tools in separation technology for biotechnological applications because of their

(a) Ease of preparation
(b) Good shelf life
(c) Lack of toxicity
(d) All above

177. The time that will be required to kill the organisms present in a fermentation medium entering in a fermenter at 75°F with a flow rate of 1000 gals/hour considering design duration 3 months and initial cell population in the medium 20×10^9 cells/gal with exit temperature of the medium from the fermenter 290°F is (Assume convention of sterilization design procedure, energy of activation 67,700 cals/gm mole and Boltzman constant $1 \times 10^{36.2}$)

(a) 5.2 secs
(b) 8.8 secs
(c) 12.2 secs
(d) 20.1 secs

178. A horizontal rotary fermenter of 30 cms diameter and one meter long rotates coaxially inside a fixed outer cylinder jacket of approximately same length of diameter of 30.5 cms. Hot water (30°C) fills the space between the cylinders to control the temperature of gluconic acid fermentation by *Ps. ovalis* B14 86. A torque of 0.25 ft lb is applied to the inner cylinder. After a constant velocity is attained what will be the power dissipated by fluid resistance ?
(ignoring end effects)

(a) 1 h.p
(b) 0.1 h.p
(c) 0.01 h.p
(d) None above

179. What will be the value of shear stress for water at ambient temperature when exposed to a shear rate of 100 seconds^{-1}? (Assume viscosity of water at ambient temperature = 1 c.p.). Evaluate in both CGS and SI systems.

	CGS	SI
(a)	0.1	0.08
(b)	0.8	0.8
(c)	1.0	0.1

(d) None above

180. In a laboratory air sterilization job an air filter is to be designed for a given fermentation which runs for 100 hours and used 1.6 cm^3 air per min. The intake air is expected to have a microbial load of 10,000 microorganisms per m^3. Assuming a reasonably safe operation i.e. low probability of a single organism for every 1000 passing the filter and that filter packing material of choice has L_{90} vlalue of 4.3 cms, how thick should the air filter be ?
(a) 25 cms
(b) 36 cms
(c) 46 cms
(d) None above

181. The pressure drop across an air sterilizer is a function of
(a) Drag coefficient
(b) Fibre diameter
(c) Void fraction
(d) All above

182. Phylogenic classifications of living being are based on
(a) Shared morphologic attributes
(b) Evolutionary relationships
(c) Shape
(d) Unusual growth characteristics

183. An intracytoplasmic granule may contain
(a) Steroids
(b) Nucleic acids
(c) Glycogen
(d) 80 s ribosomes

184. Where are porins found in Gram-negative bacteria?
(a) Cytoplasmic membrane
(b) Outer membrane
(c) Periplasm
(d) Cytoplasm

185. In commercial production of penicillin by variants of mold *Penicillium notatum* a yield was 5 mg/ml. In what way the present strain may be further improved ?
(a) By metabolic engineering
(b) By collecting the biosynthetic genes into a multicopy plasmid
(c) Pathway amplification
(d) All above

186. In lysogenic conversion, new properties are conferred on the bacterial cell by products of
(a) Bacterial genes
(b) Prophage genes
(c) Colicinogenic genes
(d) Transposons

187. The loss of activity of a protein resulting from a mutation can be at least partially restored by a second mutation at a different site (codon). Mutations of this type are called :
(a) Amber mutations
(b) Committed mutations
(c) Suppressor mutations
(d) Cryptic mutations

188. Complex bacterial cell cultivation media design contain
    (a) Many components that are well defined
    (b) Many components qualitatively not well defined
    (c) Only peptone extracts
    (d) The least number of essential components
189. The part of the bacterial growth curve that reflects an adjustment to the medium and a replenishment of the pools of metabolic intermediates is the
    (a) Lag phase
    (b) Transition phase
    (c) Exponential phase
    (d) Death phase
190. Substate (C_{SO} = 2 mol/liter) and enzyme (C_{EO} = 0.001 mol/liter) are introduced into a batch reactor. They react, conversion is 90% in 4.1 minutes, and the rate equation which represents this behavior is found to be

    $-r_A = 10^3 \frac{C_{EO} C_S}{1 + C_S}$. If one plans to

    build and operate a mixed flow reactor using a continuous feed of substrate (C_{SO} = 2 mol/liters) with enzyme (C_{EO} = 0.001 mol/liter) and assuming micro fluid system what should be the space time value to achieve 90% conversion of substrate?
    (a) 1.8 mins
    (b) 2.1 mins
    (c) 6.4 mins
    (d) 10.8 mins
191. The enzyme that catalyzes the reaction of carbonic acid from carbon dioxide and water is called
    (a) Glucose anhydrase
    (b) Carboxylase
    (c) Carbonic anhydrase
    (d) Co-carboxylase
192. Which of the given vitamins are water soluble
    (a) Vitamin B_1
    (b) Vitamin B_2
    (c) Vitamin B_6
    (d) All above
193. Which of the given vitamins are not fat soluble
    (a) Vitamin B_1
    (b) Vitamin A
    (c) Vitamin D
    (d) Vitamin K
194. Potato starch is
    (a) Pasting type
    (b) Gellying type
    (c) Cream style type
    (d) None above
195. The cell growth rate that can be expressed by the following equation

    $\frac{dx}{dt} = \mu_x \left(1 - \frac{x}{x_m}\right)$ has been called

    (a) Michaelis-Minten model
    (b) Monod's model
    (c) Logistic model
    (d) Stochastic model
196. In a cell cultivation liquid of aerobic fermentation assuming that the liquid film coefficient, K_L of air bubbles is the only variable which depend on temperature, and bubble behavior remain unaltered then under temperature variation in Newtonian cultivation liquid the value of K_L follows
    (a) Stokes-Einstein equation
    (b) Gilliland's equation
    (c) Rumford's equation
    (d) None above
197. An aerobic fermentation using *Aspergillus niger* tends to form

pellets. The average mycelial density pellets is 0.02 mg cells/mm^3 of pellet volume. If the average dissolved oxygen concentration in the bulk broth is 5 μg/ml, the specific oxygen uptake rate by the mold is 1.2 m moles of O_2/hr/gm of cells and if the oxygen diffusion coefficient is 1.8×10^{-5} cm^2/sec in fermentation broth what will be the radius of the pellet that will just cause an oxygen deficiency within the pellet.

(a) 0.125 mm
(b) 0.212 mm
(c) 0.405 mm
(d) 0.505 mm

198. In transfectional fermentation the sharing of functional viral gene products by viruses having mutations in different genes is referred to as:
(a) Complementation
(b) Recombination
(c) Cross activation
(d) Multiplicity of infection (MOI)

199. Enzymes responsible in folding of proteins are known as
(a) Chaperones
(b) Chaperonins
(c) Foldases
(d) All above

200. Proteins under the control of same operon i.e. proteins involving coordinately regulated, yet scattered, genes are termed as
(a) Transposons
(b) Regulons
(c) Positrons
(d) None above

201. Hydrofoil impellers in mixing belong to the class of
(a) Axial flow
(b) Radial flow
(c) Tangential flow
(d) None above

202. One of the methods of protection of an organism itself against its enemies is known as
(a) Antagonisis
(b) Antibiosis
(c) Antigenesis
(d) Anti serosis

203. As compared to Gram negative bacteria Gram positive bacteria possesses
(a) Thicker murein layer
(b) Thiner murein layer
(c) No murein layer
(d) No outer membrane

204. In a mixed large air bubbles and tiny air bubbles in well mixed bio-processing liquid the ratio of the rate of oxygen transfer of tiny bubbles to large bubbles is
(a) Unity
(b) $\frac{1}{2}$
(c) $\frac{3}{4}$
(d) None above

205. In haemocytometric cell density measurement if a total of 210 cells were counted in three squares the cell density per ml of the liquid would be
(a) 7×10^3
(b) 7×10^4
(c) 7×10^5
(d) None above

206. OxyR regulon belongs to the group of
(a) Transformation activator
(b) Transcriptional activator
(c) Translational activator
(d) None above

207. The expression of many of the $H_2O_2^-$ inducible genes is regulated by
    (a) SoxR regulon
    (b) OxyR regulon
    (c) OxyS system
    (d) None above
208. In maintaining a reduced environment in the *E.coli* cytosol the number of major redox systems involved is
    (a) Two
    (b) Three
    (c) Four
    (d) Five
209. The addition of the first electron to O_2 in the triplet ground state unfavourable becauses it is
    (a) Downhill limiting step
    (b) Up hill limiting step
    (c) Parallel hill step
    (d) None above
210. In DNA structure the ladder like strand is not allowed under normal solution conditions because
    (a) Straight ladder structure need a gap between bases
    (b) The faces of bases are hydrophobic
    (c) In straight structure bases would be exposed to H_2O molecule leading to DNA instability
    (d) All above
211. In helix of DNA the number of residues per turn is
    (a) 2.2
    (b) 2.5
    (c) 3.6
    (d) None above
212. Ribonucleotide reductase is essential in
    (a) Making DNA
    (b) Repairing DNA
    (c) Both (a) and (b)
    (d) None above
213. In *E. coli* cytosol main controlling factor in defense against oxidative stress is
    (a) Thioredoxin system
    (b) Glutathione-glutaredoxin system
    (c) Both (a) and (b)
    (d) None above
214. An example of a macrolide antibiotic produced by *Streptomyces* sp is
    (a) Penicillin
    (b) Streptomycin
    (c) Erythromycin
    (d) Rifamycin
215. The protein manufacturing plant in the cell is called
    (a) Mesosome
    (b) Ribosome
    (c) Cellulosome
    (d) None above
216. Cellular roughess factor can be determined by the analysis of
    (a) Scanning electron micrograph
    (b) Transmision electron micrograph
    (c) Atomic force micrograph
    (d) None above
217. The hydrolysis of ATP in a cell is
    (a) Exergonic
    (b) Endergonic
    (c) Nonthermic
    (d) None above
218. The smell/flavour of crushed garlic is
    (a) Alicin
    (b) Leucin
    (c) Isoleucin
    (d) Erythrocin
219. The smell/flavour of onion is
    (a) Diallyl disulphide
    (b) Dipropyl disulphide
    (c) Polyvinyl sulphide
    (d) None above

220. The pigeon pea is
 (a) A pulse
 (b) An impulse
 (c) Anti impulse
 (d) None above

221. Tomato plants engineered with increased levels of polyamines show
 (a) Delayed ripening of tomato
 (b) Increased levels of the antioxidant lycopene
 (c) Enhanced phytonutrient content
 (d) None above

222. In microbial adhesion process important forces include
 (a) Passive forces
 (b) Electrostatic interaction
 (c) Hydrophobic interaction
 (d) None above

223. Polyhemoglobin-superoxide dismutase-catalase function as
 (a) A blood substitute
 (b) Oxygen carrier
 (c) Antioxidant
 (d) None above

224. The following formula where L is

$$V = \frac{\pi}{4} W^2 \left(L - \frac{W}{3} \right)$$

length and W is width terms can be used to determine a bacterial cell
 (a) Perimeter
 (b) Volume
 (c) Weight
 (d) None above

225. The intrinsic ability of a microorganism/virus to cause disease is called
 (a) Inheritence
 (b) Tolerence
 (c) Virulence
 (d) None above

226. A sequence of DNA that carries the information representing a protein has been termed
 (a) mRNA
 (b) Gene
 (c) tRNA
 (d) None above

227. The unit of gene separation is called
 (a) Micron
 (b) Morgan
 (c) Meter
 (d) None above

228. The distance corresponding to unit probability of separation of two genes is
 (a) 30 Å
 (b) 10^{-5} Morgan
 (c) Only (a)
 (d) Both (a) and (b)

229. The true garlic odour is
 (a) Diethyl disulfide
 (b) Diallyl disulfide
 (c) Allyl isothiocyanate
 (d) None above

16.9 REFERENCES

1. Aiba S., A.E. Humphrey and N.F. Millis., *Biochemical Engineering*, 2nd edn., Univ. Tokyo Press, Tokyo, 1973.
2. Bailey, J.E. and D.F. Ollis., *Biochemical Engineering Fundamentals*, 2nd edn., McGraw Hill Book Co., New York, 1986.
3. Shuler, M.L. and F. Kargi, *Bioprocess Engineering: Basic Concepts*, Prentice-Hall, Englewood Cliffs, New Jersey, 1992.
4. Lee, J. *Biochemical Engineering,* Prentice Hall, Englewood Cliffs, New Jersey, 1992.
5. Ghose, T.K. (ed)., *Bioprocess Computations in Biotechnology,* Vol. I, Ellis Horwood, New York, 1990.
6. Blanch, H.W. and D.S. Clark, *Biochemical Engineering*, Marcel Dekkar, New York, 1996.
7. Atkinson, B. and F. Mavituna, *Biochemical Engineering and Biotechnology Handbook* (2nd edn.) M. Stockton Press, Hampshire, England, 1991.
8. Mukhopadhyay, S.N. and D.K. Das, *Oxygen Responses, Reactivities and Measurements in Biosystems*, CRC Press, Boca Raton, Florida, 1994.
9. Davis, B. *et al*, *Microbiology* 4th edn., Harper & Row Pub., Singapore, 1990.
10. Nielsen, J. and J. Villadsen, *Bioreaction Engineering Principles*, Plenum Press, New York, 1994.
11. Pirt, S.J., *Principles of Microbe and Cell Cultivation*, Blackwell Sci. Pubs. Oxford, 1975.
12. Mukhopadhyay A., S.N. Mukhopadhyay, and G.P. Talwar, *J. Biotechnol*. 36, pp 177-182, 1994.
13. Mukhopadhyay A., *Ph.D Thesis*, IIT Delhi, 1995.
14. Eckenfelder, W.W. and D.J. O'Connor, *Biol. Waste Tretment*., Pergamon Press, 1961.
15. Belter P.A., E.L. Cussler and W.S. Her., *Bioseparations*, John Wiley & Sons. Inc., New York, 1988.
16. Hamel, J .B. Hunter and S.K. Sikdar, "Downstream Processing and Bioseparation: Recovery and Purification of Biological Products", *Am. Chem. Soc*., Washtington DC, 1990.
17. Metcalf & Eddy, Inc. *Waste Water Engineering: Treatment, Disposal & Reuse*, 2nd edn., TMH Ltd., New Delhi, 1979.
18. Mukhopadhyay, S.N. *Ph.D. Thesis*, IIT Delhi, Feb., 1976
19. Moat, A.G., J.W. Foster and M.P. Spector, *Microbial Physiology*, pp 74, 4th edn., Wiley-Liss, A John Wiley & Sons, Inc. Pub., New York, 2002.
20. Fujio, Y. *et. al*., *J. Ferment. Technol*., pp 51, 154, 1973.

Chapter

17

SUBSTRATES FOR INDUSTRIAL PROCESS BIOTECHNOLOGY AND THEIR REFINING

17.1 INTRODUCTION

Many countries are endowed with huge natural resources. India is one of them. India's renewable resources are also enormous. In utilization of renewable waste or residue resources for process biotechnology, their pretreatment or refining is required in most cases. These substrates are usually referred to as biomass. They may serve as substrate-carbon source in industrial process biotechnology. In biomass refining philosophy both chemical processing and bio-processing or a combination of both have been used.[1,2] Commonly used substrates/resources in industrial conventional fermentation process biotechnology are as described in the following sections.[3-4]

17.2 SUBSTRATES/RESOURCES

Molasses Refining: Molasses is the most common renewable carbohydrate waste resource used for fermentative production of ethanol, baker's yeast and many other bio-products. Molasses is the syrup that is left after the recovery of crystalline sugar from the concentrated juice of sugar cane or beet. Depending on the juice resource and its processing, two kinds of molasses are produced by sugar industries. They are 'blackstrap' and 'hightest' molasses. Blackstrap molasses has been used principally in industrial alcohol production in distilleries. It usually contains 50-55% of sugars mainly sucrose. However, hightest molasses has been used for ethanol manufacture. It is an evaporated juice but most of it remains in inverted sugar form as a result of acid hydrolysis. This type of molasses is usually high in sugar content. Occasionally it may contain as high as 78% sugar. In India and some other countries, blackstrap molassess has been widely used for industrial fermentative production of ethanol. The industrial process adapted by distilleries usually consists of fermenting the diluted molasses with yeast. In many European countries, from molasses another material is produced by its concentration which is known as "Vinasses" (latin : vinaceus). Vinasses is a product from molassess through its transformation into a valuable, concentrated and marketable by – product. Vinasses has molasses like properties. An earlier estimate of vinasses production in West Europe as reported in literature is about 6.8×10^5 tons per year based on 65% dry matter. This vinasses has been termed as partly or fully de-sugared cane or beet molasses. It is also produced by desugaring process by the aid of a special method. Thus, it is clear that molasses is an industrial sugar post-treatment process by – product/residue. Its fermentable sugar serves as substrate/carbon source for a large number of microbes in producing different products by industrial microbial fermentation processes.

Molasses pretreatment/refining: In using molasses in fermentation industry in many cases for its refining, molasses is heat treated, clarified and diluted before its use. It is usually adjusted to a pH of 4.5 to 5. Next heated nearly to its boiling point. If in fermentation medium CSL (corn sleep liquor) is used, this is added to the molasses before heat treatment. Purpose of heating is to destroy a large percentage of microorganisms present and to aid in the clarification process which follows:

Also, in using molasses in fermentation industry its fermentable sugar/sucrose fraction in many cases needed to be separated from its non-sugar/sucrose salt fraction or in other words, pretreatment/refining was required. Flow sheets of molasses desugarization and desugared molasses concentration are shown in Figs. 17.1 and 17.2 respectively. This was primarily to supply carbon source in purer form by the sugars contained in molasses. In ethanol fermentation from molasses, it is well known that product yield depends upon molasses origin, i.e. molasses quality. Likewise, baker's yeast biomass production from molasses depends on its quality. The relation between degree of treatment/refining on yield or ethanol was reported as in Figs. 17.3, 17.4. In some countries, the cane juice clarification process to produce white sugar uses lime and sulfite. Fig. 17.5 shows that an inverse correlation exists between polarization (Pol) and reducing sugar in molasses. It can also be seen from this figure that the more the sulfur that is burnt for molasses, the less is the polarization.

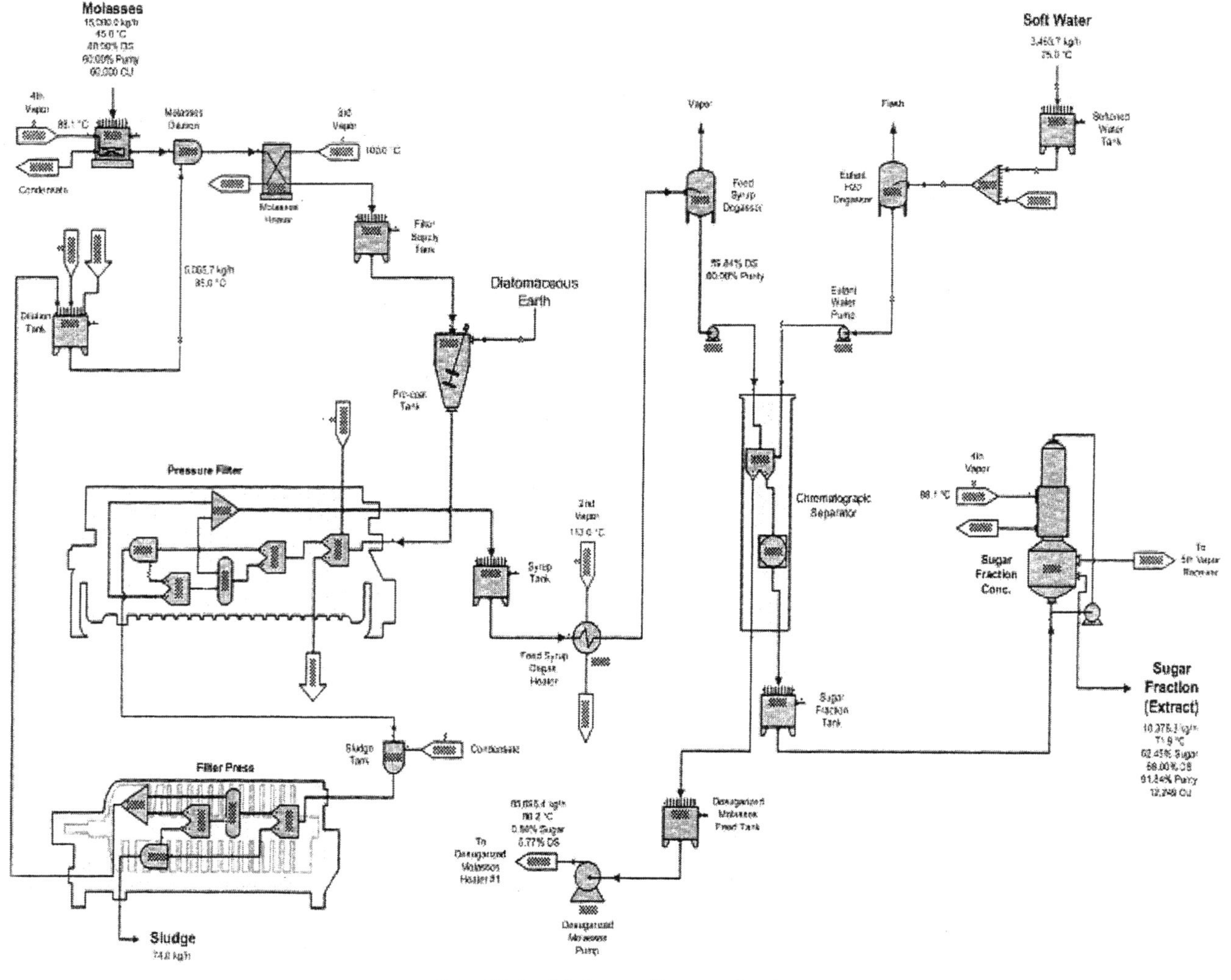

Fig, 17.1 Molasses Desugarization

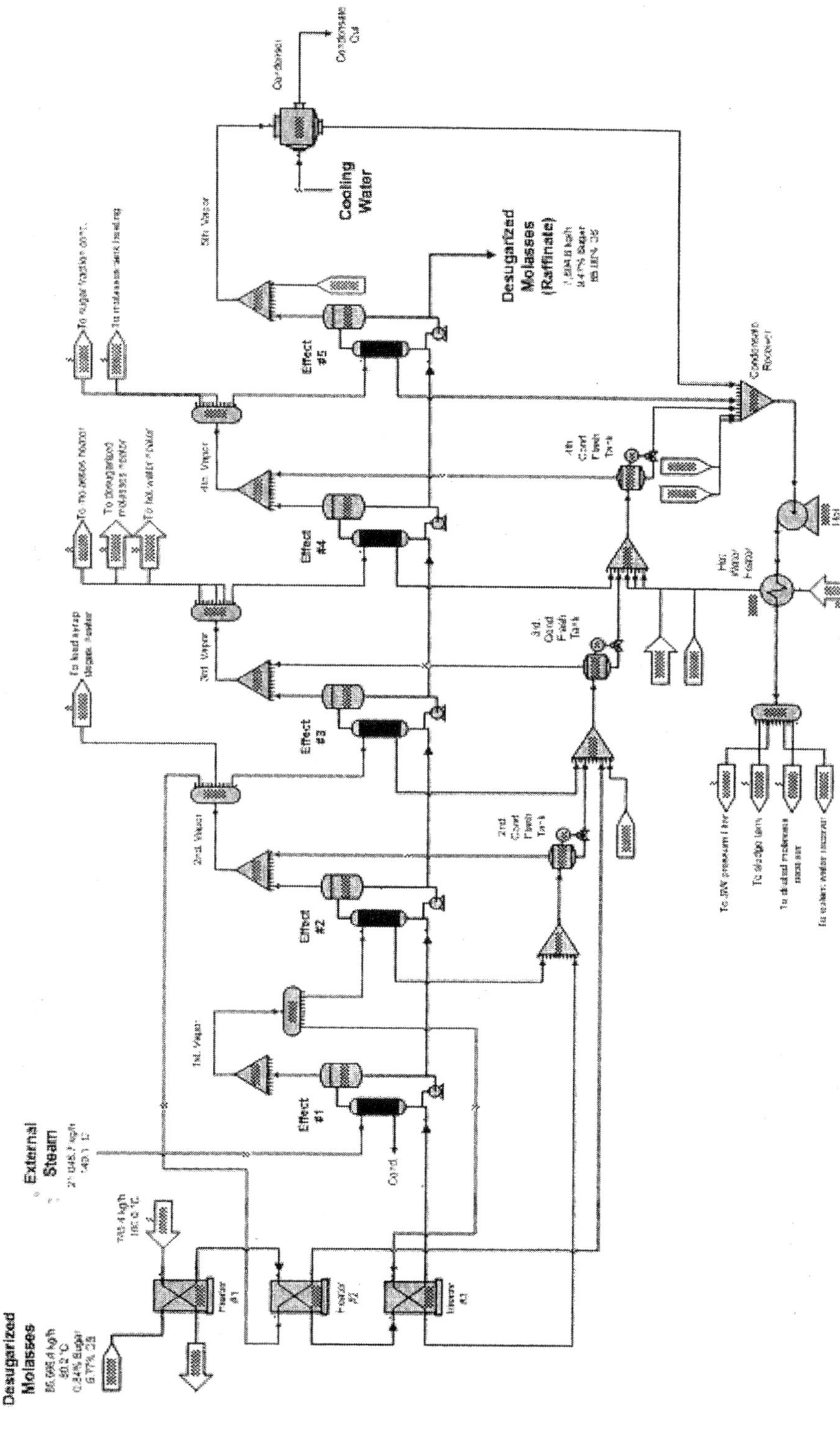

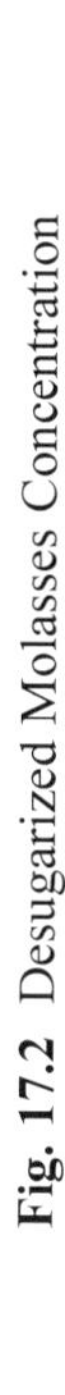

Fig. 17.2 Desugarized Molasses Concentration

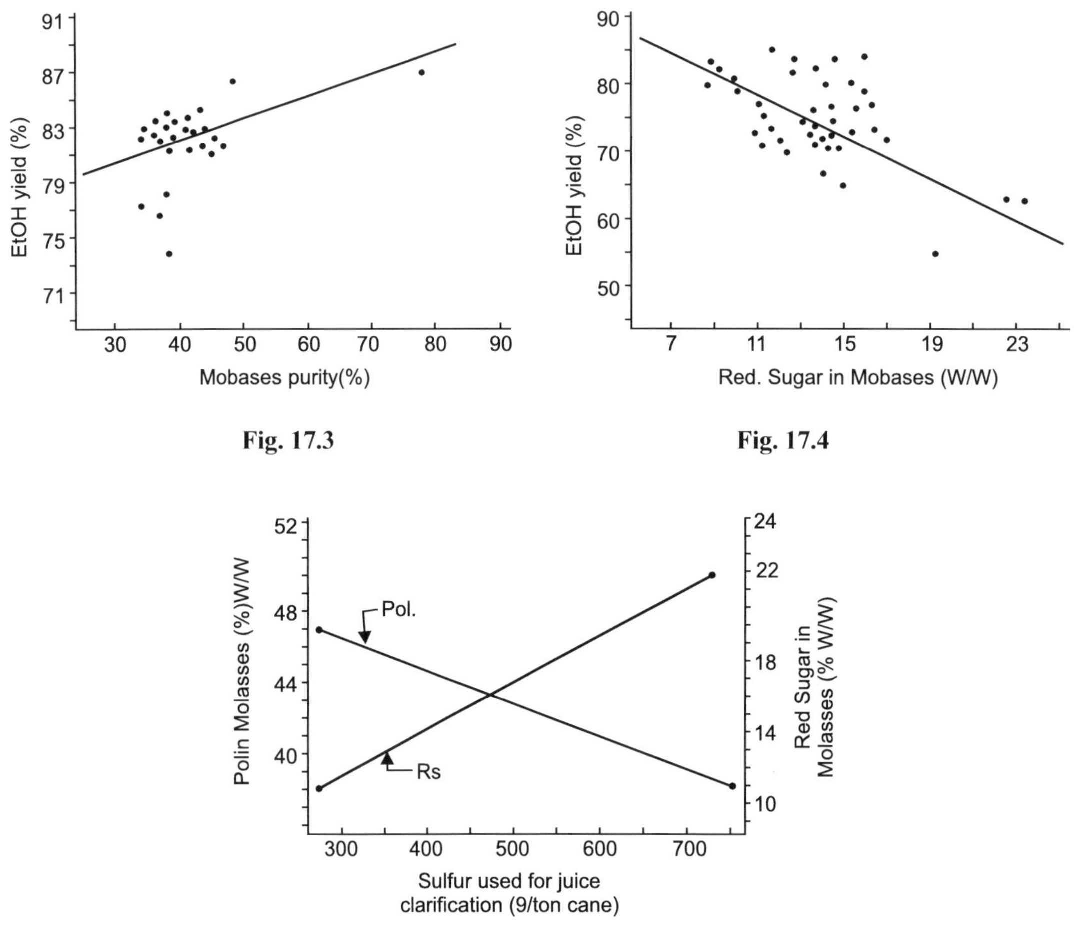

Fig. 17.3

Fig. 17.4

Fig. 17.5

Sulfite decreases the pH, and more reducing sugar/sucrose might be hydrolysed in the process. In Fig. 17.4, it can be seen that there is a negative correlation between reducing sugar in molasses and ethanol yield. By such pretreatment/refining, the ratio of sucrose/reducing sugar could also serve as an indicator of the capacity of molasses to produce ethyl alcohol. The higher the ratio, the higher is the ethanol produced by fermentation, based on total reducing sugars. The pretreatment for purity of molasses also affects the ethanol yield (Fig. 17.4). This facet agrees with the data shown in Fig. 17.8 because the higher the reducing sugar, the lower is the purity.

In more recent years, it is reported that molasses contains (1) non-conducting sucrose fraction and (2) non-sucrose salt fraction. In recovering these fractions and for abating pollution in environment, refining/pretreatment of molasses has been carried out by industrial chromatographic separation method. The efficiency of chromatographic separation of these two fraction relates strongly to the mean particle/bead size of the stationary phase. Report on the effect of mean particle size for molasses purification/separation using 5.5% cross–linked strong action exchange resins (Finex ftd, Finland) in mono-valent form indicated molasses particle size ranged from 100-500 μm. Used resin beads were of monobead type (i.e. having narrow particle size distribution). Pulse test analysis technique with water as eluant for test mixture was used in evaluation of chromatography separation for refining. One ml fraction from the effluent stream were used to analyse by HP 11OO HPLC system with Na^+ column.

In refining by chromatography the performance was characterized (Fig 17.5 to 17.13). For this, relevant column efficiency and moment analysis parameters were used. The pulse response was expressed in terms of first absolute moment as given in equation 17.1. From this the second central moment of the pulse response defined as μ_2 and given in equation 17.2. As method of moment is valid for gaussian profiles, non-gaussian profiles peak was analysed with caution in interpretation.

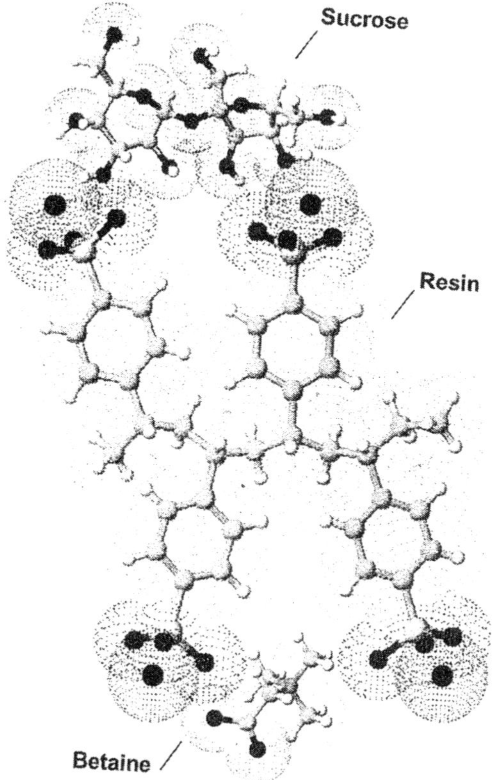

Fig. 17.6 Schematic presentation of sucrose and betaine attached to cation exchange resin in Na+ form. Colors: C = cyan, H = white, O = red, S = yellow and Na = blue

$$\mu_1 = t_r = \frac{\int_0^\infty tc(t)dt}{\int_0^\infty c(t)dt} \tag{17.1}$$

$$\mu_2 = \sigma^2 = \frac{\int_0^\infty (t-\mu_1)^2 c(t)dt}{\int_0^\infty c(t)dt} \tag{17.2}$$

The first and second moments of the peaks were applied for the calculation of bed porosity, adsorption equilibrium constant, separation factor, resolution and height equivalent to theoretical plate (HETP).

Chromatographic parameters as defined by equations 17.3 through 17.7 were used in analysing data of the experimental set up system characteristics.

Adsorption equilibrium constant
$$K = \left[\left(\mu_1 - \frac{t_0}{2}\right)\frac{u}{Z\varepsilon} - 1\right]\frac{\varepsilon}{1-\varepsilon} \tag{17.3}$$

Separation factor
$$\alpha_{A/B} = \frac{K_A}{K_B} \tag{17.4}$$

Resolution
$$R_{A/B} = \frac{2(t_{rA} - t_{rB})}{W_{bA} + W_{bB}} \tag{17.5}$$

Peak-width
$$W_b = 4\sigma \tag{17.6}$$

HETP
$$= \frac{z\mu_2}{\mu_1^{12}} \tag{17.7}$$

Experimental System

Equipment:	Chromatographic system consisting of eluant reservoir, HPLC pump, injection valve, column, column oven, temperature and pressure control, conductivity, Ri and pH detectors and fraction collector.
Column:	Steel column (diameter 2.2 cm)
Resin:	Finex CS11GC, sulfonated PS-DVB
Ionic form:	Na^+
Bed height:	26 cm
Flow rate:	3.2 ml/min
Superficial velocity:	0.5 m/h
Injection volume:	5.0 ml
Temperature:	358 K
Test mixture	
Sucrose:	120 g/*l*
Salts:	70 g/*l* (30 % Na_2SO_4, 70% K_2SO_4)
Betaine:	10 g/*l*

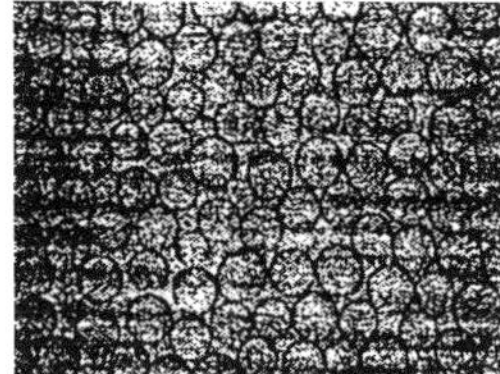

110 μm

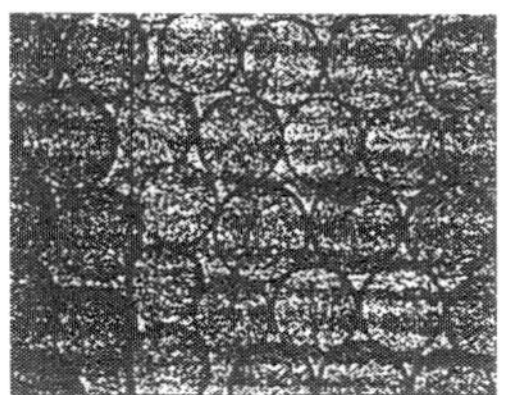

250 μm

Table 17.1 Finex CS11GC resin and bed characteristics

Mean Bead size (μm)	*Within ± 20%*	*DVB-%*	*Volume capacity H^+ -form (equiv/l)*	*H_2O-% Na^+ -form*	*Bed porosity#*
110	91.7%	5.5%	1.54	54.7	0.29
250	96.1%	5.5%	1.50	53.9	0.30
270	94.6%	5.5%	1.51	54.5	0.31
328	93.8%	5.5%	1.50	54.3	0.31
354	98.3%	5.5%	1.56	52.8	0.30
393	98.4%	5.5%	1.55	53.1	0.31
518	95.6%	5.5%	1.49	53.5	0.31

Determined with Blue Dextran 2,000,000 g/mol.

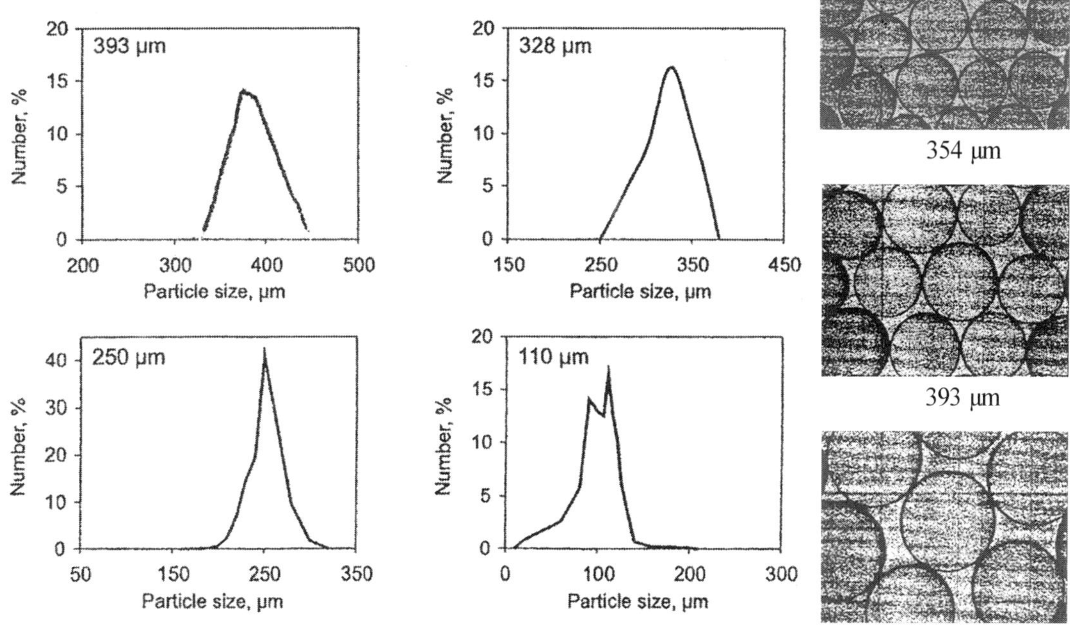

Fig. 17.7 Particle size distribution of selected fractionation resins

Table 17.2 Peak characteristics at superficial velocity of 0.5 m/h

Mean Bead size (µm)	*Salt Peak retention*[a] *(ml)*	*Sucrose Peak retention*[a] *(ml)*	*Betaine Peak retention*[a] *(ml)*	*Salt Peak Width*[c] *(ml)*	*Sucrose Peak Width*[c] *(ml)*	*Betaine Peak Width*[c] *(ml)*	*Salt Peak height (g/l)*	*Sucrose Peak height (g/l)*	*Betaine Peak height (g/l)*
110	42.0	47.8	66.0	7.52	7.48	5.88	53.7	85.7	7.77
250	43.0	47.8	66.0	8.84	8.39	10.1	50.5	76.3	4.76
270	42.4	48.1	66.4	8.53	8.76	11.5	47.6	69.3	4.41
328	43.0	47.8	67.0	8.60	10.1	13.2	49.0	61.4	4.10
354	40.9	45.7	64.0	8.85	10.0	14.1	46.8	58.4	3.77
3.93	40.1	44.9	63.2	9.67	12.2	15.7	42.6	47.8	3.31
518	34.3	43.9[b]	65.1	16.4	26.1	23.0	27.7	26.4	2.36

[a] From peak maximum. [b] Distorted peak. [c] Peak width at half height

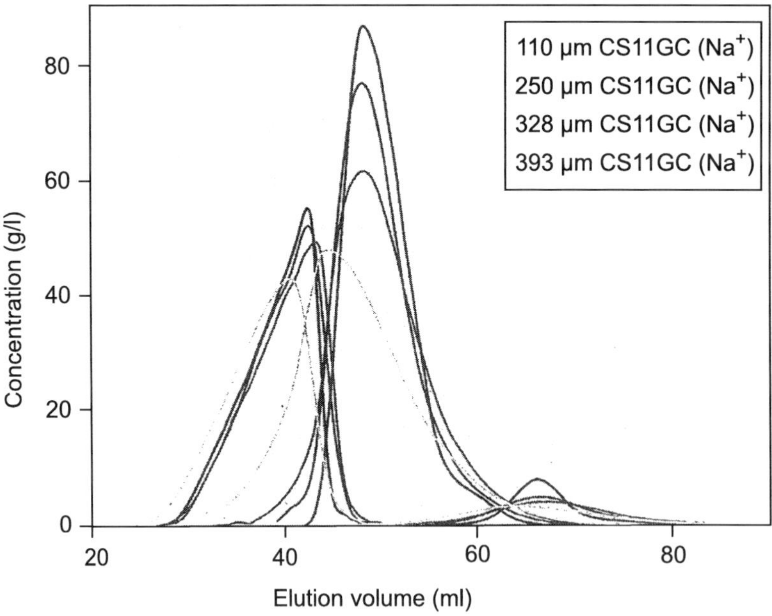

Fig. 17.8 Separation of sucrose from synthetic molasses mixture with different particle size resins. Peak groups from left: salt, sucrose, betaine.

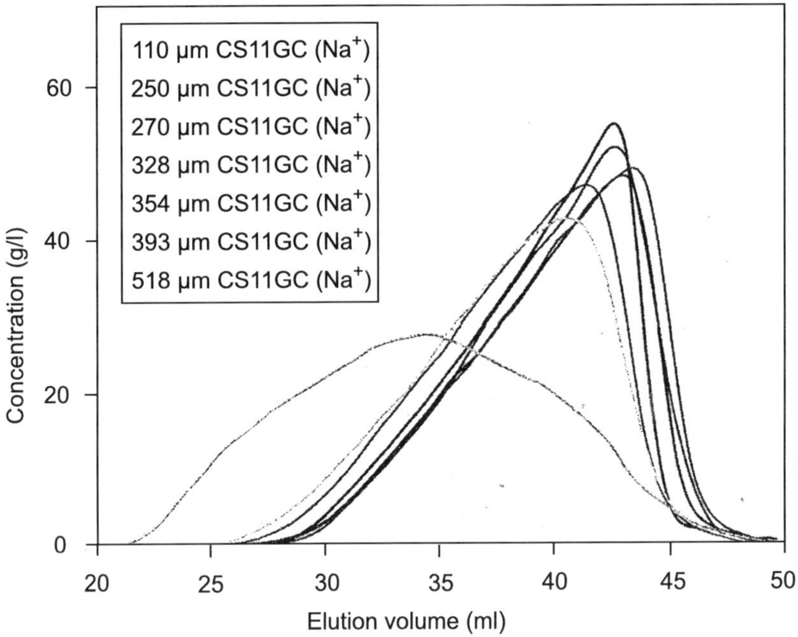

Fig. 17.9 Salt chromatograms at different particle size resins

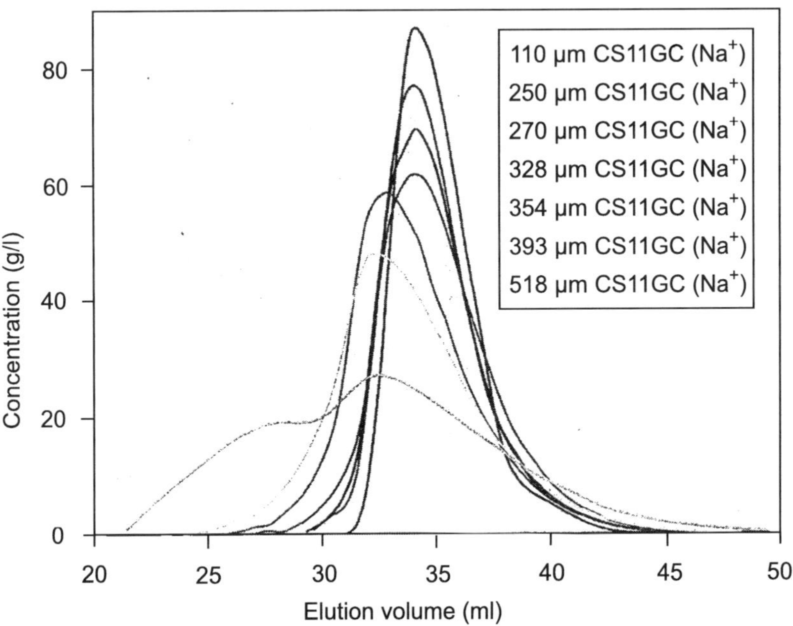

Fig. 17.10 Sucrose chromatograms at different particle size resins

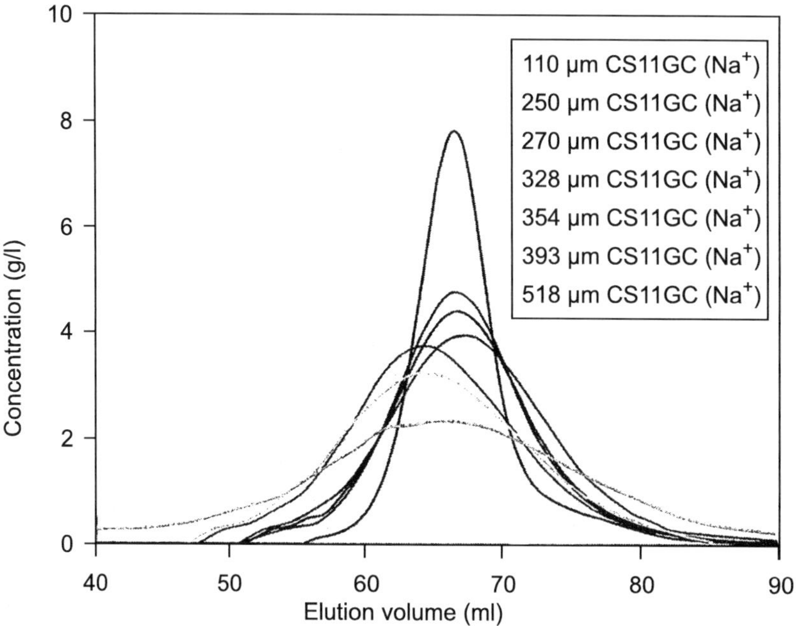

Fig. 17.11 Betaine chromatograms at different particle size resins

Table 17.3 Chromatographic parameters at superficial velocity of 0.5 m/h

Mean Bead size (µm)	*Salt K*	*Sucrose K*	*Betaine K*	*Salt HETP (cm)*	*Sucrose HETP (cm)*	*Betaine HETP (cm)*
110	0.11	0.27	0.51	0.22	0.13	0.10
250	0.11	0.26	0.51	0.22	0.19	0.17
270	0.09	0.24	0.50	0.24	0.22	0.19
328	0.10	0.25	0.51	0.24	0.27	0.23
354	0.09	0.23	0.48	0.26	0.34	0.25
393	0.07	0.21	0.47	0.30	0.50	0.30
518	0.02	0.17	0.48	0.66	1.42	0.61

[a] Distorted peak. [b] Calculated from peak area.

Table 17.4 Chromatographic parameters at superficial velocity of 0.5 m/h

Mean Bead size (μm)	*Salt Peak Purity*[b] *(%)*	*Sucrose Peak Purity*[b] *(%)*	*Betaine Peak Purity*[b] *(%)*	*Sucrose-Salt R*	*Betaine-Sucrose R*	*Sucrose-Salt α*	*Betaine-Sucrose α*
110	92.9	95.1	86.1	0.76	1.08	2.34	1.89
250	79.7	86.5	69.5	0.63	0.89	2.14	1.92
270	77.4	85.3	66.9	0.61	0.85	2.18	1.93
328	70.3	80.5	61.7	0.56	0.77	2.12	1.93
354	63.6	76.4	51.8	0.52	0.72	2.31	2.02
393	53.0	69.9	39.6	0.45	0.65	2.40	2.06
518	26.1	55.8[a]	22.0	0.33	0.51	4.17	2.51

[a] Distorted peak. [b] Calculated from peak area (100% - $X_{overlapped}$ %).

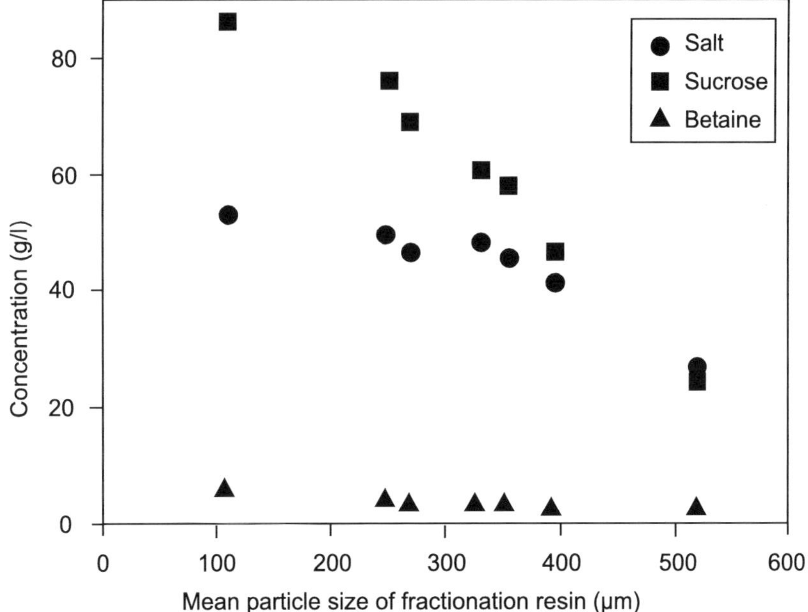

Fig. 17.12 Dependence of peak maximum concentration on the mean particle size of fractionation resin

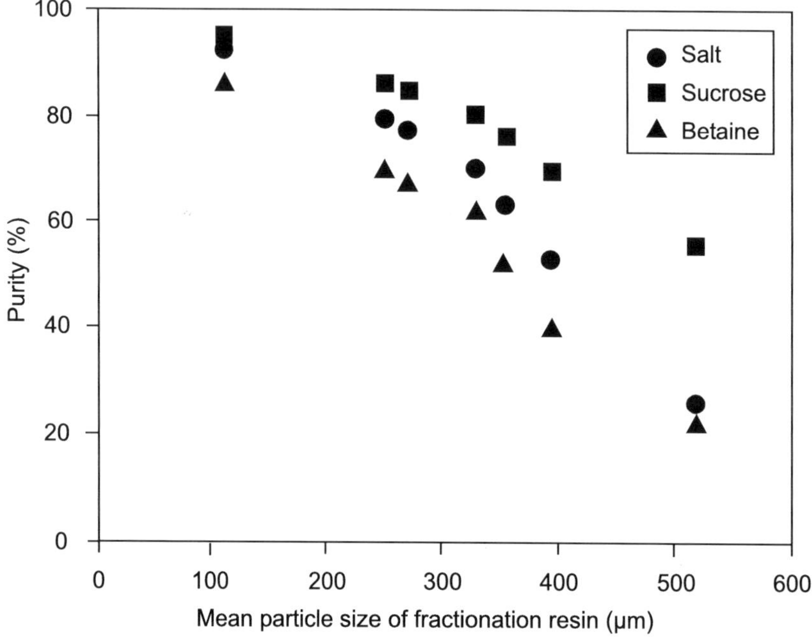

Fig. 17.13 Dependence of peak purity on the mean particle size of fractionation resin.

It is clear from the foregoing sections that customizing the mean particle size of the fractionation resin to the process allowable minimum is an effective tool for improving cost efficiency of chromatographic refining/separation processes.

For sucrose separation from synthetic molasses at the conditions in the report (0.5m/h), the bead size reduction from 328 μm to 250 μm results in:

- concentration increase for sucrose: 24%
- concentration increase for betaine: 16%
- salt peak purity increase: 13%
- sucrose peak purity increase: 7%
- betaine peak purity increase: 13%

Trace element/Mineral refining from Process Biotechnology Medium

Used Methods:

1. Adsorption
2. Chelation

1. Adsorption: Solution of the medium is mixed with an adsorbent, shakened thoroughly and allowed to settle.

Adsorbent used: $CaCO_3$

Processes: a) Medium solution + $CaCO_3$ shaken thoroughly

solution mixed up (pH 7.5)

Autoclaved (to aid coagulation of unwanted hydroxides)

Cooled

Filtered

Filtrate free from trace element contaminants

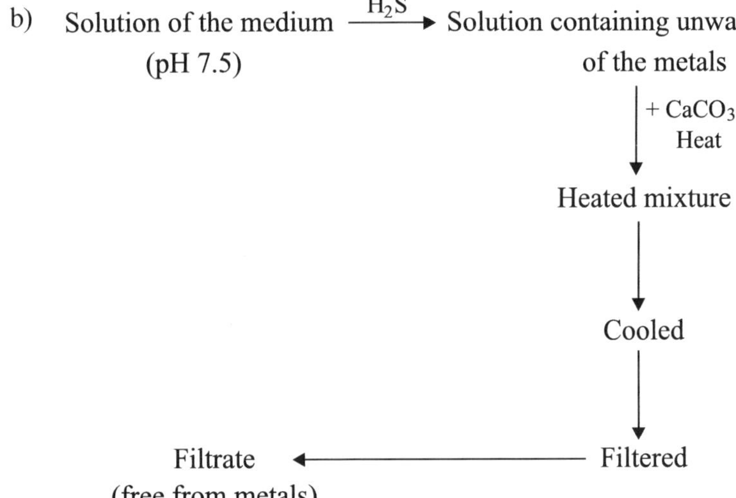

Other adsorbents used:

- Norite charcoal
- Al_2O_3
- $Al_2O_3 + H_2S$

2. Chelation Method

Chelating agents

a) Dithiazone
b) Oxime

a)

Dithiazone
NH—NH·CS·N=N
Metal solution
NH·N·CS·N=N
Chelated Complex
M
NH·N
N=N

17.2.2 Lignocellulose Refining/Pretreatment

Over the last several decades, scientists and technologists have pretreated lignocellulosic materials for its breakdown products utilization as alternate renewable resource material in process biotechnology. Treatment/refining of lignocelluloses have been carried out both by chemical processing and by bio-processing with the same objective of "biomass refining". The main components of lignocellulosics (cellulose, hemicelluloses and lignin) can be fractionated by sequential treatment to produce fraction that may be used for different product applications. One of the important feedstocks of such a category which is abundantly available and renewable is rice husks/hulls and straw. Refinining or pretreatment of such feedstocks by hydrolysis has been practiced for a long time. Catalytic agents which have been used for the hydrolysis are acid or enzyme. A comparison of activities of acid and enzyme catalysts on three cellulosic substrates at 50°C showed that 100,000 times as much acid is required to bring about the same degree of saccharification of fermentable sugars. Enzymatic saccharification of paddy hulls and bagasse have been reported. A possible process for the full utilization of biomass may start with a hydrolytic stage (carried out in aqueous media with possible addition of acids) in which hemicellulosic fraction is solubilized, while both cellulose and lignin remain in solid phase with little alteration. The liquors from the treatment (containing hemicellulose degradation products such as sugar oligomers, monosaccharides, acetic acid, furfural and hydroxymethyl furfural) are easily separated from the solid phase, which can be subjected to further processing (for example, organosolvent pulping) to achieve separation of cellulose and lignin. Refining of lignocellulosics (carbohydrate composition as in Table 17.5) thus can give its purified component which in turn, can be subjected to further modifications by alkali, solvent and biological/enzymic treatments as described and mentioned in literatures[10.10]. In more recent years, rice husk autohydrolytic refining under non-isothermal conditions using hydrothermal acid processing provided a sound basis for the kinetic interpretation of a heterogeneous system where simultaneous degradation reactions occur. It leads to several products of commercial/industrial interest[11] as well as for research and development concerns (Table 17.5). It has been reported that under the most suitable reaction condition usually employed for autohydrolytic breakdown process, sugar oligomers (mainly xylooligomers) are major breakdown products[12-17].

Table 17.5 Carbohydrates composition of lignocellulosics

Material	*%cellulose*	*% hemicellulose*	*% lignin*
Hardwoods stems	40-55	24-40	18-25
Softwoods stems	45-50	25-35	25-35
Grasses	25-40	25-50	10-30
Leaves	15-20	80-85	~0
Cotton seed hairs	80-95	5-20	~0
Newspaper	40-55	25-40	18-30
Waste papers from chemical pulps	60-70	10-20	5-10

The concentrations of the breakdown products can account for more than 50% of the initial hemicelluloses. Industrially/commercially, xylooligomers are currently used as new sweeteners or food additives[18]. In relation to human health, it has been reported that xylooligomers selectively enhance the growth of Bifidobacteria, thus promoting a favourable intestinal environment performance. Moreover, the xylooligomer solution/liquids produced in autohydrolysis can be transformed into xylose solutions by acid catalysed post hydrolysis. Availability of xylose solution by performing successive stages of autohydrolysis and post hydrolysis shows advantages for further process biotechnological conversion over the conventional single stage prehydrolysis. This is because the milder reaction conditions result in decreased content of side products causing inhibition of the microbial metabolism.

Table 17.6 Refining by non-biological and biological methods

Hydrolytic Refining Agent	*Refining/Degradation Product*		*Reference(s)*
	Constituents	*Wt.%*	*6, 12, 20*
Acid Hydrolytic Degradation	Cellulose (C)+ Hemicellulose	36.7	
	Xylan (X_n)	15.6	
	Araban (A)	1.68	
	Acetyl (Ac)	1.62	
	Lignin (L)	21.3	
	Ash (As)	14.3	
	Others (O) (by difference)	8.8	
Enzyme Hydrolytic Degradation	C	35	7-9, 13
	X_n	17	
	A	–	
	Ac	–	
	L	16	
	As	15	
	O		

Microbial Degradation	C	35.8	5, 19
	Xn	17.0	
	A	–	
	Ac	–	
	Lignin	20.6	
	Ash	16.0	

Reported above written various model schemes have been used to develop simple kinetic equations that will help in ascertaining process biotechnology parameters (Table 17.7).

Table 17.7 Reported Model schematics of acid hydrolytic degradation of cellulose/saccharides

S. No.	*Model proposer*	*Year*	*Model schematic*
1.	Saeman	1945	Cellulose → Reducing sugar → Sugar decomposition products (C)
2.	Mc Kibbins et al.	1962	G → Is → HMF → Levulinic acid; Is, HMF → Solids
3.	Reese	1965	Cellulose → Cellotrise → Cellobiose → G
4.	Conner et al.	1986	Levoglucoses ⇌ G; Ehc → G; R.c → G; G → D.P.s; G ⇌ Disaccharides; Disaccharides → Glucosides; Glucosides → G
5.	Abatzoglou et al.	1986	C → Oligo-Compounds ⇌ G → D.P.s.
6.	Bouchard et al.	1989	Anhydrosugars ⇌ G; C → 'M'.c; C → G; C → S.o → G; G → D.P.s; G ⇌ Disaccharides; Disaccharides → Glucosides; Glucosides → G
7.	Madeleine et al.	1990	1,6 Anhydroglucose ⇌ G; G ⇌ Glucose dimers; G ⇌ F, M; G → HMF; HMF → Polymers; HMF → Levo-Linic & Formic acids
8.	Mok et al.	1992	C → N.h.o; C → H.o → G → D.P.s

On treating/refining various types of lignocelluloses which contained cellulose, lignin, protein and ash as given in Table 17.6 encouraging results could be seen. In untreated and treated agroresidues and grass as seen from table, it is evident that different components of agroresidues and grass chauged a lot after refining. In case of alkali treated bagasse and rice straw, the cellulose content increased by 56 and 72 percent with a decrease in lignin content of 47 and 60 percent respectively. But in case of the butanol treatment, the percentage increase of cellulose content was less compared to the alkali-treated substrates.

Table 17.8 Chemical composition of agro-residues (untreated and treated)

Agro-	*Cemllulose (%)*			*Hemicellulose (%)*			*Lignin (%)*			*Protein (%)*	*Ash (%)*	*Extractive (%)*
residues	*RAW*	*AT*	*BT*	*RAW*	*AT*	*BT*	*RAW*	*AT*	*BT*	*RAW*	*RAW*	*RAW*
Bagasse	38.5	60	55	33	22	24	19	10.10	12	1	5	3.5
Grass	25	50	45	35	15	18.20	16.17	11.14	13	2.50	21	.33
Jute stick	45.5	70	62	31	10	16	21.34	18.37	19.50	0.50	0.80	.86
Rice husk	38	51	48	17	8.20	10	21.67	18.55	19.10	1.00	22	.33
Rice straw	36	62	56	28	10	15	16.61	6.65	9.00	2.00	17	.39

Raw = without any treatment only milled to 40—mesh. AT = alkali treatment. BT = butanol treatment

$$Xn_F \xrightarrow{K_{1F}} O_H,\quad Xn_S \xrightarrow{K_{1S}} O_H,\quad O_H \xrightarrow{K_{2H}} O_L \xrightarrow{K_{2L}} X \xrightarrow{K_3} F,\quad O_L \xrightarrow{K_4} F$$

Using rice husk, its autohydrolytic refining kinetic schemes developed more recently based on Conner and Lorenz model. This model has been represented as below. In this schematic representation, Xn_F is fast reacting xylan, Xn_s is slow reacting xylan, X is xylose, X_n is xylan, D P.s. is degradation products, F is furfural, O is oligomer, K terms are rate constants. Here,

$$K_2 = K_{2max} \exp\left[-\frac{E_{S_2}}{RT}\right]\{1 - \exp(\beta\tau)\} \tag{17.8}$$

Based on Conner and Lorenz model for degradative refining of xylan (Xn) of hemicelluloses the degradation rate equation 17.9 to 17.12 could be solved by numerical integration using fourth order Runge – Kutta method.

$$\frac{dXn_F}{d\tau} = -k_{0F} \exp\left[\frac{-E_{aF}}{RT(\tau)}\right] Xn_F \tag{17.9}$$

$$\frac{dXn_S}{d\tau} = -k_{0S} \exp\left[\frac{-E_{aS}}{RT(\tau)}\right] Xn_S \tag{17.10}$$

$$\frac{dO}{d\tau} = k_{0F} \exp\left[\frac{-E_{aF}}{RT(\tau)}\right] Xn_F + k_{0S} \exp\left[\frac{-E_{aS}}{RT(\tau)}\right] Xn_S - \tag{17.11}$$

$$k_{2\,max} \exp\left[\frac{-E_{a2}}{RT(\tau)}\right][1 - \exp(-\beta\tau)]O$$

$$\frac{dX}{d\tau} = k_{2\,max} \exp\left[\frac{-E_{a2}}{RT(\tau)}\right][1 - \exp(-\beta\tau)]O - k_{03}\, ext\left[\frac{-E_{a3}}{RT(\tau)}\right]X \tag{17.12}$$

Also, for the model given in above scheme could provide relations as given in equation 17.13 to 17.17.

$$\frac{dXn_F}{d\tau} = -k_{0F} \exp\left[\frac{-E_{aF}}{RT(\tau)}\right] Xn_F \tag{17.13}$$

$$\frac{dXn_S}{d\tau} = -k_{0S} \exp\left[\frac{-E_{aS}}{RT(\tau)}\right] Xn_S \tag{17.14}$$

$$\frac{dO_H}{d\tau} = k_{0F} \exp\left[\frac{-E_{aF}}{RT(\tau)}\right] Xn_F + k_{0S} \exp\left[\frac{-E_{aS}}{RT(\tau)}\right] Xn_S - k_{02H} \exp\left[\frac{-E_{a2H}}{RT(\tau)}\right] O_H \tag{17.15}$$

$$\frac{dO_L}{d\tau} = k_{02\,H} \exp\left[\frac{-E_{a2H}}{RT(\tau)}\right] O_H - \left\{k_{02\,L} \exp\left[\frac{-E_{a2L}}{RT(\tau)}\right] + k_{04} \exp\left[\frac{-E_{a4}}{RT(\tau)}\right]\right\} O_L \tag{17.16}$$

$$\frac{dX}{d\tau} = k_{02\,L} \exp\left[\frac{-E_{a2L}}{RT(\tau)}\right] O_L - k_{03} \exp\left[\frac{-E_{a3}}{RT(\tau)}\right] X \tag{17.17}$$

The numerical integration of above set of equations also could be worked out considering the following relations:

$$X_n = X_{n_F} + X_{n_S} \tag{17.18}$$

$$\alpha = \frac{X_{n_{Fo}}}{X_{n_o}} \tag{17.19}$$

and

$$O = O_H + O_L \tag{17.20}$$

In equation (17.20), O_H is the percentage of initial xylan converted into high molecular weight xylo-oligomers and O_L is the percentage of initial xylan converted into low molecular weight xylo-oligomers. In equations 17.9 to 17.20, k_{oF}, k_{oS}, k_{o2H}, k_{o2L}, k_{o3}, E_{aS}, E_{a2H}, F_{a2L}, E_{a3} and E_{aA} denote activation energies and $k_{2\,max}$ and β give the values of kinetic coefficient and a function of time (τ), while α is a measure of susceptible fraction of xylose in initial xylan. These treatments/ refining analysis of lignocellulosic biomass indicate the possibility of full utilization of the feedstock/ substrate in industrial process biotechnology.

Nomenclature

c	solution phase concentration (g/l)
$HETP$	height equivalent of the theoretical plate (cm)
K	adsorption equilibrium constant
$R_{A/B}$	resolution between components A and B
t	time (min)
t_r	mean retention time(min)
t_o	injection time (min)
u	superficial velocity (cm/min)
V	volume (I)
z	bed height (cm)

Greek Letters

$\alpha_{A/B}$	separation factor of component A over B
ε	bed porosity
μ_1	first absolute moment (min)
μ_2	second central moment (min^2)
σ^2	peak variance (min^2)

17.3 REFERENCES

1. S.N. Mukhopadhyay, Process Biotechnology Fundamentals (2nd edn), Viva Books Pvt. Ltd., New Delhi, 2004, Chapters ll and 13
2. H.V. Amorim and H.Campos, Molasses Quality and Ethanol yield in Brazilian Factories Proc. 6th IFS, London, Canada, Advances in Biotechnol. Vol. II, M.Moo-Young Gen Ed. Pergamon Press Canada :Std., 1981 pp 210-206.
3. S.C. Prescott and C.G. Dunn, Industrial Microbiology (3rd Edn), McGraw Hill Book Co., Inc., New York, 1959, pp-67.
4. J. Kivi et al; Effect of Mean Particle size of Fractionation Resin on Industrial Chromatographic Separation of Molasses Desugarization FINEX 127th Industrial Exhibition Congress on Chemical Engineering, Environmental Protection and Biotechnology, ACHEMA 2003, Frankfurt am main, May 23-27, 2003.
5. S.N. Mukhopadhyay (Ed.) Advanced Process Biotechnology, Viva Books Pvt. Ltd., New Delhi 2005, pp 192 (Chapter 17).
6. E.T. Reese, Enzymatic Hydrolysis of β-glycan Proc. Fifth Sympo. On Cellulases and Related enzymes, Cellulase Asso. Pub., Osaka Univ., Japan, 1965 pp 1-16.

7. T.K. Ghose and K. Das, A simplified Kinetic Approach to Cellulose-cellulase system. In Adv. Biochem. Engg. Vol 1(Ghose, T.K. and Fiechter A eds), Springer-Verlag, Berlin, 1971 pp 55-76.
8. K. Das, Ph.D. Thesis, Jadavpur University, Calcutta, 1969.
9. S.N. Mukhopadhyay, P. Ghosh and V.H. Potty, Enzymic Saccharification of Bagasse, Jr. Food Sci. & Technology 12(3), 120, 1975.
10. T.K. Ghose, Cellulose Conversion, In Advances in Food Producing systems for Arid and Semi-Arid Lands, Acad Press. Inc. Vol 1, 1981 pp 225-266.
11. S.N. Mukhopadhyay, Progress in Sci. & Technology of Cellulose Processing in Relevance to Process Biotechnology. In New Developments in Carbohydrates and Related Natural Products. (M.J. Mulky and A. Pandey eds), Oxford- IBH Pub., New Delhi, 1995, pp 80-89.
12. C.Vila, G. Garrote, H. Dominquez and J.C. Parajo, Hydrolytic processing of Rice Husks in Aqueous Media: A Kinetic Assessment, Collect. Czech. Chem. Commun 67, 509-530, 2002.
13. T.K. Ghose, Renewable Resources – Development of Biomass Conversion Technology in India. Address at IIChE 33rd Annual Session, I.I.T. Delhi, December 20, 1980.
14. J.J. Meister, J. Macromol. Sci. – Polymer Reviews, 42(2), 235-289, 2002.
15. S.N. Mukhopadhyay, TECHNORAMA A supplement to IEI News 55(T) March 2006, pp 10-20.
16. M. Saska and E. Ozer, Biotechnol Bioeng. 45, 517, 1995.
17. K. Shimizu et al. Biomass Bioenergy 14, 195, 1998.
18. G. Garrote, H. Dominguez and J.C. Parajo; J. Food Engg. 52, 211, 2002.
19. N. Toyama and K. Ogawa, Proc. Bio-conversion Symp., IIT Delhi, 373-388, 1977.
20. U.C. Banerjee and S.N. Mukhopadhyay, Ind. Chem. Engr. 32(4), 43-46, 1990.
21. A.H. Conner and L.F. Lorenz, Wood Fiber Sci. 18, 248, 1986.

INDEX